Glaucoma: Clinical Ophthalmology

Glaucoma: Clinical Ophthalmology

Edited by Collin Cruz

hayle
medical

New York

Hayle Medical,
750 Third Avenue, 9ᵗʰ Floor,
New York, NY 10017, USA

Visit us on the World Wide Web at:
www.haylemedical.com

This book contains information obtained from authentic and highly regarded sources. Copyright for all individual chapters remain with the respective authors as indicated. All chapters are published with permission under the Creative Commons Attribution License or equivalent. A wide variety of references are listed. Permission and sources are indicated; for detailed attributions, please refer to the permissions page and list of contributors. Reasonable efforts have been made to publish reliable data and information, but the authors, editors and publisher cannot assume any responsibility for the validity of all materials or the consequences of their use.

ISBN: 978-1-63241-897-5

Trademark Notice: Registered trademark of products or corporate names are used only for explanation and identification without intent to infringe.

Cataloging-in-Publication Data

Glaucoma : clinical ophthalmology / edited by Collin Cruz.
  p. cm.
Includes bibliographical references and index.
ISBN 978-1-63241-897-5
1. Glaucoma. 2. Eye--Diseases. 3. Eye--Diseases--Treatment. 4. Ophthalmology. I. Cruz, Collin.
RE871 .G53 2020
617.741--dc23

Table of Contents

Preface

Glaucoma is a group of eye diseases associated with damage to the optic nerve that may cause vision loss. Open-angle glaucoma, normal-tension glaucoma and closed-angle glaucoma are the common forms of glaucoma diseases. Open-angle glaucoma develops slowly without pain whereas closed-angle glaucoma can occur suddenly or gradually. It may involve severe eye pain, mild-dilated pupil, nausea and blurred vision. Damage of optic nerve caused by normal pressure is known as normal-tension glaucoma. The loss of vision that occurs as a result of glaucoma is permanent. High blood pressure, frequent pressure in the eye and family history are the common factors that increase the risk of glaucoma. Laser treatment, surgery or medication can cure this disease if diagnosed early. This book strives to provide a fair idea about this disease and help develop a better understanding of the latest advances within its management. From theories to research to practical applications, case studies related to all contemporary topics of relevance to this disease have been included herein. With state-of-the-art inputs by acclaimed experts of this field, this book targets students and professionals.

Significant researches are present in this book. Intensive efforts have been employed by authors to make this book an outstanding discourse. This book contains the enlightening chapters which have been written on the basis of significant researches done by the experts.

Finally, I would also like to thank all the members involved in this book for being a team and meeting all the deadlines for the submission of their respective works. I would also like to thank my friends and family for being supportive in my efforts.

Editor

1

Mapping the Structure-Function Relationship in Glaucoma and Healthy Patients Measured with Spectralis OCT and Humphrey Perimetry

Laia Jaumandreu ⓘ,[1] Francisco J. Muñoz–Negrete,[1] Noelia Oblanca,[2] and Gema Rebolleda[1]

[1]Ophthalmology Service, University Hospital Ramón y Cajal, School of Medicine and Health Science, University of Alcalá, IRYCIS, Hospital Ramón y Cajal, Ctra. Colmenar Viejo km. 9100, 28034 Madrid, Spain
[2]Ophthalmology Service, University Hospital Ramón y Cajal, IRYCIS, Hospital Ramón y Cajal, Ctra. Colmenar Viejo km. 9100, 28034 Madrid, Spain

Correspondence should be addressed to Laia Jaumandreu; laiajaumandreu@msn.com

Academic Editor: Paolo Fogagnolo

Purpose. To study the structure-function relationship in glaucoma and healthy patients assessed with Spectralis OCT and Humphrey perimetry using new statistical approaches. *Materials and Methods*. Eighty-five eyes were prospectively selected and divided into 2 groups: glaucoma (44) and healthy patients (41). Three different statistical approaches were carried out: (1) factor analysis of the threshold sensitivities (dB) (automated perimetry) and the macular thickness (μm) (Spectralis OCT), subsequently applying Pearson's correlation to the obtained regions, (2) nonparametric regression analysis relating the values in each pair of regions that showed significant correlation, and (3) nonparametric spatial regressions using three models designed for the purpose of this study. *Results*. In the glaucoma group, a map that relates structural and functional damage was drawn. The strongest correlation with visual fields was observed in the peripheral nasal region of both superior and inferior hemigrids ($r = 0.602$ and $r = 0.458$, resp.). The estimated functions obtained with the nonparametric regressions provided the mean sensitivity that corresponds to each given macular thickness. These functions allowed for accurate characterization of the structure-function relationship. *Conclusions*. Both maps and point-to-point functions obtained linking structure and function damage contribute to a better understanding of this relationship and may help in the future to improve glaucoma diagnosis.

1. Introduction

Perimetry is classically considered the "gold standard" for glaucoma diagnosis, but a significant loss of retinal ganglion cells (25–30%) occurs before any of the typical glaucomatous visual field (VF) defects are detected [1]. Several studies have found that the combination of data obtained from structural and functional tests improves the diagnostic capability of each of these tests individually [2, 3]. As a result, researchers are now focusing on exploring in depth the relationship between structure and function in glaucoma.

In 1998, Zeimer et al. [4] first suggested imaging of the macula as a potential structure for the diagnosis of

glaucoma, and it has now been widely demonstrated that thinning of the macula occurs in glaucoma as a result of the retinal ganglion cells (RGC) loss typical of this pathology [5, 6]. Several authors have studied the correlation between perimetry and macular thickness [7–13]. Most of them used simple correlation and linear regression between global indices and by sectors. We believe that this approach falls short in terms of providing an accurate explanation of the structure-function relationship. In this study, we take one more step making an analysis by regions and point to point using the macular grid given by the Spectralis OCT and novel statistical approaches. These approaches, some of which had not been employed previously in the field, may contribute to a better understanding of the relationship.

2. Materials and Methods

2.1. Subjects and Experimental Design. The research protocol followed the tenets of the Declaration of Helsinki and was approved by the ethical committee of University Hospital Ramón y Cajal, Madrid, Spain. Informed consent was obtained from each participant before enrollment after explanation of the nature and possible consequences of the study. A cohort of patients was prospectively selected according to the following inclusion criteria: between 18 and 80 years of age, best corrected visual acuity > 20/40 (Snellen) in the study eye, refractive error within ±5.00 dioptres equivalent sphere and ±2.00 dioptres astigmatism, and transparent ocular structures: crystalline lens opacity < 1 in LOCS III (Lens Opacities Classification System) [14] and availability and collaboration to perform protocol exploratory tests. Patients with any kind of retinopathy, who had previously undergone ocular surgery except phacoemulsification without complications, with a history of neuroophthalmic disorder, ocular malformations, angle or optic nerve anomalies, or who had any serious disease or current use of a medication that could affect visual field sensitivity, were excluded from the study.

The cohort of patients was divided into 2 groups: patients with glaucoma or "cases" and healthy patients or "controls." The glaucoma subjects had to meet two diagnosis criteria: (1) glaucomatous appearance of the optic disc evaluated by a glaucoma specialist, defined as focal or diffuse neuroretinal rim narrowing with concentric enlargement of the optic cup, localized notching or both [15] and (2) perimetric criteria for glaucoma: glaucoma Hemifield Test (GHT) results outside normal limits, a pattern standard deviation (PSD) with a P value < 5%, or a cluster of three or more nonedge points on the pattern deviation plot in a single hemifield with P values < 5%, one of which must have a P value < 1%.

All the patients in the study underwent the following series of tests: general anamnesis, basic eye examination, optical coherence tomography with Spectralis OCT® (Heidelberg Engineering, Heidelberg, Germany), and at least two reliable automated conventional perimetry tests of both eyes with Humphrey visual field analyzer (Carl Zeiss Meditec, Dublin, California, USA). The perimetric test was performed with SITA (Swedish interactive threshold algorithm) standard 24-2 strategy. The following reliability criteria were adopted: fixation losses, false-positive rate, and false-negative rate less than 20% [16, 17]. The last reliable perimetry test obtained was used in this study to minimize the learning effect and only reproducible visual field defects were taken into account [18, 19]. The protocol selected on the Spectralis OCT was the posterior pole asymmetry analysis which measures retinal thickness in the posterior pole using 61 lines (30°×25° OCT volume scan) for each eye in a central 20 degree area. Only the OCT scans with a signal equal to or higher than 24 that were adequately centred on the fovea and had no eye movement or blinking artefacts were considered.

2.2. Statistical Analysis. Descriptive and correlation statistical analyses were carried out using SPSS statistical software for Windows (version 20.0, IBM-SPSS, Chicago, Illinois, USA). Nonparametric regression analyses were coded in GAUSS (9.0 version, light). In order to facilitate analysis, all data were converted to left eye data. A statistical significance of $P < 0.05$ was required for all comparisons.

In order to study differences between the two groups, the following variables were compared: age, sex, laterality, test time, as well as mean and standard deviation of visual field index (VFI), mean deviation (MD), and average thickness total, superior, and inferior (ATT, ATS, ATI). The Kolmogorov-Smirnov test was used to assess the normality of distribution.

A factor analysis, principal component type, was carried out as a first approach to the study of the structure-function relationship. This was based on a previous analysis described by Ferreras et al. in 2008 [16]. We took as random variables: mean threshold sensitivities (dB) of the automated perimetry (excluding from the analysis those corresponding to the blind spot) and mean macular thickness (μm) calculated for each $3°\times 3°$ square of the macular grid. Separate analyses were carried out for each group—glaucoma and healthy patients—and for each hemifield and hemigrid individually (assuming that the superior and inferior hemifields and hemigrids are anatomically distinct). Each variable was assigned to a factor or principal component, obtaining as a result interrelated groups of variables and, thus, determining the regions. Pearson's correlation was subsequently applied to these regions (superior hemifield with inferior hemigrid and inferior hemifield with superior hemigrid) in both groups.

The second approach was nonparametric regression analysis. Nonparametric regression analysis allows the study of the relationship between two variables, x and y, when this relationship is given by an unknown function that is determined as $m(x)$ plus the prediction errors $u(y = m(x) + u)$. We used the Nadaraya-Watson estimator with standard normal kernel [20]. Threshold sensitivity (dB) was established as the dependent variable (y) and macular thickness (μm) as the independent variable (x) in all cases. Two types of regression were applied. First, nonparametric regressions were calculated for each pair of zones or regions, obtained through factor analysis, that showed significant correlation according to Pearson's correlation coefficient in the glaucoma group. Then, several nonparametric spatial regressions were calculated using three models designed by our team for the purpose of this study. The models are based on the spatial correspondence between the measuring points of threshold sensitivity in the automated perimetry and the macular thickness map, as shown in Figure 1(a), assuming the same principles of spatial correspondence than other authors [12, 13]. The study was carried out separately for the two groups (glaucoma and control). The three nonparametric spatial regression models used are summarized and explained in Figures 1(b)–1(c).

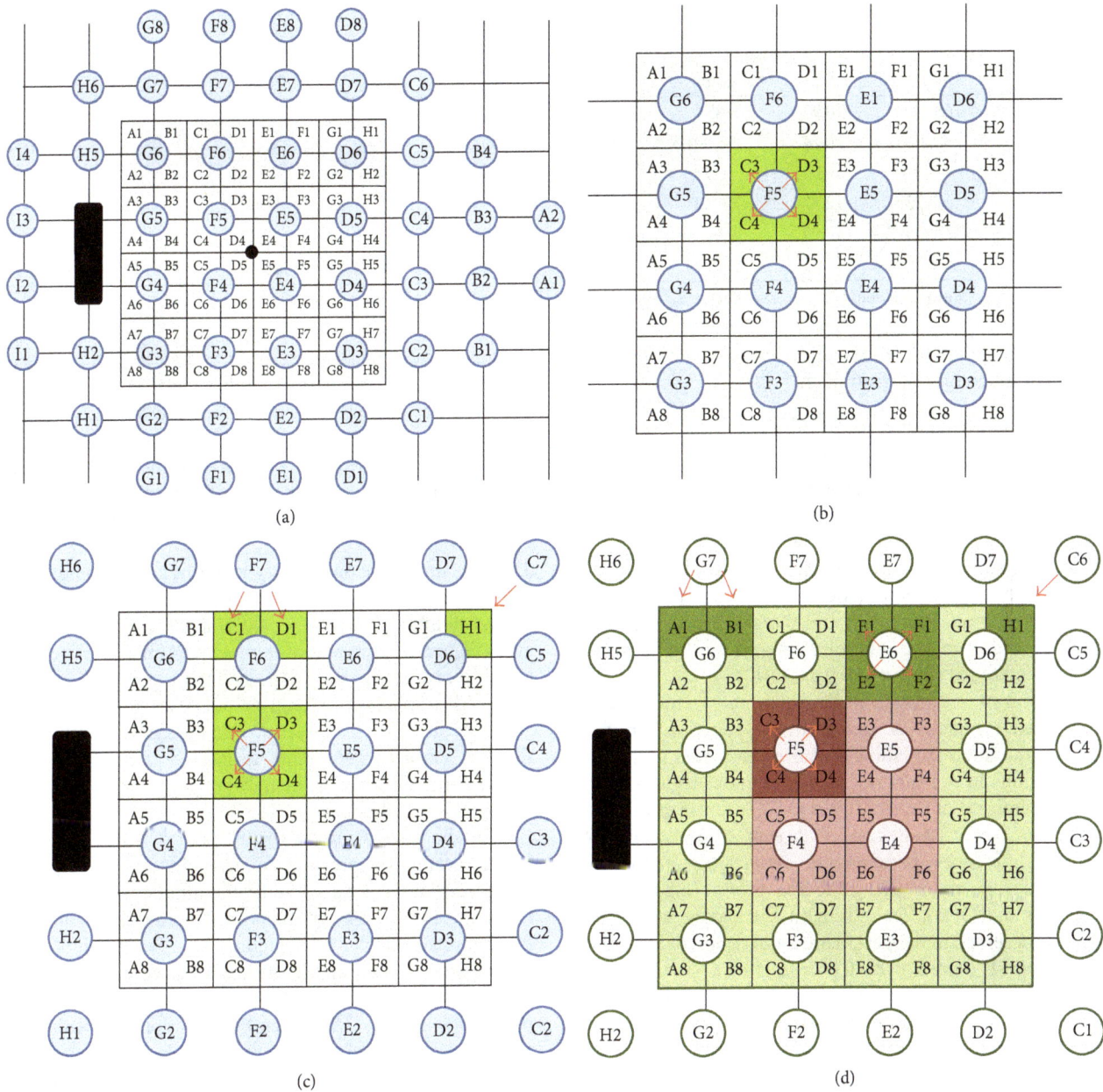

FIGURE 1: (a) Spatial correspondence between the measuring points of threshold sensitivity in the automatized perimetry (Humphrey, 24-2 program) and the macular thickness map (Spectralis OCT). (b) Graphic scheme of the first nonparametric spatial regression model. The measurements of threshold sensitivity in each of the 16 central points of the visual field are regressed on the macular thickness of the four surrounding areas. (c) Graphic scheme of the second nonparametric spatial regression model. The measurements of threshold sensitivity in each of the 34 central points of the visual field are regressed on the macular thickness of either the four surrounding areas for the 16 central points or the closest one or two areas (depending on the position) for the 18 most eccentric points. (d) Graphic scheme of the third nonparametric spatial regression model. Two separate regressions were performed: the measurements of threshold sensitivity in each of the 4 central points of the visual field on the macular thickness of the four surrounding areas (red) and the measurements in each of the other 30 points (green) on the 4, 2, or 1 (depending on the position) closest areas.

3. Results

A total of 85 eyes of 58 Caucasian patients selected according to the inclusion criteria were included in this study (44 glaucoma; 41 control). Table 1 summarizes global descriptive statistics obtained in both groups. The patients in the glaucoma group had a mean MD of -7.73 ± 5.58 dB. All the macular thickness indices analysed (ATT, ATS, and ATI) showed statistically significant differences between both groups, and their values were always lower in the glaucoma cohort. The study also revealed a significant difference between the mean macular thickness of the superior and inferior hemigrids in

TABLE 1: Demographic characteristics and global indices obtained in both groups.

	Glaucoma				Healthy				P values
	Mean	SD	Max	Min	Mean	SD	Max	Min	
Age (years)	68.43	10.93	85	35	47.93	19.24	78	24	<0.001
VFI[a]	80.84	16.24	98.00	27.00	99.0	0.95	100	96	<0.001
MD[b]	−7.73	5.58	−0.74	−23.28	−1.083	1.32	1.72	−3.39	<0.001
ATT[c]	269.75	12.77	297.00	250.00	290.00	16.77	329.00	254.00	<0.001
ATS[d]	274.34	15.02	309.00	252.00	290.68	17.46	332.00	251.00	<0.001
ATI[e]	265.39	13.81	292.00	244.00	291.10	16.30	326.00	257.00	<0.001

[a]Visual field index. [b]Mean deviation. [c]Total average thickness. [d]Superior average thickness. [e]Inferior average thickness.

the glaucoma group, while the control group did not show any significant difference between them.

3.1. Factor Analysis and Pearson's Correlation Coefficient between the Obtained Regions.
The measure of sampling adequacy (MSA), KMO (Kaiser-Meyer-Olkin) measure, was greater than 0.6 in all cases and the total variance explained by the selected components was >80%.

In the glaucoma group, the factor analysis determined 4 regions or factors in both superior and inferior hemifields of the automatized perimetry, and 5 regions in the superior hemigrid and 7 in the inferior hemigrid of the Spectralis OCT macular grid (Figures 2(b) and 3(b)).

In contrast, in the control group, the factor analysis determined 3 regions or factors in the superior hemifield and 5 in the inferior hemifield of the automated perimetry, and 3 regions in the superior hemigrid and 5 regions in the inferior hemigrid of the Spectralis OCT macular grid.

Pearson's correlation coefficients showed statistically significant differences between the associated anatomical-functional regions in the glaucoma group (Figures 2(a), 2(b), 3(a), and 3(b)). The strongest correlation with visual field was observed in the peripheral nasal region of both macular hemigrids (superior $r = 0.602$; inferior $r = 0.458$), while the temporal peripapillary and temporal peripheral regions did not show any significant correlation. In contrast, no significant correlation was found in the control group.

3.2. Nonparametric Regression between the Regions Obtained through Factor Analysis.
Figures 2(a) and 3(a) depict the regression curves between regions that showed significant correlation according to Pearson's correlation coefficient in the glaucoma group. These curves represent the mean threshold sensitivity values for each thickness value of the macular thickness map of each respective region. Only the mean threshold sensitivity values with corresponding thickness data available were plotted. Since no significant correlations between the regions were observed in the control group, we omit regression for those data. All the regression curves showed a similar pattern: an area of ascending slope (more or less steeper depending on the pair under study) that takes a shape similar to a linear function where the greater the macular thickness is, the greater the sensitivity is, and another area with a slope that is close to zero in which the threshold sensitivity is maintained more or less constant despite the increase in macular thickness. The functions

showing greater linear correlation and steeper slopes corresponded to the correlation studies between the pairs of regions that showed a stronger linear relationship (higher Pearson's correlation coefficient). The nonparametric regression curves obtained for the paracentral and peripheral regions showed similar characteristics among them. This also happened with the curves obtained for the central regions.

3.3. Nonparametric Spatial Regression.
The first model used studied the function-structure relationship between the 16 central points in the visual field and the complete macular grid (Figure 1(b)). An approximately linear ascending relationship can be observed in the glaucoma group where sensitivity (dB) increases alongside macular thickness (μm), although there are two sections of the curve in which the slope is close to zero. One is located between 220 and 240 μm and the other at the halfway point between 270 and 290 μm (Figure 4(a)).

For the second model, the 18 points in the visual field located around the previous 16 were added to the regression curve, so that the model studied the function-structure relationship between 34 central points in the visual field and the complete macular grid (Figure 1(c)). The graph obtained for the glaucoma group (Figure 4(b)) was very similar to that of the first regression model, therefore confirming the shape of the relationship. An ascending relationship with, once again, two sections in which the slope is close to zero can be observed. These two sections appear at the same point as in the first model (220 and 270 μm) but stretch slightly further in both cases.

The third model divided the data into two subgroups: the peripheral and the central macular areas (Figure 1(d)). Independent regression curves were drawn for each subgroup. The peripheral area in the glaucoma group showed an ascending relationship with two horizontal tails, while the central area showed only one ascending section (Figure 4(c)).

None of these three models revealed any significant correlation between structure and function in the control group (Figures 4(a) and 4(b)).

4. Discussion

We successfully drew a map linking functional and structural damage in the glaucoma group using Humphrey perimetry and the posterior pole asymmetry analysis of the Spectralis OCT regions, obtained completely from an objective

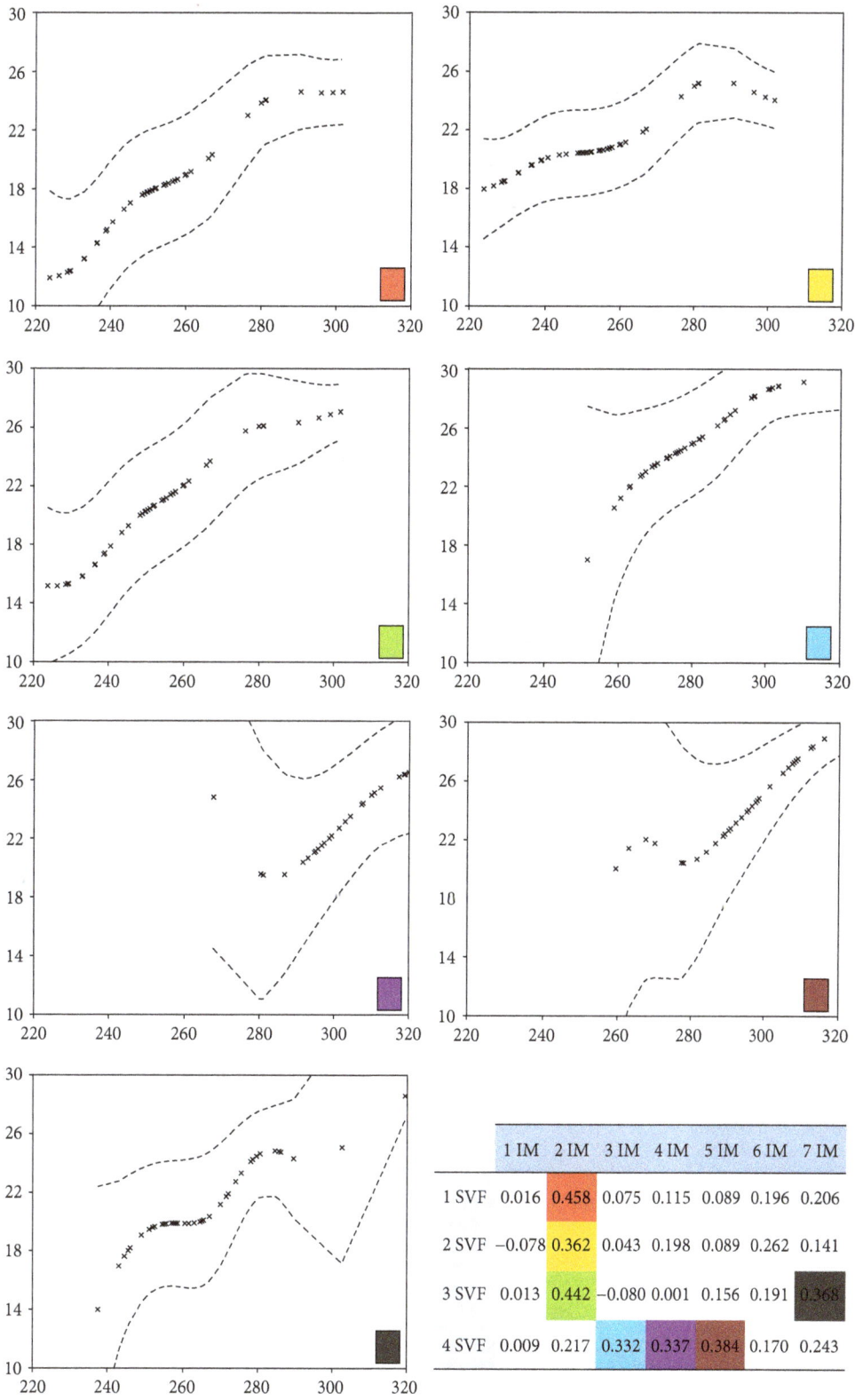

	1 IM	2 IM	3 IM	4 IM	5 IM	6 IM	7 IM
1 SVF	0.016	0.458	0.075	0.115	0.089	0.196	0.206
2 SVF	−0.078	0.362	0.043	0.198	0.089	0.262	0.141
3 SVF	0.013	0.442	−0.080	0.001	0.156	0.191	0.368
4 SVF	0.009	0.217	0.332	0.337	0.384	0.170	0.243

(a)

FIGURE 2: Continued.

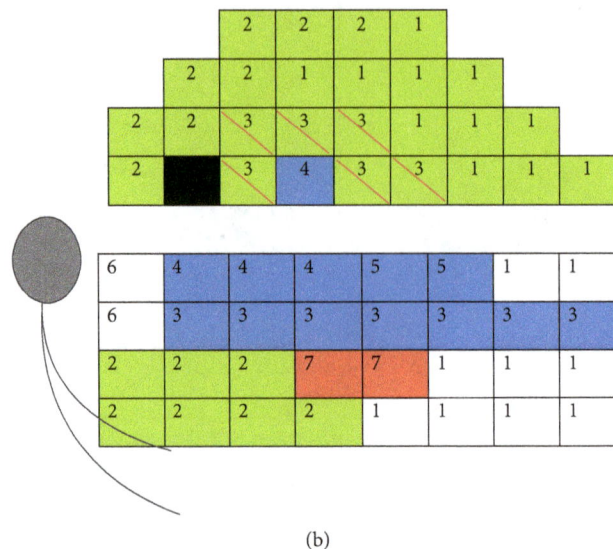

(b)

FIGURE 2: (a) Nonparametric regression between the regions of the superior hemifield (1–4 superior visual field, SVF) and inferior hemigrid (1–7 inferior macula, IM) obtained through factor analysis and that showed significant correlation according to Pearson's correlation coefficient (shown at the bottom right of the graphics) in the glaucoma group. Values of threshold sensitivity (decibels) are represented in the y-axis and values of macular thickness (microns) in the x-axis. (b) Graphic scheme of the Pearson correlations between the regions obtained through factor analysis of the superior hemifield (1–4) and factor analysis of the inferior hemigrid (1–7) in glaucoma cases. Regions that showed significant correlations are represented with the same color.

analysis, and several functions that provide the mean sensitivity that would correspond to each given macular thickness in glaucoma patients.

In contrast, consistently with previously studies, we have not found any relevant correlation between structure and function in healthy patients [17, 21, 22].

Factor analysis is a data reduction tool for statistical analysis that summarizes data supplied by a group of variables into a smaller set of representative factors. Ferreras et al. [16] first suggested the clustering of threshold points in VF testing using this technique. The advantage of establishing groups of threshold points in this way is that the cluster is not subject to anatomical knowledge of the RNFL or to any preconceived ideas about the relationships in the VF. Another advantage of carrying out factor analysis is that both direct and indirect relationships between the various threshold points are taken into consideration.

Some previous studies on the structure-function relationship maintain that the units of measurement in both must be the same (linear or logarithmic) [23]. However, we performed the study both in decibels (dB) and microns (μm), and in apostilb (asb) and μm, obtaining equivalent outcomes. In this paper, we present the results maintaining the values of the perimetric variables in dB and the macular thickness values in μm because this allows for a more intuitive interpretation of the data and the relationships.

Our VF maps, although with some differences, are overall similar to those obtained in previous studies in which factor analysis of the visual field was carried out [16, 24]. As far as we know, such an analysis has not been previously carried out for the macular hemigrids. The regions obtained were different in the two groups analysed and asymmetrical

between hemifields and hemigrids. However, a general similar pattern was observed in all of them.

All the global parameters used to measure total macular thickness (ATT, ATS, and ATI) were significantly lower in the glaucoma group than in the control group. This agrees with previous studies [25–28] and demonstrates the thinning of the macula in glaucoma patients. Mathers et al. [9], also using the Spectralis OCT posterior pole asymmetry analysis, found that patients with a mean macular thickness greater than 300 μm showed practically normal VF. In our study, the mean total macular thickness in the control group was 290.95 μm.

Although most of previous studies agree that the inferior hemimacula shows the strongest correlation with the VF, they do not agree that the peripheral nasal region has the strongest correlation [21, 29, 30]. Only Kim et al. [12], that analysed the point-wise relationship between VF and macular retinal thickness with the posterior pole asymmetry analysis, found that it was stronger in the central and nasal test points (range $r = 0.14$–0.38). Rolle et al. [13], also with this protocol, obtained the strongest correlation in nasal inferior ($r = 0.55$) and temporal inferior quadrant ($r = 0.57$). In the protocols to map the thickness of the macular and the inner retinal layers heretofore used, the nasal and papillomacular bundles are assessed in the same sector. It has been established that the papillomacular bundle is only affected in the advanced stages of glaucoma [28, 31, 32]. This fact may have caused masking of stronger correlations in the nasal peripheral sector in the results obtained until now. In our study, the regions established through factor analysis distinguish between the temporal peripapillary and peripheral nasal regions, and we analyse them separately. The results obtained

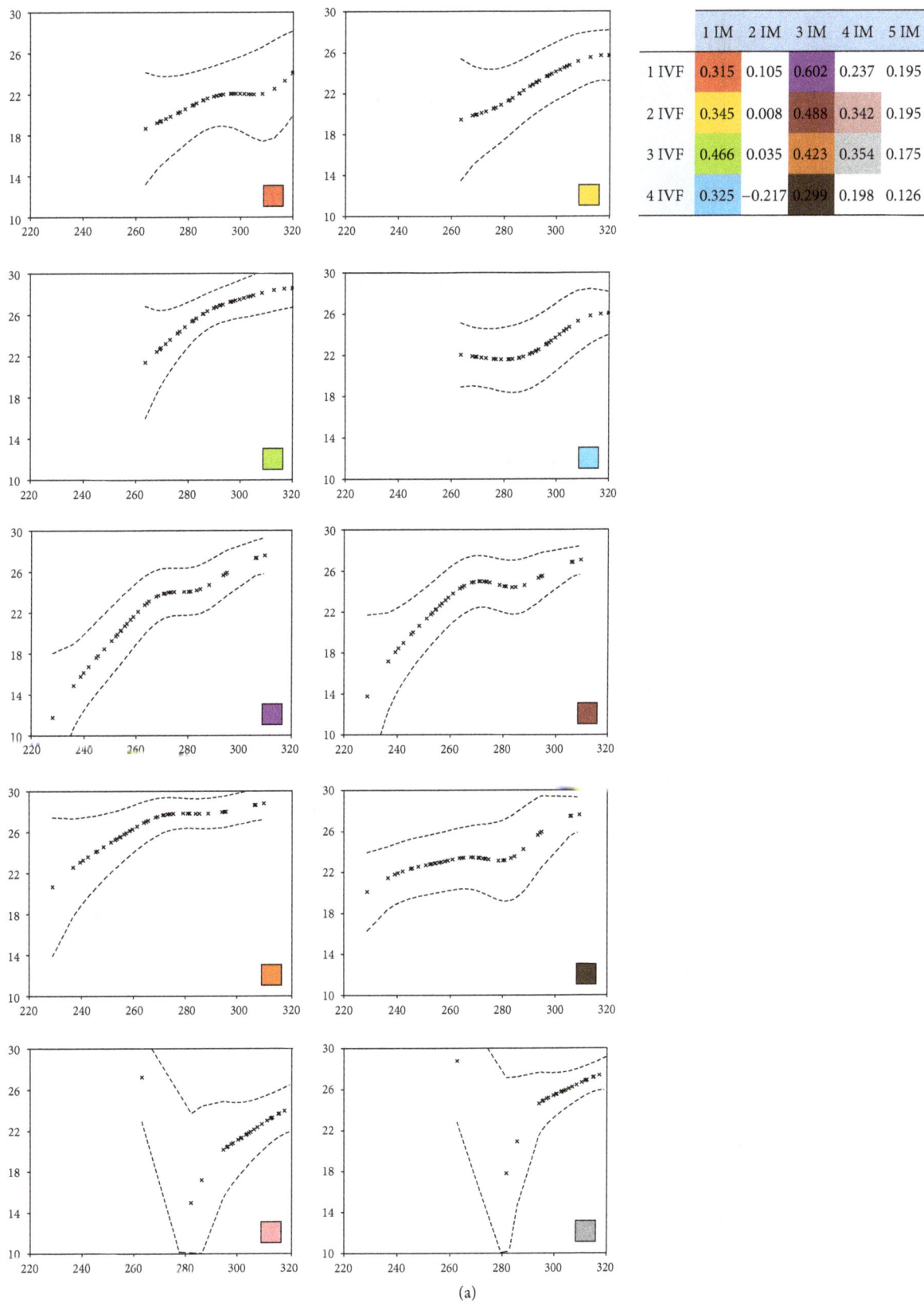

	1 IM	2 IM	3 IM	4 IM	5 IM
1 IVF	0.315	0.105	0.602	0.237	0.195
2 IVF	0.345	0.008	0.488	0.342	0.195
3 IVF	0.466	0.035	0.423	0.354	0.175
4 IVF	0.325	−0.217	0.299	0.198	0.126

(a)

FIGURE 3: Continued.

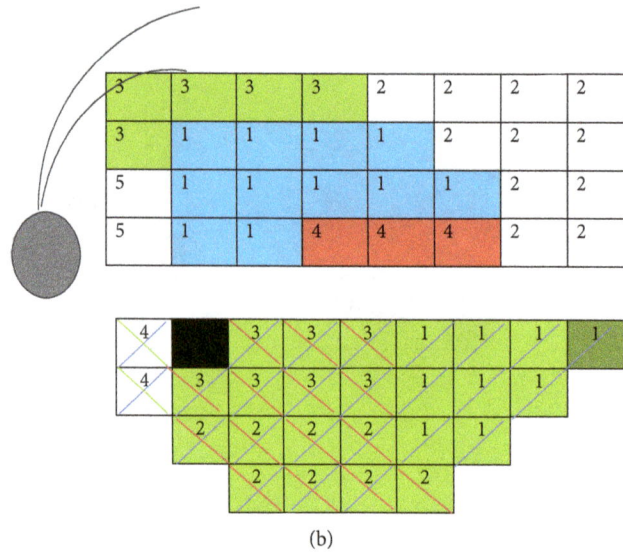

(b)

FIGURE 3: (a) Nonparametric regression between the regions of the inferior hemifield (1–4 inferior visual field, IVF) and superior hemigrid (1–5 superior macula, SM) obtained through factor analysis and that showed significant correlation according to Pearson's correlation coefficient (shown at the top right of the graphics) in the glaucoma group. Values of threshold sensitivity (decibels) are represented in the *y*-axis and values of macular thickness (microns) in the *x*-axis. (b) Graphic scheme of the Pearson correlations between the regions obtained though factor analysis of the inferior hemifield (1–4) and factor analysis of the superior hemigrid (1–5) in glaucoma cases. Regions that showed significant correlations are represented with the same color. Correlations with $P < 0.05$ are represented by colored thin strips.

showed that no significant correlation existed between both hemimacular of the peripapillary temporal region (through which the fibers of the papillomacular bundle would enter) and any of the field regions. By contrast, the peripheral nasal region showed the strongest correlation with VF.

Further studies with protocols to map both regions separately, in different populations and with larger samples, are required in order to confirm whether this region indeed presents better structure-function correlation than the temporal region.

The application of nonparametric regression analysis between each pair of areas that had shown a significant Pearson correlation allowed for the confirmation, quantification, and accurate detection of the characteristics of this relationship. All pairs displayed similar characteristics, especially in the relationships between peripheral and central regions, although some distinctive features were also observed. The shape of the curve resembles the "hockey" or "broken stick" statistical model used by several authors to determine the cut-off point at which peripapillary RNFL thickness begins to show correlation with visual field defects [17, 33, 34].

Nonparametric spatial regression is the third approach to assess structure-function correlation that is suggested in this study. This approach moves away from the principles of classic statistical analysis towards more recent trends and innovations in the field, and it allows for the adoption of a novel perspective to the study of the structure-function relationship. The three nonparametric spatial regression models applied offer an alternative approach that bypasses the need to factor analysis and estimates on average an unknown relationship that is presupposed to exist in all the patients. The estimated function provides the mean sensitivity that would

correspond to each given macular thickness, both in glaucoma patients and in healthy ones.

The earliest studies on the structure-function relationship were carried out using statistical models that in one or another way tried to explain this relationship in a linear manner [23]. However, researchers found that good linear correlation only appeared in certain intervals but not throughout, and that often the relationship obtained fitted better a curve rather than a line. For example, Kim et al. [12] found that the global structure-function association was better explained with a quadratic regression model than the linear regression. Garway-Heath et al. [35, 36] suggested that this trend could be the consequence of measuring the dimensions using units that had very different characteristics but this does not fully explain the relationships obtained to the present. Gonzalez-Hernandez et al. [22] correlating the standard automated perimetry mean sensitivity and the global mean RNFL throughout different stages of glaucoma found that the curvilinear relationship between the morphologic and perimetric results may be due to the wide variability in normal morphology and limitations in the dynamic range of the morphologic tests in cases with moderate and severe defects.

There are several facts that suggest a priori that the structure-function relationship at macular level may adjust better to a curvilinear model than to linear regression.

On the one hand, it has been demonstrated that there is a "floor effect" or residual thickness, which has been studied extensively in perimetry-peripapillary RNFL correlations. This concept can also be applied to the measurement of macular thickness if understood from a wider perspective.

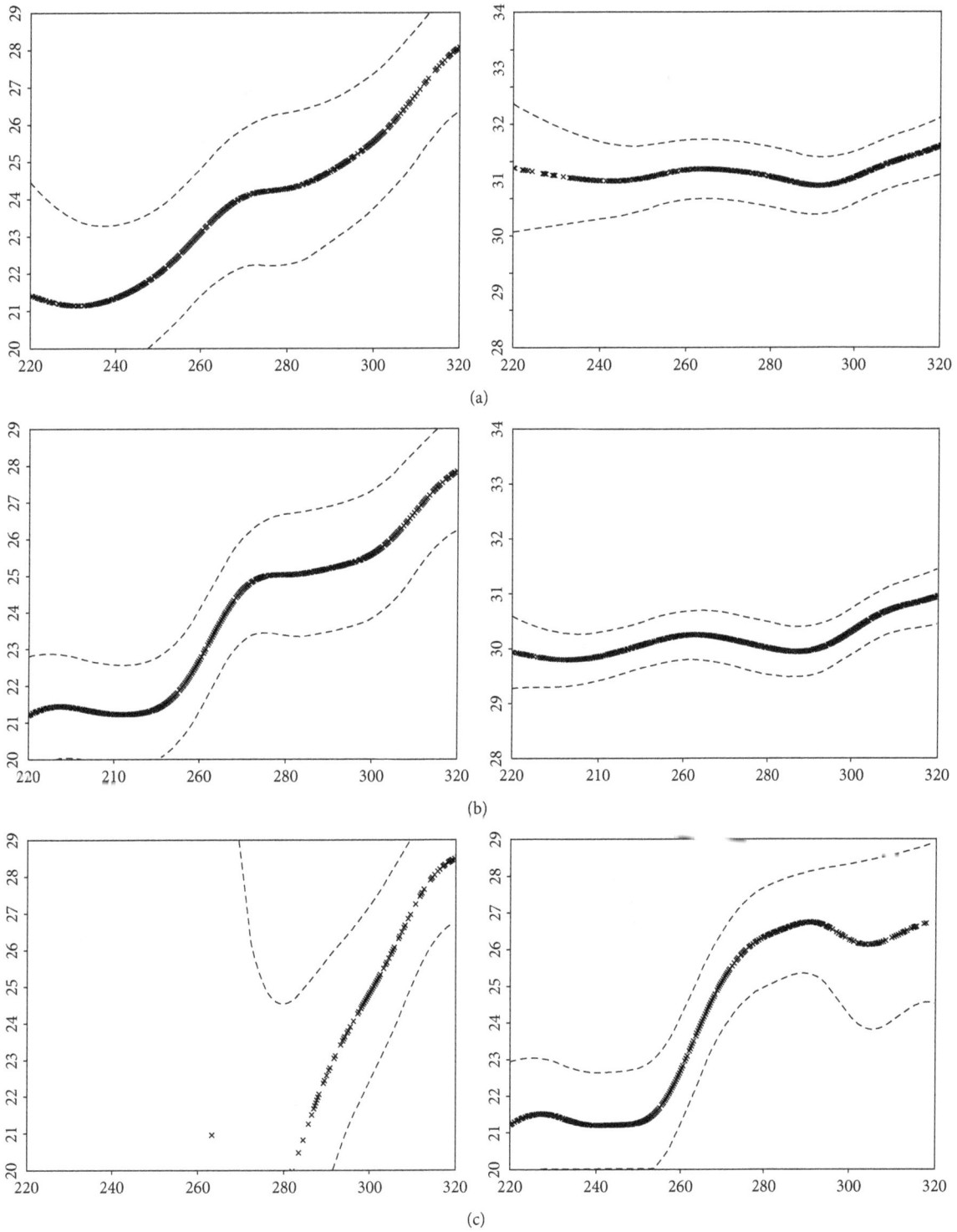

Figure 4: (a) Regression curves obtained with the application of the first model in the glaucoma (left) and control (right) groups. Dashed lines represent 90% confidence intervals. Values of threshold sensitivity (decibels) are represented in the y-axis and values of macular thickness (microns) in the x-axis. (b) Regression curves obtained with the application of the second model in the glaucoma (left) and control (right) groups. (c) Regression curves for centre (left) and periphery (right), obtained with the application of the third model in the glaucoma group.

On the other hand, several studies suggest that structural defects precede alterations in the visual field [37, 38]. It is also important to consider that early diagnosis depends on the resolution of the system used. Over the past ten years, OCT models have significantly improved in resolution power and accuracy of measurements, while automated perimetry has not changed significantly in the last twenty years. If we accept a linear correlation model for the relationship between structure and function, we would be suggesting that neither parameter affects the other earlier than the other, but rather that the effect is simultaneous.

Other authors [39, 40] have also described linear relationships with varying slope as retinal eccentricity increases, which could point to the appearance of nonlinear relationships in the global analysis of the data.

In conclusion, none of the statistical models currently available fits or can explain thoroughly the characteristics of the relationship between structure and function in glaucoma.

The nonparametric spatial regression models suggested in this study try to resolve many of the weakness in previous studies. Their greatest advantage is that no preestablished functional form is imposed on the data, therefore allowing for the data to determine and draw both linear and nonlinear relationships. They also allow for the use of the most commonly used units of measurement and enable the use of all the values obtained in the analysis of both tests. The relationships can be spatially mapped in order to explore correspondences in more depth than through the application of global parameters or point averages in specific regions. We obtain a function than provides the mean sensitivity that would correspond to each given macular thickness in glaucoma patients improving our understanding of the structure-function relationship.

Although carrying out the correlation study between structure and function using the posterior pole asymmetry analysis provided with Spectralis OCT has several advantages, it is limited by the fact that it can only measure the total thickness of the macula and not the specific layers that are usually more affected in glaucoma (retinal ganglion cell layer). This can increase data noise and the results can also be affected by other eye conditions. This protocol adjusts better to the 24-2 pattern than other systems and we chose this pattern because it is the most often used in clinic in the diagnosis and monitoring of glaucoma; however, it is possible that some relevant information was lost, especially in the centremost points in the visual field [41].

Another limitation of this study is that statistically significant differences in age were found between the two groups. Patients were obtained prospectively and included in one or another group according to the inclusion criteria. The fact that glaucoma is a more frequent pathology in elderly people and that for being included in the control group it was required to lack any other ophthalmic pathology explains this difference. Previous studies have shown that RNFL thickness and visual field sensitivity decrease with age [42–45]. This could induce some bias when comparing the results between both groups. However, because our research focuses on studying separately the correlation between structure and function in glaucomatous or healthy eyes, we think this difference does not imply a distortion in the interpretation of the data.

5. Conclusions

This study explores the relationship between structure and function in glaucoma, using novel statistical approaches,

and some of which had not been employed previously in this field. The VF test point measures show significant correlation with the corresponding macular thickness points, varying across different regions. The map linking structural damage and functional damage and the corresponding point-to-point functions can be used in the future to improve glaucoma diagnosis and be an additional structural assessment tool.

Further work is necessary in order to confirm these results. The development of more powerful image resolution and better analytical algorithms as well as better functional tests will eventually allow for more accuracy in the assessment of these relationships.

Conflicts of Interest

The authors declare that there is no conflict of interest regarding the publication of this article.

Acknowledgments

The authors are grateful to Jordi Jaumandreu for his assistance and contribution to the statistical analysis of this report.

References

[1] L. A. Kerrigan-Baumrind, H. A. Quigley, M. E. Pease, D. F. Kerrigan, and R. S. Mitchell, "Number of ganglion cells in glaucoma eyes compared with threshold visual field tests in the same persons," *Investigative Ophthalmology & Visual Science*, vol. 41, no. 3, pp. 741–748, 2000.

[2] A. S. Raza, X. Zhang, C. G. V. de Moraes et al., "Improving glaucoma detection using spatially correspondent clusters of damage and by combining standard automated perimetry and optical coherence tomography," *Investigative Ophthalmology & Visual Science*, vol. 55, no. 1, pp. 612–624, 2014.

[3] A. J. Tatham, R. N. Weinreb, and F. A. Medeiros, "Strategies for improving early detection of glaucoma: the combined structure–function index," *Clinical Ophthalmology*, vol. 8, pp. 611–621, 2014.

[4] R. Zeimer, S. Asrani, S. Zou, H. Quigley, and H. Jampel, "Quantitative detection of glaucomatous damage at the posterior pole by retinal thickness mapping. A pilot study," *Ophthalmology*, vol. 105, no. 2, pp. 224–231, 1998.

[5] C. K. S. Leung, W. M. Chan, W. H. Yung et al., "Comparison of macular and peripapillary measurements for the detection of glaucoma: an optical coherence tomography study," *Ophthalmology*, vol. 112, no. 3, pp. 391–400, 2005.

[6] F. A. Medeiros, L. M. Zangwill, C. Bowd, R. M. Vessani, R. Susanna Jr., and R. N. Weinreb, "Evaluation of retinal nerve fiber layer, optic nerve head, and macular thickness measurements for glaucoma detection using optical coherence tomography," *American Journal of Ophthalmology*, vol. 139, no. 1, pp. 44–55, 2005.

[7] W. Boling, D. WuDunn, L. B. Cantor, J. Hoop, M. James, and V. Nukala, "Correlation between macular thickness and glaucomatous visual fields," *Journal of Glaucoma*, vol. 21, no. 8, pp. 505–509, 2012.

[8] F. N. Kanadani, D. C. Hood, T. M. Grippo et al., "Structural and functional assessment of the macular region in patients

with glaucoma," *The British Journal of Ophthalmology*, vol. 90, no. 11, pp. 1393–1397, 2006.

[9] K. Mathers, J. A. Rosdahl, and S. Asrani, "Correlation of macular thickness with visual fields in glaucoma patients and suspects," *Journal of Glaucoma*, vol. 23, no. 2, pp. e98–104, 2014.

[10] D. S. Greenfield, H. Bagga, and R. W. Knighton, "Macular thickness changes in glaucomatous optic neuropathy detected using optical coherence tomography," *Archives of Ophthalmology*, vol. 121, no. 1, pp. 41–46, 2003.

[11] Y. Nakatani, T. Higashide, S. Ohkubo, H. Takeda, and K. Sugiyama, "Evaluation of macular thickness and peripapillary retinal nerve fiber layer thickness for detection of early glaucoma using spectral domain optical coherence tomography," *Journal of Glaucoma*, vol. 20, no. 4, pp. 252–259, 2011.

[12] J. M. Kim, K. R. Sung, Y. C. Yoo, and C. Y. Kim, "Point-wise relationships between visual field sensitivity and macular thickness determined by spectral-domain optical coherence tomography," *Current Eye Research*, vol. 38, no. 8, pp. 894–901, 2013.

[13] T. Rolle, L. Manerba, P. Lanzafame, and F. M. Grignolo, "Diagnostic power of macular retinal thickness analysis and structure-function relationship in glaucoma diagnosis using SPECTRALIS OCT," *Current Eye Research*, vol. 41, no. 5, pp. 667–675, 2016.

[14] L. T. Chylack Jr., J. K. Wolfe, D. M. Singer et al., "The lens opacities classification system III," *Archives of Ophthalmology*, vol. 111, no. 6, pp. 831–836, 1993.

[15] A. Tuulonen and P. J. Airaksinen, "Initial glaucomatous optic disk and retinal nerve fiber layer abnormalities and their progression," *American Journal of Ophthalmology*, vol. 111, no. 4, pp. 485–490, 1991.

[16] A. Ferreras, L. E. Pablo, D. F. Garway-Heath, P. Fogagnolo, and J. García-Feijoo, "Mapping standard automated perimetry to the peripapillary retinal nerve fiber layer in glaucoma," *Investigative Ophthalmology & Visual Science*, vol. 49, no. 7, pp. 3018–3025, 2008.

[17] T. Alasil, K. Wang, F. Yu et al., "Correlation of retinal nerve fiber layer thickness and visual fields in glaucoma: a broken stick model," *American Journal of Ophthalmology*, vol. 157, no. 5, pp. 953–959.e2, 2014.

[18] A. Heijl, A. Lindgren, and G. Lindgren, "Test-retest variability in glaucomatous visual fields," *American Journal of Ophthalmology*, vol. 108, no. 2, pp. 130–135, 1989.

[19] B. C. Chauhan and C. A. Johnson, "Test-retest variability of frequency-doubling perimetry and conventional perimetry in glaucoma patients and normal subjects," *Investigative Ophthalmology & Visual Science*, vol. 40, no. 3, pp. 648–656, 1999.

[20] M. P. J. Wand and M. C. Jones, "Kernel smoothing," in *Monographs on Statistics and Applied Probability*, pp. 97–103, Chapman & Hall, London, UK, 1995.

[21] S. Kim, J. Y. Lee, S. O. Kim, and M. S. Kook, "Macular structure–function relationship at various spatial locations in glaucoma," *The British Journal of Ophthalmology*, vol. 99, no. 10, pp. 1412–1418, 2015.

[22] M. Gonzalez-Hernandez, L. E. Pablo, K. Armas-Dominguez, R. R. de la Vega, A. Ferreras, and M. G. de la Rosa, "Structure--function relationship depends on glaucoma severity," *The British Journal of Ophthalmology*, vol. 93, no. 9, pp. 1195–1199, 2009.

[23] R. Malik, W. H. Swanson, and D. F. Garway-Heath, "'Structure–function relationship' in glaucoma: past thinking

[24] B. Monsalve, A. Ferreras, A. P. Khawaja et al., "The relationship between structure and function as measured by OCT and Octopus perimetry," *The British Journal of Ophthalmology*, vol. 99, no. 9, pp. 1230–1235, 2015.

[25] K. R. Sung, G. Wollstein, N. R. Kim et al., "Macular assessment using optical coherence tomography for glaucoma diagnosis," *The British Journal of Ophthalmology*, vol. 96, no. 12, pp. 1452–1455, 2012.

[26] V. Guedes, J. S. Schuman, E. Hertzmark et al., "Optical coherence tomography measurement of macular and nerve fiber layer thickness in normal and glaucomatous human eyes," *Ophthalmology*, vol. 110, no. 1, pp. 177–189, 2003.

[27] M. Tanito, N. Itai, A. Ohira, and E. Chihara, "Reduction of posterior pole retinal thickness in glaucoma detected using the retinal thickness analyzer," *Ophthalmology*, vol. 111, no. 2, pp. 265–275, 2004.

[28] O. Tan, V. Chopra, A. T. H. Lu et al., "Detection of macular ganglion cell loss in glaucoma by Fourier-domain optical coherence tomography," *Ophthalmology*, vol. 116, no. 12, pp. 2305–2314.e2, 2009.

[29] Y. Kotera, M. Hangai, F. Hirose, S. Mori, and N. Yoshimura, "Three-dimensional imaging of macular inner structures in glaucoma by using spectral-domain optical coherence tomography," *Investigative Ophthalmology & Visual Science*, vol. 52, no. 3, pp. 1412–1421, 2011.

[30] J. S. Jeong, M. G. Kang, C. Y. Kim, and N. R. Kim, "Pattern of macular ganglion cell-inner plexiform layer defect generated by spectral-domain OCT in glaucoma patients and normal subjects," *Journal of Glaucoma*, vol. 24, no. 8, pp. 583–590, 2015.

[31] D. C. Hood, P. Thienprasiddhi, V. C. Greenstein et al., "Detecting early to mild glaucomatous damage: a comparison of the multifocal VEP and automated perimetry," *Investigative Ophthalmology & Visual Science*, vol. 45, no. 2, pp. 492–498, 2004.

[32] A. Anton, N. Yamagishi, L. Zangwill, P. A. Sample, and R. N. Weinreb, "Mapping structural to functional damage in glaucoma with standard automated perimetry and confocal scanning laser ophthalmoscopy," *American Journal of Ophthalmology*, vol. 125, no. 4, pp. 436–446, 1998.

[33] C. Ajtony, Z. Balla, S. Somoskeoy, and B. Kovacs, "Relationship between visual field sensitivity and retinal nerve fiber layer thickness as measured by optical coherence tomography," *Investigative Ophthalmology & Visual Science*, vol. 48, no. 1, pp. 258–263, 2007.

[34] G. Wollstein, L. Kagemann, R. A. Bilonick et al., "Retinal nerve fibre layer and visual function loss in glaucoma: the tipping point," *The British Journal of Ophthalmology*, vol. 96, no. 1, pp. 47–52, 2012.

[35] D. F. Garway-Heath, J. Caprioli, F. W. Fitzke, and R. A. Hitchings, "Scaling the hill of vision: the physiological relationship between light sensitivity and ganglion cell numbers," *Investigative Ophthalmology & Visual Science*, vol. 41, no. 7, pp. 1774–1782, 2000.

[36] D. F. Garway-Heath, M. J. Greaney, and J. Caprioli, "Correction for the erroneous compensation of anterior segment birefringence with the scanning laser polarimeter for glaucoma diagnosis," *Investigative Ophthalmology & Visual Science*, vol. 43, no. 5, pp. 1465–1474, 2002.

[37] P. J. Airaksinen and H. I. Alanko, "Effect of retinal nerve fibre loss on the optic nerve head configuration in early glaucoma," *Graefe's Archive for Clinical and Experimental Ophthalmology*, vol. 220, no. 4, pp. 193–196, 1983.

[38] A. J. Vingrys, K. A. Helfrich, and G. Smith, "The role that binocular vision and stereopsis have in evaluating fundus features," *Optometry and Vision Science*, vol. 71, no. 8, pp. 508–515, 1994.

[39] R. S. Harwerth and H. A. Quigley, "Visual field defects and retinal ganglion cell losses in patients with glaucoma," *Archives of Ophthalmology*, vol. 124, no. 6, pp. 853–859, 2006.

[40] N. Drasdo, K. E. Mortlock, and R. V. North, "Ganglion cell loss and dysfunction: relationship to perimetric sensitivity," *Optometry and Vision Science*, vol. 85, no. 11, pp. 1036–1042, 2008.

[41] D. C. Hood, A. S. Raza, C. G. V. de Moraes, J. M. Liebmann, and R. Ritch, "Glaucomatous damage of the macula," *Progress in Retinal and Eye Research*, vol. 32, pp. 1–21, 2013.

[42] R. S. Parikh, S. R. Parikh, G. C. Sekhar, S. Prabakaran, J. G. Babu, and R. Thomas, "Normal age-related decay of retinal nerve fiber layer thickness," *Ophthalmology*, vol. 114, no. 5, pp. 921–926, 2007.

[43] T. Alasil, K. Wang, P. A. Keane et al., "Analysis of normal retinal nerve fiber layer thickness by age, sex, and race using spectral domain optical coherence tomography," *Journal of Glaucoma*, vol. 22, no. 7, pp. 532–541, 2013.

[44] H. Hirasawa, A. Tomidokoro, M. Araie et al., "Peripapillary retinal nerve fiber layer thickness determined by spectral-domain optical coherence tomography in ophthalmologically normal eyes," *Archives of Ophthalmology*, vol. 128, no. 11, pp. 1420–1426, 2010.

[45] P. G. D. Spry and C. A. Johnson, "Senescent changes of the normal visual field: an age-old problem," *Optometry and Vision Science*, vol. 78, no. 6, pp. 436–441, 2001.

2

Cyanin Chloride Inhibits Hyperbaric Pressure-Induced Decrease of Intracellular Glutamate-Aspartate Transporter in Rat Retinal Müller Cells

Xiaomin Chen, Yue Wang, Fangfang Han, and Min Ke

Department of Ophthalmology, Zhongnan Hospital, Wuhan University, Wuhan, China

Correspondence should be addressed to Min Ke; keminyk@163.com

Academic Editor: Biju B. Thomas

Purpose. Glaucoma is the leading cause of irreversible blindness throughout the world. The pathogenesis of glaucoma is complex, and neuroprotection is a crucial aspect of therapy. High concentrations of extracellular glutamate are toxic to the optic nerve. The glutamate-aspartate transporter (GLAST) in retinal Müller cells is involved in the development of glaucoma. Anthocyanin has been reported to protect retinal neurons. We hypothesize that cyanin chloride, a type of anthocyanin, can inhibit hyperbaric pressure-induced GLAST decreases in cultured rat retinal Müller cells and may serve as a potential neuroprotective agent in glaucoma treatment. *Materials and Methods.* Sprague Dawley rat Müller cells were cultured in a hyperbaric pressure device at 60 mmHg additional pressure and treated with cyanin chloride (10 μmol/L, 30 μmol/L, or 50 μmol/L) or vehicle for 2 hours. Cell survival rates (SRs) were evaluated by an MTT assay. GLAST mRNA and protein expression were determined by western blot and RT-PCR analyses, respectively. *Results.* Cell SR was significantly decreased in the 60 mmHg additional hyperbaric pressure group compared to the control group ($P < 0.01$). Cyanin chloride treatment significantly improved SR under 60 mmHg additional pressure ($P < 0.01$). GLAST mRNA and protein expression levels in Müller cells were significantly reduced in the 60 mmHg hyperbaric pressure group compared to the control group ($P < 0.01$), but cyanin chloride significantly inhibited hyperbaric pressure-induced decreases in GLAST expression ($P < 0.01$). *Conclusion.* Our results support our hypothesis and demonstrate that cyanin chloride can protect rat retinal Müller cells from hyperbaric pressure-induced decreases of GLAST.

1. Introduction

Glaucoma, characterized by the death of retinal ganglion cell neurons and subsequent visual dysfunction, is the leading cause of irreversible blindness worldwide [1]. The pathogenesis of glaucoma is complex and not fully elucidated. A series of pathological changes contribute to the development of the disease, including obstruction of retrograde transport of axial plasma flow, caused by high intraocular pressure; ischemia and reperfusion injury; oxidative stress; glutamate excitatory toxicity; abnormal immune response; and glial activation [2–7]. Clinically, glaucoma is primarily treated by reducing intraocular pressure (IOP). However, it is commonly known that both retinal ganglion cell (RGC) death and optic nerve damage can occur independently of IOP, and loss of RGCs can continue despite IOP reduction in

some patients [8, 9]. Recently, neuroprotective approaches against excitotoxic glutamate have been investigated as potential therapy for optic neuropathies [10, 11].

Glutamate is one of the most important excitatory neurotransmitters in the mammalian central nervous system (CNS), including the retina [12]. However, its accumulation in extracellular spaces is excitotoxic to neurons through activation of glutamate receptors [13]. Glutamate excitotoxicity has been proposed to be an important contributor to the death of CNS neurons in conditions ranging from acute ischemic stroke to chronic neurodegenerative diseases such as Alzheimer's disease [14, 15]. In the eye, glutamate excitotoxicity has been implicated in RGC death in glaucoma and ischemia-related conditions such as diabetic retinopathy [16–21]. Researchers have detected excessive levels of glutamate in glaucoma [8, 22]. Dreyer et al. investigated elevated glutamate concentrations in the vitreous body of both humans and monkeys with glaucoma [22], and Brooks et al. showed that eyes from dogs with primary glaucoma also had high vitreal glutamate expression [8]. Furthermore, experiments support the idea that excessive glutamate induces RGC death both *in vivo* and *in vitro* [23–26]. However, the exact mechanism of glutamate-induced RGC death with elevated IOP remains to be elucidated. One of the leading hypotheses is that ocular hypertension causes glutamate transporter dysfunction, leading to the excessive glutamate increase in the extracellular space. This induces excessive increases in intracellular calcium-ion concentration or oxidative stress and leads to apoptosis [27–31].

In the retina, glutamate is metabolized via the glutamate-glutamine cycle between the neurons and glial cells. Müller cells, the principal retinal glial cells, play an important role in maintaining normal retina morphology and function, including supporting nerve cells in the retina, regulating the retinal environment, and transmitting and integrating retinal nerve signals [17, 32]. Glutamate transporters play a key role in the glutamate-glutamine cycle. To date, five excitatory amino acid transporters (EAAT1–5) have been identified that may be significant in the clearance of glutamate in the nervous system [33, 34]. In the retina, EAAT1, also referred to as GLAST, is found in Müller cells [34]. If excessive extracellular glutamate is implicated in neuronal loss, the possibility of a transporter abnormality should be considered. Some studies have shown decreased GLAST concentration both in human patients with glaucoma and in a rat model of glaucoma [27, 35]. Therefore, reduced GLAST function may contribute to the elevated glutamate found in the vitreous of patiens with glaucoma.

In contrast to the damaging effects of decreased GLAST, several lines of evidence have shown that anthocyanin can protect retinal neurons *in vivo* and *in vitro* [36, 37]. In our former study, cyanin chloride (a type of anthocyanin) improved GLAST expression in rat retinal Müller cells cultured in high glucose [38]. We hypothesize that cyanin chloride can protect against decreased GLAST activity and may serve as a potential neuroprotective agent in glaucoma treatment. We propose to test this hypothesis by culturing rat retinal Müller cells in a hyperbaric chamber, to simulate the effects of increased IOP.

2. Materials and Methods

2.1. Cell Culture. Müller cells were obtained from the College of Life Sciences, Wuhan University (Wuhan, China). The cells were cultured in Dulbecco's modified Eagle's medium (DMEM; Gibco Life Technologies, Carlsbad, CA, USA) supplemented with 100 U/ml penicillin, 100 μg/ml streptomycin, and 10% fetal bovine serum (FBS; Gibco Life Technologies) in a 25 cm² culture flask.

In our previous studies, different hyperbaric pressure levels (15 mmHg additional pressure/30 mmHg additional pressure/45 mmHg additional pressure/60 mmHg additional pressure) were used to test Müller cell survival and GLAST protein expression. Our data showed that 60 mmHg additional pressure exhibited the most pronounced effect on

cell survival and GLAST protein levels, compared with the atmospheric pressure control [39].

The cells were cultured in five groups. When they reached 80–90% confluence, the cells were exposed to atmospheric or hyperbaric pressure for 2 h. Then, the cells exposed to hyperbaric pressure were treated with the different concentrations of cyanin chloride, and the cells were cultured for an additional 3 days: Group A (control group): 0 mmHg additional pressure without cyanin chloride treatment; Group B (hyperbaric group): 60 mmHg additional pressure; Group C: 60 mmHg additional pressure and 10 μmol/L cyanin chloride; Group D: 60 mmHg additional pressure and 30 μmol/L cyanin chloride; and Group E: 60 mmHg additional pressure and 50 μmol/L cyanin chloride.

2.2. Pressure Device. A T25 culture flask (Corning, USA) was equipped with a manometer (Yueqing City Supreme Electric Co. Ltd., Shanghai, China) and placed in an incubator at 37°C. A mixture of 95% air and 5% CO₂ was pumped into the chamber to obtain 60 mmHg pressure. The pressure was adjusted every 10 min for the 2-hour exposure period to maintain a constant pressure of 60 mmHg.

2.3. Cell Morphology. The cells were viewed under an Axio microscope (Zeiss, Oberkochen, Germany), and images were acquired with a digital camera (Canon, Tokyo, Japan).

2.4. MTT. The cells from each group were seeded in 96-well plates at a density of 5 × 10⁵ cells per well. After overnight culture, MTT (Sigma-Aldrich, USA) was added to each well at a concentration of 0.5 mg/ml and incubated for an additional 4 h. A 150 μL aliquot of DMSO was added for 10 min to induce a reaction. The absorbance was measured at a wavelength of 570 nm in a microplate spectrophotometer (Multiskan MK3, Thermo Fisher Scientific, USA).

2.5. Real-Time PCR. RNA was extracted from Müller cells using the Trizol reagent (Invitrogen) according to the manufacturer's protocol and stored at −80°C. The concentration and purity of the RNA preparations were determined by measuring the absorbance at 260/280 nm. RNA was reverse transcribed into complementary DNA using a reverse transcription kit (Fermentas, Canada). SYBR Real-Time PCR Master Mix (Fermentas) was used to conduct real-time PCR analyses. The following primer pairs were used: 5'-GGGGAACTCCGTGATTGA-3' (sense) and 5'-CATCTTGGTTTCGCTGTCT-3' (antisense) for GLAST and 5'-CACGATGGAGGGGCCGGACTCATC-3' (sense) and 5'-TAAAGACCTCTATGCCAACACAGT-3' (antisense) for β-actin. The reactions were performed in triplicates. The comparative Ct (ΔΔCt) method was used to obtain quantitative data of relative gene expression according to the manufacturer's instructions. Relative GLAST expression levels were normalized to β-actin.

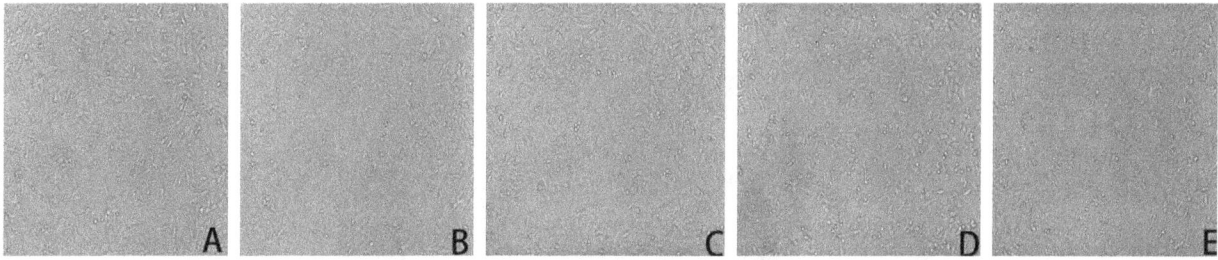

FIGURE 1: Cell morphology observed under inverted-phase microscopy (×100). Müller cells were cultured to 80–90% confluence and exposed to hyperbaric or atmospheric pressure for two hours and then to varying concentrations of cyanin chloride (or vehicle) for three days before images were captured. (A) Group A: 0 mmHg; (B) Group B: 60 mmHg; (C) Group C: 60 mmHg + 10 μmol/L cyanin chloride; (D) Group D: 60 mmHg + 30 μmol/L cyanin chloride; (E) Group E: 60 mmHg + 50 μmol/L cyanin chloride.

2.6. Western Blot Analysis. The cells were homogenized in the RIPA lysis buffer (Bigtime, China) containing a protease inhibitor cocktail (Beyotime, China) and PMSF (Bigtime, China). Proteins were separated on 12% SDS-PAGE gels (Sigma-Aldrich, St. Louis, MO, USA) and transferred to nitrocellulose filter membranes. Membranes were blocked in Tris-buffered saline containing 5% fat-free milk and incubated overnight at 4°C with antibodies against GLAST (1 : 200; ab416, Abcam). The membranes were then incubated with horseradish peroxidase-linked secondary antibodies against rabbit IgG (1 : 5000; Invitrogen) for 1 h at room temperature in the dark. Bands were visualized by exposure to the Kodak X-ray film. Image analysis and densitometry were performed by ImageJ.

2.7. Statistical Analysis. Statistical analyses were performed using SPSS 19.0 statistical software (IBM SPSS, Chicago, IL, USA). One way ANOVA was used to compare differences among three or more groups. P value <0.05 was considered statistically significant.

3. Results

Under the light microscope, normal Müller cell bodies appeared oblong, star shaped, spindled, and pyramidal (Figure 1(a)). Cell morphology did not change significantly after exposure to either hyperbaric pressure (Figure 1(b)) or cyanin chloride (Figures 1(c)–1(e)).

The MTT assay was used to evaluate the cell survival rate (SR). The cell SRs of Groups A to E, respectively, were 1.2665 ± 0.0399, 0.5129 ± 0.0259, 0.6232 ± 0.0247, 0.8987 ± 0.0389, and 1.0293 ± 0.0421, and accordingly, the relative values were 100%, 40.33%, 49.33%, 71%, and 81%. The relative SR was significantly decreased in Group B (+60 mmHg additional pressure) compared to Group A (atmospheric pressure) ($P < 0.01$; Figure 2), but treatment with cyanin chloride increased survival in Groups C, D, and E compared to Group B, and the effect was dose-dependent ($P < 0.01$; Figure 2).

We investigated the effect of cyanin chloride on GLAST mRNA and protein expression in cultured retinal Müller cells under hyperbaric pressure. The mRNA analysis revealed nearly a 50% reduction in GLAST mRNA expression in the cells exposed to 60 mmHg additional pressure (Group B), compared with the control (Group A). This

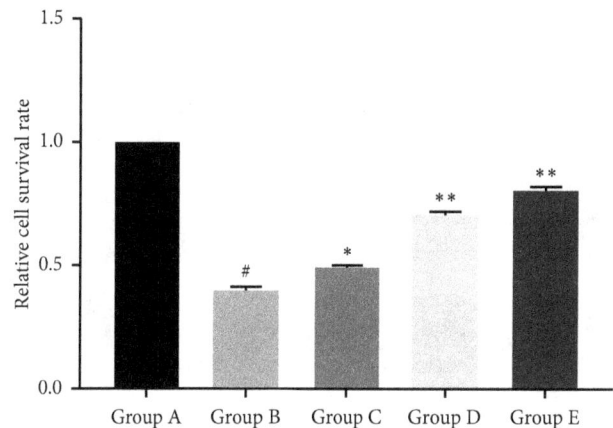

FIGURE 2: Relative cell survival rate in Müller cells. The cells were treated as described in Figure 1 and then incubated with MTT to determine the relative survival rate. $^{\#}P < 0.0001$, compared with Group A (0 mmHg additional pressure); $^{*}P < 0.0005$ and $^{**}P < 0.0001$, compared with Group B (60 mmHg additional pressure). Data from one experiment are shown as a representative of three studies performed under the same conditions. Group A: 0 mmHg; Group B: 60 mmHg; Group C: 60 mmHg + 10 μmol/L cyanin chloride; Group D: 60 mmHg + 30 μmol/L cyanin chloride; Group E: 60 mmHg + 50 μmol/L cyanin chloride.

effect was reversed in a dose-dependent manner in the treatment groups (Figure 3). Western blot analyses revealed a similar but not identical picture. GLAST protein expression was decreased by 70% in the cells exposed to hyperbaric pressure (Group B), compared to control (Group A) ($P < 0.05$; Figure 4). While GLAST protein expression was significantly elevated in Groups D and E ($P < 0.05$; Figure 4), 10 μmol/L cyanin chloride did not rescue GLAST expression.

4. Discussion

Our results confirm our hypothesis that cyanin chloride, a type of anthocyanin, can improve the GLAST level in hyperbaric pressure-cultured rat retinal Müller cells. In the present study, we found that hyperbaric pressure inhibited the GLAST level and was accompanied with Müller cell death, and cyanin chloride reversed this effect. Our findings suggest that cyanin chloride may be a potential therapeutic agent for glaucoma.

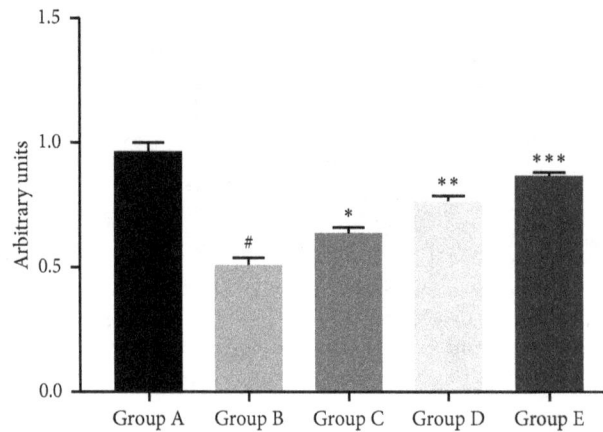

FIGURE 3: RT-PCR analysis of GLAST mRNA expression levels in retinal Müller cells. The cells were treated as described in Figure 1. #$P < 0.0001$, compared with Group A (0 mmHg additional pressure); *$P < 0.05$, **$P < 0.001$, and ***$P < 0.0001$, compared with Group B (60 mmHg additional pressure). Data from one experiment are shown as a representative of three studies performed under the same conditions. Group A: 0 mmHg; Group B: 60 mmHg; Group C: 60 mmHg + 10 μmol/L cyanin chloride; Group D: 60 mmHg + 30 μmol/L cyanin chloride; Group E: 60 mmHg + 50 μmol/L cyanin chloride.

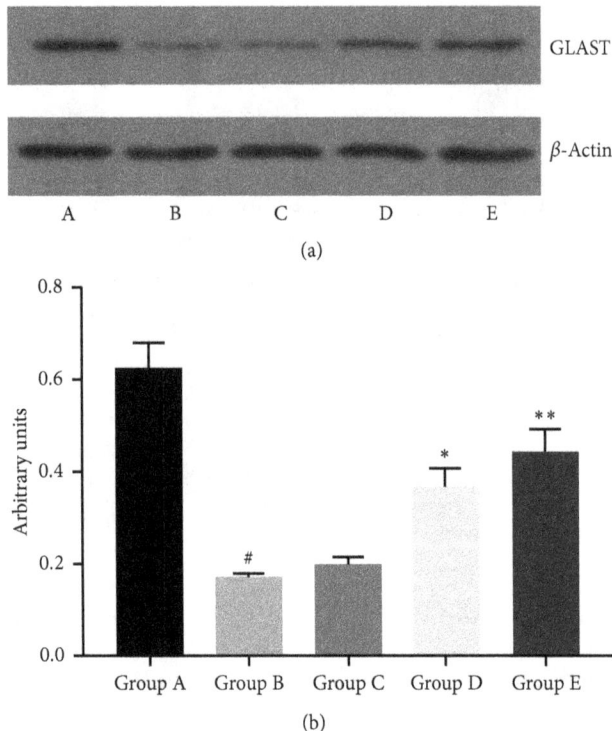

FIGURE 4: GLAST protein expression levels in retinal Müller cells. The cells were treated as described in Figure 1. (a) Representative western blot shows GLAST expression; (b) quantification of GLAST protein expression. #$P < 0.0001$, compared with Group A (0 mmHg additional pressure); *$P < 0.01$ and **$P < 0.001$, compared with Group B (60 mmHg additional pressure). Data from one experiment are shown as a representative of three studies performed under the same conditions. Group A: 0 mmHg; Group B: 60 mmHg; Group C: 60 mmHg + 10 μmol/L cyanin chloride; Group D: 60 mmHg + 30 μmol/L cyanin chloride; Group E: 60 mmHg + 50 μmol/L cyanin chloride.

Anthocyanins belong to the most common class of phenolic compounds, which is the group of water-soluble pigments [40]. These plant pigments that are widely distributed in berries, dark grapes, and other pigmented fruits and vegetables [40] and anthocyanins have numerous protective effects, including antioxidant, anti-inflammatory, antiproliferative, antimutagenic, antimicrobial, antiallergic, and anticarcinogenic effects; protect from cardiovascular damage; improve microcirculation; prevent diabetes; and improve vision [40–43].

In some observational and clinical trials, consumption of high amounts of fruits and vegetables rich in phenolics is associated with a reduced risk of major age-related eye diseases such as cataracts, glaucoma, and age-related macular degeneration (AMD) [44]. Anthocyanins can also help prevent diabetic retinopathy and retinitis pigmentosa [45]. It has been reported that anthocyanin exerts its retinoprotective effect by scavenging free radicals [46]. In addition, anthocyanins have been shown to reduce N-methyl-N-nitrosourea-induced retinal degeneration in rats [37]. Furthermore, oral administration of black currant anthocyanins induced a significant decrease in IOP levels in glaucoma patients [47].

In our study, 30 μmol/L and 50 μmol/L cyanin chloride increased GLAST protein levels in Müller cells exposed to hyperbaric pressure. GLAST is a sodium-dependent transporter that transports extracellular glutamate into Müller cells using free energy established by the Na$^+$-K$^+$-ATPase [48]. Since ATP production is reduced as hyperbaric pressure increases [49], the extracellular glutamate level increasing by Müller cells is reduced, leading to an increase in extracellular glutamate concentration. Consistent with our findings, it has been reported that hyperbaric pressure increases glutamate toxicity to RGCs [23]. Increased extracellular glutamate may be responsible for the decreased survival of Müller cells exposed to hyperbaric pressure. Increased GLAST levels may promote metabolism of extracellular glutamate into Müller cells, thereby preventing glutamate excitotoxicity. In addition, we found that hyperbaric pressure significantly decreased the GLAST level, suggesting that increased pressure may also lead to decreased metabolism capacity by the cells.

The mechanism by which anthocyanin increases the GLAST level under hyperbaric pressure has not yet been elucidated. GLAST expression can be regulated via DNA transcription, mRNA splicing and degradation, and protein synthesis and localization [23]. Oxygen-free radicals can oxidize the glutamate transporter proteins [50]. Increasing evidence suggests possible involvement of oxidative alterations to glutamate transporters in specific pathologies of excitotoxic neurodegeneration [51]. Thus, the antioxidant effect of anthocyanin may contribute to its role in GLAST regulation. Future studies are warranted to identify the mechanisms underlying GLAST regulation in Müller cells under hyperbaric pressure. The limitation of our study is that we did not test the effect of anthocyanin on Müller cells under atmospheric pressure condition. The reason is that we were trying to imitate the glaucomatic condition *in vivo* and were focused on observing the protective effect of the drug under high-pressure conditions. The biotinylation experiments and functional assays will be done to further investigate the transportation of flats [52].

In conclusion, we have demonstrated that cyanin chloride prevents hyperbaric pressure-induced decreases in survival of cultured Müller cells, and this effect is mirrored by the increased GLAST level. Our findings suggest that cyanin chloride may be a useful therapeutic approach in the management of glaucoma and other diseases mediated by chronic excitotoxicity.

5. Conclusion

The results support our hypothesis and demonstrate that cyanin chloride can protect rat retinal Müller cells from hyperbaric pressure-induced decreases in the GLAST level.

Conflicts of Interest

The authors declare that they have no conflicts of interest.

Acknowledgments

The authors acknowledge Yang Liu. This work was supported by the Provincial Natural Science Foundation of Hubei (no. 2015CFB540).

References

[1] J. W. Cheng, S. W. Cheng, X. Y. Ma, J. P. Cai, Y. Li, and R. L. Wei, "The prevalence of primary glaucoma in mainland China: a systematic review and meta-analysis," *Journal of Glaucoma*, vol. 22, no. 4, pp. 301–306, 2013.

[2] D. Krizaj, D. A. Ryskamp, N. Tian et al., "From mechano-sensitivity to inflammatory responses: new players in the pathology of glaucoma," *Current Eye Research*, vol. 39, no. 2, pp. 105–119, 2014.

[3] D. J. Calkins, "Critical pathogenic events underlying progression of neurodegeneration in glaucoma," *Progress in Retinal and Eye Research*, vol. 31, no. 6, pp. 702–719, 2012.

[4] N. G. Strouthidis and M. J. Girard, "Altering the way the optic nerve head responds to intraocular pressure-a potential approach to glaucoma therapy," *Current Opinion in Pharmacology*, vol. 13, no. 1, pp. 83–89, 2013.

[5] M. Vidal-Sanz, M. Salinas-Navarro, F. M. Nadal-Nicolas et al., "Understanding glaucomatous damage: anatomical and functional data from ocular hypertensive rodent retinas," *Progress in Retinal and Eye Research*, vol. 31, no. 1, pp. 1–27, 2012.

[6] E. C. Johnson and J. C. Morrison, "Friend or foe? Resolving the impact of glial responses in glaucoma," *Journal of Glaucoma*, vol. 18, no. 5, pp. 341–353, 2009.

[7] A. J. Payne, S. Kaja, Y. Naumchuk, N. Kunjukunju, and P. Koulen, "Antioxidant drug therapy approaches for neuroprotection in chronic diseases of the retina," *International Journal of Molecular Sciences*, vol. 15, no. 2, pp. 1865–1886, 2014.

[8] D. E. Brooks, G. A. Garcia, E. B. Dreyer, D. Zurakowski, and R. E. Franco-Bourland, "Vitreous body glutamate concentration in dogs with glaucoma," *American Journal of Veterinary Research*, vol. 58, no. 8, pp. 864–867, 1997.

[9] A. Doozandeh and S. Yazdani, "Neuroprotection in glaucoma," *Journal of Ophthalmic and Vision Research*, vol. 11, no. 2, pp. 209–220, 2016.

[10] N. Bai, T. Aida, M. Yanagisawa et al., "NMDA receptor subunits have different roles in NMDA-induced neurotoxicity in the retina," *Molecular Brain*, vol. 6, no. 1, p. 34, 2013.

[11] H. Hayashi, Y. Eguchi, Y. Fukuchi-Nakaishi et al., "A potential neuroprotective role of apolipoprotein E-containing lipoproteins through low density lipoprotein receptor-related protein 1 in normal tension glaucoma," *Journal of Biological Chemistry*, vol. 287, no. 30, pp. 25395–25406, 2012.

[12] L. Hertz, "The glutamate-glutamine (GABA) cycle: importance of late postnatal development and potential reciprocal interactions between biosynthesis and degradation," *Frontiers in Endocrinology*, vol. 4, p. 59, 2013.

[13] D. W. Choi, "Glutamate neurotoxicity and diseases of the nervous system," *Neuron*, vol. 1, no. 8, pp. 623–634, 1988.

[14] D. W. Choi and S. M. Rothman, "The role of glutamate neurotoxicity in hypoxic-ischemic neuronal death," *Annual Review of Neuroscience*, vol. 13, no. 1, pp. 171–182, 1990.

[15] A. G. Chapman, "Glutamate and epilepsy," *Journal of Nutrition*, vol. 130, no. 4, pp. 1043S–1045S, 2000.

[16] C. K. Park, J. Cha, S. C. Park et al., "Differential expression of two glutamate transporters, GLAST and GLT-1, in an experimental rat model of glaucoma," *Experimental Brain Research*, vol. 197, no. 2, pp. 101–109, 2009.

[17] A. Bringmann, T. Pannicke, B. Biedermann et al., "Role of retinal glial cells in neurotransmitter uptake and metabolism," *Neurochemistry International*, vol. 54, no. 3-4, pp. 143–160, 2009.

[18] R. J. Casson, "Possible role of excitotoxicity in the pathogenesis of glaucoma," *Clinical and Experimental Ophthalmology*, vol. 34, no. 1, pp. 54–63, 2006.

[19] C. Kaur, W. S. Foulds, and E. A. Ling, "Hypoxia-ischemia and retinal ganglion cell damage," *Clinical Ophthalmology*, vol. 2, no. 4, pp. 879–889, 2008.

[20] C. Hernandez and R. Simo, "Neuroprotection in diabetic retinopathy," *Current Diabetes Reports*, vol. 12, no. 4, pp. 329–337, 2012.

[21] L. L. Kusner, V. P. Sarthy, and S. Mohr, "Nuclear translocation of glyceraldehyde-3-phosphate dehydrogenase: a role in high glucose-induced apoptosis in retinal Muller cells," *Investigative Ophthalmology & Visual Science*, vol. 45, no. 5, pp. 1553–1561, 2004.

[22] E. B. Dreyer, D. Zurakowski, R. A. Schumer, S. M. Podos, and S. A. Lipton, "Elevated glutamate levels in the vitreous body of humans and monkeys with glaucoma," *Archives of Ophthalmology*, vol. 114, no. 3, pp. 299–305, 1996.

[23] M. Aihara, Y. N. Chen, S. Uchida, M. Nakayama, and M. Araie, "Hyperbaric pressure and increased susceptibility to glutamate toxicity in retinal ganglion cells in vitro," *Molecular Vision*, vol. 20, pp. 606–615, 2014.

[24] N. J. Sucher, S. A. Lipton, and E. B. Dreyer, "Molecular basis of glutamate toxicity in retinal ganglion cells," *Vision Research*, vol. 37, no. 24, pp. 3483–3493, 1997.

[25] C. K. Vorwerk, M. S. Gorla, and E. B. Dreyer, "An experimental basis for implicating excitotoxicity in glaucomatous optic neuropathy," *Survey of Ophthalmology*, vol. 43, no. 1, pp. S142–S150, 1999.

[26] T. Harada, C. Harada, K. Nakamura et al., "The potential role of glutamate transporters in the pathogenesis of normal tension glaucoma," *Journal of Clinical Investigation*, vol. 117, no. 7, pp. 1763–1770, 2007.

[27] R. Naskar, C. K. Vorwerk, and E. B. Dreyer, "Concurrent downregulation of a glutamate transporter and receptor in glaucoma," *Investigative Ophthalmology & Visual Science*, vol. 41, no. 7, pp. 1940–1944, 2000.

[28] C. K. Vorwerk, R. Naskar, F. Schuettauf et al., "Depression of retinal glutamate transporter function leads to elevated intravitreal glutamate levels and ganglion cell death," *Investigative Ophthalmology & Visual Science*, vol. 41, no. 11, pp. 3615–3621, 2000.

[29] K. R. Martin, H. Levkovitch-Verbin, D. Valenta, L. Baumrind, M. E. Pease, and H. A. Quigley, "Retinal glutamate transporter changes in experimental glaucoma and after optic nerve transection in the rat," *Investigative Ophthalmology & Visual Science*, vol. 43, no. 7, pp. 2236–2243, 2002.

[30] P. Marcaggi, N. Hirji, and D. Attwell, "Release of L-aspartate by reversal of glutamate transporters," *Neuropharmacology*, vol. 49, no. 6, pp. 843–849, 2005.

[31] R. K. Sullivan, E. Woldemussie, L. Macnab, G. Ruiz, and D. V. Pow, "Evoked expression of the glutamate transporter GLT-1c in retinal ganglion cells in human glaucoma and in a rat model," *Investigative Ophthalmology & Visual Science*, vol. 47, no. 9, pp. 3853–3859, 2006.

[32] M. Garcia and E. Vecino, "Role of Muller glia in neuroprotection and regeneration in the retina," *Histology and Histopathology*, vol. 18, pp. 1205–1218, 2003.

[33] S. Eliasof, J. L. Arriza, B. H. Leighton, M. P. Kavanaugh, and S. G. Amara, "Excitatory amino acid transporters of the salamander retina: identification, localization, and function," *Journal of Neuroscience*, vol. 18, no. 2, pp. 698–712, 1998.

[34] T. Rauen, J. D. Rothstein, and H. Wassle, "Differential expression of three glutamate transporter subtypes in the rat retina," *Cell and Tissue Research*, vol. 286, no. 3, pp. 325–336, 1996.

[35] G. Tezel and M. B. Wax, "Glial modulation of retinal ganglion cell death in glaucoma," *Journal of Glaucoma*, vol. 12, no. 1, pp. 63–68, 2003.

[36] N. Matsunaga, S. Imai, Y. Inokuchi et al., "Bilberry and its main constituents have neuroprotective effects against retinal neuronal damage in vitro and in vivo," *Molecular Nutrition and Food Research*, vol. 53, no. 7, pp. 869–877, 2009.

[37] S. S. Paik, E. Jeong, S. W. Jung et al., "Anthocyanins from the seed coat of black soybean reduce retinal degeneration induced by N-methyl-N-nitrosourea," *Experimental Eye Research*, vol. 97, no. 1, pp. 55–62, 2012.

[38] Z. Qian and M. Ke, "Effect of Anthocyanin on the expression of L-glutamate and L-aspartate transporter in high glucose cultured retina Müller cells," *Chinese Journal of Ocluar Fundus Diseases*, vol. 27, pp. 170–173, 2011.

[39] F. Han, X. Chen, M. Ke, and Y. Wang, "Expression of GLAST under different pressure in Müller cell in vitro," *Medical Journal of Wuhan University*, vol. 37, no. 3, pp. 386–389, 2016.

[40] D. Ghosh and T. Konishi, "Anthocyanins and anthocyanin-rich extracts: role in diabetes and eye function," *Asia Pacific Journal of Clinical Nutrition*, vol. 16, no. 2, pp. 200–208, 2007.

[41] S. Zafra-Stone, T. Yasmin, M. Bagchi, A. Chatterjee, J. A. Vinson, and D. Bagchi, "Berry anthocyanins as novel antioxidants in human health and disease prevention," *Molecular Nutrition & Food Research*, vol. 51, no. 6, pp. 675–683, 2007.

[42] B. N. Ames, M. K. Shigenaga, and T. M. Hagen, "Oxidants, antioxidants, and the degenerative diseases of aging," *Proceedings of the National Academy of Sciences*, vol. 90, no. 17, pp. 7915–7922, 1993.

[43] Y. Levy and Y. Glovinsky, "The effect of anthocyanosides on night vision," *Eye*, vol. 12, no. 6, pp. 967–969, 1998.

[44] M. Rhone and A. Basu, "Phytochemicals and age-related eye diseases," *Nutrition Reviews*, vol. 66, no. 8, pp. 465–472, 2008.

[45] S. Lamy, M. Blanchette, J. Michaud-Levesque et al., "Delphinidin, a dietary anthocyanidin, inhibits vascular endothelial growth factor receptor-2 phosphorylation," *Carcinogenesis*, vol. 27, no. 5, pp. 989–996, 2006.

[46] R. Chen, M. Hollborn, A. Grosche et al., "Effects of the vegetable polyphenols epigallocatechin-3-gallate, luteolin, apigenin, myricetin, quercetin, and cyanidin in primary cultures of human retinal pigment epithelial cells," *Molecular Vision*, vol. 20, pp. 242–258, 2014.

[47] H. Ohguro, I. Ohguro, and S. Yagi, "Effects of black currant anthocyanins on intraocular pressure in healthy volunteers and patients with glaucoma," *Journal of Ocular Pharmacology and Therapeutics*, vol. 29, no. 1, pp. 61–67, 2013.

[48] K. Namekata, C. Harada, K. Kohyama, Y. Matsumoto, and T. Harada, "Interleukin-1 stimulates glutamate uptake in glial cells by accelerating membrane trafficking of Na$^+$/K$^+$-ATPase via actin depolymerization," *Molecular and Cellular Biology*, vol. 28, no. 10, pp. 3273–3280, 2008.

[49] N. C. Danbolt, "Glutamate uptake," *Progress in Neurobiology*, vol. 65, no. 1, pp. 1–105, 2001.

[50] H. J. Reis, M. V. Gomez, E. Kalapothakis et al., "Inhibition of glutamate uptake by Tx3-4 is dependent on the redox state of cysteine residues," *NeuroReport*, vol. 11, no. 10, pp. 2191–2194, 2000.

[51] D. Trotti, N. C. Danbolt, and A. Volterra, "Glutamate transporters are oxidant-vulnerable: a molecular link between oxidative and excitotoxic neurodegeneration?," *Trends in Pharmacological Sciences*, vol. 19, no. 8, pp. 328–334, 1998.

[52] O. Sery, N. Sultana, M. A. Kashem, D. V. Pow, and V. J. Balcar, "GLAST but not least—distribution, function, genetics and epigenetics of L-glutamate transport in brain—focus on GLAST/EAAT1," *Neurochemical Research*, vol. 40, no. 12, pp. 2461–2472, 2015.

3

The Association between Female Reproductive Factors and Open-Angle Glaucoma in Korean Women: The Korean National Health and Nutrition Examination Survey V

Yong Un Shin ⒾⒹ, Eun Hee Hong ⒾⒹ, Min Ho Kang ⒾⒹ, Heeyoon Cho ⒾⒹ, and Mincheol Seong ⒾⒹ

Department of Ophthalmology, Hanyang University College of Medicine, Seoul, Republic of Korea

Correspondence should be addressed to Mincheol Seong; goddns76@hanmail.net

Academic Editor: Gonzalo Carracedo

Purpose. We investigated associations between female reproductive factors and open-angle glaucoma (OAG) in Korean females using the Korea National Health and Nutrition Examination Survey (KNHANES). *Methods*. A nationwide, population-based, cross-sectional study was conducted. We enrolled 23,376 participants from the KNHANES who had undergone ophthalmologic exams from 2010 through 2012. Associations between undiagnosed OAG and female reproductive factors such as age at menarche and menopause, parity, history of lactation, and administration of oral contraceptives (OC) or hormone replacement therapy (HRT) were determined using stepwise logistic regression analyses. *Results*. Of the enrolled participants, 6,860 participants (397 with OAG and 6,163 without OAG) met our study criteria and were included in the analyses. In the multivariate logistic regression analysis after adjusting for all potential confounding factors, only early menopause (younger than 45 years) was significantly associated with OAG in participants with natural menopause (OR 2.28, 95% CI 1.17–4.46). Age at menarche, parity, history of lactation, and administration of OC or HRT were not significantly associated with OAG. *Conclusions*. Only early menopause was associated with an increased risk of OAG in our study, in contrast to previous Western studies reporting both early menopause and late menarche as associated factors.

1. Introduction

Glaucoma, the second leading cause of blindness worldwide [1], is a neurodegenerative disease characterized by the loss of retinal ganglion cells (RGCs) and their axons [2]. Among known risk factors, including elevated intraocular pressure (IOP), family history, older age and African American ethnicity [1], elevated IOP is the major risk factor for developing the disease and the only confirmed modifiable risk factor. However, visual field loss and RGC death also occur and progress in cases of controlled or normal IOP [3]. Furthermore, therapies aimed at lowering IOP are not always successful and early detection does not always lead to prevention of visual impairment because of the lack of highly effective treatments. Accordingly, complementary strategies targeting alternate modifiable glaucoma risk factors other than IOP are needed to manage and screen for the disease.

There is some emerging evidence that estrogen plays an important role in the pathogenesis of open-angle glaucoma (OAG). Several previous population-based studies conducted in Caucasians have found a relationship between factors associated with exposure to estrogen such as age at menopause or menarche, use of hormone replacement therapy (HRT) in postmenopausal women, or use of oral contraceptives (OC) and the risk of OAG [4–7]. However, only two population-based studies have examined associations between female reproductive factors and OAG in Asian populations: one in a rural Indian population [8] and the other in a population with Malay ethnicity [9].

The Korea National Health and Nutrition Examination Survey (KNHANES) includes extensive data on health and socioeconomic status from a large population in Korea [10]. Using the raw data from KNHANES, we conducted a population-based study to describe the effects of female reproductive factors on OAG in Korean females.

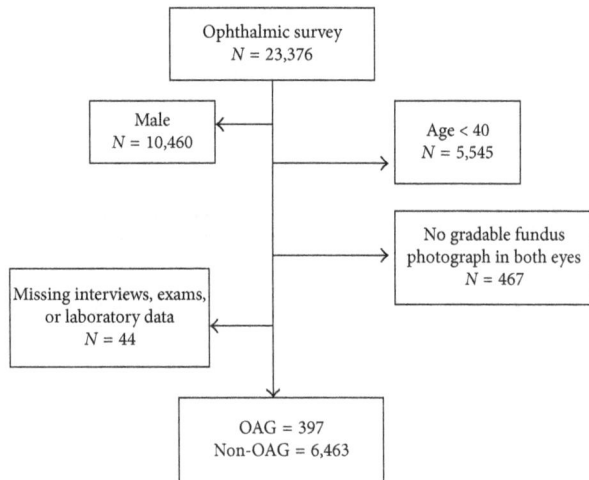

FIGURE 1: Flow chart for selection of the study participants. A total of 16,516 participants were excluded due to male sex, age < 40 years old, and ungradable.

2. Materials and Methods

2.1. Study Population. The KNHANES is a population-based, cross-sectional survey conducted in South Korea by the Division of Chronic Disease Surveillance of the Korea Centers for Disease Control and Prevention and the Korean Ministry of Health and Welfare. The KNHANES uses a complex, multistage, stratified, probability-clustered sampling method to analyze a representative, civilian, noninstitutionalized South Korean population. The details of the KNHANES have been described previously [11, 12]. We examined data obtained from a representative sample in the period between 2010 and 2012, using the fifth Korea National Health and Nutrition Examination Survey (KNHANES-V, 2010–2012), which employed stratified multistage sampling based on geographical area, sex, and age group [11].

The KNHANES consists of three parts: the Health Interview Survey, the Health Examination Survey, and the Nutritional Survey. Ophthalmologic interviews and exams were only conducted in participants ≥19 years old. The present study included the data from a randomly chosen eye of 23,376 individuals from the KNHANES between 2010 and 2012 who met the following inclusion criteria: were women 40 years of age or older; received the ophthalmology survey; and had a gradable fundus photograph and frequency-doubling technology (FDT) perimetry test result for at least one eye. Participants with missing data or unreliable examination results were excluded (Figure 1).

The survey adhered to the tenets of the Declaration of Helsinki, and written informed consent was obtained from all KNHANES participants. The survey protocol and study design were reviewed and approved by the Institutional Review Board (IRB) of the Korean Centers for Diseases Control and Prevention.

2.2. Measurements. We obtained data from the Health Interview Survey and Health Examination Survey. In the Health Interview Survey, participants responded to questions about

female health: age at menarche, age at menopause and whether it was natural or artificial, parity, history of lactation, administration and duration of OC, and administration of HRT.

The Health Examination Survey included blood pressure (BP), physical examination, and basic laboratory tests. Physical examinations were performed by trained investigators following a standardized procedure. Body weight and height were measured in light indoor clothing without shoes to the nearest 0.1 kg and 0.1 cm. Body mass index (BMI) was calculated as the ratio of weight/height [2] (kg/m^2). Systolic blood pressure (SBP) and diastolic blood pressure (DBP) were measured on the right arm using a standard Mercury sphygmomanometer (Baumanometer, Baum, Copiague, NY, USA). We calculated final blood pressure by averaging the second and third blood pressure measurements. For the routine blood test, blood samples were collected after at least an eight-hour fasting period and analyzed within 24 hours after transport to a certified laboratory using a Hitachi 7600-110 chemistry analyzer (Hitachi, Tokyo, Japan). Fasting plasma glucose (FPG) was also analyzed.

Ophthalmology-focused interviews were performed using self-reported questionnaires, including past or current medical or surgical conditions relevant to ophthalmology, such as a history of cataract surgery. Subjects underwent a detailed eye examination, which included visual acuity measurements; autorefraction using an autorefractor keratometer (KR8800, Topcon, Tokyo, Japan); slit-lamp examination, including assessment of peripheral anterior chamber depth by the Van Herick method (Haag-Streit model BQ-900; Haag-Streit AG, Koeniz, Switzerland); IOP, measured by Goldmann applanation tonometry (GAT; Haag-Streit, Haag-Streit AG) by ophthalmologists; and fundus photographs with a nonmydriatic 45° digital fundus camera (TRC-NW6S, Topcon) and a Nikon D-80 digital camera (Nikon, Tokyo, Japan). These ophthalmologic examinations were performed in a mobile examination unit by a trained ophthalmologist or ophthalmology resident. In addition, visual field testing using the N-30-1 screening program (Humphrey Matrix frequency-doubling perimeter, Carl Zeiss Meditec, Inc., Dublin, CA, USA) was performed on participants who had elevated IOP (≥22 mmHg), a horizontal or vertical cup-to-disc ratio ≥ 0.5, violation of the ISNT rule (neuroretinal rim broadest in the inferior area in the normal eye, followed by the superior, nasal, and temporal areas), an optic disc hemorrhage, or a retinal nerve fiber layer (RNFL) defect. The test location was deemed abnormal if not identified on two attempts at a contrast level identified by 99% of the healthy population. Frequency doubling technology was repeated if the rate of fixation errors was more than 0.33 or if the false-positive rate was greater than 0.33. An FDT with greater than a 0.33 rate of fixation errors or 0.33 rate of false positives was deemed invalid and was not used as criteria for glaucoma classification and required either International Society of Geographical and Epidemiological Ophthalmology (ISGEO) category 2 criteria (described below) for a glaucoma diagnosis.

2.3. Variable Definition. We defined several new variables in this study from KNHANES raw data. Early menarche was defined as age at menarche younger than or at 12 years old and late menarche as older than or at 17 years old. Early menopause was defined as age at menopause younger than 45 years old. The reproductive years were defined as the period between age at menarche and age at menopause. The duration of OC use was categorized into 2 groups: <3 years of OC use and ≥3 years of OC use, as in a previous study [13]. Hypertension presence was defined as systolic pressure ≥ 140 mmHg, diastolic pressure ≥ 90 mmHg, or a current prescription for antihypertensive medication. Diabetes presence was defined as fasting glucose ≥126 mg/dL or a current prescription for antiglycemic medication. Myopia was defined as a spherical equivalent less than or equal to −1.00 diopters (D).

The definition of open-angle glaucoma (OAG) was based on ISGEO criteria and a previous study [14, 15]. Patients were defined as having open-angle glaucoma if an open angle (peripheral anterior chamber depth > 1/4 corneal thickness) was present along with any one of the following category diagnostic criteria. Category I criteria: the presence of FDT testing results and fixation error and false-positive error ≤ 1: (i) loss of neuroretinal rim with vertical or horizontal cup : disc ratio ≥ 0.6, or asymmetry of vertical cup : disc ratio ≥ 0.2 (both values determined by ≥97.5th percentile for the normal population in the KNHANES), or a retinal nerve fiber layer defect; and (ii) the presence of an abnormal FDT testing result (at least one location of reduced sensitivity). Category II criteria: the absence of FDT testing results or fixation error or false-positive error ≥ 2: (i) loss of neuroretinal rim with vertical cup: disc ratio ≥ 0.9 or asymmetry of vertical cup: disc ratio ≥ 0.3 (both values determined by ≥99.5th percentile for the normal population in the KNHANES), or (ii) the presence of a retinal nerve fiber layer defect with violation of the ISNT rule (the neuroretinal rim thickness order of inferior > superior > nasal > temporal). Category III (when no visual field testing or optic disc exam was available) required a visual acuity < 20/400 and an IOP greater than 21 mmHg.

2.4. Statistical Analysis. Statistical analyses for a complex sampling design were performed using SPSS 21.0 Version (IBM, Armonk, NY, USA). According to statistical guidelines from the Korea Centers for Disease Control and Prevention, survey sample weights were used in all analyses to produce an integrated new dataset from the 3-year data that was representative of the noninstitutionalized civilian Korean population. Baseline characteristics of the study participants were expressed as either weighted means ± standard error (SE) for continuous variables or numbers and percentage (%) ± SE for categorical variables as appropriate for total participants and were compared using the Student's t-test and the chi-square test, respectively, between the OAG and non-OAG groups. To determine which factors had significant associations with OAG, potential associated factors for OAG were investigated via univariate logistic regression analysis. This step was performed in both the study population as a whole and participants with natural menopause, respectively, and in each group we also performed age-adjusted analyses. In the next step, multivariate adjusted logistic regression analyses were conducted to examine the odds ratio (OR) and 95% confidence interval

(CI) for the association between OAG and associated factors, adjusting for age and all other confounders (DM, HTN, myopia, BMI, OC, and HRT in Model I; addition of early menopause, age at menarche, lactation, and parity in Model II). Factors that yielded a P value < 0.05 were considered statistically significant.

3. Results

3.1. Baseline Characteristics. After application of exclusion criteria, 6,860 participants were eligible for this study (397 participants with OAG and 6,463 participants without OAG). Of all the participants who underwent an ophthalmic survey, we excluded 16,516 participants due to male sex, age < 40 years old, ungradable fundus image on either eye or missing survey data (Figure 1). Overall, the mean age of all participants in this study was 56.09 ± 0.2 years. Among the included participants, 36.6 ± 0.8% had hypertension and 11.0 ± 0.5% had diabetes. The mean body mass index was 24.0 ± 0.06 kg/m^2. Among female reproductive factors, mean age at menarche and menopause was 15.5 ± 0.1 years and 48.7 ± 0.1 years, respectively. The mean number of parity and reproductive years was 4.3 ± 0.01 and 32.7 ± 0.1 years, respectively. Natural menopause occurred in 86.2 ± 0.7% of participants with menopause. The percentage of participants who took OC and HRT was 17.6 ± 0.6% and 10.9 ± 0.5%, respectively. A history of lactation was reported by 82.6% of participants. The percentage of participants with myopia was 23.0 ± 0.7%. Differences in demographic characteristics according to the presence of OAG are shown in Table 1. Participants with OAG were more likely to be older (62.7 ± 0.8 versus 55.8 ± 0.2 years, P < 0.001) and to have hypertension (53.8 ± 3.4 versus 35.7 ± 0.8%, P < 0.001) or diabetes (20.4 ± 2.8 versus 10.5 ± 0.5%, P < 0.001) than participants without OAG. Among female reproductive factors, both the proportion of participants with early menopause and parity were significantly different between participants with and without OAG. There was no significant difference in the proportion of age at menarche, natural menopause, OC use, HRT, or history of lactation. The proportion of participants with myopia was similar between the two groups.

3.2. Association of OAG with Female Reproductive Factors. The prevalences of OAG (presented as mean ± standard error) for the different age groups, 40 to 49 years, 50 to 59 years, 60 to 69 years, and 70 years or older, were 2.4 ± 0.4%, 3.8 ± 0.5%, 6.4 ± 0.7%, and 9.9 ± 0.9%, respectively. Table 2 shows OAG-associated factors as determined by logistic regression analysis. In univariate logistic regression analyses, the following factors were significantly associated with OAG: old age (OR 1.04 per 1 year, 95% CI 1.03–1.06), early menopause (OR 1.56, 95% CI 1.03–2.35), parity (OR 1.15 per one pregnancy, 95% CI 1.10–1.20), and the presence of hypertension (OR 2.10, 95% CI 1.59–2.76) and diabetes (OR 2.17, 95% CI 1.53–3.07). In the age-adjusted logistic regression analysis, the presence of diabetes (OR 1.54, 95% CI 1.07–2.22) and the presence of myopia (OR 1.69, 95% CI 1.24–2.31) were significantly associated with OAG (Table 2).

TABLE 1: Descriptive statistics for demographics and clinical characteristics of the study participants.

	Open-angle glaucoma ($n = 397$)	Non-open-angle glaucoma ($n = 6463$)	P value
Age, years	62.7 ± 0.8	55.8 ± 0.2	$<0.001^a$
Age at menarche, years			
≤12 years (%)	5.5 ± 1.8	5.8 ± 0.4	0.224^a
13–16 years (%)	58.4 ± 3.1	63.7 ± 0.9	
≥17 years (%)	36.1 ± 2.9	30.5 ± 0.8	
Age at menopause, years	49.0 ± 0.3	48.7 ± 0.1	0.700^b
Early menopause (<45 years) (%)	19.1 ± 3.1	13.2 ± 0.7	0.033^a
Natural menopause (%)	90.2 ± 2.0	85.8 ± 0.7	0.07^a
Parity	5.0 ± 0.1	4.3 ± 0.0	0.013^b
Reproductive years, years	32.8 ± 0.4	32.7 ± 0.1	0.898^b
Hypertension (%)	53.8 ± 3.4	35.7 ± 0.8	$<0.001^a$
Diabetes mellitus (%)	20.4 ± 2.8	10.5 ± 0.5	$<0.001^a$
Oral contraceptives use (ever, %)	16.0 ± 2.3	17.7 ± 0.6	0.515^a
≥3 years (%)	23.0 ± 7.0	21.9 ± 1.6	0.882^a
Hormone replacement (ever, %)	9.9 ± 1.9	10.9 ± 0.5	0.625^a
Myopia (%)	26.6 ± 2.9	23.0 ± 0.7	0.209^a
Body mass index	23.9 ± 0.2	24.0 ± 0.1	0.545^b
Lactation (ever, %)	85.1 ± 2.6	82.5 ± 0.6	0.355^a

Values are presented as weighted mean ± standard error. P value is calculated by the chi-square test[a] or independent t-test[b] within the complex sample analysis method.

TABLE 2: Univariate and age-adjusted logistic regression analyses for the association between factors and open-angle glaucoma in all participants and participants with natural menopause.

All participants	Univariate		Age-adjusted	
	OR (95% CI)	P value	OR (95% CI)	P value
Age, per year	1.04 (1.03–1.06)	<0.001		
Age at menarche, years				
13–16 years	Reference	0.145	Reference	0.126
≤12 years	1.03 (0.53–2.03)		1.39 (0.70–2.74)	
≥17 years	1.29 (1.00–1.67)		0.80 (0.62–1.04)	
Early menopause (<45 years) (%)	1.56 (1.03–2.35)	0.035	1.41 (0.91–2.16)	0.122
Parity	1.15 (1.10–1.20)	<0.001	1.01 (0.96–1.07)	0.627
Reproductive years	1.00 (0.97–1.03)	0.804	1.01 (0.98–1.04)	0.396
Hypertension (%)	2.10 (1.59–2.76)	<0.001	1.33 (0.99–1.80)	0.015
Diabetes mellitus (%)	2.17 (1.53–3.07)	<0.001	1.54 (1.07–2.22)	0.021
Oral contraceptives use (ever, %)	0.89 (0.63–1.26)	0.515	0.75 (0.52–1.06)	0.099
≥3 years	1.06 (0.48–2.36)	0.882	0.94 (0.42–2.11)	0.875
Hormone replacement (ever, %)	0.90 (0.58–1.39)	0.625	0.90 (0.58–1.39)	0.623
Myopia (%)	1.21 (0.90–1.64)	0.210	1.69 (1.24–2.31)	0.001
Body mass index	0.99 (0.95–1.03)	0.552	0.98 (0.95–1.02)	0.390
Lactation (ever, %)	1.21 (0.85–1.83)	0.259	0.68 (0.45–1.04)	0.106
Participants with natural menopause				
Age, per year	1.04 (1.02–1.05)	<0.001		
Age at menarche, years				
13–16 years	Reference	0.335	Reference	0.041
≤12 years	1.70 (0.74–3.90)		1.94 (0.85–4.47)	
≥17 years	0.94 (0.70–1.26)		0.79 (0.59–1.06)	
Early menopause (<45 years) (%)	2.40 (1.50–3.83)	<0.001	1.88 (1.11–3.19)	0.019
Number of parity	1.08 (1.03–1.14)	0.003	1.01 (0.95–1.07)	0.808
Reproductive years, years	1.00 (0.96–1.03)	0.846	1.01 (0.98–1.05)	0.439
Hypertension (%)	1.57 (1.15–2.13)	0.005	1.24 (0.89–1.73)	0.200
Diabetes mellitus (%)	1.47 (0.95–2.28)	0.085	1.27 (0.82–1.98)	0.114
Oral contraceptives use (ever, %)	0.82 (0.56–1.19)	0.286	0.80 (0.55–1.16)	0.239
≥3 years	1.04 (0.45–2.40)	0.936	1.02 (0.44–2.37)	0.961
Hormone replacement (ever, %)	0.86 (0.54–1.37)	0.522	1.06 (0.66–1.70)	0.805
Myopia (%)	1.53 (1.06–2.21)	0.022	1.59 (1.10–2.32)	0.015
Body mass index	0.98 (0.94–1.03)	0.486	0.99 (0.94–1.03)	0.587
Lactation (ever, %)	0.92 (0.53–1.60)	0.775	0.68 (0.38–1.19)	0.176

CI = confidence interval.

TABLE 3: Multivariate logistic regression analyses for the association between open-angle glaucoma and age at menarche, early menopause, and parity.

		All		Natural menopause	
		OR (95% CI)	P value	OR (95% CI)	P value
Age at menarche, years					
13–16 years	Model I	Reference	0.506	Reference	0.397
≤12 years		0.99 (0.45–2.15)		1.10 (0.40–3.02)	
≥17 years		0.83 (0.60–1.14)		0.79 (0.56–1.13)	
13–16 years	Model II	Reference	0.425	Reference	0.279
≤12 years		1.01 (0.38–2.65)		1.10 (0.39–3.15)	
≥17 years		0.80 (0.56–1.13)		0.75 (0.52–1.09)	
Early menopause <45 years					
	Model I	1.50 (0.96–2.34)	0.073	2.05 (1.22–3.50)	0.009
	Model II	1.60 (0.94–2.73)	0.082	2.28 (1.17–4.46)	0.016
Parity					
	Model I	1.03 (0.97–1.09)	0.415	1.02 (0.96–1.08)	0.556
	Model II	1.02 (0.95–1.10)	0.631	1.02 (0.94–1.11)	0.686

CI = confidence interval. Model I, adjusted for age, diabetes mellitus, hypertension, myopia, body mass index, oral contraceptive use, and hormone replacement. Model II, adjusted for age, diabetes mellitus, hypertension, myopia, body mass index, oral contraceptive use, hormone replacement, and female reproductive factors (age at menarche, early menopause, lactation history, and parity).

In participants who had natural menopause, old age (OR 1.04 per year, 95% CI 1.02–1.05), early menopause (OR 2.40, 95% CI 1.50–3.83), parity (OR 1.08 per pregnancy, 95% CI 1.03–1.14), the presence of hypertension (OR 1.57, 95% CI 1.15–2.13), and myopia (OR 1.53, 95% CI 1.06–2.21) were significantly associated with OAG in univariate logistic regression analyses. Age-adjusted logistic regression analysis found that early menopause (OR 1.88, 95% CI 1.11–3.19) and myopia (OR 1.59, 95% CI 1.10–2.32) were significantly associated with OAG.

In multivariate logistic regression analysis after adjusting for all potential confounding factors, early menopause was significantly associated with OAG only in participants with natural menopause (OR 1.60, 95% CI 0.94–2.73 in all participants versus OR 2.28, 95% CI 1.17–4.46 in participants with natural menopause) (Table 3). Multivariate logistic regression analysis did not show a statistically significant association between early menarche and OAG (OR 1.01, 95% CI 0.38–2.65 in all participants and OR 1.10, 95% CI 0.39–3.15 in participants with natural menopause) or between parity and OAG (OR 1.02, 95% CI 0.95–1.10 in all participants and OR 1.02, 95% CI 0.95–1.08 in participants with natural menopause).

4. Discussion

According to a previous population-based prevalence study in Korea using KNHANES data, the primary OAG prevalences for the different age groups, 40 to 49 years, 50 to 59 years, 60 to 69 years, 70 to 79 years, and 80 years or older, were 3.6%, 5.9%, 7.3%, 8.8%, and 10.5% in men, and 2.0%, 3.3%, 5.1%, 7.7%, and 8.1% in women, respectively [16]. Our data showed similar prevalences in each age group of female. Although our study did not reveal the incidence of OAG, in a previous cohort study in Korea, the 5-year incidences of primary OAG among women aged 40 to 49, 50 to 59, 60 to 69, and 70 years or older were 0.32%, 0.50%, 1.45%, and 3.45%, respectively [17]. Several risk factors of OAG have

been mentioned in these epidemiological studies in Korea. However, population-based studies of female reproductive factors as risk factors for OAG were lacking. In this population-based study of Korean women, we found that early natural menopause was associated with an increased risk of OAG. There was no significant association between OAG and age at menarche, reproductive duration, parity, or use of OC or HRT among Korean women.

Our findings agree with many previous population-based studies showing that early menopause might increase the risk of OAG. In the Rotterdam Study, the first population-based study about OAG and early menopause, the risk of OAG was higher in women who entered menopause before 45 years of age (odds ratio (OR) 2.6; 95% CI 1.5–4.8) [7]. According to secondary analysis of the Nurses' Health Study (NHS), the risk of OAG was 50% lower in women who underwent menopause at age ≥ 54 years than at age < 54 years (relative risk (RR) 0.53; 95% CI 0.32–0.89) over more than 20 years of follow-up [4]. In the Singapore Malay Eye study, women who had menopause at a younger age were more likely to have glaucoma (before age 53 years, OR 3.54; 95% CI 1.24–10.12) [9]. On the contrary, the risk of OAG was not associated with early menopause in the Blue Mountains Study [5], and the Aravind Comprehensive Eye Survey also did not find significant associations between early menopause and the risk of OAG [8].

In our study, both early and late menarche were not associated with the risk of OAG. Some previous population-based studies have reported that early menarche may decrease the risk of OAG because of the longer duration of estrogen exposure over a lifetime. In the Blue Mountains Study, the risk of OAG was significantly higher in women who reported late menarche (after age 13 years, OR 2.0; 95% CI 1.0–3.9) [5]. Recently, a population-based study in the United States also found that older age at menarche was significantly associated with a higher prevalence of self-reported glaucoma or ocular hypertension using data from the National Health and Nutrition Examination Survey

(NHANES) (OR 1.13; 95% CI 1.03–1.22) [13]. However, in a cohort study with more than 25 years of follow-up in the NHS, there was no significant relationship between age at menarche and OAG [18], in agreement with our findings.

We assumed that estrogen in the menopausal period may help protect against OAG. Although the exact mechanism of the protective effect of estrogen has not been elucidated, some mechanisms have been suggested. Estrogen enhances ocular blood flow, and it has been demonstrated that aging and age-related declines in female sex hormones negatively affect ocular blood flow [18]. Toker et al. showed that serum estrogen has beneficial effects on blood flow velocities and resistive indices in the retrobulbar arteries [6], which might result from vascular smooth muscle relaxation [19–21]. Estrogen is also known to reduce IOP in women [22–26]. 17β-estradiol augments the activity of endothelial nitric oxide synthase (NOS) [27], which in turn mediates vasodilation and vascular tone to modulate blood flow to the optic nerve [28] and might potentially influence IOP by regulating both aqueous production and aqueous outflow through receptors located in the ciliary body and the outflow system [25, 29]. Additionally, the neuroprotective effects of estrogen on the optic nerve are supported by clinical, epidemiological, and basic science evidence [30–37].

Among female reproductive factors, only early menopause was significantly associated with OAG in this study, while age at menarche was not. We offer several reasons for these findings in our study. First, the protective role of estrogen against OAG is more effective in menopausal women because the prevalence of OAG is much higher in old age, and the development of glaucoma is a degenerative aging process. A recent clinical study suggested that in postmenopausal women, estrogen deficiency is a causative factor for increased susceptibility to glaucomatous damage with age [30] and use of HRT protects the retinal nerve fiber layer [38]. Previous studies have also shown that postmenopausal women with glaucoma suffer from more serious damage of optic nerves than younger women with glaucoma, even at the same level of IOP [39]. Second, the relationship between myopia and age at menarche may influence our results. According to a recent Korean population-based study, later age at menarche is associated with a decreased risk of moderate to high myopia [40], and the effects of female sex hormones on ocular structures (e.g., the change of axial length) may mediate this relationship. Late menarche reduces the duration of estrogen exposure, which may lead to the development of OAG, as reported in Western studies, while decreased risk of myopia development in late menarche may help protect against OAG. Therefore, in Korean women, age at menarche was not associated with OAG due to these conflicting reasons.

The use of OC or HRT was not associated with the risk of OAG in this study. In recent Caucasian population-based studies, OC use for more than 3 years was associated with a greater risk of self-reported glaucoma or ocular hypertension [13], and OC use for more than 5 years was associated with a modestly increased risk of OAG [18]. In addition, HRT improves ocular blood flow in postmenopausal women [38], reduces vascular resistance in the central retinal artery and posterior ciliary artery [25, 41], and

decreases IOP [42, 43]. In some studies, estrogen-only treatment was more effective at lowering IOP than the combination of estrogen and progesterone [24]. In contrast, in the Rotterdam [7] and Blue Mountains Eye studies [5], the risk of OAG did not significantly reduce the odds in Caucasian women who had used HRT. Similarly, in the Singapore Malay Eye study and a recent Korean study regarding ocular benefits after HRT, no significant association was observed between the use of HRT and OAG [9, 44].

The strength of our study is that the data were collected from a nationwide survey in Korea. Unlike previous similar Asian studies [8, 9], ours is the first nationwide general population-based study of the association between female reproductive factors and OAG conducted in Asian women. Second, the KNHANES data underwent rigorous quality control of study procedures. Third, OAG was diagnosed in this study according to standard protocols, allowing us to include all undiagnosed OAG patients; in some studies, the OAG group has only included those previously diagnosed with OAG.

Several issues should be considered during interpretation of our results. First, because the KNHANES used self-reported interview data for age at menopause and menarche, as well as the cause of menopause, recall bias could be important. Second, the retrospective and cross-sectional design makes it difficult to explain the causality between female reproductive factors and risk of OAG. Future studies are needed to assess cause-effect relationships in the Korean population. Third, although the KNHANES provides a large, robust database, relatively few participants fit our criteria, limiting the power of the analysis. A larger study could better elucidate the role of female reproductive factors. Fourth, the definition of open angle was made basically by Van Herick method rather than standard gonioscopy, which might misclassify some angle closure glaucoma (such as cases with plateau iris) as OAG. Finally, the KNHANES did not distinguish between estrogen-only treatment or a combination of estrogen and progestin for the type of HRT.

Previous Western studies have found that early menopause and late menarche, as well as the use of OC or HRT in some studies, are associated with OAG. Our data from a representative population of Korean women indicate that, among female reproductive factors, only early menopause was associated with OAG, consistent with the results of a previous study in Singapore. This result may suggest not only a protective effect of estrogen against the development of OAG in old age, but also genetic or ethnic differences between Western and Asian women. Causative relationships and the role of other female reproductive factors in OAG in Asians should be confirmed by additional studies.

Conflicts of Interest

None of the authors have any proprietary interests or conflicts of interest related to this submission.

Authors' Contributions

Yong Un Shin and Eun Hee Hong contributed equally to this work.

Acknowledgments

This research was supported by the research fund of Hanyang University (HY-201800000000614). The authors would like to thank Eunwoo Nam, PhD (Biostatistical Consulting and Research Lab, Hanyang UniversityUnassigned, Seoul, Korea), for assistance with statistical analysis.

References

[1] H. A. Quigley and A. T. Broman, "The number of people with glaucoma worldwide in 2010 and 2020," *British Journal of Ophthalmology*, vol. 90, no. 3, pp. 262–267, 2006.

[2] K. G. Schmidt, H. Bergert, and R. H. Funk, "Neurodegenerative diseases of the retina and potential for protection and recovery," *Current Neuropharmacology*, vol. 6, no. 2, pp. 164–178, 2008.

[3] S. K. Vasudevan, V. Gupta, and J. G. Crowston, "Neuroprotection in glaucoma," *Indian Journal of Ophthalmology*, vol. 59, no. 7, pp. S102–S113, 2011.

[4] L. R. Pasquale, B. A. Rosner, S. E. Hankinson et al., "Attributes of female reproductive aging and their relation to primary open-angle glaucoma: a prospective study," *Journal of Glaucoma*, vol. 16, no. 7, pp. 598–605, 2007.

[5] A. J. Lee, P. Mitchell, E. Rochtchina et al., "Female reproductive factors and open angle glaucoma: the Blue Mountains Eye Study," *British Journal of Ophthalmology*, vol. 87, no. 11, pp. 1324–1328, 2003.

[6] E. Toker, O. Yenice, I. Akpinar et al., "The influence of sex hormones on ocular blood flow in women," *Acta Ophthalmologica Scandinavica*, vol. 81, no. 6, pp. 617–624, 2003.

[7] C. A. Hulsman, I. C. Westendorp, R. S. Ramrattan et al., "Is open-angle glaucoma associated with early menopause? The Rotterdam Study," *American Journal of Epidemiology*, vol. 154, no. 2, pp. 138–144, 2001.

[8] P. K. Nirmalan, J. Katz, A. L. Robin et al., "Female reproductive factors and eye disease in a rural South Indian population: the Aravind Comprehensive Eye Survey," *Investigative Ophthalmology and Visual Science*, vol. 45, no. 12, pp. 4273–4276, 2004.

[9] J. S. Lam, W. T. Tay, T. Aung et al., "Female reproductive factors and major eye diseases in Asian women–the Singapore Malay Eye Study," *Ophthalmic Epidemiology*, vol. 21, no. 2, pp. 92–98, 2014.

[10] Korea Centers for Disease Control and Prevention, *Korean National Health and Nutrition Examination Survey*, 2013, http://knhanes.cdc.go.kr/.

[11] S. Kweon, Y. Kim, M. J. Jang et al., "Data resource profile: the Korea National Health and Nutrition Examination Survey (KNHANES)," *International Journal of Epidemiology*, vol. 43, no. 1, pp. 69–77, 2014.

[12] W. J. Lee, L. Sobrin, M. J. Lee et al., "The relationship between diabetic retinopathy and diabetic nephropathy in a population-based study in Korea (KNHANES V-2, 3)," *Investigative Ophthalmology and Visual Science*, vol. 55, no. 10, pp. 6547–6553, 2014.

[13] Y. E. Wang, C. Kakigi, D. Barbosa et al., "Oral contraceptive use and prevalence of self-reported glaucoma or ocular hypertension in the United States," *Ophthalmology*, vol. 123, no. 4, pp. 729–736, 2016.

[14] M. J. Kim, M. J. Kim, H. S. Kim et al., "Risk factors for open-angle glaucoma with normal baseline intraocular pressure in a young population: the Korea National Health and Nutrition Examination Survey," *Journal of Clinical and Experimental Ophthalmology*, vol. 42, no. 9, pp. 825–832, 2014.

[15] P. J. Foster, R. Buhrmann, H. A. Quigley et al., "The definition and classification of glaucoma in prevalence surveys," *British Journal of Ophthalmology*, vol. 86, no. 2, pp. 238–242, 2002.

[16] K. E. Kim, M. J. Kim, K. H. Park et al., "Prevalence, awareness, and risk factors of primary open-angle glaucoma: Korea National Health and Nutrition Examination Survey 2008–2011," *Ophthalmology*, vol. 123, no. 3, pp. 532–541, 2016.

[17] Y. K. Kim, H. J. Choi, J. W. Jeoung et al., "Five-year incidence of primary open-angle glaucoma and rate of progression in health center-based Korean population: the Gangnam Eye Study," *PloS One*, vol. 9, no. 12, Article ID e114058, 2014.

[18] L. R. Pasquale and J. H. Kang, "Female reproductive factors and primary open-angle glaucoma in the Nurses' Health Study," *Eye*, vol. 25, no. 5, pp. 633–641, 2011.

[19] T. Mikkola, L. Viinikka, and O. Ylikorkala, "Estrogen and postmenopausal estrogen/progestin therapy: effect on endothelium-dependent prostacyclin, nitric oxide and endothelin-1 production," *European Journal of Obstetrics and Gynecology and Reproductive Biology*, vol. 79, no. 1, pp. 75–82, 1998.

[20] A. J. Proudler, A. I. Ahmed, D. Crook et al., "Hormone replacement therapy and serum angiotensin-converting-enzyme activity in postmenopausal women," *The Lancet*, vol. 346, no. 8967, pp. 89-90, 1995.

[21] J. B. Salom, M. C. Burguete, F. J. Pérez-Asensio et al., "Relaxant effects of 17-β-estradiol in cerebral arteries through Ca2+ entry inhibition," *Journal of Cerebral Blood Flow and Metabolism*, vol. 21, no. 4, pp. 422–429, 2001.

[22] I. Qureshi, "Intraocular pressure: association with menstrual cycle, pregnancy and menopause in apparently healthy women," *Chinese Journal of Physiology*, vol. 38, no. 4, pp. 229–234, 1994.

[23] B. A. Siesky, A. Harris, C. Patel et al., "Comparison of visual function and ocular hemodynamics between pre- and postmenopausal women," *European Journal of Ophthalmology*, vol. 18, no. 2, pp. 320–323, 2008.

[24] G. Uncu, R. Avci, Y. Uncu et al., "The effects of different hormone replacement therapy regimens on tear function, intraocular pressure and lens opacity," *Gynecological Endocrinology*, vol. 22, no. 9, pp. 501–505, 2006.

[25] O. Altintas, Y. Caglar, N. Yuksel et al., "The effects of menopause and hormone replacement therapy on quality and quantity of tear, intraocular pressure and ocular blood flow," *Ophthalmologica*, vol. 218, no. 2, pp. 120–129, 2004.

[26] P. Affinito, A. Di Spiezio Sardo, C. Di Carlo et al., "Effects of hormone replacement therapy on ocular function in postmenopause," *Menopause*, vol. 10, no. 5, pp. 482–487, 2003.

[27] K. L. Chambliss and P. W. Shaul, "Estrogen modulation of endothelial nitric oxide synthase," *Endocrine Reviews*, vol. 23, no. 5, pp. 665–686, 2002.

[28] R. F. Furchgott and J. V. Zawadzki, "The obligatory role of endothelial cells in the relaxation of arterial smooth muscle by acetylcholine," *Nature*, vol. 288, no. 5789, pp. 373–376, 1980.

[29] S. B. Ogueta, S. D. Schwartz, C. K. Yamashita et al., "Estrogen receptor in the human eye: influence of gender and age on gene expression," *Investigative Ophthalmology and Visual Science*, vol. 40, no. 9, pp. 1906–1911, 1999.

[30] T. S. Vajaranant and L. R. Pasquale, "Estrogen deficiency accelerates aging of the optic nerve," *Menopause*, vol. 19, no. 8, pp. 942–947, 2012.

[31] R. Russo, F. Cavaliere, C. Watanabe et al., "17Beta-estradiol prevents retinal ganglion cell loss induced by acute rise of intraocular pressure in rat," *Progress in Brain Research*, vol. 173, pp. 583–590, 2008.

[32] X. Zhou, F. Li, J. Ge et al., "Retinal ganglion cell protection by 17-beta-estradiol in a mouse model of inherited glaucoma," *Developmental Neurobiology*, vol. 67, no. 5, pp. 603–616, 2007.

[33] J. Guo, S. P. Duckles, J. H. Weiss et al., "17beta-Estradiol prevents cell death and mitochondrial dysfunction by an estrogen receptor-dependent mechanism in astrocytes after oxygen-glucose deprivation/reperfusion," *Free Radical Biology and Medicine*, vol. 52, no. 11-12, pp. 2151–2160, 2012.

[34] K. Prokai-Tatrai, H. Xin, V. Nguyen et al., "17beta-estradiol eye drops protect the retinal ganglion cell layer and preserve visual function in an in vivo model of glaucoma," *Molecular Pharmaceutics*, vol. 10, no. 8, pp. 3253–3261, 2013.

[35] X. Chen, M. Zhang, C. Jiang et al., "Estrogen attenuates VEGF-initiated blood-retina barrier breakdown in male rats," *Hormone and Metabolic Research*, vol. 43, no. 9, pp. 614–618, 2011.

[36] S. Kaja, S. H. Yang, J. Wei et al., "Estrogen protects the inner retina from apoptosis and ischemia-induced loss of Vesl-1L/ Homer 1c immunoreactive synaptic connections," *Investigative Ophthalmology and Visual Science*, vol. 44, no. 7, pp. 3155–3162, 2003.

[37] R. D. Spence and R. R. Voskuhl, "Neuroprotective effects of estrogens and androgens in CNS inflammation and neurodegeneration," *Frontiers in Neuroendocrinology*, vol. 33, no. 1, pp. 105–115, 2012.

[38] M. C. Deschenes, D. Descovich, M. Moreau et al., "Postmenopausal hormone therapy increases retinal blood flow and protects the retinal nerve fiber layer," *Investigative Ophthalmology and Visual Science*, vol. 51, no. 5, pp. 2587–2600, 2010.

[39] N. M. Guttridge, "Changes in ocular and visual variables during the menstrual cycle," *Ophthalmic and Physiological Optics*, vol. 14, no. 1, pp. 38–48, 1994.

[40] I. J. Lyu, M. H. Kim, S.-Y. Baek et al., "The association between menarche and myopia: findings from the Korean National Health and Nutrition Examination, 2008–2012 association between menarche and myopia," *Investigative Ophthalmology and Visual Science*, vol. 56, no. 8, pp. 4712–4718, 2015.

[41] T. S. Vajaranant, S. Nayak, J. T. Wilensky et al., "Gender and glaucoma: what we know and what we need to know," *Current Opinion in Ophthalmology*, vol. 21, no. 2, pp. 91–99, 2010.

[42] M. O. Sator, E. A. Joura, P. Frigo et al., "Hormone replacement therapy and intraocular pressure," *Maturitas*, vol. 28, no. 1, pp. 55–58, 1997.

[43] M. O. Sator, J. Akramian, E. A. Joura et al., "Reduction of intraocular pressure in a glaucoma patient undergoing hormone replacement therapy," *Maturitas*, vol. 29, no. 1, pp. 93–95, 1998.

[44] K. S. Na, D. H. Jee, K. Han et al., "The ocular benefits of estrogen replacement therapy: a population-based study in postmenopausal Korean women," *PLoS One*, vol. 9, no. 9, Article ID e106473, 2014.

Washout Duration of Prostaglandin Analogues

Vlad Diaconita ⓘ,[1,2] **Matthew Quinn,**[2,3] **Dania Jamal,**[4] **Brad Dishan,**[5]
Monali S. Malvankar-Mehta ⓘ,[1,6] **and Cindy Hutnik**[1,2]

[1]*Ivey Eye Institute, London, ON, Canada*
[2]*Schulich School of Medicine and Dentistry, Western University, London, ON, Canada*
[3]*Queen's University, Ophthalmology Department, Kingston, ON, Canada*
[4]*King Abdulaziz University, Saudi Arabia*
[5]*St. Joseph's Health Care, London, ON, Canada*
[6]*Department of Epidemiology and Biostatistics, Schulich School of Medicine and Dentistry, Western University, London, ON, Canada*

Correspondence should be addressed to Vlad Diaconita; vdiaconi@uwo.ca

Academic Editor: Michele Figus

Topic. Prostaglandin analogues (PGAs) are first-line medical therapy for primary open angle glaucoma (POAG) and ocular hypertension (OHT). Intraocular pressure (IOP) lowering effects in full responders are known to be 25–33% for this class; however, partial responders and nonresponders do exist. In clinical trials or prospective series, discontinuation and washout of PGAs is necessary to evaluate true change in IOP from novel surgeries and medical therapies. *Clinical Relevance.* To identify all relevant papers with pertinent data on washout of PGAs and quantify the duration and long-term effect of reported PGA washout periods in glaucoma and OHT patients. *Methods.* A systematic review and meta-analysis was conducted to investigate the long-term effects on IOP after discontinuation of topical PGAs POAG and OHT patients. The main search was conducted in MEDLINE/PubMed, EMBASE, Cochrane Library, CINAHL, Web of Science, and BIOSIS Previews and conference proceedings. *Results.* 1055 papers were identified, 548 were independently screened by two physicians., and 56 papers were analyzed for washout durations. The mean washout was found to be 4.56 weeks (±1.25), with the mode and median being 5 weeks. Five studies were analyzed as randomized control trials in which latanoprost was discontinued for 4 weeks prior to restarting another intraocular pressure-lowering drug. Meta-analysis revealed a 4-week discontinuation of latanoprost, on average, subjects returned to their baseline IOP. *Conclusion.* A significant IOP-lowering effect of latanoprost was not observed beyond 4 weeks, suggesting this may be an appropriate washout period for latanoprost. We could not identify appropriate washout periods for either travoprost or bimatoprost, although a majority of articles had 4-week washout durations for the two drugs. Despite the widespread use of this class of medication, there is a paucity of literature on the effects of PGA washout in patients that are treatment naïve to other topical medications.

1. Background

Intraocular pressure (IOP) is the only known modifiable risk factor for glaucoma. In the mid 1990s, prostaglandin analogues (PGAs) were introduced and are now recognized as first-line topical medical therapy for primary open angle glaucoma and ocular hypertension [1–3]. In Canada, latanoprost (generic and Xalatan, Pfizer, New York, NY, USA),

travoprost (generic and Travatan, Alcon, Fort Worth, TX, USA), and bimatoprost (generic and Lumigan, Allergan, Irvine, CA, USA) are the widely available PGAs. IOP-lowering effects are known to be in the 25–33% range for this class, mostly by increasing uveoscleral outflow and minimally by increasing trabecular meshwork outflow [4–13]

Jampel and colleagues performed a retrospective analysis of discontinuation of IOP-lowering medication. They showed that the largest change in IOP was observed after discontinuation of the first medication (33%) as compared to the second medication (9%) or third (13%). This difference was not class dependent. They concluded that the effectiveness of IOP-lowering medications may be significantly lower than that in ideal conditions [14]. The PGA class is dosed once daily, and during clinical trials, the typical washout period for prostaglandin analogues varies between 2 weeks and 8 weeks, with most trials using a 4-week washout. Lingering effects of medications beyond a presumed washout period could lead to erroneous conclusions about the efficacy and responder rates to subsequent medications, laser trabeculoplasty, minimally invasive, and/or filtering surgeries either alone or combined with cataract extraction. This would be true for both clinical practice as well as in clinical trials designed to evaluate new IOP-lowering drugs and devices.

It is for these reasons that the purpose of this study was to investigate if sufficient evidence exists to determine the long-term effects on IOP after discontinuation of topical PGAs in glaucoma or ocular hypertension patients (OHT). A systematic review and meta-analysis was conducted of the available literature.

2. Methods

2.1. Search Strategy. The effects of prostaglandins on the eye were first reported in 1985 by Giuffre [15]. The review therefore considered studies published in English between 1985 and 2016. Since clinical prostaglandin analogue use began after 1996, most papers were published between 1996 and 2016.

A preliminary search was conducted in MEDLINE to identify relevant MeSH terms and keywords. Then, a comprehensive search was completed using identified index terms and keywords and was adapted accordingly to different databases. The main search was conducted in six (6) databases: MEDLINE/PubMed, EMBASE, Cochrane Library, CINAHL, Web of Science, and BIOSIS Previews. Conference proceedings were included as found in EMBASE and Web of Science. The main search was conducted in May 2014, with a follow-up search on the years 2014–2016 conducted in October 2016. A medical librarian, experienced in systematic review searching, designed the search strategy and conducted the searches. The reference lists of included studies were searched to identify additional studies that may meet inclusion criteria.

Index terms used in the search were (adjusted by database) open angle glaucoma, Primary glaucoma, Ocular hypertension, Intraocular hypertension, Intraocular pressure, and prostaglandins.

Keyword terms used in the search were open angle glaucoma, POAG, OAG, (intra)ocular hypertension, Intraocular pressure Discontinu*, stop*, withdraw*, washout, prostaglandins, bimatoprost, travoprost, latanoprost, and tafluprost.

2.4. Systematic Review. Title screening was performed by two independent reviewers familiar with systematic reviews. Papers that were agreed upon by both reviewers were included in the next phase of analysis. Disagreements were reanalyzed by both reviewers, and agreement was reached by consensus. The inclusion/exclusion criteria are listed in Table 1 and the algorithm is shown in Figure 1.

2.5. Quality Assessment of Included Articles. All included articles were scored for quality using the Downs and Black checklist [16]. A quality check was performed to ensure completeness of our methodology.

2.6. Statistical Analysis. The primary outcome was the mean and standard deviation (SD) of pre- and postwashout IOP. Meta-analysis was completed on the primary outcome of interest using STATA v. 15.0 (STATA Corporation, College Station, TX). The extracted mean of the IOP at baseline and end point was used to compute the mean IOP reduction (IOPR) and percentage of IOP reduction (IOPR%) using the equations below [17]:

$$IOPR = IOP_{baseline} - IOP_{endpoint}, \quad (1)$$

$$IOPR\% = \frac{IOPR}{IOP_{baseline}}. \quad (2)$$

For continuous scale outcomes such as mean values, standardized mean difference (SMD) was calculated as the treatment effect or effect size. SMD was chosen as the treatment effect since it is a mean difference standardized across all studies. To compute SMD for each study, the difference between the mean pre- and postoperative values for outcome measure (i.e., IOP) was divided by the SD for that same outcome measure. Weights were assigned to each SMD according to the inverse of its variance, and then average was computed. SMD for each study was then aggregated using the fixed- or random-effect model based on the presence of heterogeneity to estimate the summary effect.

To test heterogeneity, I^2 statistics, Z-value, and χ^2 statistics were computed. An I^2 value of less than 50% implies low heterogeneity, and in these cases, a fixed-effect model was computed. An I^2 statistics of 50% or more represents high heterogeneity, and in these cases, a random-effect model was calculated. Additionally, a high Z-value, a low P value (<0.01), and a large χ^2 value imply significant heterogeneity, and therefore, a random-effect model using DerSimonian and Laird methods was computed. A forest plot was generated to display the statistics. A funnel plot was generated to check publication bias.

3. Results

3.1. Search Results. 1055 papers that met the search strategy were identified. 507 were removed as duplicates. The remaining 548 records were screened according to their title and abstract by two independent physicians. 424 were removed through the screening process. 213 were excluded due to study design: 66 were studies without a diagnosis of POAG or OHT, 62 were irrelevant papers to our search, 56 did not have prostaglandin analogue medications in the study protocol, 16 had an enrolment age of less than 18

TABLE 1: Inclusion and exclusion criteria.

Inclusion	Exclusions
Population of study >18 years of age	Non-English papers
Diagnosis of POAG, OHT	Nonhuman studies
Treatment with prostaglandin analogue or prostamide or combination drug which includes prostaglandin analogue or prostamide	Diagnosis of normotensive glaucoma
	Study design: meta-analyses, opinion papers, reviews

years, 10 were nonhuman studies, and 1 was a non-English study without available translation (Figures 1 and 2).

In total, 56 of the 74 papers which were analyzed listed washout durations for the prostaglandin analogues. Of the 56, 32 had a washout period listed of 4 weeks (57.1%). Seven had a washout of less than 4 weeks (12.5%), and 19 had a washout period of more than 4 weeks (33.3%) of which most were washouts of 6-week duration. The mean was 4.56 weeks with a standard deviation of 1.25 weeks. Both the median and mode washout period was 4 weeks (Figure 3).

3.2. Study Characteristics. Eight studies were identified that reported both means and standard errors/standard deviations for intraocular pressure. All eight studies were prospective, of which five were randomized control trials in which latanoprost was discontinued for 4 weeks prior to restarting another intraocular pressure-lowering drug. For each of those five papers, IOP was measured and documented prewashout (on latanoprost) and 4- week postwashout (off latanoprost). Each study had differing inclusion and exclusion criteria. Overall, studied participants varied greatly with respect to previous laser (SLT/ALT) treatment, phakic status, or previous medication history. Comparison between the two measurements was used to determine change in IOP due to the 4-week washout (Table 2).

3.3. Publication Bias. A funnel plot was generated to check publication bias. Visual inspection of the funnel plot for both pre- and postwashout IOP (Figure 4) did not reveal any asymmetry. Additionally, publication bias is only one of the numerous possible explanations for funnel plot asymmetry.

3.4. Impact on Primary Outcome. A forest plot was created of five studies which yielded data (Figure 5). Figure 5 summarizes the results for the outcome measure IOP. Five studies (178 subjects) considered the impact on IOP due to discontinuation of topical PGAs in glaucoma or ocular hypertension patients at week four. Two studies showed a sustained IOP-lowering effect relative to pretreatment baseline after four weeks after washout. Heterogeneity between studies that investigated the impact on IOP ($I^2 = 89.3\%$) was significantly ($p = 0.0$) high. In studies examining the impact of washout or discontinuation of topical latanoprost (SMD = −0.53, CI = −1.22, 0.17), IOP change was not different as compared to baseline.

3.5. Analysis. This study reviewed 548 papers of which 56 met the study criteria. We found that the washout duration between studies varied from 4-5 days to 8 weeks. Seven of the fifty-six articles had a washout duration which was less than 4 weeks, ranging between 4-5 days and 3 weeks. Their year of publication ranged between 1996 and 2015, demonstrating no apparent standard duration of washout of PGA in the setting of clinical trials. The mean washout period in the reviewed articles was 4.56 (±1.25) weeks, with the median and mode both being 4 weeks (Figure 3).

Our analysis of eight articles found that the difference between baseline IOP (pretreatment) and postwashout IOP was statistically significant in only 3 studies. Aung et al. [18] discontinued monotherapy PGA prior to starting a crossover trial of either unoprostone and latanoprost. Sit et al. [23] washed out a heterogenous group of patients (some naïve and others on previous therapy) and then administered only with travoprost for 4 weeks. These participants were washed out for 41–63 hours, after which their IOP was re-measured. Meanwhile, the findings of Kobayashi and colleagues showed that after a 4-week discontinuation of latanoprost, patients who had remained on beta-blockers and brinzolamide did not have an expected increase of 25–33% of pretreatment IOP, but only a 15.4% of baseline IOP increase. As expected, the IOP did not return to baseline as patients remained on at least one other IOP-lowering medication.

The remainder of the analyzed studies did not show a statistically significant effect. Larsson et al. [20] showed that treatment naïve OHT patients who were treated with latanoprost for 4 weeks and then washed out for 4 weeks, returned to their pre-treatment IOPs. Linden et al. [21] found that in patients treated with monotherapy latanoprost for at least 6 months, with most greater than 1 year, experienced a significantly lower IOP of 1.3 mmHg compared to baseline measurements following a 14-day washout period. Sehi et al. [22] analyzed the washout results from a cohort of patients. A four-week washout showed an IOP of 18.0 mmHg which was lower than untreated baseline of 18.8 mmHg. Stewart et al. [22, 23] had an open label assessment of a four-week latanoprost washout in patients who had previously been treated with various classes of IOP-lowering medications. There were inadequate data in the published data to draw specific conclusions regarding washout duration. Finally, Walters et al. looked at 4-week discontinuation of PGA in patients previously treated with IOP-lowering medication and found no statistically significant change after washout. All participants had already discontinued other ocular medications prior to the study.

In a prospective analysis of 603 patients, Jampel and colleagues showed that the IOP changes caused by removing a medication was significantly less than the historically reported maximal IOP changes observed in monotherapy published trials, following discontinuation of a second or third medication class [14]. This finding highlights the complexity of understanding the true IOP effects of single-agent washout in clinical settings where patients are subject to multiple drug classes.

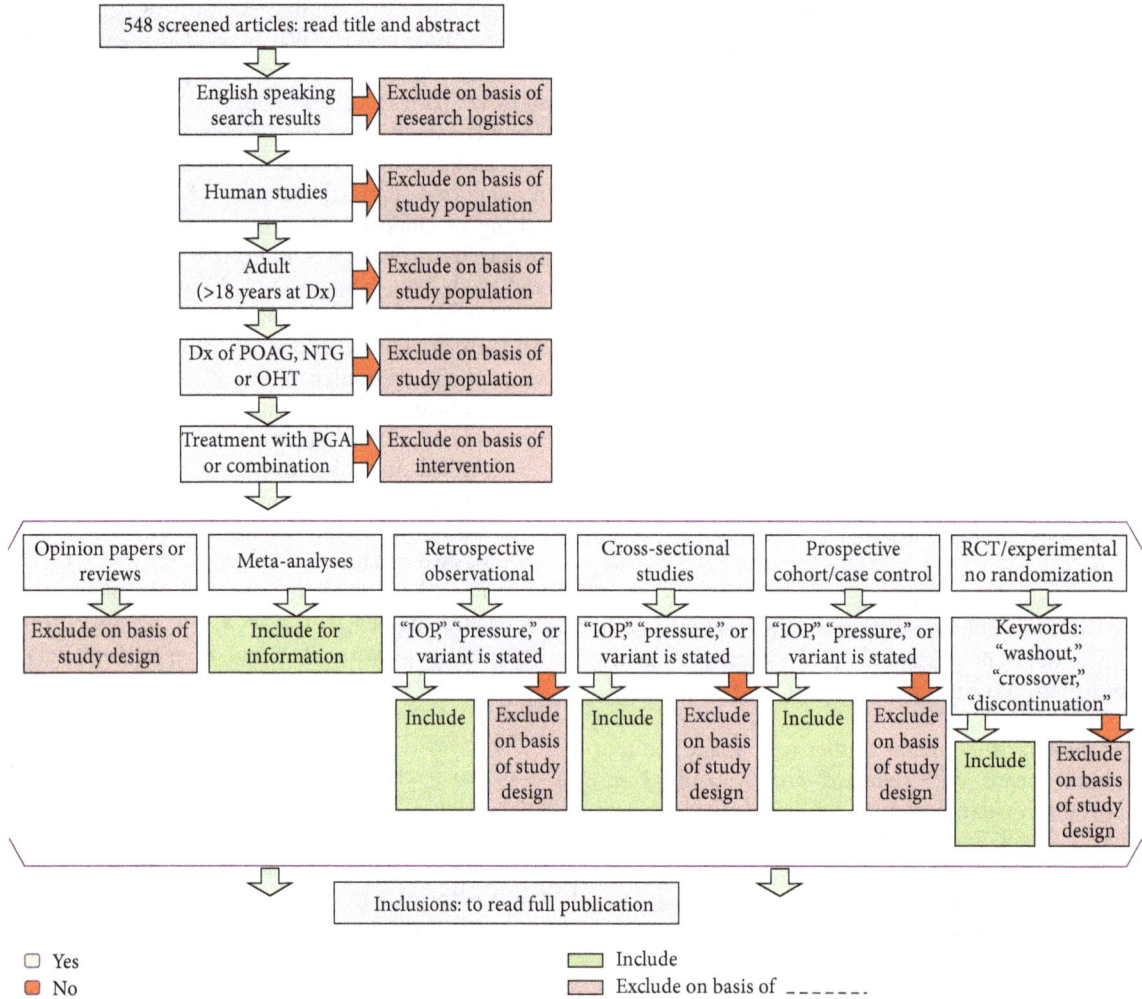

FIGURE 1: Inclusion and exclusion algorithm for screening articles.

Of the five articles included in the meta-analysis, all except Kobayashi [19] showed a return to baseline IOP following a washout of 3 or 4 weeks. Participants in the study by Kobayashi [19] continued on their other intraocular medications, while the other studies had participants discontinue their previous drops prior to the start of each study [18–22]. Stewart et al. were the first to identify that there may be a variation in the time to return to baseline IOP following washout in individuals being treated with latanoprost. Moreover, they showed that the washout effect is longer than that of brimonidine. They concluded that latanoprost washout periods were often greater than 4 weeks (Stewart et al. 2000).

In an open-label pilot study, Dubiner and colleagues showed that travoprost can have lasting IOP-lowering effects even up to 84 hours after initial dosing. Subsequently, they studied 34 open-angle glaucoma patients and concluded that IOP-lowering effects were identified up to 44 hours after use of travoprost drops [25]. Sit and colleagues also showed that travoprost IOP lowering persisted up to 63 hours after the final dose [23], while Kurtz and Shemesh found that in a certain group of 20 OHT patients, dosing latanoprost once weekly was noninferior to daily use of the medication. Their

results were not statistically different up to 3 months of follow-up [26].

4. Discussion

Meta-analysis of existing literature demonstrated that after washout, IOP returned to baseline values, with a maximum of 17% IOP reduction (IOPR%) from baseline occurring at 4-weeks after washout. Of the eight articles which met the study criteria, the difference between baseline IOP (pretreatment) and postwashout IOP was statistically significant in only 3 studies [18, 19, 23]. A 4-week discontinuation of latanoprost in patients who had remained on beta-blockers and brinzolamide did not have an expected increase of 25–33% of pretreatment IOP, but only a 15.4% of baseline IOP increase. As expected, the IOP did not return to baseline, as patients remained on at least one other IOP-lowering medication. This suggests that the effectiveness of PGAs is not as high as expected, especially in the setting of using multiple drug classes [14, 19] (Stewart et al. 2000). It is also possible that full responders, partial responders, and nonresponders to the PGA drug class were pooled in these studies, which the mean IOP values would not adequately reflect.

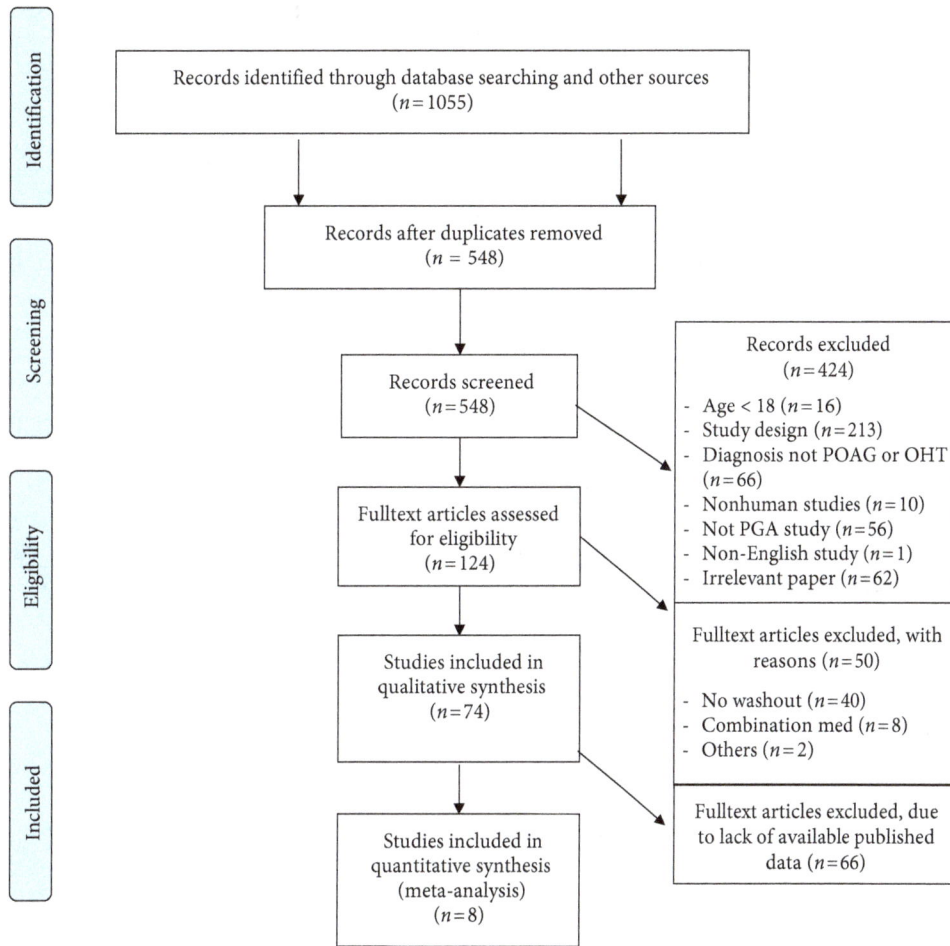

FIGURE 2: Prisma 2009 flow diagram.

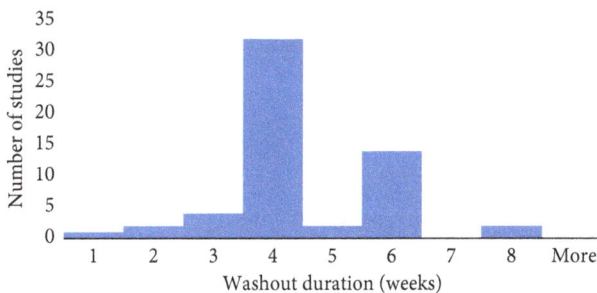

FIGURE 3: Washout duration of prostaglandin analogues and prostamides in research studies 1996–2016 ($n = 56$). Mean = 4.56 weeks; SD = 1.25; median = 4 weeks; mode = 4 weeks.

The analysis reveals that there is no standard for PGA washout in reported studies although 4 weeks appears to be the most common period. The analysis also reveals that the various members of the PGA class may differ in the duration of their effectiveness after washout, with some patients having lingering effects to all of the PGA medications. If inappropriate washout is conducted, lingering effects of a PGA drug may influence conclusions regarding subsequent IOP-lowering interventions. As an example,

minimally invasive glaucoma surgeries (MIGS) are being suggested as a treatment option to reduce dependency on medical therapy. Lingering IOP effects following an insufficient washout period may prevent the observation of the true IOP-lowering effect of MIGS. This has relevance not only with respect to potential erroneous conclusions from MIGS clinical trials but also can lead to a false security of the effectiveness of MIGS in the clinical setting, the latter resulting in insufficient monitoring after surgery.

The Ocular Hypertension Study found that to achieve target IOP, nearly 40% of patients had to be on at least two IOP-lowering medications [27]. As such, a large portion of glaucoma and OHT patients are on multiple drug classes to control IOP. The findings of Jampel et al. highlight the complexity of the interactions of the IOP-lowering agents when used in combination [14].

The lingering IOP-lowering effects following an insufficient washout may also influence clinical trials designed to evaluate new drugs and/or devices. In clinical trials designed to study the effectiveness of a new IOP-lowering strategy, treatment naive patients would be preferred to avoid the confounding effects of other current or previous interventions. The results of this meta-analysis revealed a paucity of such studies. Only Larsson et al. [20] studied treatment naive participants, with Sit et al. [23] looking at

Table 2: Pre-and postwashout IOP of prostaglandin analogues in research studies 1997–2012, $n = 8$ studies.

References	Study design	Study location	Medication	N	Treatment (weeks)	Washout (weeks)	IOP Baseline Mean	Baseline SD	Afterwashout Mean	Afterwashout SD	P value
Aung et al. [18]	RCT	Singapore	Latanoprost	27	4	3	22.8	2.08	22.2	3.12	0.4095
			Unoprostone	29	4	3	24.3	3.23	20.9	2.70	<0.001
Kobayashi et al. [19]	RCT	Japan	Latanoprost	20	13.3 ± 5.6	4	23.6	1.6	19.5	1.2	<0.001
Larsson [20]	RCT	Sweden	Latanoprost	27	4	4	23.6	1.04	23.8	1.04	0.4830
Linden et al. [21]	Prospective case series	Sweden	Latanoprost	26	26–52	2	—	—	—	—	—
Sehi et al. [22]	RCT	US	Latanoprost	68	—	4	18.8	4.7	18.0	4.3	0.3023
Sit et al. [23]	Prospective open label	US	Travoprost	20	—	41–63 (hrs)	21.5	2.9	19.6	2.6	0.0354
Stewart et al. [22, 23]	Prospective open label	US	Latanoprost	17	—	4	—	—	—	—	—
Walters et al. [24]	RCT	US	Latanoprost	36	—	4	23.6	2.1	23.6	0.3	1
			Bimatoprost	37	—	4	24.1	2.6	24.1	0.1	1

RCT: randomized control trial; P value: Student's t test comparing pre- and postwashout IOP.

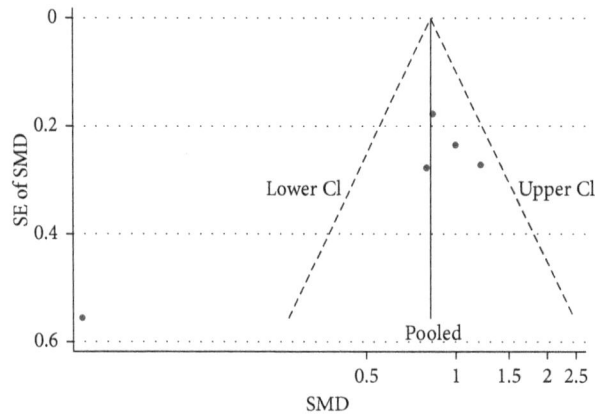

Figure 4: Visual inspection of funnel plot for both pre- and postwashout IOP (Figure 4) did not reveal any asymmetry.

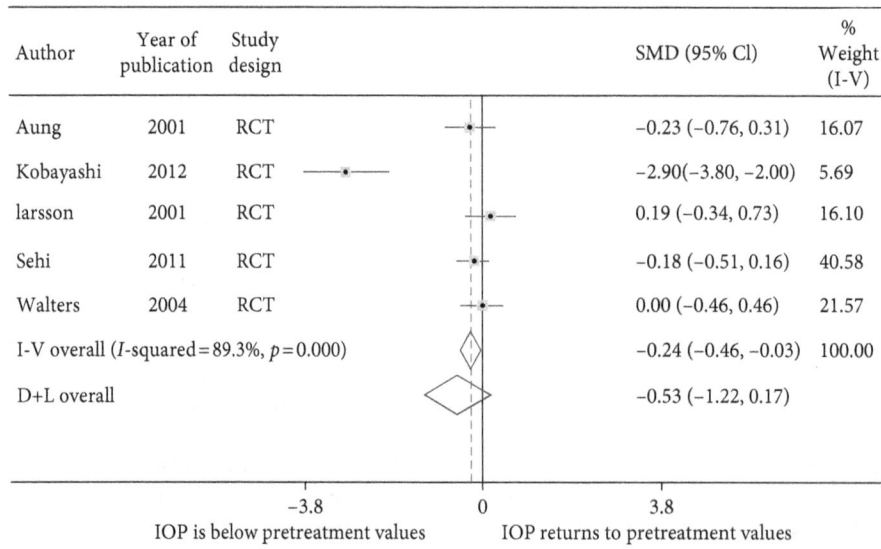

Figure 5: Forest plot of 5 studies of latanoprost washout.

a mix of treatment naive and previously treated patients. Without a thorough understanding of the impact of previous and current topical antiglaucoma medication use, it is not possible to gauge the true efficacy of adjunctive medications, SLT, and/or surgical interventions such as cataract extraction with or without MIGS.

This review was limited by the number of available studies with published data. Only five studies had washout IOP as the main outcome measured [14, 19, 22, 23], with only one study [19] publishing data that could be analyzed for PGAs. A majority of studies were crossover studies which included a discontinuation period.

Another limitation was the considerable amount of heterogeneity among the five studies examining the impact of washout on IOP. This reflected different study populations, demographics, inclusion/exclusion criteria, study location, washout technique, surgeon's experience, available facilities to perform washout, rates of complications, the year washout was performed, and the year the study was conducted. Of note is that there may exists intra-rater and inter rater IOP measurement differences between the various studies. Random-effect computations showed a nonsignificantly controlled and lowered IOP after washout of latanoprost.

In this meta-analysis the Downs and Black checklist [16] was employed to assess the quality of the included studies. This revealed a significant variation in quality scoring with high-, medium-, and poor-quality studies having been reported. Nevertheless, as only five studies were available for analysis, all were included. This is a recognized but necessary limitation due to the few clinical studies currently available. Meta-analysis of RCTs is influenced by inherent biases in the included articles [28]. For example, a multitude of other factors such as level of education, ethnicity, income status, socioeconomic status, previous ocular and nonocular surgeries, family history, other ocular and nonocular diseases, preoperative and postoperative medications, number of medications and comorbidities (e.g., high blood pressure, diabetes, stroke, heart conditions, etc.) could influence the estimates in the original studies.

The results of this quantitative synthesis of the currently available literature suggest that more studies need to be reported to better understand the optimal role of washout in IOP management and topical glaucoma medication management. Washout periods of medications are important to patients, researchers, and physicians. Accurate dosing is key in maintaining IOP to slow or halt progression of glaucomatous changes. Physicians need to know how often to prescribe medications, whether it is safe to discontinue one class and to have guidance when it is appropriate to stop treatment altogether. Researchers, on the other hand, should know the effects of IOP-lowering agents when investigating new therapies or surgical procedures and devices. If the sustained effect of prostaglandin analogues on IOP are not known, baseline IOP measurements cannot be accurately determined in patients previously treated with this drug class.

This meta-analysis demonstrates very little published evidence exists describing the washout effects of prostaglandin

drugs on intraocular pressure. Most of the available data are retrospective and confounded by heterogeneity due to exposure to multiple drug classes. Further, confounding factors such as the phakic state and previous laser trabeculoplasty are rarely addressed. Accepting these limitations, four weeks may be a sufficient washout period for many patients who have been subjected to multiple drug therapy. However, the evidence is inconclusive and insufficient to apply to all patients. To address this gap in knowledge, consideration may be given to conduct a prospective, masked study specifically designed to determine the washout period for patients on monotherapy prostaglandin medications. This will be useful to provide guidance to both clinicians and researchers as to when and how to assess the effects of adjunctive therapies in patients previously exposed to first-line prostaglandin medical management.

Conflicts of Interest

The authors declare that there are no conflicts of interest regarding the publication of this paper.

References

[1] C. B. Camras, A. Alm, P. Watson, and J. Stjernschantz, "Latanoprost, a prostaglandin analog, for glaucoma therapy. Efficacy and safety after 1 year of treatment in 198 patients. Latanoprost study groups," *Ophthalmology*, vol. 103, no. 11, pp. 1916–1924, 1996.

[2] E. J. Higginbotham, J. S. Schuman, I. Goldberg et al., "One-year, randomized study comparing bimatoprost and timolol in glaucoma and ocular hypertension," *Archives of Ophthalmology*, vol. 120, no. 10, pp. 1286–1293, 2002.

[3] Canadian Opthalmology Association, "Canadian ophthalmological society evidence-based clinical practice guidelines for the management of glaucoma in the adult eye," *Canadian Journal of Ophthalmology*, vol. 44, pp. S7–S54, 2009.

[4] A. Alm, "PhXA34, a new potent ocular hypotensive drug," *Archives of Ophthalmology*, vol. 109, no. 11, pp. 1564–1568, 1991.

[5] N. Ziai, J. W. Dolan, R. D. Kacere, and R. F. Brubaker, "The effects on aqueous dynamics of PhXA41, a new prostaglandin F2α analogue, after topical application in normal and ocular hypertensive human eyes," *Archives of Ophthalmology*, vol. 111, no. 10, pp. 1351–1358, 1993.

[6] A. Alm and J. Stjernschantz, "Effects on intraocular pressure and side effects of 0.005% latanoprost applied once daily, evening or morn- ing: a comparison with timolol," *Ophthalmology*, vol. 102, no. 12, pp. 1743–1752, 1995.

[7] C. B. Camras, "Comparison of latanoprost and timolol in patients with ocular hypertension and glaucoma: a six-month masked, multicenter trial in the United States. The United States latanoprost study group," *Ophthalmology*, vol. 103, no. 1, pp. 138–147, 1996.

[8] H. K. Mishima, K. Masuda, Y. Kitazawa, and I. A. M. Azuma, "A comparison of latanoprost and timolol in primary open-angle glaucoma and ocular hypertension A 12-week study," *Archives of Ophthalmology*, vol. 114, no. 8, pp. 929–932, 1996.

[9] P. Watson, J. Stjernschantz, L. Beck et al., "A six-month, randomized, double-masked study comparing latanoprost with timolol in open-angle glaucoma and ocular hypertension," *Ophthalmology*, vol. 103, no. 1, pp. 126–137, 1996.

[10] S. Gandolfi, S. T. Simmons, R. Sturm, K. Chen, and A. M. VanDenburgh, "Three-month comparison of bimatoprost and latanoprost in patients with glaucoma and ocular hypertension," *Advances in Therapy*, vol. 18, no. 13, pp. 110–121, 2001.

[11] R. S. Noecker, M. S. Dirks, N. T. Choplin, P. Bernstein, A. L. Batoosingh, and S. M. Whitcup, "A six-month randomized clinical trial comparing the intraocular pressure-lowering efficacy of bimatoprost and latanoprost in patients with ocular hypertension or glaucoma," *American Journal of Ophthalmology*, vol. 135, no. 1, pp. 55–63, 2003.

[12] W. C. Stewart, D. G. Day, J. A. Stewart, J. Schuhr, and K. E. Latham, "The efficacy and safety of latanoprost 0.005% once daily versus brimonidine 0.2% twice daily in open-angle glaucoma or ocular hypertension," *American Journal of Ophthalmology*, vol. 131, no. 5, pp. 631–635, 2001.

[13] W. C. Stewart, K. T. Holmes, and M. A. Johnson, "Washout periods for brimonidine 0.2% and latanoprost 0.005%," *American Journal of Ophthalmology*, vol. 131, no. 6, pp. 798-799, 2001.

[14] H. D. Jampel, B. H. Chon, R. Stamper et al., "Effectiveness of intraocular pressure-lowering medication determined by washout," *JAMA Ophthalmology*, vol. 132, no. 4, pp. 390–395, 2014.

[15] G. Giuffrè, "The effects of prostaglandin F2a in the human eye," *Graefe's Archive for Clinical and Experimental Ophthalmology*, vol. 222, no. 3, pp. 139–141, 1985.

[16] S. H. Downs and N. Black, "The feasibility of creating a checklist for the assessment of the methodological quality both of randomised and non-randomised studies of health care interventions," *Journal of Epidemiology and Community Health*, vol. 52, no. 6, pp. 377–384, 1998.

[17] M. S. Malvankar-Mehta, Y. Chen, Y. Iordanous, W. Wang, and C. Hutnik, "iStent as a solo procedure for glaucoma patients: a systematic review and meta-analysis," *PLoS One*, vol. 10, no. 5, Article ID e0128146, 2015.

[18] T. Aung, P. T. Chew, C. C. Yip et al., "A randomized double-masked crossover study comparing latanoprost 0.005% with unoprostone 0.12% in patients with primary open-angle glaucoma and ocular hypertension," *American Journal of Ophthalmology*, vol. 131, no. 5, pp. 636–642, 2001.

[19] H. Kobayashi, "Efficacy of single glaucoma medication in combined latanoprost and timolol xe therapy in patients with open-angle glaucoma and ocular hypertension: a discontinuation study," *Journal of Ocular Pharmacology and Therapeutics*, vol. 28, no. 4, pp. 387–391, 2012.

[20] L. I. Larsson, "Intraocular pressure over 24 hours after repeated administration of latanoprost 0.005% or timolol gel-forming solution 0.5% in patients with ocular hypertension," *Ophthalmology*, vol. 108, no. 8, pp. 1439–1444, 2001.

[21] C. Linden, E. Nuija, and A. Alm, "Effects on IOP restoration and blood-aqueous barrier after long-term treatment with latanoprost in open angle glaucoma and ocular hypertension," *British Journal of Ophthalmology*, vol. 81, no. 5, pp. 370–372, 1997.

[22] M. Sehi, D. S. Grewal, W. J. Feuer, and D. S. Greenfield, "The impact of intraocular pressure reduction on retinal ganglion cell function measured using pattern electroretinogram in eyes receiving latanoprost 0.005% versus placebo," *Vision Research*, vol. 51, no. 2, pp. 235–242, 2011.

[23] A. J. Sit, R. N. Weinreb, J. G. Crowston, D. F. Kripke, and J. H. K. Liu, "Sustained effect of travoprost on diurnal and nocturnal intraocular pressure," *American Journal of Ophthalmology*, vol. 141, no. 6, pp. 1131–1133, 2006.

[24] T. R. Walters, H. B. DuBiner, S. P. Carpenter, B. Khan, and A. M. VanDenburgh, "24-hour IOP control with once-daily bimatoprost, timolol gel-forming solution, or latanoprost: A 1-month, randomized, comparative clinical trial," *Survey of Ophthalmology*, vol. 49, no. 2, pp. S26–S35, 2004.

[25] H. B. Dubiner, M. D. Sircy, T. Landry et al., "comparison of the diurnal ocular hypotensive efficacy of travoprost and latanoprost over a 44-hour period in patients with elevated intraocular pressure," *Clinical Therapeutics*, vol. 26, no. 1, pp. 84–91, 2004.

[26] S. Kurtz and G. Shemesh, "The efficacy and safety of once-daily versus once-weekly latanoprost treatment for increased intraocular pressure," *Journal of Ocular Pharmacology and Therapeutics*, vol. 20, no. 4, pp. 321–327, 2004.

[27] M. Kass, C. A. Johnson, J. L. Keltner, J. P. Miller, R. K. P. Ii, and M. R. Wilson, "The ocular hypertension treatment study," *Journal of Glaucoma*, vol. 120, 1994.

[28] M. Egger, G. D. Smith, M. Schneider, and C. Minder, "Bias in meta-analysis detected by a simple, graphical test," *BMJ*, vol. 315, no. 7109, pp. 629–634, 1997.

5

Ocular Biometric Characteristics of Chinese with History of Acute Angle Closure

Wei-ran Niu ⓘ, Chun-qiong Dong, Xi Zhang, Yi-fan Feng ⓘ, and Fei Yuan ⓘ

Department of Ophthalmology, Zhongshan Hospital of Fudan University, Shanghai 200032, China

Correspondence should be addressed to Fei Yuan; yuanfei_zs@126.com

Academic Editor: Usha P. Andley

Purpose. To investigate the biometric characteristics of Chinese patients with a history of acute angle closure (AAC). *Methods.* In this clinic-based, retrospective, observational, cross-sectional study, biometric parameters of eyes were acquired from a general population of Chinese adults. The crowding value (defined as lens thickness (LT); central corneal thickness (CCT); anterior chamber depth (ACD)/axial length (AL)) was calculated for each patient. Logistic regression analysis was performed to identify risk factors for AAC. Receiver operating characteristic (ROC) curves were plotted, and biometric variables were compared to compile a risk assessment for AAC. *Result.* This study included 1500 healthy subjects (2624 eyes, mean age of 66.54 ± 15.82 years) and 107 subjects with AAC (202 eyes, mean age of 70.01 ± 11.05 years). Eyes with AAC had thicker lens ($P \leq 0.001$), shallower anterior chamber depth ($P \leq 0.001$), and shorter axial length ($P \leq 0.001$) than healthy eyes. Logistic regression analysis and ROC curve analysis indicated that a crowding value above 0.13 was a significant ($P < 0.05$) risk factor for the development of AAC. *Conclusions.* Biometric parameters were significantly different between the eyes from the AAC group to the normal group. Ocular crowding value might be a new noncontact screening method to assess the risk of AAC in adults.

1. Introduction

Glaucoma is a leading cause of ocular morbidity and blindness worldwide [1]. It is estimated that by 2020, there will be 79.6 million people suffering from glaucoma, of which 26% will have primary angle closure glaucoma (PACG) [2]. Previous studies have stated that PACG is responsible for nearly half the cases of glaucoma-related blindness in the world, and the prevalence of this condition is highest in China [2, 3].

In the Primary Angle Closure Preferred Practice Pattern® (PPP) guidelines (2016), acute angle closure crisis (AACC) is described as a suddenly occluded angle with symptomatic high IOP [4]. Acute angle closure (AAC) can occur rapidly, recur, and cause permanent vision loss or blindness [5–7]. Eyes with optic neuropathy caused by AAC will be diagnosed as primary angle-closure glaucoma. Since approximately half of fellow eyes of acute angle-closure patients can develop AACCs within 5 years, the fellow eye is also at high risk of AAC [4]. Preventive interventions can be effective in the treatment of patients with AAC [8, 9];

managing AACC successfully has been one of the main clinic objectives of PAC and, it is of paramount importance to assess the risk of AAC properly.

Notably, many ways have been used for detecting a closed angle to diagnose primary angle closure disease (PACD) instead of assessing the risk of AAC. For example, gonioscopy examination is the current gold standard for the detection of PACD [10], and is not so suitable for case-finding or large-scale population screening; Van Herick's method has been used as a substitutive assessment method of gonioscopy [11, 12], screening results of which may vary from one ophthalmologist to another [13].

Knowledge of biometric parameters is essential for understanding the development of ocular growth and AAC pathologies. Some ocular anatomical characteristics such as short axial length and shallow anterior chamber depth have been reported to be major risk factors of AAC [14–18], and in other words, the "small eyes" are at a higher risk of developing AAC. However, the traditional biometric parameters such as anterior chamber depth or lens vault are not strong predictors of ACC [19–21]. We speculate that the crowding condition of the eye would be a more important factor to trigger an AAC, and thus the parameters describing the condition should be more appropriate predictors for AAC.

It remains difficult to investigate the in-depth pathologies of AAC; but there may be a way to assess the risk of it. With identification of high-risk individuals, the development of AAC could be interrupted at the right time. Towards this end, we collected the ocular biometric parameters of Chinese subjects with an AAC history and compared those of AAC eyes to healthy eyes to identify a new method to assess the risk of AAC.

2. Materials and Methods

This retrospective, observational, cross-sectional study was approved by the Department of Ophthalmology, Zhongshan Hospital, Fudan University, Shanghai, China, and conducted in accordance with the Declaration of Helsinki.

2.1. Study Population. Here, 1810 subjects were recruited consecutively between October 2013 and April 2015. The subjects were either outpatients or inpatients in the Department of Ophthalmology, Zhongshan Hospital, Fudan University, Shanghai, China. All subjects were over 18 years old and from the ethnic Chinese Han population. Both healthy eyes and those with a history of AAC were selected; both eyes of each patient were included in the study. The healthy group included patients who presented at our clinic for glasses, minor external ocular discomfort, or cataracts with normal angles and optic nerve head. Patients with an AAC history should be clinic silent and intraocular pressures (IOPs) should be maintained in a normal range.

Data from subjects with AAC who were surgically treated for glaucoma or had a laser treatment such as laser peripheral iridotomy (LPI) or were in the acute stage, with a history of ocular surgery, trauma, tumor, and pathologies such as detachment of retina or second glaucoma were excluded. Subjects younger than 18 years were also excluded. Pilocarpine treatment was discontinued at least one day before the examination, and IOP were measured during the examining period.

2.2. Study Design. All subjects underwent a thorough ophthalmic examination, which included slit-lamp biomicroscopy, IOP measurement by applanation tonometry, fundus examination, and measurements of other ocular biometrics. Central corneal thickness (CCT), lens thickness (LT), anterior chamber depth (ACD), and axial length (AL) were measured using a LENSTAR LS 900 (Haag-Streit, Koeniz, Switzerland). The associated measurements were carried out by the same investigator, and the LENSTAR LS 900 measurement procedure has previously been described in detail elsewhere [22].

2.3. Statistical Analysis. All statistical analyses were performed using SPSS (Windows ver. 20.0; SPSS Inc., Chicago, IL, USA). Basic descriptive statistics were calculated on all

data reported as mean value ± standard deviation. Categorical data were compared using the chi-squared test, and numerical data were compared employing one-way ANOVA and Student's t-test. Numerical data of eyes from one subject were compared using the paired sample t-test. All tests were two-tailed, and P values were considered statistically significant at $P < 0.05$.

Biometric parameters with statistically significant differences between the study group and the control group were used to build a binary conditional logistic regression analysis model to assess the risk of AAC. Receiver operating characteristic (ROC) curves were plotted using crowding values (defined in Results) to obtain a suitable cutoff value to separate healthy from eyes at risk of AAC. The best sensitivity/specificity relationship was determined using the cutoff point extrapolated from the area under ROC curves and predicted probabilities.

3. Results

3.1. The Demographic Characteristics of all Subjects. Complete data were available for 107 subjects with an AAC history (202 eyes) and 1500 subjects (2624 eyes) in the control group (Table 1). The IOP of all the subjects were in the normal range from 10.0 to 21.0 mmHg.

3.2. Differences between the Biometric Parameters in the AAC and Control Groups and between Right and Left Eyes. AAC cases were significantly older (70 ± 11 years) than the control group (67 ± 16 years) ($P = 0.026$). There were statistically more females in the AAC group compared with the control group ($P = 0.021$), and there were no significant differences in all four biometric parameters between the right and left eyes of the AAC group (Table 2). The CCT, LT, and AL of two groups were significantly different (Table 3).

3.3. Correlation between AAC Biometric Parameters Based on Logistic Regression Analysis. Shallower ACD and shorter AL as well as LT were significantly associated with the prediction of AAC by binary conditional logistic regression analysis, after adjustment for age and sex (Table 4). After adjusting for all other parameters, older age (ORs 1.018; $P < 0.0001$) was shown to be significantly associated with AAC by conditional logistic regression analysis.

3.4. Crowding Value and Receiver Operating Characteristic Curves. A crowding value was calculated from the following equation which was created based on our results:

$$\text{crowding value} = \frac{(\text{CCT} + \text{LT} - \text{ACD})}{\text{AL}}. \quad (1)$$

ROC curves were then plotted using crowding values to assess the risk of AAC. ROC curve analysis showed that the optimal probability cutoff for the assessment of AAC was a crowding value over 0.13, with the area under the curve being 0.899 ± 0.009 (Figure 1). The corresponding sensitivity and specificity of crowding measurement were 86.6% and 80.6%, respectively. ROC curves using other formulas previously reported in the literature to determine the risk of

TABLE 1: Demographic characteristics of subject groups.

Parameter	AAC group (n = 107)	Control group (n =1500)	P value
Female sex, n (%)	72 (67.3)	837 (55.8)	0.021
Mean age ± SD (y)	70.0 ± 11.1	66.5 ± 15.8	0.026
Right eye, n (%)	105 (52.0)	1411 (53.8)	0.661

TABLE 2: Comparison of biometric parameters between right and left eyes in the AAC and the control groups.

	AAC group				Control group			
	Right eye (mean ± SD)	Left eye (mean ± SD)	N (right/left)	P value (paired Sample t- test)	Right eye	Left eye	N (right/left)	P value (paired Sample t-test)
CCT, μm	544.93 ± 41.82	539.89 ±35.80	87/87	0.155	538.03 ± 34.87	539.72 ±36.05	1112/1112	0.000
AD, mm	1.82 ± 0.32	1.86 ± 0.39	87/87	0.274	2.69 ± 0.51	2.67 ± 0.51	1112/1112	0.134
LT, mm	4.89 ± 0.42	4.89 ± 0.42	87/87	0.915	4.37 ± 0.47	4.38 ± 0.48	1112/1112	0.050
AL, mm	22.89 ± 1.45	22.94 ± 1.61	87/87	0.336	24.80 ± 2.44	24.70 ± 2.37	1112/1112	0.000

CCT = central corneal thickness; ACD = anterior chamber depth; LT = lens thickness; AL = axial length.

TABLE 3: Comparison of biometric parameters between the AAC and the control groups.

	AAC (mean ± SD)	Control group (mean ± SD)	P value (Student's t-test)
CCT, μm	544.25 ± 38.97	539.17 ± 36.02	0.055
ACD, mm	1.85 ± 0.37	2.65 ± 0.50	0.000
LT, mm	4.88 ± 0.41	4.40 ± 0.47	0.000
AL, mm	22.88 ± 1.45	24.70 ± 2.40	0.000

CCT = central corneal thickness; ACD = anterior chamber depth; LT = lens thickness; AL = axial length.

TABLE 4: Results of binary logistic regression analysis of biometric parameters for the prediction of AAC.

	Adjusted odds ratios	P value	95% confidence interval
CCT	1.005	0.077	1.000–1.009
ACD	0.014	0.000	0.009–0.031
LT	1.796	0.065	0.974–2.351
AL	0.872	0.017	0.745–0.972

CCT = central corneal thickness; ACD = anterior chamber depth; LT = lens thickness; AL = axial length.

angle closure were also plotted (Table 5). Results of simple crowding value (calculated as (LT − ACD)/AL) are also listed in Table 5.

4. Discussion

The Asian population has a high prevalence of AAC [2, 3, 23, 24]. Although AAC is well-studied, the pathological processes of AAC remains poorly understood. In the present study, we investigate the biometric characteristic of Han Chinese subjects with a history of AAC.

In many studies, only biometric data from one eye, commonly the right eye, were measured [19, 25]. PACD is a bilateral disease. Although 90% of AACs are unilateral, approximately half of fellow eyes of acute angle-closure patients can develop AACCs within 5 years; therefore, the contralateral eye of patients with a monocular AAC would

be at high risk for AAC [18, 26, 27]. For this reason, biometric data from contralateral eyes were important for this analysis; accordingly data from both eyes were collected and analyzed.

There was no significant difference between the biometric parameters of the right eye and the left eye for patients in the AAC group, a finding which disagrees with previous study [28]. We presume that there might be two reasons for this contradictory finding. Firstly, the data from patients in the acute stage of AAC were excluded from this study, and data from patients in poor condition who underwent surgery or LPI were also excluded. Removal of these confounding factors led to a more homogenous AAC group.

In the present study, there were more females and older subjects in the AAC group in agreement with previous research [3, 29]. We found that the eyes of the AAC group had a shorter AL, shallower ACD, and thicker LT than normal eyes, consistent with other publications [15,30–32]. There was no difference in CCT between the 2 groups; however, in our opinion, it would be too thin a cornea for eyes with a short AL in AAC group.

Earlier studies failed to identify an eye with AAC simply by the value of ACD [20, 27], LT [20,33–35], AL [21,36–38], and CCT [19, 39]. It was reported that patients with an ACD < 2.55 mm and a LT > 4.66 mm were at higher risk of APAC, with sensitivity of 60% and 67.6% and specificity of 65.3% and 60.5%, respectively [40].

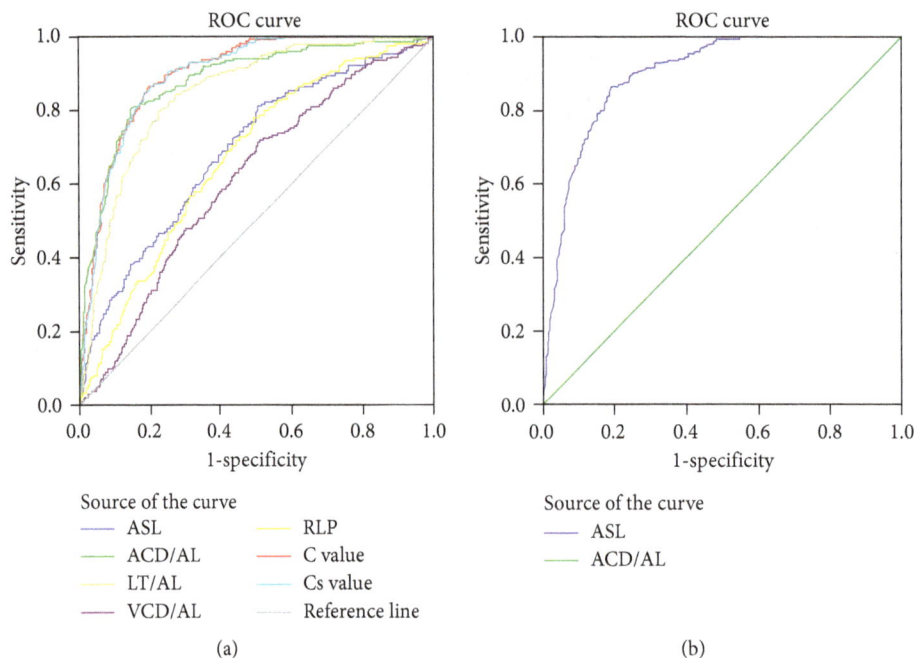

(a)   (b)

Figure 1: ROC curves plotting sensitivity against one-specificity (Az ROC: area under the ROC curve). In our study, a cutoff of 0.13 for crowding value seems to be the best value to separate healthy eyes from those at risk of AAC.

Table 5: Area under the receiver operating characteristic curve (AUROC), sensitivity, specificity, and cutoff value in healthy and AAC Subjects.

	AUROC	Sensitivity, specificity	Cutoff
ASL, mm	0.690	48.5%, 81.7%	≤7.58
Ratio (ACD/AL)	0.879	84.8%, 81.2%	≤0.09
Ratio (LT/AL)	0.845	85.5%, 77.1%	≥0.20
Ratio (VCD/AL)	0.669	72.0%, 42.7%	≤0.89
Ratio (RLP)	0.611	50.2%, 78.2%	≤0.19
Ratio (crowding value)	0.899	86.6%, 80.6%	≥0.13
Ratio (simple crowding value)	0.897	84.7%, 81.8%	≥0.11

ACD = anterior chamber depth; LT = lens thickness; AL = axial length; ASL = anterior segment length; RLP = relative lens position; simple crowding value = (LT - ACD)/AL. $P < 0.05$ was considered statistically significant.

Formulas were used to assess the risk of angle closure such as anterior segment length (ASL: summation of CCT, ACD, and LT) [19], the contribution of individual ocular components to the total axial (ACD/AL, LT/AL, VCD vitreous chamber depth/AL) [41], and the relative lens position (RLP: calculated as (ACD + 1/2LT)/AL) [42].

In the present study, we calculated a crowding value as follows: (LT+CCT-ACD)/AL according to the results of the logistic regression model. All four biometric parameters were shown to play a role in the development of AAC.

All these variables were calculated based on the recorded results of biometric parameters in the present study. The crowding value had the highest AUROC which means it is more sensitive and more specific than all the other variables mentioned in previous studies to assess the risk of AAC [40].

Changes in eyes with age such as an increase in LT make the structure of eyes more crowded, and a record of crowding value may help us to understand the development of ocular growth and AAC pathologies.

The results of our study should be interpreted with some limitations in mind. Firstly, because all patients were of Han Chinese descent and were recruited from the Department of Ophthalmology, Zhongshan Hospital, the results of this study may not be applicable to other racial groups and may not be generalizable to the larger population. Secondly, some studies have shown that cortical or nuclear cataracts may also be associated with angle closure [41]. However, the presence of severe cataracts makes measurements of LT and AL difficult, so such patients were excluded. Thirdly, because not all patients should be examined with gonioscopy, PACS eyes without any complaints, special biometric parameters, and medical history might be included in the healthy participants although studies suggest that the majority of patients with PACS will not develop either PAC or PACG [8, 43]. Lastly, we excluded patients who had accepted laser peripheral iridotomy treatment or surgery as this might have led to unnatural biometric differences between the right and left eyes.

5. Conclusions

In conclusion, ACC eyes have higher crowding values in terms of biometric parameters. Determination of ocular crowding value using ocular biometric parameters may represent a novel and rapid method to assess the risk of AAC. Future studies with a larger population representing different ethnic groups are needed to test the reliability and repeatability of our findings.

Conflicts of Interest

The authors have no proprietary or commercial interest in any materials discussed in this paper.

Acknowledgments

We thank for Yuan Yuan-zhi, MD for his suggestions and support. This study was supported by the Youth Foundation of Zhongshan Hospital (Grant no. 2017ZSQN47)

References

[1] B. Thylefors, A. D. Negrel, R. Pararajasegaram, and K. Y. DaGdzie, "Global data on blindness," *Bulletin of the World Health Organization*, vol. 73, no. 1, pp. 115–121, 1995.

[2] H. A. Quigley and A. T. Broman, "The number of people with glaucoma worldwide in 2010 and 2020," *British Journal of Ophthalmology*, vol. 90, no. 3, pp. 262–267, 2006.

[3] P. J. Foster and G. J. Johnson, "Glaucoma in China: how big is the problem?," *British Journal of Ophthalmology*, vol. 85, no. 11, pp. 1277–1282, 2001.

[4] B. E. Prum Jr., L. W. Herndon Jr., S. E. Moroi et al., "Primary angle closure preferred practice pattern((r)) guidelines," *Ophthalmology*, vol. 123, no. 1, pp. P112–P151, 2016.

[5] L. P. Ang, T. Aung, W. H. Chua, L. W. Yip, and P. T. Chew, "Visual field loss from primary angle-closure glaucoma: a comparative study of symptomatic and asymptomatic disease," *Ophthalmology*, vol. 111, no. 9, pp. 1636–1640, 2004.

[6] R. N. Weinreb, T. Aung, and F. A. Medeiros, "The pathophysiology and treatment of glaucoma: a review," *JAMA*, vol. 311, no. 18, pp. 1901–1911, 2014.

[7] American Academy of Ophthalmolog and Preferred Practice Patterns Committee, *The Primary Angle Closure Preferred Practice Pattern® Guidelines*, Elsevier Inc., New York, NY, USA, 2015, http://www.aao.org/ppp.

[8] R. Thomas, R. George, R. Parikh, J. Muliyil, and A. Jacob, "Five year risk of progression of primary angle closure suspects to primary angle closure: a population based study," *British Journal of Ophthalmology*, vol. 87, no. 4, pp. 450–454, 2003.

[9] R. Thomas and M. J. Walland, "Management algorithms for primary angle closure disease," *Clinical & Experimental Ophthalmology*, vol. 41, no. 3, pp. 282–292, 2013.

[10] M. E. Nongpiur, X. Wei, L. Xu et al., "Lack of association between primary angle-closure glaucoma susceptibility loci and the ocular biometric parameters anterior chamber depth and axial length," *Investigative Ophthalmology & Visual Science*, vol. 54, no. 8, pp. 5824–5828, 2013.

[11] E. W. Chan, X. Li, Y. C. Tham et al., "Glaucoma in Asia: regional prevalence variations and future projections," *British Journal of Ophthalmology*, vol. 100, no. 1, pp. 78–85, 2015.

[12] S. B. Park, K. R. Sung, S. Y. Kang, J. W. Jo, K. S. Lee, and M. S. Kook, "Assessment of narrow angles by gonioscopy, Van Herick method and anterior segment optical coherence tomography," *Japanese Journal of Ophthalmology*, vol. 55, no. 4, pp. 343–350, 2011.

[13] R. Thomas, T. George, A. Braganza, and J. Muliyil, "The flashlight test and van Herick's test are poor predictors for occludable angles," *Australian and New Zealand Journal of Ophthalmology*, vol. 24, no. 3, pp. 251–256, 1996.

[14] A. Tomlinson and D. A. Leighton, "Ocular dimensions in the heredity of angle-closure glaucoma," *British Journal of Ophthalmology*, vol. 57, no. 7, pp. 475–486, 1973.

[15] R. F. Lowe, "Aetiology of the anatomical basis for primary angle-closure glaucoma. Biometrical comparisons between normal eyes and eyes with primary angle-closure glaucoma," *British Journal of Ophthalmology*, vol. 54, no. 3, pp. 161–169, 1970.

[16] M. E. Nongpiur, L. M. Sakata, D. S. Friedman et al., "Novel association of smaller anterior chamber width with angle closure in Singaporeans," *Ophthalmology*, vol. 117, no. 10, pp. 1967–1973, 2010.

[17] M. E. Nongpiur, M. He, N. Amerasinghe et al., "Lens vault, thickness, and position in Chinese subjects with angle closure," *Ophthalmology*, vol. 118, no. 3, pp. 474–479, 2011.

[18] X. Sun, Y. Dai, Y. Chen et al., "Primary angle closure glaucoma: what we know and what we don't know," *Progress in Retinal and Eye Research*, vol. 57, pp. 26–45, 2017.

[19] S. W. Cheung and P. Cho, "Validity of axial length measurements for monitoring myopic progression in orthokeratology," *Investigative Ophthalmology & Visual Science*, vol. 54, no. 3, pp. 1613–1615, 2013.

[20] Y. W. Lan, J. W. Hsieh, and P. T. Hung, "Ocular biometry in acute and chronic angle-closure glaucoma," *Ophthalmologica*, vol. 221, no. 6, pp. 388–394, 2007.

[21] J. H. Sun, K. R. Sung, S. C. Yun et al., "Factors associated with anterior chamber narrowing with age: an optical coherence tomography study," *Investigative Ophthalmology & Visual Science*, vol. 53, no. 6, pp. 2607–2610, 2012.

[22] H. J. Shammas and K. J. Hoffer, "Repeatability and reproducibility of biometry and keratometry measurements using a noncontact optical low-coherence reflectometer and keratometer," *American Journal of Ophthalmology*, vol. 153, no. 1, pp. 55.e2–61.e2, 2012.

[23] T. Y. Wong, S. C. Loon, and S. M. Saw, "The epidemiology of age related eye diseases in Asia," *British Journal of Ophthalmology*, vol. 90, no. 4, pp. 506–511, 2006.

[24] Y. C. Tham, X. Li, T. Y. Wong, H. A. Quigley, T. Aung, and C. Y. Cheng, "Global prevalence of glaucoma and projections of glaucoma burden through 2040: a systematic review and meta-analysis," *Ophthalmology*, vol. 121, no. 11, pp. 2081–2090, 2014.

[25] R. Iribarren, I. G. Morgan, V. Nangia, and J. B. Jonas, "Crystalline lens power and refractive error," *Investigative Ophthalmology & Visual Science*, vol. 53, no. 2, pp. 543–550, 2012.

[26] S. K. Seah, P. J. Foster, P. T. Chew et al., "Incidence of acute primary angle-closure glaucoma in Singapore: an island-wide survey," *Archives of Ophthalmology*, vol. 115, no. 11, pp. 1436–1440, 1997.

[27] D. S. Friedman, G. Gazzard, P. Foster et al., "Ultrasonographic biomicroscopy, Scheimpflug photography, and novel provocative tests in contralateral eyes of Chinese patients initially seen with acute angle closure," *Archives of Ophthalmology*, vol. 121, no. 5, pp. 633–642, 2003.

[28] J. R. Lee, K. R. Sung, and S. Han, "Comparison of anterior segment parameters between the acute primary angle closure eye and the fellow eye," *Investigative Ophthalmology & Visual Science*, vol. 55, no. 6, pp. 3646–3650, 2014.

[29] R. Thomas, K. Mengersen, A. Thomas, and M. J. Walland, "Understanding the causation of primary angle closure disease using the sufficient component cause model," *Clinical &*

Experimental Ophthalmology, vol. 42, no. 6, pp. 522–528, 2014.

[30] R. George, P. G. Paul, M. Baskaran et al., "Ocular biometry in occludable angles and angle closure glaucoma: a population based survey," *British Journal of Ophthalmology*, vol. 87, no. 4, pp. 399–402, 2003.

[31] G. Marchini, A. Pagliarusco, A. Toscano, R. Tosi, C. Brunelli, and L. Bonomi, "Ultrasound biomicroscopic and conventional ultrasonographic study of ocular dimensions in primary angle-closure glaucoma," *Ophthalmology*, vol. 105, no. 11, pp. 2091–2098, 1998.

[32] R. J. Casson, "Anterior chamber depth and primary angle-closure glaucoma: an evolutionary perspective," *Clinical & Experimental Ophthalmology*, vol. 36, no. 1, pp. 70–77, 2008.

[33] Z. Mimiwati and J. Fathilah, "Ocular biometry in the subtypes of primary angle closure glaucoma in University Malaya Medical Centre," *Medical Journal of Malaysia*, vol. 56, no. 3, pp. 341–349, 2001.

[34] M. C. Lim, L. S. Lim, G. Gazzard et al., "Lens opacity, thickness, and position in subjects with acute primary angle closure," *Journal of Glaucoma*, vol. 15, no. 3, pp. 260–263, 2006.

[35] J. F. Salmon, S. A. Swanevelder, and M. A. Donald, "The dimensions of eyes with chronic angle-closure glaucoma," *Journal of Glaucoma*, vol. 3, no. 3, pp. 237–243, 1994.

[36] F. Aptel and P. Denis, "Optical coherence tomography quantitative analysis of iris volume changes after pharmacologic mydriasis," *Ophthalmology*, vol. 117, no. 1, pp. 3–10, 2010.

[37] C. Y. Cheung, S. Liu, R. N. Weinreb et al., "Dynamic analysis of iris configuration with anterior segment optical coherence tomography," *Investigative Ophthalmology & Visual Science*, vol. 51, no. 8, pp. 4040–4046, 2010.

[38] N. G. Congdon, Q. Youlin, H. Quigley et al., "Biometry and primary angle-closure glaucoma among Chinese, white, and black populations," *Ophthalmology*, vol. 104, no. 9, pp. 1489–1495, 1997.

[39] P. Y. Chang and S. W. Chang, "Corneal biomechanics, optic disc morphology, and macular ganglion cell complex in myopia," *Journal of Glaucoma*, vol. 22, no. 5, pp. 358–362, 2013.

[40] M. R. Razeghinejad and M. Banifatemi, "Ocular biometry in angle closure," *Journal of Ophthalmic & Vision Research*, vol. 8, no. 1, pp. 17–24, 2013.

[41] I. Debert, M. Polati, D. L. Jesus, E. C. Souza, and M. R. Alves, "Biometric relationships of ocular components in esotropic amblyopia," *Arquivos Brasileiros de Oftalmologia*, vol. 75, no. 1, pp. 38–42, 2012.

[42] R. V. Merula, S. Cronemberger, A. Diniz Filho, and N. Calixto, "New comparative clinical and biometric findings between acute primary angle-closure and glaucomatous eyes with narrow angle," *Arquivos Brasileiros de Oftalmologia*, vol. 73, no. 6, pp. 511–516, 2010.

[43] J. T. Wilensky, P. L. Kaufman, D. Frohlichstein et al., "Follow-up of angle-closure glaucoma suspects," *American Journal of Ophthalmology*, vol. 115, no. 3, pp. 338–346, 1993.

6

The Impact of Adherence and Instillation Proficiency of Topical Glaucoma Medications on Intraocular Pressure

Tesfay Mehari Atey,[1] **Workineh Shibeshi,**[2] **Abeba T. Giorgis,**[3] **and Solomon Weldegebreal Asgedom**[1]

[1]Clinical Pharmacy Unit, School of Pharmacy, College of Health Sciences, Mekelle University, Mekelle, Tigray, Ethiopia
[2]Department of Pharmacology and Clinical Pharmacy, School of Pharmacy, College of Health Sciences, Addis Ababa University, Addis Ababa, Ethiopia
[3]Department of Ophthalmology, School of Medicine, College of Health Sciences, Addis Ababa University, Addis Ababa, Ethiopia

Correspondence should be addressed to Tesfay Mehari Atey; tesfay.mehari@mu.edu.et

Academic Editor: Kazuyuki Hirooka

Background. The possible sequel of poorly controlled intraocular pressure (IOP) includes treatment failure, unnecessary medication use, and economic burden on patients with glaucoma. *Objective.* To assess the impact of adherence and instillation technique on IOP control. *Methods.* A cross-sectional study was conducted on 359 glaucoma patients in Menelik II Hospital from June 1 to July 31, 2015. After conducting a Q-Q analysis, multiple binary logistic analyses, linear regression analyses, and two-tailed paired t-test were conducted to compare IOP in the baseline versus current measurements. *Results.* Intraocular pressure was controlled in 59.6% of the patients and was relatively well controlled during the study period (mean (M) = 17.911 mmHg, standard deviation (S) = 0.323) compared to the baseline ($M = 20.866$ mmHg, $S = 0.383$, t (358) = −6.70, $p < 0.0001$). A unit increase in the administration technique score resulted in a 0.272 mmHg decrease in IOP ($p = 0.03$). Moreover, primary angle-closure glaucoma (adjusted odds ratio (AOR) = 0.347, 95% confidence interval (CI): 0.144–0.836) and two medications (AOR = 1.869, 95% CI: 1.259–9.379) were factors affecting IOP. *Conclusion.* Good instillation technique of the medications was correlated with a reduction in IOP. Consequently, regular assessment of the instillation technique and IOP should be done for better management of the disease.

1. Introduction

Glaucoma is a type of eye disorder resulting from optic neuropathy and leads to a progressive loss of retinal ganglion cell axons and ultimately irreversible blindness if left untreated [1–3]. It is the foremost cause of blindness among blacks [4] and the second leading cause of blindness globally next to cataract [5]. Worldwide, about 64 million people were affected by glaucoma in 2013 and this prevalence is expected to reach 76.0 and 111.8 million by 2020 and 2040, respectively [2]. Glaucoma inexplicably affects more Africans and Asians than whites [6] and it is considered as a public health problem in sub-Saharan Africa [7].

Because elevated intraocular pressure (IOP) is a major risk and causal factor for glaucoma [3], hence, hypotensive medications are prescribed as primary medications to control this pressure [8, 9]. Different studies proved that an elevated IOP hastens optic nerve head damage and waning of the visual field unless good adherence and appropriate instillation proficiency of topical glaucoma medications are strictly followed by the patients [10, 11].

During application of topical glaucoma medications into the eye, the administered dose could be lost through leakage and the punctum route. Approximately 80% of the administered drug could be removed from this route and go into the systemic circulation. Accordingly, the eyelid should be closed and the punctum route should be occluded in order to maximize the ocular bioavailability and to minimize the adverse systemic effects of these topically applied medications. Both these techniques serve to increase the therapeutic index of these eye drops and minimize dosage requirements [12, 13].

Previous studies showed that a large proportion of patients improperly administer their eye drops. For instance, a multicenter study from ten centers across Canada showed that over 50% of the patients were either nonadherent or demonstrated improper instillation proficiency [14]. A study conducted by Sleath et al. also found that 44% of the patients reported frequently missing the eye during attempted drop application [15]. A further study by Stone et al. also found that 17%–25% of patients were unable to effectively apply eye drop medications to their eye [16].

There are many factors that lead to poor control of IOP. Uncontrolled IOP could be due to poor adherence and/or incorrect instillation technique such as missing the eye during application. Possible sequel of poorly controlled IOP includes treatment failure, unnecessary use of additional medications, and economic burden on the patients [17–19]. The goal of every efficient antiglaucoma therapy is the attainment of target IOP. Target IOP is the level of IOP that is related to an insignificant likelihood of optic nerve damage and/or visual field loss. An association between the curve of IOP decrease and glaucoma progression is demonstrated in previous studies. In general, better protection from the loss of vision and visual field impairment in glaucoma patients could be achieved through reduced level of IOP [20]. Consequently, this study was done to assess the impact of adherence and instillation proficiency of topically applied medications on intraocular pressure among patients attending the glaucoma clinic of Menelik II Hospital.

2. Methods

The study was conducted at the glaucoma clinic of Menelik II Hospital (Addis Ababa, Ethiopia) using a cross-sectional study design. Patients, who attended the clinic from June 1, 2015, to July 31, 2015, were enrolled in the study to determine their level of intraocular pressure. Their medical records were reviewed for the type and severity of glaucoma and intraocular pressure in the baseline and current measurements. Baseline measurements and current measurements were extracted from the patients' record and were referring to the measurements of IOP during the first visit in the hospital and at the end of the data collection period, respectively. All glaucoma patients who were obtaining services at the clinic during the study period were considered as the study population. To select samples from the study population, a systematic random sampling technique was used in this study.

To estimate the minimum sample size required for the study, a single population estimating formula [21], accompanied by a conservative sample estimate (since there was no information from similar studies, past studies, or studies done on similar populations and no pilot study about the proportion was done), was used. The following points were taken into consideration during the sample size calculation: 95% confidence interval, 80% power of the study, 5% margin

of error, 10% attrition, and 0.5 prevalence. Therefore, the number of study samples for this study was found to be 359. On average, 2110 patients were being served at the clinic per two months (statistics office of the hospital). Accordingly, the sampling interval (k) was calculated to be six ($k = 2120/359 = 6$). A starting number (i.e., two) was chosen randomly and blindly from number one to six so that patients were recruited in this study at every second interval from a list of six patients.

Besides the above methodological aspects, the following inclusion and exclusion criteria were applied in the study. Patients who were 18 years and older, diagnosed with glaucoma or ocular hypertension, were on eye drops for at least six months, had a regular follow-up, and had not undergone either laser or glaucoma surgery in the past three months were included in the study. Glaucoma patients with postoperative follow-up without having any medications and who were not willing to give informed written consent were excluded from the study.

An appropriate two-day training was given to three ophthalmic nurses before data collection. The data collectors had more than three years of work experience at the clinic, but neither recently nor currently working at the clinic during the study period. The data collection tool was pretested in 18 patients (5% of the sample size) to maximize the quality of data. Adherence to topical glaucoma medications and instillation technique were measured using the Morisky Medication Adherence Scale-8 [21–25] and a World Health Organization (WHO) recommended Eye Drop Instillation Technique [2, 9, 12, 26]. The IOP was measured in the hospital using a standardized and calibrated tonometry. Notwithstanding differences in the control of IOP among studies, a favorable strategy to achieve IOP control is 20% reduction from the initial IOP or below 18 mmHg in an advanced stage of glaucoma. In patients with initial glaucoma, 25% reduction from the initial IOP will slow down the disease progression by 45% [20]. Accordingly, in this study, an IOP was deemed to be controlled if there was more than 20% reduction for moderate and advanced glaucoma, and more than 25% in early glaucoma or the target IOP (10–21 mmHg) have been achieved.

Data were entered using Epi Info™ version 3.5.3 and analyzed using SPSS® version 21. Factors affecting controlled IOP were identified using multiple logistic regression. Likewise, multiple linear regression was done, after incorporating variables that were statistically significant at $p < 0.2$ during the bivariate analysis, to relate intraocular pressure with the level of adherence and instillation technique. After conducting Q-Q plots to determine the distribution normality of the IOP, a two-tailed paired t-test was also employed to assess the level of IOP control in the baseline versus the current measurements of IOP. Statistical significance for the aforementioned analyses was declared at $p < 0.05$.

3. Results

3.1. Sociodemographic and Clinical Characteristics. The response rate in this study was found to be 100%. Concerning the sociodemographic characteristic of the patients, more than two-thirds (69%) of the patients were males. The mean

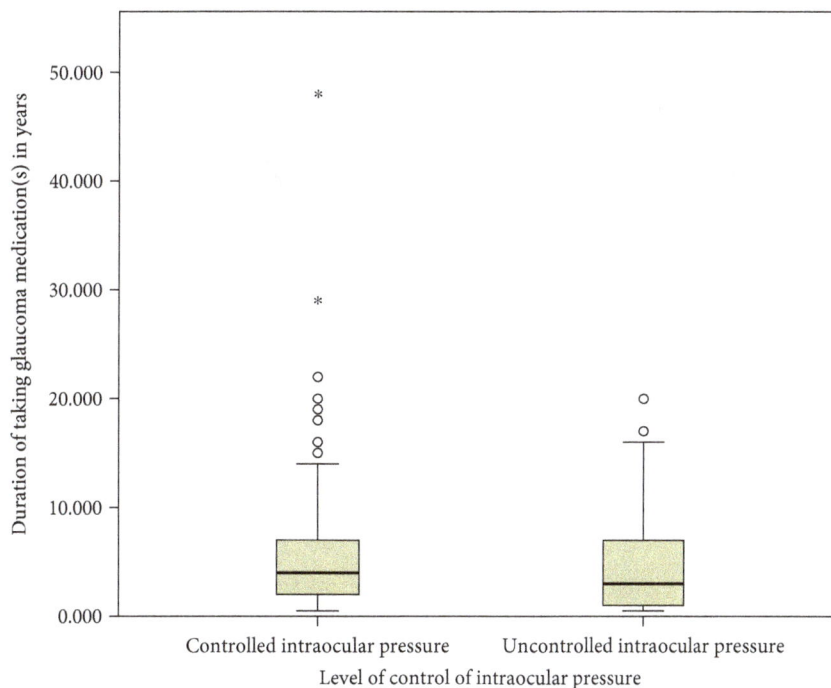

FIGURE 1: Level of intraocular pressure by the duration of taking glaucoma medications in Menelik II Hospital, 2015. *Outliers.

age of the participants was found to be about 61 ± 12.34 years ranging from 18 to 88 years. Furthermore, approximately one in three (32%) of the patients was retired. Despite the fact that a large proportion (90%) of the patients was living in urban areas, a lower educational level accounted for 64% of the patients. The sociodemographic data of these patients have been previously published [27, 28].

The mean duration of taking topical glaucoma medications for patients who had uncontrolled and controlled IOP were 4.92 years (standard error of mean (SE): ± 0.40; 95% CI: 4.13–5.71; range: half a year to 20 years) and 5.61 years (SE: ± 0.38; 95% CI: 4.87–6.35; range: half a year to 48 years) (Figure 1).

The severity of glaucoma in these patients showed that advanced, moderate, and early glaucoma accounted for about 24%, 64%, and 12% of the patients, respectively. The most common type of glaucoma was pseudoexfoliative glaucoma, responsible for about 41% of the disease followed by primary open-angle glaucoma (27%) Figure 2.

In this study, based upon the international council of ophthalmology's classification for visual acuity [29], about 34%, 37%, and 32% of the patients were having (near) normal vision, low vision, and (near) blindness.

3.2. Eyelid Closure and Nasolacrimal Occlusion. Almost all of the study participants (98%) claimed that they were not occluding their nasolacrimal route during the application of glaucoma medications. In contrast, approximately 91% of the patients claimed the closure of their eyelid (Figure 3).

3.3. Level of Intraocular Pressure Control. The mean IOP, in mmHg, in the right eye and left eye was 17.8 (SD: ± 7.7; range: 8 to 52) and 18.3 (SD: ± 8.8; range: 6 to 61), respectively. For more than half of the patients, their IOP in the left eye (59%), right eye (57%), and both eyes (60%) were controlled using the glaucoma medications. The overall level of controlled IOP was found to be about 60% (Figure 4).

To test normality of the mean IOP of the patients for the purpose of linear regression analysis and paired t-test, a Q-Q plot was made. The Q-Q plots of IOP revealed that the pressure was almost normally distributed with a slight skewness to the left (-0.523 ± 0.129).

Figure 5 shows a relationship of a percentage of difference IOP (reduction or increment) from the baseline in relation to the duration of taking glaucoma medication by a number of medications (panel a) and types of glaucoma medications (panel b). Generally, there was a greater reduction of intraocular pressure as the time of medications increased, as expected. A relatively slightly better IOP was controlled for patients taking timolol and pilocarpine compared to other medications (Figure 5).

Of the 113 patients who claimed to be highly adherent to their topical glaucoma medications, 57% of them had controlled IOP and the remaining (43%) had uncontrolled IOP. Likewise, among 62 patients who were appropriately instilling their topical glaucoma medications, 61% of them had controlled IOP compared to 39% of them whose IOP was not controlled.

Adherence status was found to be statistically associated with the instillation technique of topical glaucoma medications. Accordingly, the odds of appropriately instilling glaucoma medications were about 68% (crude odds ratio (COR) = 0.318, 95% CI: 0.174–0.579, $p < 0.0001$) and 76% (COR = 0.245, 95% CI: 0.096–0.621, $p < 0.003$) lower for patients with medium and low level of adherence, respectively, compared to those with high level of adherence (Table 1).

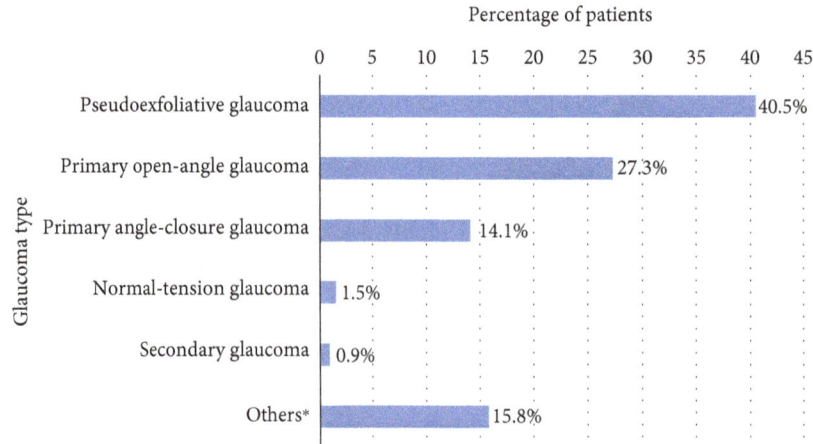

FIGURE 2: Profile of diagnosis of glaucoma among patients attending the glaucoma clinic of Menelik II Hospital, 2015. *Ocular hypertension, juvenile glaucoma.

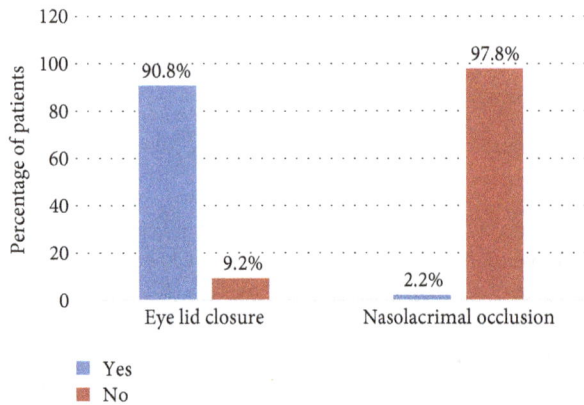

FIGURE 3: Percentage of practice of eyelid closure and nasolacrimal route occlusion among patients attending the glaucoma clinic of Menelik II Hospital, 2015.

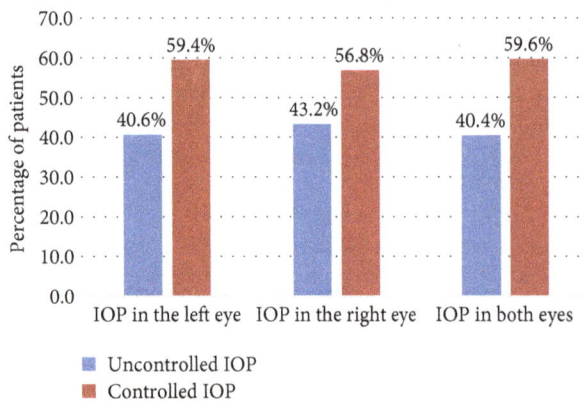

FIGURE 4: Comparison of the percentage of controlled intraocular pressure in the left, right, and both eyes among glaucoma patients in Menelik II Hospital, 2015.

Regarding the association of the status of adherence with IOP, a unit increase in the score of nonadherence results in a 0.026 mmHg increase in IOP ($p = 0.665$). Concerning the administration technique, a unit increase in the score of administration technique results in a 0.272 mmHg decrease in IOP ($p = 0.03$) (Table 2).

The glaucoma patients had also a lower score of IOP during the study period (mean (M) = 17.911, standard error (S) = 0.323) compared to the baseline measurements ($M = 20.866$, $S = 0.383$, t (358) = −6.70, $p < 0.0001$).

3.4. Factors Associated with Intraocular Pressure. The list of factors associated with the IOP is summarized in Figure 6. Accordingly, the glaucoma type and the number of glaucoma medications were found to be factors that were significantly associated with controlled IOP. Patients with primary angle-closure glaucoma were having 65% (adjusted odds ratio (AOR) = 0.347, 95% confidence interval (CI): 0.144–0.836, $p < 0.018$) lower odds of controlled IOP compared to patients with pseudoexfoliative glaucoma. Furthermore, the odds of having controlled IOP in patients who were taking two medications were almost twofold (AOR = 1.869, 95% CI: 1.259–9.379, $p < 0.047$) more compared to patients who were taking only one medication (Figure 6).

4. Discussions

This study assessed the impact of glaucoma medications on the level of IOP control. In the previous publications, 42.6% of the patients were found to be adherent to their prescribed hypotensive agents [27] and the rate of the appropriate administration technique was also found to be 17.3% [28]. Despite the importance of assessing the adherence behavior towards the prescribed medications and administration technique of eye drops in glaucoma management, their effect on the treatment outcome of glaucoma, that is, intraocular pressure should be determined. Accordingly, for about 60% of the study participants, their IOP was controlled using the glaucoma medications. This finding might be substandard as substantiated by the findings that the majority (57%) of the patients were being nonadherent to their medications and most (83%) of the patients were not appropriately

(a)

(b)

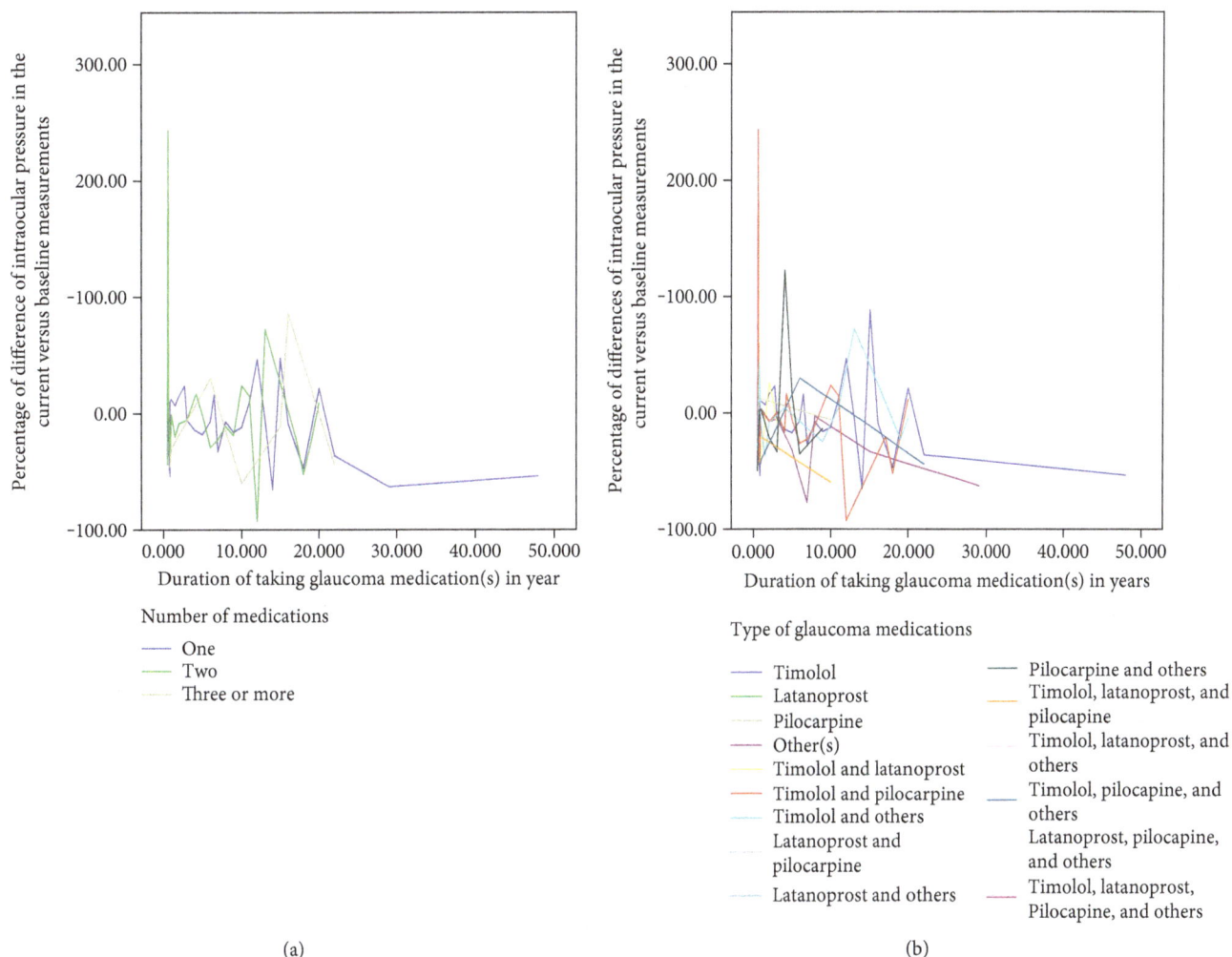

FIGURE 5: Relationship of intraocular pressure with the type and number of medications among glaucoma patients in Menelik II Hospital, 2015. (a) By the number of medications; and (b) by the type of medications.

TABLE 1: Association of medication adherence with instillation proficiency among patients attending the glaucoma clinic of Menelik II Hospital, 2015.

| Adherence | Instillation proficiency, n (%) | | COR (95% CI) | p value |
	Inappropriate	Appropriate		
High adherence	79 (69.9)	34 (30.1)	ref	
Medium adherence	161 (88.0)	22 (12.0)	0.318 (0.174–0.579)	0.0001
Low adherence	57 (90.5)	6 (9.5)	0.245 (0.096–0.621)	0.003

CI: confidence interval; COR: crude odds ratio.

TABLE 2: Association of intraocular pressure with adherence and administration technique among patients attending the glaucoma clinic of Menelik II Hospital, 2015.

Variable	Beta estimate (SE)	CI (p value)
Adherence	0.026 (0.325)	−0.613 to 0.665 (0.936)
Administration technique	−0.272 (0.214)	−0.692 to −0.149 (0.03)

CI: confidence interval; SE: standard error of mean.

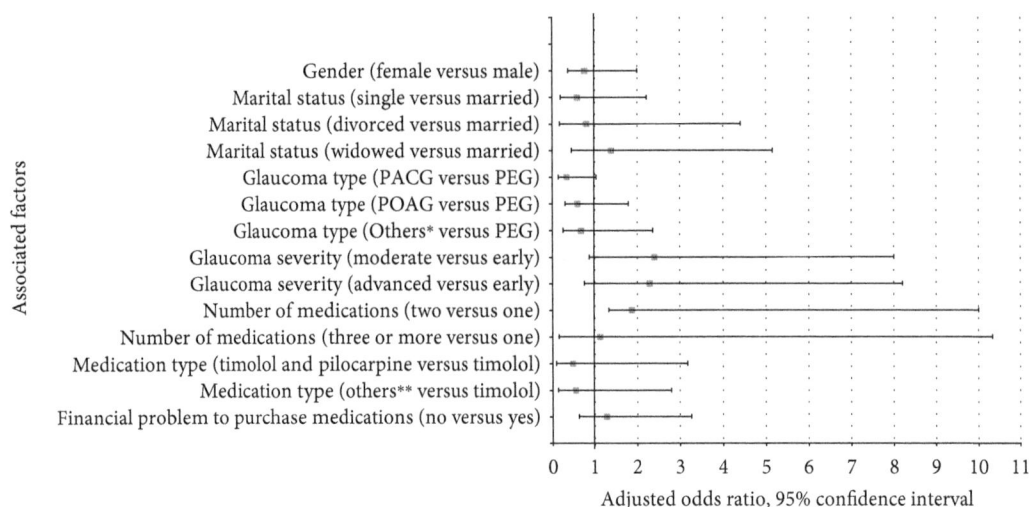

FIGURE 6: Factors associated with controlled intraocular pressure among patients attending the glaucoma clinic of Menelik II Hospital, 2015. The following factors were used in the logistic regression model: age, sex, marital status, ethnicity, educational level, residence, religion, occupation, monthly family income, type and severity of glaucoma, duration of the glaucoma in years, duration of taking medications in years, average follow-up period per year, the presence of previous surgery or laser treatment, major comorbidities, side effects of medications, acquisition of the medications (free of charge or not), financial problem to purchase the medications, the presence of other types of eye drops, adherence towards the medications, and instillation proficiency of the eye drops. The factors were assumed statistically significant at $p < 0.05$ and the end of the bar graph shows the odds ratio. PACG: primary angle-closure glaucoma; PEG: pseudoexfoliative glaucoma; POAG: primary open-angle glaucoma. *Secondary glaucoma, ocular hypertension, normal tension glaucoma, juvenile glaucoma **latanoprost; pilocarpine; timolol and latanoprost; timolol with other types of eye drops; pilocarpine with other types of eye drops; latanoprost with other types of eye drops; timolol, latanoprost, and pilocarpine; timolol and latanoprost with other types of eye drops; timolol and pilocarpine with other types of eye drops.

administering their topical glaucoma medications, according to the WHO guide. In this study, almost 60% of the study participants were neither adherent nor properly administered their eye drops, which was similar to studies that reported analogous rates in the USA [30], Greece [10], and Canada [14].

Besides the above findings, the present study also revealed that 77.2% of the study participants closed their eyes, but only 2.2% of them occluded their punctum route for at least two minutes during the administration procedure. Nevertheless, this result deviated from a study done in India that indicated a prevalence rate of about 29% of eyelid closure and 6% for punctum occlusion [18]. This difference might be instigated from discrepancies in patient education and awareness regarding instillation of eye drops and from variations in study methods. The practice of punctum occlusion was much poorer in the present study and almost all of the study participants admitted that they never occluded the punctum route. This poor practicing might be emanating from the poor patient education system and the unavailability of posters and brochures regarding instillation proficiency in the study center.

Among the patients who claimed to be adherent and who were appropriately instilling their medications, about two-thirds of them had controlled IOP. Being adherent and applying eye drops correctly maximize the intraocular concentration of the medications and minimize the systemic adverse effects. This could lead to a cumulative effect of better control of IOP. Furthermore, patients with high level of adherence were more likely to accurately administer their

eye drops compared to patients with a low and medium level of adherence. This finding was attributable to the more cautious nature of the adherent patients in the correct instillation of their medications. This implied that adherence and instillation proficiencies are interconnected and poor practicing in instillation proficiency could jeopardize adherence and vice versa.

Another finding of this study also showed that a unit increase in a score of the nonadherence and in a score of the administration technique results in a 0.026 mmHg increase and a 0.272 mmHg decrease in the IOP, respectively. Improper instillation proficiency and poor adherence increase failure to deliver the desired drug to the eye and in turn lead to wasted medication. This, in turn, leads to poor IOP control and eventually augments frequent changes in the types of prescribed medications and more frequent hospital visits [31]. In contrast, enhancement of drug delivery, improvement in treatment effectiveness, and reduction of the number of patient visits to the hospital could be achieved through good adherence and proper instillation technique of the medications [31]. Thus, eye care providers and other stakeholders should give more emphasis on the proper education of adherence, instillation technique, and their effect on IOP control.

Glaucoma patients had better controlled IOP at the end of the study period compared to the baseline measurements. Despite the poor instillation proficiency and suboptimal adherence observed among the study participants, application of these medications results in the overall reduction of the IOP through their pharmacodynamic mechanism.

The number of medications and type of glaucoma were statistically associated with the level of IOP control. Accordingly, patients who were taking two glaucoma medications were more likely to have a controlled IOP compared to patients who were taking only one medication. Applying different medications with a different mechanism of action will effectively lower IOP more than a single medication. On the contrary, patients with primary angle-closure glaucoma had lower odds of controlled IOP compared to patients with pseudoexfoliative glaucoma and this might be attributable to the aggressive nature of the latter disease (i.e., pseudoexfoliative glaucoma) which tied to more attention and close follow-up for patients with this disease. On the other hand, the characteristics of the study participants might affect the nonexistence of a relationship observed among controlled IOP with sociodemographic factors, adherence level, and instillation proficiency. Demographic factors might have less influence on the level of IOP because of a longer duration of glaucoma (with a mean of 5.6 years) and a lengthy period of taking the topical glaucoma medications (with a mean of 5.4 years).

The present study has certain limitations. Primarily, the nature of the design, that is, cross-sectional, did not allow a longitudinal follow-up of the study participants to comprehensively identify the factors contributing for uncontrolled IOP. Secondly, two measurements, the baseline and current, were used to assess IOP control. The baseline measurement—which was assumed as the first measurement recorded during their first follow-up in the hospital—might not necessarily mean the actual baseline measurements as some of the patients might be referred from other eye care centers with medications. Besides this, variability in IOP measurements can occur as a function of instrumentation or even in patients' own diurnal variation. Thirdly, the value of controlled IOP depends on the pretreatment level of IOP and other factors. However, these factors were difficult to assess during the study period and hence, future studies should be done considering these factors. Lastly, self-reported adherence has been shown to be poorly predictive of adherence compared to objective measurements such as electronic monitoring. Therefore, objective measurements of adherence using drug concentrations and with longer assessment follow-up periods should be planned in future studies.

5. Conclusion

There was a substandard level of controlled intraocular pressure in the tertiary referral hospital. Good instillation technique of topical glaucoma medications is correlated with a reduction in intraocular pressure. Applying two topical glaucoma medications is found to be a contributing factor for having a controlled intraocular pressure. Consequently, regular assessment of the patients' instillation technique and intraocular pressure should be done for better management of the disease.

Abbreviations

AOR: Adjusted odds ratio
CI: Confidence interval
COR: Crude odds ratio
df: Degree of freedom
IOP: Intraocular pressure
M: Mean
mmHg: Millimeters of mercury
SD: Standard deviation
SE (S): Standard error of mean.

Conflicts of Interest

The authors report no conflicts of interest.

Acknowledgments

The authors would like to acknowledge all participants of the study.

References

[1] K. A. McVeigh and G. Vakros, "The eye drop chart: a pilot study for improving administration of and compliance with topical treatments in glaucoma patients," *Clinical Ophthalmology*, vol. 9, pp. 813–819, 2015.

[2] Y. C. Tham, X. Li, T. Y. Wong, H. A. Quigley, T. Aung, and C. Y. Cheng, "Global prevalence of glaucoma and projections of glaucoma burden through 2040: a systematic review and meta-analysis," *Ophthalmology*, vol. 121, pp. 2081–2090, 2014.

[3] R. N. Weinreb and P. T. Khaw, "Primary open-angle glaucoma," *Lancet*, vol. 363, pp. 1711–1720, 2004.

[4] A. Sommer, J. M. Tielsch, J. Katz et al., "Racial differences in the cause-specific prevalence of blindness in East Baltimore," *The New England Journal of Medicine*, vol. 325, p. 1412, 1991.

[5] S. Kingman, "Glaucoma is second leading cause of blindness globally," *Bulletin of the World Health Organization*, vol. 82, p. 887, 2004.

[6] F. Kyari, M. M. Abdull, A. Bastawrous, C. E. Gilbert, and H. Faal, "Epidemiology of glaucoma in sub-Saharan Africa: prevalence, incidence and risk factors," *Middle East African Journal Ophthalmology*, vol. 20, pp. 111–125, 2013.

[7] M. Alemu, L. A. Nelson, B. Kruft, J. A. Stewart, and W. C. Stewart, "Epidemiology of glaucoma in central Ethiopia," *International Journal Ophthalmology*, vol. 2, pp. 168–173, 2009.

[8] P. P. Lee, J. W. Walt, L. C. Rosenblatt, L. R. Siegartel, and L. S. Stern, "Association between intraocular pressure variation and glaucoma progression: data from a United States chart review," *American Journal of Ophthalmology*, vol. 144, pp. 901–907, 2007.

[9] T. Tsai, A. L. Robin, and J. P. Smith, "An evaluation of how glaucoma patients use topical medications: a pilot study," *Transactions of the American Ophthalmological Society*, vol. 105, pp. 29–35, 2007.

[10] G. P. Konstas, G. Maskaleris, S. Gratsonidis, and C. Sardelli, "Compliance and viewpoint of glaucoma patients in Greece," *Eye*, vol. 14, pp. 752–756, 2000.

[11] W. C. Stewart, A. G. P. Konstas, and N. Pfeiffer, "Patient and ophthalmologist attitudes concerning compliance and dosing in glaucoma treatment," *Journal of Ocular Pharmacology and Therapeutics*, vol. 20, pp. 461–469, 2004.

[12] T. P. G. M. Vries, R. H. Henning, H. V. Hogerzeil, and D. A. Fresle, *Guide to Good Prescribing: A Practical Manual*, World Health Organization, Geneva, Switzerland, 1st edition, 2009.

[13] J. Flach, "The importance of eyelid closure and nasolacrimal occlusion following the ocular instillation of topical glaucoma medications, and the need for the universal inclusion of one of these techniques in all patient treatments and clinical studies," *Transactions of the American Ophthalmological Society*, vol. 106, pp. 138–145, 2008.

[14] R. Kholdebarin, R. J. Campbell, Y. P. Jin, and Y. M. Buys, "Multicenter study of compliance and drop administration in glaucoma," *Canadian Journal of Ophthalmology*, vol. 43, pp. 454–461, 2008.

[15] B. Sleath, A. L. Robin, D. Covert, J. E. Byrd, G. Tudor, and B. Svarstad, "Patient reported behavior and problems in using glaucoma medications," *Ophthalmology*, vol. 113, pp. 431–436, 2006.

[16] J. L. Stone JL, A. L. Robin, G. D. Novack, D. W. Covert, and G. D. Cagle, "An objective evaluation of eyedrop instillation in patients with glaucoma," *Archives of Ophthalmology*, vol. 127, pp. 732–736, 2009.

[17] J. Lacey, H. Cate, and D. C. Broadway, "Barriers to adherence with glaucoma medications: a qualitative research study," *Eye*, vol. 23, pp. 924–932, 2009.

[18] R. Gupta, B. Patil, B. M. Shah, S. J. Bali, S. K. Mishra, and T. Dada, "Evaluating eye drop instillation technique in glaucoma patients," *Journal of Glaucoma*, vol. 21, pp. 189–192, 2012.

[19] B. Sleath, S. Blalock, D. Covert et al., "The relationship between glaucoma medication adherence, eye drop technique, and visual field defect severity," *Ophthalmology*, vol. 118, pp. 2398–2402, 2011.

[20] S. Popović-Suić, J. Sikić, N. Vukojević, B. Cerovski, M. Nasić, and R. Pokupec, "Target intraocular pressure in the management of glaucoma," *Collegium Antropologicum*, vol. 29, Supplement 1, pp. 149–151, 2005.

[21] W. W. Daniel and L. C. Cross, *Biostatistics: A Foundation for Analysis in the Health Sciences*, John Wiley and Sons Inc., Hoboken, NJ, USA, 8th edition, 2005.

[22] D. E. Morisky, A. Ang, M. Krousel-Wood, and H. J. Ward, "Predictive validity of a medication adherence measure in an outpatient setting," *Journal of Clinical Hypertension*, vol. 10, pp. 384–354, 2008.

[23] D. E. Morisky, A. Ang, M. Krousel-Wood, and H. Ward, "Predictive validity of a medication adherence measure for hypertension control," *Journal of Clinical Hypertension*, vol. 10, pp. 348–354, 2008.

[24] M. A. Krousel-Wood, T. Islam, L. S. Webber, R. S. Re, D. E. Morisky, and P. Muntner, "New medication adherence scale versus pharmacy fill rates in seniors with hypertension," *The American Journal of Managed Care*, vol. 15, pp. 59–66, 2009.

[25] D. E. Morisky and M. R. DiMatteo, "Improving the measurement of self-reported medication nonadherence: final response," *Journal of Clinical Epidemiology*, vol. 64, pp. 262-263, 2011.

[26] M. Shaw, "How to administer eye drops and ointments,"

[27] T. Mehari, A. T. Giorgis, and W. Shibeshi, "Level of adherence to ocular hypotensive agents and its determinant factors among glaucoma patients in Menelik II Referral Hospital, Ethiopia," *BMC Opthalmology*, vol. 16, p. 131, 2016.

[28] T. Mehari, A. T. Giorgis, and W. Shibeshi, "Appropriateness and determinants of proper administration technique of ocular hypotensive agents among glaucoma patients in Menelik II Referral Hospital, Ethiopia," *Journal of Clinical Experimental Ophthalmology*, vol. 7, p. 554, 2016.

[29] C. August, "Visual standards: aspects and ranges of vision loss," in *Proceedings of the International Council of Ophthalmology*, 2002.

[30] S. A. Taylor, S. M. Galbraith, and R. P. Mills, "Causes of non-compliance with drug regimens in glaucoma patients: a qualitative study," *Journal of Ocular Pharmacology and Therapeutics*, vol. 18, pp. 401–409, 2002.

[31] J. Tatham, U. Sarodia, F. Gatrad, and A. Awan, "Eye drop instillation technique in patients with glaucoma," *Eye*, vol. 27, pp. 1293–1298, 2013.

Nursing Times, vol. 110, pp. 16–18, 2014.

7

Eye-Tracking as a Tool to Evaluate Functional Ability in Everyday Tasks in Glaucoma

Enkelejda Kasneci,[1] Alex A. Black,[2] and Joanne M. Wood[2]

[1]*Department of Computer Science, University of Tübingen, Sand 14, 72076 Tübingen, Germany*
[2]*School of Optometry and Vision Science, Institute of Health and Biomedical Innovation, Queensland University of Technology, Brisbane, QLD, Australia*

Correspondence should be addressed to Enkelejda Kasneci; enkelejda.kasneci@uni-tuebingen.de

Academic Editor: Antonio M. Fea

To date, few studies have investigated the eye movement patterns of individuals with glaucoma while they undertake everyday tasks in real-world settings. While some of these studies have reported possible compensatory gaze patterns in those with glaucoma who demonstrated good task performance despite their visual field loss, little is known about the complex interaction between field loss and visual scanning strategies and the impact on task performance and, consequently, on quality of life. We review existing approaches that have quantified the effect of glaucomatous visual field defects on the ability to undertake everyday activities through the use of eye movement analysis. Furthermore, we discuss current developments in eye-tracking technology and the potential for combining eye-tracking with virtual reality and advanced analytical approaches. Recent technological developments suggest that systems based on eye-tracking have the potential to assist individuals with glaucomatous loss to maintain or even improve their performance on everyday tasks and hence enhance their long-term quality of life. We discuss novel approaches for studying the visual search behavior of individuals with glaucoma that have the potential to assist individuals with glaucoma, through the use of personalized programs that take into consideration the individual characteristics of their remaining visual field and visual search behavior.

1. Introduction

Glaucoma is one of the main causes of visual field loss in older populations [1], affecting approximately 60 million people worldwide, with the numbers estimated to increase significantly in the future as the population ages [2, 3]. For this reason, the impact of glaucoma on everyday activities such as reading, walking, shopping, or driving, and quality of life has been the focus of numerous research studies [4–12]. Nevertheless, the relationship between functional measures and patients' visual disability in everyday life is still not well understood and requires further research [13].

Many studies have assessed the impact of glaucomatous vision loss on everyday activities through questionnaires or patient-reported outcome measures [8, 9, 14–19], simulators [20–22], or under laboratory conditions [23–26], and some

have incorporated measures of visual search behavior. Results from these studies suggest that visual search behavior plays a key role in the ability of individuals with glaucoma to complete everyday activities. More specifically, several studies have reported that some individuals with glaucoma process visual information differently than controls during everyday tasks. For example, Wiecek et al. [27] reported that patients with glaucomatous visual field loss tend to ignore the region of the computer-based image where their scotoma is located, rather than making more eye movements to compensate for their loss. Conversely, another study demonstrated that when viewing dynamic movies of road traffic scenes, glaucoma patients made more fixations and saccades than controls [23]. In a recent study, Crabb et al. [28] showed that visual scanpaths, derived from a passive watching task, can be used to differentiate between individuals with glaucomatous visual field loss and those with no visual field loss. In less dynamic tasks, glaucomatous visual field loss was associated with restricted eye movements; that is, patients performed fewer saccades than controls and viewed different locations of static naturalistic scenes than controls [25, 29]. However, the most valid approach to assessing the functional impairment of patients with glaucoma in everyday activities is by conducting real-world experiments (i.e., observing the person undertaking a particular activity in a field-based environment). However, since such experiments are expensive, time-consuming, and often difficult to standardize, to date few everyday activities have been investigated. Indeed, most of the work on everyday activities has focused on assessing the driving ability and safety of individuals with glaucoma [5–7, 10, 16, 21, 30–32].

Importantly, while the methodological approaches of these studies have varied, they have reached similar conclusions: (1) task performance varies among individuals, (2) glaucomatous field loss does not always lead to poorer performance, and (3) visual field defects related to glaucoma can be compensated for in some individuals through effective head and eye movement strategies. Furthermore, it has been suggested that the results of different studies may relate specifically to that set of circumstances and not reflect individuals' visual behavior in other everyday activities, given that compensatory gaze patterns are highly specific and intrinsically related to the specific task [33]. Furthermore, there appears to be a wide degree of variability in patients' compensatory strategies that are adopted during activities of daily living.

One approach to evaluate the real-world impact of glaucomatous loss and potential compensatory strategies is through assessment of visual search and scanning during daily activities. Assessment of visual search in this way also enables better understanding of the link between visual function and ability, as well as providing a basis for designing training strategies for improvement of daily functioning, and the development of assessment tools for use in a clinical setting.

Eye movements are important in directing gaze and attention towards important task-relevant areas within the visual scene, in order to guide subsequent actions when completing everyday activities [34]. Gaze position identifies where foveal vision is directed towards, known as overt attention. At the same time, attention can also be directed towards peripheral areas of the visual field without reorientating gaze, known as covert attention [35]; when something important is identified in peripheral vision, overt attention can be shifted via a corresponding eye movement. While eye-tracking analysis provides information specifically regarding overt attention, it is also the key technology that helps us in the understanding of visual search and scanning behaviors during daily activities. Importantly, patients with glaucoma may have impaired covert attention capacity, relative to the extent of their visual field loss. Indeed, the ability to simultaneously extract central and peripheral visual information within a single glance, as measured with attentional or useful field of view tests, has been shown to be reduced among older adults with glaucoma, compared to normally sighted controls [36, 37].

Incorporating eye movement analysis in settings that reflect everyday activities is becoming an increasingly popular approach, given that several studies have reported that the ability of patients with glaucoma to perform these activities of daily living is only weakly associated with the extent of their visual field defects, but may be mediated through the complex interaction between field loss and visual scanning strategies. The study of eye movements in glaucoma, particularly in comparison to participants with normal visual fields, is also becoming more common, with advances in eye-tracking technology and analytical approaches making it a more practical approach, particularly for assessing task performance while individuals complete everyday tasks in natural environments.

In this paper, we review existing methods that quantify the effect of glaucomatous visual field defects on the ability to undertake everyday activities through the use of eye movement analysis. Although there is a large body of work investigating eye movements in those with glaucoma, the focus of this narrative review is on studies that have employed eye-tracking while participants complete everyday tasks such as reading, mobility and walking, and driving. We also discuss studies that explored the gaze patterns of individuals with glaucoma while shopping [38], during a face recognition task [26], and making a sandwich [39]. Published studies in peer-reviewed journals were identified through searches using Google Scholar and searches of MEDLINE, PubMed, and Cochrane databases using the following combinations of keywords and phrases: "glaucoma", "visual field loss", "eye-tracking", "eye movements", "visual search", "scanpath", "everyday tasks", "driving", "mobility", "walking", "stepping", and "shopping". Studies of other eye conditions causing visual field loss were also considered, where appropriate, to inform future research directions. Relevant studies from these searches were sourced and reviewed and are discussed as appropriate; only studies that were published in English were included.

2. Eye-Tracking Technology

The use of eye-tracking as a tool to assess and analyze visual search strategies under real-world conditions is growing, given improvements in eye-tracking technology which make it increasingly applicable to the study of both simple and complex scenarios. Video-based eye-tracking is available as head-mounted and remote technology. Recent developments in head-mounted, mobile eye-tracking technology (e.g., Dikablis Mobile eye-tracker, Pupil Labs eye-tracker, SMI Glasses, and Tobii Glasses) have enabled the study of visual perception and visual behavior in natural environments. Some of these eye-trackers, such as the Dikablis Mobile system, can be worn with spectacles, thus interfering only minimally with the participant's natural viewing behavior. On the other hand, observation and monitoring of scanning behavior can benefit from the use of non-intrusive systems, where cameras are positioned remotely at some distance from the participant.

While eye-tracking can be accomplished successfully under laboratory conditions, many studies report difficulties

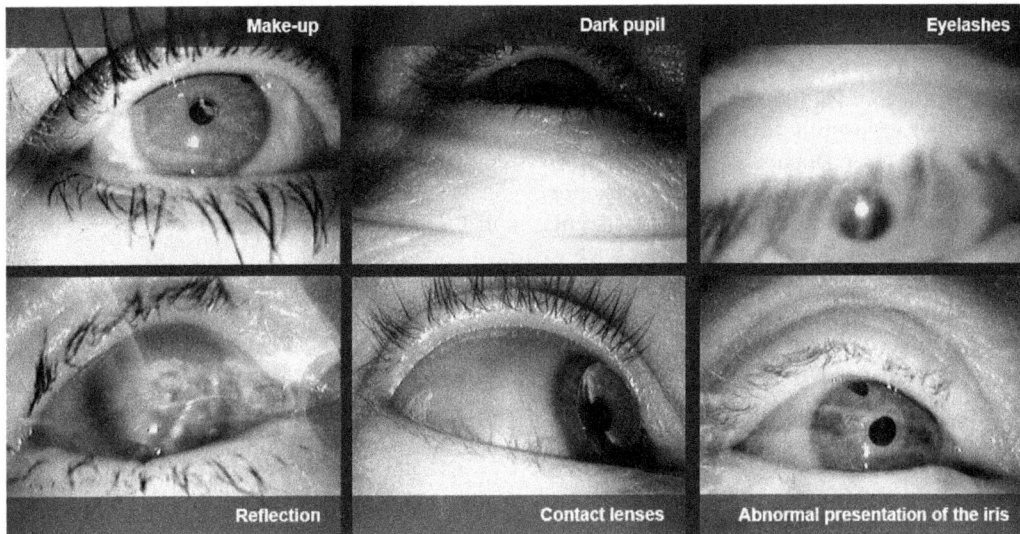

FIGURE 1: Eye images recorded by mobile, head-mounted eye-trackers in outdoor experiments.

when video-based eye-trackers are employed in natural environments, such as driving [21, 30, 40], shopping [38, 41], or simply walking [42]. The main source of error in such settings is a non-robust pupil signal which primarily arises from challenges in the image-based detection of the pupil. More specifically, a variety of difficulties may occur when using eye-trackers, such as changing illumination (especially problematic when walking outside during the daytime), motion blur, recording errors, and eyelashes covering the pupil (Figure 1). Rapidly changing illumination conditions arise primarily in tasks where the participant is moving rapidly (e.g., while driving), or where the participant rotates relative to unequally distributed light sources. Particularly for older populations, it is important to test the tracking quality of the eye-tracker with the participant's spectacles. Often the tracking rate (i.e., the percentage of video frames where pupil information can be extracted, and consequently, the gaze position can be calculated) and accuracy are significantly degraded when strong illumination and reflections on the spectacle lenses are present. A further issue arises due to the off-axis position of the eye camera in head-mounted eye-trackers. Therefore, studies based on eye-tracking in uncontrolled environments frequently report low pupil detection rates. As a consequence, the data collected in such studies has to be manually post-processed, which is laborious and time-consuming.

Recently, several algorithms have been introduced to tackle these challenges and report very high pupil detection rates in both head-mounted [43–45] and remote eye-tracking [46] technology. Among the state-of-the art algorithms for head-mounted and remote eye-tracking, ExCuSe [43] and ElSe [44], two decision-based approaches based on edge detection and ellipse fitting, show very high accuracy combined with real-time processing capability. When eye-trackers with low sampling rates up to 60 Hz are incorporated, the PupilNet algorithm based on advanced machine learning techniques (i.e., Convolutional Neural Networks),

achieves even higher robustness with regard to the above-mentioned sources of noise [47]. The tracking rate is an important parameter and is reported as the proportion of frames where the pupil is detected. It can easily be computed and is usually also reported by the manufacturer's software. The second important parameter is the calibration accuracy, that is, how exactly the position of the participant's gaze is projected into world coordinates (or pixel coordinates in a video for head-mounted devices). Contrary to the tracking rate, a dedicated calibration measurement during the experiment has to be performed, for example, by instructing the participant to fixate on specific markers. As calibration quality is likely to decrease over the duration of the experiment, it is important to assess accuracy before and after the experiment.

Given a reliable eye-tracking signal, several processing steps have to be applied on top of the raw data stream to derive information about visual search behavior. As mentioned in the introductory section, several studies have collected eye movement data on glaucoma patients while they complete everyday tasks, in order to identify their exploratory search patterns. The data recorded in these studies has been mainly analyzed manually and post-experimentally. Basic fixation filters are then applied to extract fixation locations and saccades.

Eye-tracking technology, however, has huge potential beyond that of simply measuring eye movements. Online analysis of eye-tracking data could help to design gaze-based interactive and assistive systems for patients with impaired vision, such as in glaucoma. A crucial prerequisite towards the development of such interactive systems is a robust data analysis pipeline. The first processing step in this pipeline addresses the automated detection of the eye movement type (i.e., fixation, saccade, or smooth pursuit), to extract the spatiotemporal sequence of eye movements (also known as the visual scanpath). Other movements, such as smooth pursuits, microsaccades, ocular drifts, and microtremor, are usually ignored, since it is difficult to extract them from the eye-tracking signal, especially when recorded at low sampling rates (below 120 Hz). For some tasks, information on gaze density in specific areas of interest is sufficient. Such information can be derived from heatmap visualization, as provided by most eye-tracking data analysis software. More sophisticated methods require the examination of a fixation sequence in combination with information from the scene. Several algorithms are available for event detection, such as [54–56], and have been applied in some studies with glaucoma patients. For example, Sippel et al. [38] used advanced data analysis to identify characteristic visual exploration patterns of glaucoma patients during a shopping task. In Kübler et al. [21], such methods were used to investigate eye movement patterns in patients with glaucoma while driving.

To date, most eye movement analytical approaches are based on time-integrated measures, such as the average fixation duration, or the number of fixations directed towards a specific region of interest. Several studies have described such exploratory eye movement patterns in glaucoma patients during everyday tasks. But extracting these at the scanpath level (i.e., the sequence of fixations and saccades) from the large amount of data generated is highly challenging. A manual analysis is very laborious and only applicable to experiments of short duration involving static stimuli (e.g., such as in reading). Dynamic activities such as walking or driving, where the scene is changing with the ego perspective, require automated methods to compare eye-tracking data of different participants (or even more demanding, that of different participant groups), in order to identify common patterns of eye movements, as well as those that differentiate between participant groups. Only a few approaches, such as those based on string similarity [57] which compare scanpaths as a whole, or in segments as described by Kübler et al. [51, 58], can be applied to the analysis of eye-tracking data derived while completing interactive tasks. Such methods are only rudimentarily implemented in most analysis software, yet determining gaze patterns that distinguish between two experimental groups can be highly valuable.

A major issue that needs to be considered prior to undertaking eye-tracking experiments, is the reference coordinate system that the eye-tracker works within. Head-mounted devices record the gaze position relative to the head position (scene video image), which can be challenging to analyze automatically. If the participants move their head, the position of the objects in the video image also changes. Placing easily traceable markers for further image analysis close to relevant objects can speed up data analysis significantly. Remote trackers more commonly provide a gaze vector in a world reference system. Therefore, the exact position of relevant objects with regard to the eye-tracker is helpful to automatically determine whether a certain object was looked at. A relevant issue for recording naturalistic viewing behavior is that the areas over which head movements can be recorded are limited. For tasks that require a large freedom of head movement and rotation, it is possible to combine multiple remote cameras or a head-mounted device and a head tracker. Some eye-trackers also measure head position and orientation within a limited area; for example,

the EyeLink tracker can detect a marker placed on the participant's forehead, while Smart Eye fits a head model to multiple camera perspectives.

Recently, eye-tracking has been integrated into virtual reality devices. These have enormous potential to study eye movements in glaucoma, through the provision of ecologically valid measures to individually assess viewing behavior in a well-circumscribed environment.

3. Eye Movements and Glaucoma in Everyday Tasks

Table 1 provides a summary of eye-tracking studies that have investigated eye movements of individuals with glaucoma, or other relevant conditions causing visual field loss, while undertaking a range of everyday tasks. The main findings from these studies will be discussed in more detail in the following subsections.

3.1. Insights from Reading Experiments. Reading is an everyday task that requires good central vision. Although glaucoma is mainly associated with impaired peripheral vision, many patients also experience paracentral and central visual field loss and difficulties with reading are commonly reported [8, 9, 11, 59, 60]. In support of these self-reported reading difficulties, studies that have measured reading performance in individuals with glaucoma report reduced reading speeds compared to those with normal vision for small size text [61], at low contrast levels [48], or when reading for sustained periods of time [9]. Those individuals with central glaucomatous field loss [62], or who have advanced field loss [9, 63], are also particularly impaired in terms of reading ability. Importantly, as outlined by Crabb [13] in his viewpoint on glaucoma, the reading capacity of those with glaucomatous field loss varies considerably between individuals; studies of eye movements and reading by his research group suggest that differences in eye movement patterns in those with glaucomatous loss may account for some of this variability [48, 49].

Smith et al. [49] reported that reading performance was significantly worse in the eye with more glaucomatous field loss compared to the better eye in a given individual, but that this was not related to the extent of field loss, but rather to measures of contrast sensitivity and visual acuity. Furthermore, those individuals, whose reading speeds were particularly affected in their worse eye, made a larger proportion of backward saccades and "unknown" eye movements (not adhering to expected reading patterns) when reading with this eye in comparison to the better eye [49]. A study by the same research group [50] demonstrated that some of the variability in reading speed in those with advanced glaucomatous loss could be explained by eye movement patterns. A significant association was found between increased saccadic frequency in those with higher reading speeds (for short passages of text) in individuals with glaucoma, which suggested the adoption of compensatory mechanisms to improve task performance. In addition, those who read more slowly tended to read every word in a line (termed text saturation) compared to those with higher reading speeds

TABLE 1: Summary of eye-tracking studies referenced in this work with regard to their participants and eye-tracking devices.

Study	Cohort demographics	Eye-tracker (fps)	Main findings
Burton et al. [48]	53 bilateral glaucoma (mean age 66 ± 9); 40 controls (mean age 69 ± 8)	EyeLink 1000 (1000)	Reduction in reading speed for lower contrast text was greater in glaucoma patients than controls.
Smith et al. [49]	14 bilateral glaucoma (median age 69, IQR 64 to 81)	EyeLink 1000 (1000)	Slower performance and more regression when reading with the worse eye, compared to better eye. Differences in performance not related to magnitude of difference in VF mean deviation index between eyes.
Burton et al. [50]	18 advanced bilateral glaucoma (mean age 71 ± 7); 39 controls (mean age 67 ± 8)	EyeLink 1000 (500)	Similar reading speeds between groups. Some glaucoma patients read slower than controls, partly explained by differences in eye movement behavior.
Prado Vega et al. [20]	23 glaucoma (mean age 65 ± 12); 12 controls (mean age 65.7 ± 9.4)	Smart Eye (60)	Glaucoma patients missed more peripherally projected stimuli during driving in a simulator than controls. Glaucoma patients did not use compensatory visual search patterns.
Kübler et al. [21]	6 binocular glaucoma (mean age 62 ± 7); 8 controls (mean age 602 ± 10)	Dikablis (25)	Glaucoma patients who passed the driving test in the simulator showed increased number of head and gaze movements toward eccentric regions of the VF in comparison to patients who failed.
Crabb et al. [23]	9 binocular glaucoma (mean age 67.6 ± 9.3); 10 controls (mean age 64.4 ± 11.4)	EyeLink (250)	Patients showed different eye movement characteristics (more saccades) than controls when viewing driving scenes in a hazard perception test.
Kasneci et al. [30]	10 binocular glaucoma (mean age 61 ± 9); 10 controls (mean age 60 ± 9)	Dikablis (25)	Patients who passed the on-road driving test focused longer on the central VF and performed more glances towards the area of their VF defect than patients who failed.
Kübler et al. [51]	10 binocular glaucoma (mean age 61 ± 9); 10 controls (mean age 60 ± 9)	Dikablis (25)	Patients can be identified based on their visual scanpath while driving above chance levels.
Sippel et al. [38]	10 binocular glaucoma (mean age 61 ± 9); 10 controls (mean age 60 ± 9)	Dikablis (25)	Patients who showed good performance during supermarket shopping made more glances towards the VF defect area.
Vargas-Martín and Peli [52]	5 retinitis pigmentosa (mean age 58 ± 16); 3 controls (mean age 67 ± 5)	ISCAN (60)	Retinitis pigmentosa patients exhibited narrower scanning strategy than controls.
Ivanov et al. [53]	25 retinitis pigmentosa (mean age 54 ± 13)	Tobii Glasses (30)	An exploratory saccadic training improved search performance, as well as mobility performance.
Dive et al. [39]	12 bilateral glaucoma (mean age 64 ± 15); 13 controls (mean age 73 ± 9)	iViewX^{TM} (50)	Glaucoma patients took longer to complete the task, with longer fixations and more eye and head movements, than controls.
Smith et al. [24]	20 bilateral glaucoma (mean age 67 ± 10); 20 controls (mean age 67 ± 11)	EyeLink II (500)	Glaucoma patients took longer to find targets in photographs.
Crabb et al. [28]	44 glaucoma (median age 69, IQR 63–77); 32 controls (median age 70, IQR 64–75)	EyeLink 1000 (1000)	Differences in signature scanpath patterns when watching television could separate glaucoma from controls.

and controls; these effects were exacerbated during longer periods of sustained reading.

In summary, the incorporation of eye-tracking provides a useful experimental approach for exploring differences in reading performance in those with glaucoma and better understanding of the mechanisms underlying these reading difficulties.

3.2. Glaucoma, Mobility, and Walking. Peripheral vision is important for spatial orientation, balance control, and efficient navigation when walking, particularly guiding obstacle avoidance, locomotion planning, and foot placement. Adults with glaucomatous visual field loss have been shown to demonstrate altered balance control when standing [64, 65], along with impaired mobility performance when walking, including slower walking speeds and increased contacts with obstacles, especially in those with bilateral visual field loss [4, 12]. Impaired balance and mobility performance in those with glaucoma is likely to negatively impact on the health and well-being of older adults. For example, greater glaucomatous visual field loss has been linked to reductions in physical activity levels [66], greater levels of fear of falling [67], and increased risk of falls and injuries [5, 68].

Studies have also explored whether specific areas of the visual field are more important for mobility and falls in adults with glaucoma. Murata et al. [69] reported significant associations between central and inferior hemifield regions and self-reported walking difficulties. Other studies also highlight the importance of the inferior visual field region for postural stability [64] and falls risk [68] in glaucoma. These associations are likely to reflect natural human gaze behavior when walking. In uncluttered environments, such as an unobstructed level footpath, gaze is generally directed several steps ahead in the direction of travel to guide route planning and to scan for potential hazards [70, 71]; therefore the inferior visual field area is used to provide important information guiding foot placement and detection of hazards. In more challenging or cluttered environments, where precise foot placement is important for safety, gaze tends to shift towards the stepping locations to optimize stepping accuracy [72].

While inefficient visual scanning of the environment is likely to be an important factor linking visual field loss and impaired mobility and falls in adults with glaucoma, there have been few studies that have assessed the link between eye movements and gaze behavior while walking in individuals with glaucoma. Eye-tracking studies have been undertaken in other ocular conditions with peripheral visual field loss, such as retinitis pigmentosa (RP). Patients with RP have been shown to exhibit narrower horizontal scanning patterns when walking in real environments compared to healthy controls [52], potentially due to the absence of peripheral visual stimulation to trigger eye movements and attention towards these areas. Indeed, recent research using saccadic training has shown promise in improving mobility for RP patients, by consciously directing eye movements and attention outside of the seeing region of the visual field [53]. Further research using robust eye-tracking technology and advanced data analysis, with respect to the dynamic nature of walking, is needed to better understand the eye movement patterns of adults with glaucomatous visual field loss, and explore potential saccadic training paradigms to improve their mobility and quality of life.

3.3. Glaucoma and Driving. A large body of work has been conducted over the last two decades to investigate the impact of glaucoma on driving, which has drawn a range of conclusions regarding the impact of glaucoma on driving ability and safety, as summarized in a recent review [73]. Glaucoma has been shown to be an important risk factor for self-reported crashes over the previous 10 years [74–76] and state-recorded crashes [5, 77–80]; however, the underlying reasons for this increased crash risk are unclear. Simulator-based assessments have revealed equivocal results, with some

studies reporting increased simulator crashes [81], while others reveal only small differences in performance between those with glaucoma and age-matched controls [20, 21]. On-road performance is also impaired in some drivers with glaucoma compared to those without glaucoma [6, 30–32], with drivers with glaucoma demonstrating difficulties in observation, maintaining their lane position, changing lanes, and planning ahead [31]. Interestingly, while some studies report links between the extent of field loss and driving ability and safety [77, 80, 81], others have failed to find a link [21, 30, 82]. Importantly, few studies have investigated the eye movement patterns of individuals with glaucoma while undertaking driving tasks, which might provide insight into the link between visual field loss and driving ability. Indeed, specific eye movement patterns might act as a compensatory mechanism for the loss of visual function and ultimately provide the basis for effective visual rehabilitation and coping strategies.

In the few on-road studies that have involved eye movements, those glaucoma patients who were rated as safe to drive showed increased exploration activity, in terms of more eccentric head movements, compared to those drivers with glaucoma who were rated as unsafe to drive [21, 30, 83]. Indeed, in a recent study conducted in a driving simulator, driving behavior and gaze patterns of a small group of participants with bilateral glaucoma were investigated by employing recently developed mobile eye- and head-tracking technology [21]. Results from this study demonstrated that those drivers scored as unsafe displayed less eye movements (shorter saccade amplitudes, longer fixation durations, and less fixations), a gaze bias to the right, and a more straight-ahead eye position [21]. The effect of head movements has been shown to be most important in realistic experimental setups and in those driving simulations with a wide field of view which were more representative of the driving scene. Simple driving simulations with a narrow field of view and relatively simple tasks are unlikely to reflect naturalistic viewing behaviors. Differences in eye movement patterns have also been reported in those with glaucoma compared to controls when completing video-based hazard perception tasks [23]. A reduction in saccade rates and smaller number of fixations indicates decreased eye scanning activity, and longer fixation durations appear to be associated with an inability to acquire visual information in a quick and effective manner, as observed in patients who passed the driving assessment in the study by Kübler et al. [21]. Because new information is acquired during fixations, the finding that patients who failed the driving test made fewer saccades suggests that they were unable to process as much of the visual scene as those patients who passed the test. The finding that unsafe glaucoma drivers showed a gaze bias to the right [21] is also in line with Prado Vega et al. [20], who attributed this finding to the optimal control theory of manned-vehicle systems. A possible explanation is that safe glaucoma drivers pay more attention to avoiding traffic hazards (by gaze scanning), whereas unsafe glaucoma drivers attempt to maintain a stable lane position but fail to recognize traffic hazards because of limited gaze compensatory reserves.

3.4. Other Everyday Tasks. Very few studies have investigated the link between task performance and eye movements in other everyday tasks.

Glen et al. [26] studied the performance of individuals with advanced glaucoma in a face recognition task and demonstrated that some patients showed good task performance despite their visual field defects. More specifically, the authors found that in patients with bilateral visual defects in the central 10° of their visual field, larger saccades led to better face recognition performance [26]. In contrast, the authors found no significant association between saccade amplitude and task performance in people with normal vision. These findings are in line with several studies described previously, which report that some individuals with glaucomatous visual field loss adopt compensatory eye movements during visual tasks.

Two recent studies, involving the everyday tasks of shopping and sandwich making, provide further interesting insight into this issue. In a real-world shopping task, Sippel et al. [38] compared the functional ability and eye movements of 10 patients with bilateral glaucomatous field loss in comparison to 10 normally sighted subjects. Overall, the glaucoma group took longer to complete the task, yet 8 of the glaucoma patients were able to successfully complete the task within a time frame commensurate with the controls, and showed a significantly higher number of glances towards their visual field defect area. Therefore, systematic exploration of the area of visual field defects seems to be a "time-effective" compensatory mechanism during supermarket shopping, which mirrors the results of on-road driving for those with hemianopic field defects [30, 84].

Recently, Dive et al. [39] showed that while patients with glaucoma were slower than controls to complete naturalistic tasks, such as making a sandwich, as well as an unfamiliar task of building a model, they could still complete these tasks efficiently. Assessment of eye movements while doing these tasks revealed that the glaucoma participants made more head and eye movements and had longer fixation durations compared to the controls; the authors suggested that this may have been a strategy to compensate for reduced visibility when key targets fell within their visual field defects.

4. Eye-Tracking as a Means to Assist Individuals with Glaucoma

An interesting research question that arises from the study of eye movements in glaucoma, is whether specific training procedures can assist in the adoption of compensatory gaze patterns in patients with glaucoma that are effective in improving task performance. However, since gaze patterns are task-dependent, it is unclear to what extent eye movement patterns that have been adopted during training on a specific visual search task, can be transferred to real-world tasks, such as driving, walking around, or shopping. For example, Kasneci et al. [30] reported that safe drivers with glaucoma employed a similar viewing strategy in an on-road setting as in a simulated drive [21]. More specifically, the viewing strategy of glaucoma patients who passed the driving tests

concentrated on the central 20° visual field area and was combined with frequent but short gazes towards their field defect area and the peripheral visual field. Furthermore, the authors reported that those glaucoma patients who failed the on-road driving test tended to also fail the simulator drive. These researchers investigated task performance and gaze patterns of the same glaucoma group in comparison to normally sighted subjects during a shopping task. Interestingly, there was very high agreement between "good performers" in the driving task and "good performers" in the shopping task, although the compensation strategy employed during shopping differed from that adopted during driving.

In light of these findings, we propose that new methods need to be developed to assess task performance and train and assist glaucoma patients. This is an area where eye-tracking technology could be extremely beneficial. In particular, the combination of eye-tracking and virtual reality offers the potential for evaluating functional ability in glaucoma in complex, yet standardized tasks that mimic everyday tasks. Particularly, in the driving context, this technology could facilitate the systematic assessment of driving safety and viewing behavior during driving. Furthermore, measurements of the visual field could be used to assess individual viewing behavior with respect to the impaired areas in the visual field in an automated way. In this way, personalized training could be developed, for example, by guiding the gaze of an individual towards specific regions through visual or acoustic stimuli.

Moreover, in the driving context, driving assistance systems could utilize unique information regarding an individual driver's eye movements and visual field defects. The design and implementation of such systems is, however, highly challenging, since the visual search behavior (i.e., the visual scanpath) of the driver has to be analyzed in real-time in alignment with objects presented in the dynamically changing driving scene. Kasneci et al. [85] recently introduced a framework based on several machine learning methods to explore hazard perception based on eye movements, where a reliable alignment of gaze and the scene provides the foundation for detection of potentially overlooked traffic hazards. For those cases where the system predicts that the driver has not seen the upcoming hazard, the driver's gaze could be guided towards the hazard by means of visual or acoustic stimuli. If the driver does not react in time, the system should intervene to avoid the collision. Gaze guidance for drivers with visual impairments is particularly challenging, however, as it has to be performed taking into consideration the specific type and location of visual field loss.

In summary, eye-tracking technology is currently a research tool that provides insights into how glaucoma alters attention and viewing behavior. There is huge potential for further development, especially due to advanced analytics that might enable the detection of visual field defects from eye movement recordings during everyday tasks. In recent work, Crabb et al. [28] showed that it might be possible to detect glaucoma during a simple everyday task, such as watching television. Beyond the diagnosis aspects and knowledge of gaze behavior adaptation, it may be possible to design assistive systems that help individuals with glaucomatous visual field loss to maintain or even improve their performance on everyday tasks, increase their independence, and hence improve their long-term quality of life.

5. Conclusion

Visual search behavior plays a key role in the ability of individuals with glaucoma to complete everyday activities. With the development of more sophisticated eye-tracking technology, assessment of eye movements is transitioning out of the laboratory to encompass activities such as walking, driving, or other real-world tasks and, hence, provides a powerful tool for better understanding the visual search mechanisms of individuals with glaucoma and their implications for everyday tasks. Combined with virtual reality technology, eye-tracking offers the possibility for focused eye movement research under standardized experimental conditions and the development of personalized solutions to assist glaucoma patients.

Competing Interests

The authors declare that there is no conflict of interests regarding the publication of this paper.

Acknowledgments

The authors acknowledge the support from Deutsche Forschungsgemeinschaft and Open Access Publishing Fund of University of Tübingen.

References

[1] R. S. Ramrattan, R. C. W. Wolfs, S. Panda-Jonas et al., "Prevalence and causes of visual field loss in the elderly and associations with impairment in daily functioning: the Rotterdam Study," *Archives of Ophthalmology*, vol. 119, no. 12, pp. 1788–1794, 2001.

[2] H. Quigley and A. T. Broman, "The number of people with glaucoma worldwide in 2010 and 2020," *British Journal of Ophthalmology*, vol. 90, no. 3, pp. 262–267, 2006.

[3] H. A. Quigley, "Glaucoma," *The Lancet*, vol. 377, no. 9774, pp. 1367–1377, 2011.

[4] D. S. Friedman, E. Freeman, B. Munoz, H. D. Jampel, and S. K. West, "Glaucoma and mobility performance: the Salisbury Eye Evaluation Project," *Ophthalmology*, vol. 114, no. 12, pp. 2232–2237.e1, 2007.

[5] S. A. Haymes, R. P. LeBlanc, M. T. Nicolela, L. A. Chiasson, and B. C. Chauhan, "Risk of falls and motor vehicle collisions in glaucoma," *Investigative Ophthalmology & Visual Science*, vol. 48, no. 3, pp. 1149–1155, 2007.

[6] S. A. Haymes, R. P. LeBlanc, M. T. Nicolela, L. A. Chiasson, and B. C. Chauhan, "Glaucoma and on-road driving performance," *Investigative Ophthalmology & Visual Science*, vol. 49, no. 7, pp. 3035–3041, 2008.

[7] C. A. Johnson and J. L. Keltner, "Incidence of visual field loss in 20,000 eyes and its relationship to driving performance," *Archives of Ophthalmology*, vol. 101, no. 3, pp. 371–375, 1983.

[8] P. Nelson, P. Aspinall, and C. O'Brien, "Patients' perception of visual impairment in glaucoma: a pilot study," *British Journal of Ophthalmology*, vol. 83, no. 5, pp. 546–552, 1999.

[9] P. Ramulu, "Glaucoma and disability: which tasks are affected, and at what stage of disease?" *Current Opinion in Ophthalmology*, vol. 20, no. 2, pp. 92–98, 2009.

[10] J. P. Szlyk, C. L. Mahler, W. Seiple, D. P. Edward, and J. T. Wilensky, "Driving performance of glaucoma patients correlates with peripheral visual field loss," *Journal of Glaucoma*, vol. 14, no. 2, pp. 145–150, 2005.

[11] A. C. Viswanathan, A. I. McNaught, D. Poinoosawmy et al., "Severity and stability of glaucoma: patient perception compared with objective measurement," *Archives of Ophthalmology*, vol. 117, no. 4, pp. 450–454, 1999.

[12] K. A. Turano, G. S. Rubin, and H. A. Quigley, "Mobility performance in glaucoma," *Investigative Ophthalmology & Visual Science*, vol. 40, no. 12, pp. 2803–2809, 1999.

[13] D. P. Crabb, "A view on glaucoma—are we seeing it clearly?" *Eye*, vol. 30, no. 2, pp. 304–313, 2016.

[14] A. Béchetoille, B. Arnould, A. Bron et al., "Measurement of health-related quality of life with glaucoma: validation of the Glau-QoL© 36-item questionnaire," *Acta Ophthalmologica*, vol. 86, no. 1, pp. 71–80, 2008.

[15] H. D. Jampel, D. S. Friedman, H. Quigley, and R. Miller, "Correlation of the binocular visual field with patient assessment of vision," *Investigative Ophthalmology and Visual Science*, vol. 43, no. 4, pp. 1059–1067, 2002.

[16] G. McGwin Jr., A. Mays, W. Joiner, D. K. DeCarlo, S. McNeal, and C. Owsley, "Is glaucoma associated with motor vehicle collision involvement and driving avoidance?" *Investigative Ophthalmology & Visual Science*, vol. 45, no. 11, pp. 3934–3939, 2004.

[17] G. Noe, J. Ferraro, E. Lamoureux, J. Rait, and J. E. Keeffe, "Associations between glaucomatous visual field loss and participation in activities of daily living," *Clinical and Experimental Ophthalmology*, vol. 31, no. 6, pp. 482–486, 2003.

[18] G. Spaeth, J. Walt, and J. Keener, "Evaluation of quality of life for patients with glaucoma," *American Journal of Ophthalmology*, vol. 141, no. 1, pp. 3–14, 2006.

[19] K. J. Warrian, G. L. Spaeth, D. Lankaranian, J. F. Lopes, and W. C. Steinmann, "The effect of personality on measures of quality of life related to vision in glaucoma patients," *British Journal of Ophthalmology*, vol. 93, no. 3, pp. 310–315, 2009.

[20] R. Prado Vega, P. M. van Leeuwen, E. Rendón Vélez, H. G. Lemij, and J. C. F. de Winter, "Obstacle avoidance, visual detection performance, and eye-scanning behavior of glaucoma patients in a driving simulator: A Preliminary Study," *PLoS ONE*, vol. 8, no. 10, Article ID e77294, 2013.

[21] T. C. Kübler, E. Kasneci, W. Rosenstiel et al., "Driving with glaucoma: task performance and gaze movements," *Optometry & Vision Science*, vol. 92, no. 11, pp. 1037–1046, 2015.

[22] T. C. Kübler, E. Kasneci, W. Rosenstiel, U. Schiefer, K. Nagel, and E. Papageorgiou, "Stress-indicators and exploratory gaze for the analysis of hazard perception in patients with visual field loss," *Transportation Research Part F: Traffic Psychology and Behaviour*, vol. 24, pp. 231–243, 2014.

[23] D. P. Crabb, N. D. Smith, F. G. Rauscher et al., "Exploring eye movements in patients with glaucoma when viewing a driving scene," *PLoS ONE*, vol. 5, no. 3, Article ID e9710, 2010.

[24] N. D. Smith, D. P. Crabb, and D. F. Garway-Heath, "An exploratory study of visual search performance in glaucoma,"

Ophthalmic & Physiological Optics, vol. 31, no. 3, pp. 225–232, 2011.

[25] N. D. Smith, D. P. Crabb, F. C. Glen, R. Burton, and D. F. Garway-Heath, "Eye movements in patients with glaucoma when viewing images of everyday scenes," *Seeing & Perceiving*, vol. 25, no. 5, pp. 471–492, 2012.

[26] F. C. Glen, N. D. Smith, and D. P. Crabb, "Saccadic eye movements and face recognition performance in patients with central glaucomatous visual field defects," *Vision Research*, vol. 82, pp. 42–51, 2013.

[27] E. Wiecek, L. R. Pasquale, J. Fiser, S. Dakin, and P. J. Bex, "Effects of peripheral visual field loss on eye movements during visual search," *Frontiers in Psychology*, vol. 3, article 472, 2012.

[28] D. P. Crabb, N. D. Smith, and H. Zhu, "What's on TV? Detecting age-related neurodegenerative eye disease using eye movement scanpaths," *Frontiers in Aging Neuroscience*, vol. 6, article 312, 2014.

[29] N. D. Smith, F. C. Glen, and D. P. Crabb, "Eye movements during visual search in patients with glaucoma," *BMC Ophthalmology*, vol. 12, no. 1, article no. 45, 2012.

[30] E. Kasneci, K. Sippel, K. Aehling et al., "Driving with binocular visual field loss? A study on a supervised on-road parcours with simultaneous eye and head tracking," *PLoS ONE*, vol. 9, no. 2, Article ID e87470, 2014.

[31] J. M. Wood, A. A. Black, K. Mallon, R. Thomas, and C. Owsley, "Glaucoma and driving: on-road driving characteristics," *PLoS ONE*, vol. 11, no. 7, Article ID e0158318, 2016.

[32] A. Bowers, E. Peli, J. Elgin, G. McGwin Jr., and C. Owsley, "On-road driving with moderate visual field loss," *Optometry & Vision Science*, vol. 82, no. 8, pp. 657–667, 2005.

[33] S. Schuett, R. W. Kentridge, J. Zihl, and C. A. Heywood, "Adaptation of eye-movements to simulated hemianopia in reading and visual exploration: transfer or specificity?" *Neuropsychologia*, vol. 47, no. 7, pp. 1712–1720, 2009.

[34] M. Hayhoe and D. Ballard, "Eye movements in natural behavior," *Trends in Cognitive Sciences*, vol. 9, no. 4, pp. 188–194, 2005.

[35] M. P. Eckstein, "Visual search: a retrospective," *Journal of Vision*, vol. 11, no. 5, article 14, 2011.

[36] S. A. Bentley, R. P. LeBlanc, M. T. Nicolela, and B. C. Chauhan, "Validity, reliability, and repeatability of the useful field of view test in persons with normal vision and patients with glaucoma," *Investigative Ophthalmology & Visual Science*, vol. 53, no. 11, pp. 6763–6769, 2012.

[37] P. N. Rosen, E. R. Boer, C. P. B. Gracitelli et al., "A portable platform for evaluation of visual performance in glaucoma patients," *PLoS ONE*, vol. 10, no. 10, Article ID e0139426, 2015.

[38] K. Sippel, E. Kasneci, K. Aehling et al., "Binocular glaucomatous visual field loss and its impact on visual exploration—a supermarket study," *PLoS ONE*, vol. 9, no. 8, Article ID e106089, 2014.

[39] S. Dive, J. F. Rouland, Q. Lenoble, S. Szaffarczyk, A. M. McKendrick, and M. Boucart, "Impact of peripheral field loss on the execution of natural actions: a study with glaucomatous patients and normally sighted people," *Journal of Glaucoma*, vol. 25, no. 10, pp. e889–e896, 2016.

[40] C. Braunagel, E. Kasneci, W. Stolzmann, and W. Rosenstiel, "Driver-activity recognition in the context of conditionally autonomous driving," in *Proceedings of the 18th IEEE International Conference on Intelligent Transportation Systems (ITSC '15)*, pp. 1652–1657, IEEE, Gran Canaria, Spain, September 2015.

[41] E. Kasneci, K. Sippel, M. Heister et al., "Homonymous visual field loss and its impact on visual exploration: a supermarket

study," *Translational Vision Science & Technology*, vol. 3, no. 6, article no. 2, 2014.

[42] Y. Sugano and A. Bulling, "Self-calibrating head-mounted eye trackers using egocentric visual saliency," in *Proceedings of the 28th Annual ACM Symposium on User Interface Software and Technology (UIST '15)*, pp. 363–372, ACM, Daegu, South Korea, November 2015.

[43] W. Fuhl, T. Kübler, K. Sippel, W. Rosenstiel, and E. Kasneci, "ExCuSe: robust pupil detection in real-world scenarios," *Lecture Notes in Computer Science (including subseries Lecture Notes in Artificial Intelligence and Lecture Notes in Bioinformatics)*, vol. 9256, pp. 39–51, 2015.

[44] W. Fuhl, T. C. Santini, T. Kübler, and E. Kasneci, "ElSe: ellipse selection for robust pupil detection in real-world environments," in *Proceedings of the 9th Biennial ACM Symposium on Eye Tracking Research and Applications (ETRA '16)*, pp. 123–130, Charleston, SC, USA, March 2016.

[45] W. Fuhl, M. Tonsen, A. Bulling, and E. Kasneci, "Pupil detection for head-mounted eye tracking in the wild: an evaluation of the state of the art," *Machine Vision and Applications*, vol. 27, no. 8, pp. 1275–1288, 2016.

[46] W. Fuhl, D. Geisler, T. Santini, W. Rosenstiel, and E. Kasneci, "Evaluation of state-of-the-art pupil detection algorithms on remote eye images," in *Proceedings of the ACM International Joint Conference on Pervasive and Ubiquitous Computing and Proceedings of the ACM International Symposium on Wearable Computers (ACM 1'6)*, pp. 1716–1725, Heidelberg, Germany, September 2016.

[47] W. Fuhl, T. Santini, G. Kasneci, and E. Kasneci, "PupilNet: convolutional neural networks for robust pupil detection," https://arxiv.org/abs/1601.04902.

[48] R. Burton, D. P. Crabb, N. D. Smith, F. C. Glen, and D. F. Garway-Heath, "Glaucoma and reading: exploring the effects of contrast lowering of text," *Optometry & Vision Science*, vol. 89, no. 9, pp. 1282–1287, 2012.

[49] N. D. Smith, F. C. Glen, V. M. Mönter, and D. P. Crabb, "Using eye tracking to assess reading performance in patients with glaucoma: a within-person study," *Journal of Ophthalmology*, vol. 2014, Article ID 120528, 10 pages, 2014.

[50] R. Burton, N. D. Smith, and D. P. Crabb, "Eye movements and reading in glaucoma: observations on patients with advanced visual field loss," *Graefe's Archive for Clinical and Experimental Ophthalmology*, vol. 252, no. 10, pp. 1621–1630, 2014.

[51] T. C. Kübler, C. Rothe, U. Schiefer, W. Rosenstiel, and E. Kasneci, "SubsMatch 2.0: scanpath comparison and classification based on subsequence frequencies," *Behavior Research Methods*, pp. 1–17, 2016.

[52] F. Vargas-Martín and E. Peli, "Eye movements of patients with tunnel vision while walking," *Investigative Ophthalmology & Visual Science*, vol. 47, no. 12, pp. 5295–5302, 2006.

[53] I. V. Ivanov, M. Mackeben, A. Vollmer, P. Martus, N. X. Nguyen, and S. Trauzettel-Klosinski, "Eye movement training and suggested gaze strategies in tunnel vision—a randomized and controlled pilot study," *PLoS ONE*, vol. 11, no. 6, Article ID e0157825, 2016.

[54] E. Kasneci, G. Kasneci, T. C. Kübler, and W. Rosenstiel, "Online recognition of fixations, saccades, and smooth pursuits for automated analysis of traffic hazard perception," in *Artificial Neural Networks*, vol. 4 of *Springer Series in Bio-/Neuroinformatics*, pp. 411–434, Springer International, Cham, Switzerland, 2015.

[55] E. Tafaj, G. Kasneci, W. Rosenstiel, and M. Bogdan, "Bayesian online clustering of eye movement data," in *Proceedings of the*

7th Eye Tracking Research and Applications Symposium (ETRA '12), pp. 285–288, Santa Barbara, Calif, USA, March 2012.

[56] E. Tafaj, T. Kübler, G. Kasneci, W. Rosenstiel, and M. Bogdan, "Online classification of eye tracking data for automated analysis of traffic hazard perception," in *Artificial Neural Networks and Machine Learning ICANN 2013*, vol. 8131, pp. 442–450, Springer, Berlin, Germany, 2013.

[57] D. Noton and L. Stark, "Scanpaths in eye movements during pattern perception," *Science*, vol. 171, no. 3968, pp. 308–311, 1971.

[58] T. C. Kübler, E. Kasneci, and W. Rosenstiel, "SubsMatch: scanpath similarity in dynamic scenes based on subsequence frequencies," in *Proceedings of the 8th Symposium on Eye Tracking Research and Applications (ETRA '14)*, pp. 319–322, ACM, Safety Harbor, Fla, USA, March 2014.

[59] P. A. Aspinall, Z. K. Johnson, A. Azuara-Blanco, A. Montarzino, R. Brice, and A. Vickers, "Evaluation of quality of life and priorities of patients with glaucoma," *Investigative Ophthalmology & Visual Science*, vol. 49, no. 5, pp. 1907–1915, 2008.

[60] E. E. Freeman, B. Muñoz, S. K. West, H. D. Jampel, and D. S. Friedman, "Glaucoma and quality of life: the Salisbury Eye Evaluation," *Ophthalmology*, vol. 115, no. 2, pp. 233–238, 2008.

[61] U. Altangerel, G. L. Spaeth, and W. C. Steinmann, "Assessment of function related to vision (AFREV)," *Ophthalmic Epidemiology*, vol. 13, no. 1, pp. 67–80, 2006.

[62] K. Fujita, N. Yasuda, K. Oda, and M. Yuzawa, "Reading performance in patients with central visual field disturbance due to glaucoma," *Nippon Ganka Gakkai Zasshi*, vol. 110, no. 11, pp. 914–918, 2006.

[63] M. Ishii, M. Seki, R. Harigai, H. Abe, and T. Fukuchi, "Reading performance in patients with glaucoma evaluated using the MNREAD charts," *Japanese Journal of Ophthalmology*, vol. 57, no. 5, pp. 471–474, 2013.

[64] A. A. Black, J. M. Wood, J. E. Lovie-Kitchin, and B. M. Newman, "Visual impairment and postural sway among older adults with glaucoma," *Optometry & Vision Science*, vol. 85, no. 6, pp. 489–497, 2008.

[65] A. Kotecha, G. Richardson, R. Chopra, R. T. A. Fahy, D. F. Garway-Heath, and G. S. Rubin, "Balance control in glaucoma," *Investigative Ophthalmology & Visual Science*, vol. 53, no. 12, pp. 7795–7801, 2012.

[66] P. Y. Ramulu, E. Maul, C. Hochberg, E. S. Chan, L. Ferrucci, and D. S. Friedman, "Real-world assessment of physical activity in glaucoma using an accelerometer," *Ophthalmology*, vol. 119, no. 6, pp. 1159–1166, 2012.

[67] P. Y. Ramulu, S. W. Van Landingham, R. W. Massof, E. S. Chan, L. Ferrucci, and D. S. Friedman, "Fear of falling and visual field loss from glaucoma," *Ophthalmology*, vol. 119, no. 7, pp. 1352–1358, 2012.

[68] A. A. Black, J. M. Wood, and J. E. Lovie-Kitchin, "Inferior field loss increases rate of falls in older adults with glaucoma," *Optometry & Vision Science*, vol. 88, no. 11, pp. 1275–1282, 2011.

[69] H. Murata, H. Hirasawa, Y. Aoyama et al., "Identifying areas of the visual field important for quality of life in patients with glaucoma," *PLoS ONE*, vol. 8, no. 3, Article ID e58695, 2013.

[70] D. S. Marigold, "Role of peripheral visual cues in online visual guidance of locomotion," *Exercise & Sport Sciences Reviews*, vol. 36, no. 3, pp. 145–151, 2008.

[71] A. E. Patla, "Understanding the roles of vision in the control of human locomotion," *Gait & Posture*, vol. 5, no. 1, pp. 54–69, 1997.

[72] R. F. Reynolds and B. L. Day, "Visual guidance of the human foot during a step," *The Journal of Physiology*, vol. 569, no. 2, pp. 677–684, 2005.

[73] J. M. Wood and A. A. Black, "Ocular disease and driving," *Clinical & Experimental Optometry*, vol. 99, no. 5, pp. 395–401, 2016.

[74] S. Tanabe, K. Yuki, N. Ozeki et al., "The association between primary open-angle glaucoma and motor vehicle collisions," *Investigative Ophthalmology & Visual Science*, vol. 52, no. 7, pp. 4177–4181, 2011.

[75] L. W. Mccloskey, T. D. Koepsell, M. E. Wolf, and D. M. Buchner, "Motor vehicle collision injuries and sensory impairments of older drivers," *Age & Ageing*, vol. 23, no. 4, pp. 267–273, 1994.

[76] D. J. Foley, R. B. Wallace, and J. Eberhard, "Risk factors for motor vehicle crashes among older drivers in a rural community," *Journal of the American Geriatrics Society*, vol. 43, no. 7, pp. 776–781, 1995.

[77] G. McGwin Jr., A. Xie, A. Mays et al., "Visual field defects and the risk of motor vehicle collisions among patients with glaucoma," *Investigative Ophthalmology & Visual Science*, vol. 46, no. 12, pp. 4437–4441, 2005.

[78] C. Owsley, G. McGwin Jr., and K. Ball, "Vision impairment, eye disease, and injurious motor vehicle crashes in the elderly," *Ophthalmic Epidemiology*, vol. 5, no. 2, pp. 101–113, 1998.

[79] P. S. Hu, D. A. Trumble, D. J. Foley, J. W. Eberhard, and R. B. Wallace, "Crash risks of older drivers: a panel data analysis," *Accident Analysis & Prevention*, vol. 30, no. 5, pp. 569–581, 1998.

[80] M. Kwon, C. Huisingh, L. A. Rhodes, G. McGwin, J. M. Wood, and C. Owsley, "Association between glaucoma and at-fault motor vehicle collision involvement among older drivers: A Population-based Study," *Ophthalmology*, vol. 123, no. 1, pp. 109–116, 2016.

[81] S. Kunimatsu-Sanuki, A. Iwase, M. Araie et al., "An assessment of driving fitness in patients with visual impairment to understand the elevated risk of motor vehicle accidents," *BMJ Open*, vol. 5, no. 2, Article ID e006379, 2015.

[82] T. Ono, K. Yuki, S. Awano-Tanabe et al., "Driving self-restriction and motor vehicle collision occurrence in glaucoma," *Optometry & Vision Science*, vol. 92, no. 3, pp. 357–364, 2015.

[83] T. R. M. Coeckelbergh, W. H. Brouwer, F. W. Cornelissen, P. Van Wolffelaar, and A. C. Kooijman, "The effect of visual field defects on driving performance: A driving simulator study," *Archives of Ophthalmology*, vol. 120, no. 11, pp. 1509–1516, 2002.

[84] J. M. Wood, G. McGwin Jr., J. Elgin et al., "Hemianopic and quadrantanopic field loss, eye and head movements, and driving," *Investigative Ophthalmology & Visual Science*, vol. 52, no. 3, pp. 1220–1225, 2011.

[85] E. Kasneci, G. Kasneci, T. C. Kübler, and W. Rosenstiel, "Online recognition of fixations, saccades, and smooth pursuits for automated analysis of traffic hazard perception," in *Artificial Neural Networks*, vol. 4 of *Springer Series in Bio-/Neuroinformatics*, pp. 411–434, Springer International, Cham, Switzerland, 2015.

8

Short-Term Observation of Ultrasonic Cyclocoagulation in Chinese Patients with End-Stage Refractory Glaucoma

Dongpeng Hu ⓘ, Shu Tu, Chengguo Zuo, and Jian Ge ⓘ

State Key Laboratory of Ophthalmology, Zhongshan Ophthalmic Center, Sun Yat-sen University, 54 Xianlie Road, Guangzhou 510060, China

Correspondence should be addressed to Jian Ge; gejian@mail.sysu.edu.cn

Academic Editor: Michele Figus

Purpose. To assess the efficacy and safety of HIFU-based ultrasonic cyclocoagulation in Chinese patients with end-stage refractory glaucoma. *Method.* Patients were recruited consecutively from May 2016 to May 2017 in the Zhongshan Ophthalmic Center. Ultrasonic cyclocoagulation was performed on every patient, using the EyeOP1 ultrasound emitting device. Return visits were set at 1 day, 7 days, 1 month, and 3 months after the treatment. An intraocular pressure (IOP) reduction of ≥20% while IOP ≥ 5 mmHg was deemed as success. Mean IOP change was assessed. Efficacy of two modes (6 sectors and 8 sectors) was also compared. Complications were recorded for safety evaluation. *Results.* 61 eyes were treated in this study. The baseline IOP (mean ± SD) was 41.11 ± 10.65 mmHg. The percentage of IOP reduction after treatment was 29.2%, 43.2%, 34.8%, and 23.1% at 1 day, 7 days, 1 month, and 3 months, respectively. Overall success rate at 3 months was 50.0% (26/52). No significant difference was found between the 6 sectors group and the 8 sectors group in terms of the success rate (48.6% vs. 52.9%, $p = 0.768$) as well as IOP reduction ($p = 0.417$) at 3 months. Primary angle-closure glaucoma (PACG) had the highest success rate (80.0%, 12/15). Scleral thinning existed in 12 eyes, among which 2 developed hypotony (2 mmHg and 3 mmHg). Average pain score decreased massively compared with baseline data. *Conclusion.* With high percentage of IOP reduction and a good safety profile observed in our study, HIFU-based ultrasonic cyclocoagulation might become a promising alternative to cyclodestructive methods. Long-term efficacy and safety need further assessment. The study was registered with Chinese Clinical Trial Registry (http://www.chictr.org.cn; Registration number: ChiCTR-OOC-17014028).

1. Introduction

High-intensity-focused ultrasound (HIFU) technology is being used to destroy target tissue with HIFU focused onto a small point, where the temperature will go up critically due to thermal effect of ultrasound [1]. With great accuracy, it can effectively avoid damage to the surrounding tissue. HIFU has been widely adopted in the treatment of prostate cancer [2], breast cancer [3], and liver cancer [4]. The application of this technology in glaucoma can be traced back to the 1980s. By coagulating part of the ciliary body, whose epithelium can secrete aqueous humor, HIFU-based ultrasonic cyclocoagulation is regarded as a potential way to reduce intraocular pressure (IOP). The 1-year success rate of

ultrasonic cyclocoagulation reported in some literature was about 50% in 1980s [5]. However, due to technical limitations at that time, the ultrasound emitting device was somewhat bulky and complicated to operate. IOP spikes (or major IOP increases) and scleral thinning often happened after the procedure. Occurrence of other severe complications such as scleral perforation, severe hypotony, or phthisis after the treatment was also hard to avoid. Thus, the treatment was gradually abandoned two decades ago [6].

Thanks to advances in technology, ultrasonic cyclocoagulation has made a comeback in recent years. With a miniaturized probe and intelligent operating system, ultrasonic cyclocoagulation can be performed much easily and safely on the eye [7]. Florent Aptel was the first to use miniaturized HIFU device for the treatment of advanced refractory glaucoma, reporting a 1-year success rate of 10/12, and a mean IOP drop of 33.9% [8]. A multicenter clinical study published in 2016 showed that 30 open-angle glaucoma patients without filtering surgery history had a 1-year success rate of 63% (30% mean IOP reduction) after ultrasonic cyclocoagulation and did not present serious complications, suggesting that it is a safe and effective method to reduce IOP [9].

However, because there is a clear distinction between China and European countries in terms of glaucoma types, for example, PACG accounts for about 50% of glaucoma types in China [10] while only 9% [11] in Europe, it cannot be extrapolated that the therapeutic effect of ultrasonic cyclocoagulation still remain the same for Chinese. Although this treatment has been officially approved by China Food and Drug Administration (CFDA) for glaucoma treatment last year, there is no publication regarding the effect of ultrasonic cyclocoagulation in Chinese patients until now. Therefore, in this study, we reviewed records of patients with end-stage glaucoma who underwent ultrasonic cyclocoagulation in the Zhongshan Ophthalmic Center from May 2017 to September 2017, assessing the clinical outcomes of this treatment.

2. Patients and Methods

2.1. Patients. Glaucoma patients who received ultrasonic cyclocoagulation in the Zhongshan Ophthalmic Center were consecutively recruited from May 2017 to September 2017. The specific inclusion criteria were as follows: (1) end-stage glaucoma according to the Glaucoma Severity Staging (GSS) system [12], (2) IOP ≥ 21 mmHg despite the use of glaucoma medications, and (3) age >18 years and <90 years. Patients were excluded if they met the following criteria: (1) previous cyclophotocoagulation or other cyclodestructive surgery, (2) the presence of glaucoma drainage device, (3) ocular infection, (4) other diseases that can affect intraocular pressure (such as choroidal detachment and subluxation of the lens), or (5) pregnancy or serious systemic disease.

2.2. HIFU Device. EyeOP1 device developed by Eye Tech Care company was used in the study. The device consists of three major parts, namely, the control module, coupling cone, and ultrasound emitting probe. Before the treatment, some parameters should be set in the control module. After routine surgical disinfection and topical anesthesia, the coupling cone is firmly attached to the eye via vacuum aspiration, making sure that the position of the pupil is right at the center. Later the ultrasound-emitting probe is placed in the coupling cone, using sterile saline as a coupling agent and cooling agent. After all these steps, treatment procedure can be started. In this study, 8 seconds (2 W) of ultrasound exposure time per sector (6 sectors in total on the probe) and a 20-second interval (sequential sector activation during treatment) were applied. The entire procedure lasts 2 minutes and 28 seconds. In this article, there were two modes (6 sectors and 8 sectors activated) being used for the

treatment. 43 patients received 6-sectors activated modality in the early recruitment, while the following patients (18) were treated with 8-sectors, activated, ultrasonic cyclocoagulation. The 8 sectors mode can be achieved easily by rotating the probe to another position. Detailed structure and operation instructions were mentioned in some relevant literature [7, 9].

2.3. Methods. This study was approved by the independent Institute Research Ethics Committee at Zhongshan Ophthalmic Center (ZOC, Guangzhou, P. R. China), and written consents were obtained from all participants. Before the treatment, the following baseline information was collected: best-corrected visual acuity, automatic optometry, slit-lamp biomicroscopy with gonioscopy, Goldmann applanation tonometry with three measurements (obtained at 8 am to 9 am), ultrasound pachymetry, and ultrasound biomicroscopy (UBM). Here, UBM is aimed at measuring the diameter of the circle where the ciliary processes are placed, determining the optimal size of the ultrasound emitting probe (10 mm, 11 mm, 12 mm, and 13 mm) for individuals. To be specific, four cross-sections of UBM scan (0°–180°, 45°–225°, 90°–270°, and 135°–315°) were taken into account to calculate the average diameter. All procedures were performed by a senior doctor (Jian Ge) with the assistance of a resident (Shu Tu). Posttreatment follow-up contain corresponding examination data, which were recorded at 1 day, 7 days, 1 month, and 3 months after the treatment. At each visit, photographs of the anterior segment were taken for comparison. One ophthalmologist (Chengguo Zuo) from glaucoma department was in charge of the eye examination and data recording. The number of ocular hypotensive agents was included for analysis. In addition, we used the 0–10 numeric rating scale (NRS) to record the severity of local pain at each follow-up, strictly following the instructions of NRS practice [13].

2.4. Outcome Evaluation. In terms of efficacy, the success rate and mean IOP reduction after the treatment were calculated. Success was defined as IOP reduced by ≥20% but still ≥5 mmHg (despite the presence of ocular hypotensive agents), consistent with some related literature [8, 9, 14–20].

Safety assessment depended on the occurrence of posttreatment complications, including pain, bleeding, vision acuity decrease, scleral thinning, hypotony, choroidal detachment, retinal detachment, and phthisis.

2.5. Statistical Analysis. Line chart and scatter plot were adopted to present mean IOP trend and individual IOP change, respectively. W test was used to analyze the normality of data. Student's t-test and analysis of variance were used to compare means, and chi-squared tests or Fisher's exact tests were used for the analysis of dichotomous variables like success rate. Statistical significance was set at $p < 0.05$. Statistical software (SPSS version 17.0; SPSS Inc., Chicago, IL, USA) was used for data analysis.

3. Results

3.1. Patient Characteristics. The characteristics of 61 glaucoma patients (43 in 6 sectors group/18 in 8 sectors group) were listed in Table 1. Nine of them (9/61, 14.8%) were lost to follow-up at 3 months. Only one eye underwent ultrasonic cyclocoagulation for each patient. One subject received cyclophotocoagulation during follow-up and was seen as failure at 3 months (9 mmHg). Patients could be divided into four groups in our study: primary open-angle glaucoma (POAG) (10/61; 16.4%), primary angle closure glaucoma (PACG) (18/61; 29.5%), neovascular glaucoma (NVG) (29/61; 47.5%), and traumatic glaucoma (4/61; 6.6%). 55 patients presented no light perception visual acuity, while the rest (6 patients) ranged from finger count to light perception.

3.2. IOP Trend for all Patients. The baseline mean IOP ± SD (standard deviation) was 41.11 ± 10.65 mmHg (Figure 1). The percentage of IOP reduction after the treatment was 29.2% (29.11 ± 10.13 mmHg), 43.2% (23.37 ± 11.37 mmHg), 34.8% (26.79 ± 12.35 mmHg), and 23.1% (31.63 ± 14.59 mmHg) at 1 day, 7 days, 1 month, and 3 months, respectively. Success rate at 3 months was 50.0% (26/52) (Figure 2). The greatest IOP reduction was noted at 7 days. Thereafter, IOP increased slowly while no plateau appeared during follow-up.

3.3 IOP Comparison between 6 Sectors and 8 Sectors Groups. There was no significant difference between the 6 sectors and 8 sectors groups in terms of age ($p = 0.130$), diagnosis ($p = 0.867$), and surgery history (Table 1). No significant difference ($p = 0.241$) of baseline IOP levels was revealed between the two groups (40.07 ± 10.18 mmHg vs. 43.59 ± 11.62 mmHg) (Table 2). However, when it came to mean IOP reduction change (Figure 3), we found that the extent of IOP reduction was much more dramatic in the 8 sectors group at the early stage but not at 3 months (8.81 ± 11.96 mmHg vs. 12.42 ± 19.79, $p = 0.417$). In addition, no significant difference of the success rate (48.6% vs. 52.9%, $p = 0.768$) was found between the two groups at 3 months (Figure 2).

3.4. Different Outcomes among Glaucoma Types. We then conducted subgroup analyses and found out that there was difference in success rate among glaucoma types ($p = 0.013$). Interestingly, PACG had the greatest percentage of IOP reduction (36.1%) and the highest success rate (12/15; 80.0%), while NVG seemed to be less responsive to treatment (18.6% of IOP reduction) with the success rate of only 29.2% at 3 months. The success rate for POAG and traumatic glaucoma was 55.6% (5/9) and 50.0% (2/4), respectively. Those who had previous glaucoma surgery (12/52; 11 had a history of trabeculectomy, and 1 had anterior chamber paracentesis) presented a success rates of 75.0% (9/12). For detailed figures across two modalities (6 sectors and 8 sectors), please refer to Table S1. There was no significant

TABLE 1: Patient demographics.

Groups	6 sectors	8 sectors	All	p
Number of patients	43	18	61	—
Age, mean (range), y	59.2 (27–86)	52.5 (22–77)	57.2 (22–86)	0.130
Sex (male/female)	28/15	6/12	34/27	0.023
Diagnosis (n (%))				
POAG	7 (16.3)	3 (16.7)	10 (16.4)	0.867*
PACG	14 (32.6)	4 (22.2)	18 (29.5)	—
NVG	19 (44.2)	10 (55.6)	29 (47.5)	—
Traumatic	3 (7.0)	1 (5.6)	4 (6.6)	—
Glaucoma surgery				0.360*
Trabeculectomy	10	2	12	—
AC penetration	1	0	1	—
Vision acuity				
NLP	37	18	55	—
CF-LP	6	0	6	—
Follow-up completed	35/43 (81.4)	17/18 (94.4)	52/61 (85.2)	—

POAG: primary open-angle glaucoma; PACG: primary angle closure glaucoma; NVG: neovascular glaucoma; AC: anterior chamber; NLP: no light perception; CF: count finger; LP: light perception. *Fisher's exact test.

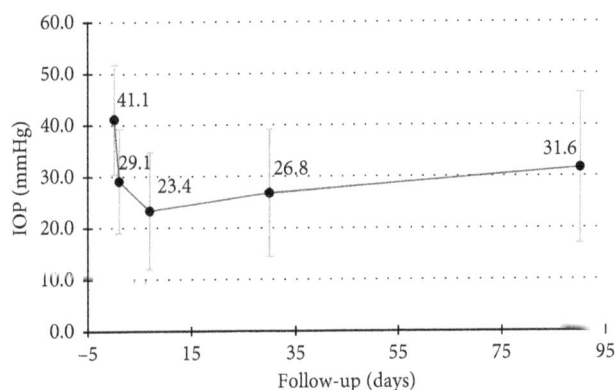

FIGURE 1: Mean IOP levels at 1 day, 7 days, 1 month, and 3 months after the treatment. Error bars represent standard deviation.

difference between patients with and without glaucoma surgery before (17/40; 42.5%) ($p = 0.100$; χ^2 continuity correction) (Table 3).

3.5. Safety. The intraoperative and postoperative complications are shown in Table 4. The minor complications were pain, conjunctival hyperemia, anterior chamber reaction, keratic precipitates, bulbar conjunctival edema, and subconjunctival hemorrhage. Most of the signs disappeared within 1 month. Twelve subjects had scleral thinning during follow-up. Typical photographs of anterior segment at each visit and scleral thinning are shown in Supplementary Figure S1. One case showed astigmatism increased from −0.5 diopters to −4.5 diopters. Two patients developed hypotony (2 mmHg and 3 mmHg) (Figure 2), and one of them even presented retinal detachment at last follow-up (Figure S1). However, without b-ultrasound examination of the fundus before the treatment, we had not been able to rule out

Month 3 follow-up

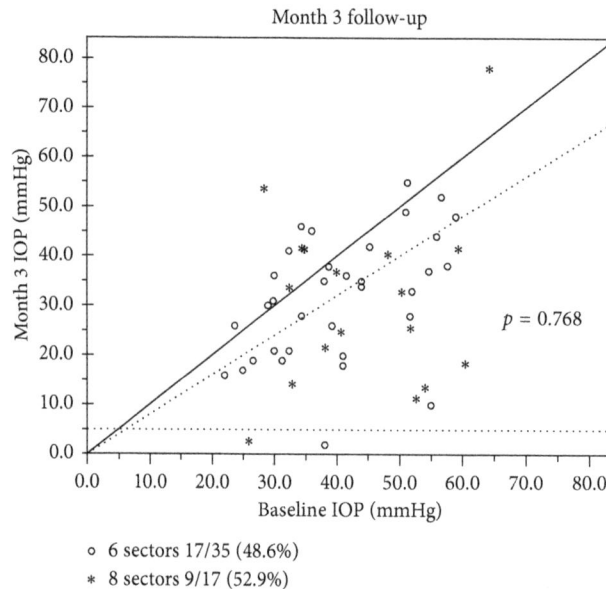

○ 6 sectors 17/35 (48.6%)
* 8 sectors 9/17 (52.9%)

FIGURE 2: Scatter diagram of IOP changes at 3 months. 50% of cases located in the triangular area (below the oblique dash line $y = 0.8x$ and above the horizontal dash line $y = 5$) were seen as success cases after the treatment because the IOP reduction was more than 20% but no less than 5 mmHg.

TABLE 2: IOP levels at return visits for two groups of patients.

Groups	FU	N	IOP (mmHg)	p	IOP range	IOP reduction (%)	Number of medications	p^*
6 sectors	Baseline	43	40.07 ± 10.18	—	22–59	—	2.6 ± 1.1	—
	D1	41	30.91 ± 10.09	<0.001	11–55	22.20	2.6 ± 1.1	1
	D7	43	25.42 ± 11.14	<0.001	8–48.3	36.60	2.6 ± 1.1	1
	M1	42	28.34 ± 12.92	<0.001	8.3–57.7	29.40	2.6 ± 1.2	0.589
	M3	34	31.65 ± 12.56	<0.001	2–55	22	2.4 ± 1.2	0.34
8 sectors	Baseline	18	43.59 ± 11.62	—	26–64	—	2.7 ± 0.7	—
	D1	18	25.02 ± 9.24	<0.001	5–36	42	2.7 ± 0.7	1
	D7	18	18.46 ± 10.66	<0.001	4.3–36.7	57.70	2.7 ± 0.7	1
	M1	17	22.98 ± 10.15	<0.001	9–40.3	50.20	2.6 ± 0.7	0.317
	M3	17	31.59 ± 18.44	0.019	3–79	28.50	2.3 ± 1.1	0.038

D1: day 1; D7: day 7; M1: month 1; M3: month 3; IOP: intraocular pressure. [&]Paired t-test, compared to baseline IOP; *Wilcoxon's test.

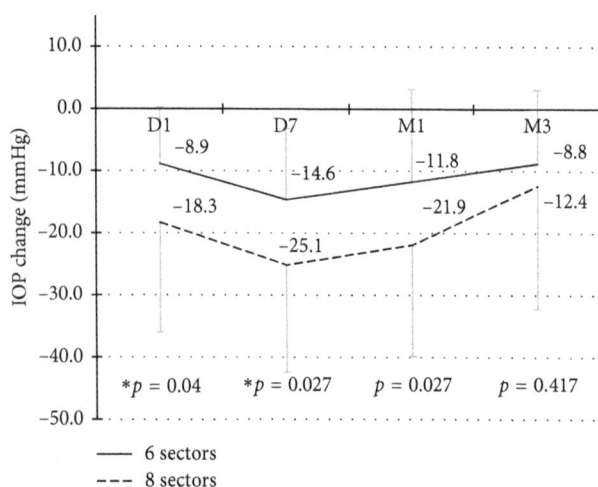

FIGURE 3: IOP reduction comparison between 6 sectors group and 8 sectors group.

a possibly preexistent retinal detachment because of the serious cataract. When it came to visual acuity, we found no obvious deterioration due to treatment among six patients with CF-LP VA (Table S2).

3.6. Pain Score Decreased Massively. All patients involved in our study were end-stage glaucoma patients with severely damaged visual function. A remarkable feature of these patients was the complaint of local pain due to uncontrollable high IOP, in spite of maximal hypotensive agents being administered. In this study, the baseline pain score on average was 1.0, with 14 patients presenting local pain. Although on the day after the treatment, both numbers rose slightly (1.3 points; 21), downward trend was conspicuous afterward. At 3 months, the average pain score was only 0.1 points, and the number of patients with local pain fell to 1 (Figure 4). Statistical significance was detected between baseline and 3 months' average pain score ($p = 0.002$). Corneal edema existed in about half of patients complaining of local pain (Table S3).

TABLE 3: Subgroup analyses.

Subgroups	N	Baseline IOP (mmHg)	IOP reduction at M3 (mmHg)	Percentage of IOP reduction (%)	Success rate		p
POAG	9	37.84 ± 9.20	6.69 ± 8.21	17.7	5/9	55.6%	0.013
PACG	15	43.99 ± 11.88	15.90 ± 13.66	36.1	12/15	80.0%	—
NVG	24	41.77 ± 11.11	7.78 ± 17.05	18.6	7/24	29.2%	—
Traumatic	4	39.28 ± 14.21	8.50 ± 15.20	21.6	2/4	50.0%	—
No surgery	40	41.14 ± 11.11	8.98 ± 15.93	21.8	17/40	42.5%	0.100*
Surgery	12	42.86 ± 11.66	13.37 ± 10.46	31.2	9/12	75.0%	—
Total	52	41.11 ± 10.65	9.99 ± 14.87	24.3	26/52	50%	—

POAG: primary open-angle glaucoma; PACG: primary angle closure glaucoma; NVG: neovascular glaucoma; IOP: intraocular pressure. [&]Fisher's exact probability; *chi-squared tests with correction for continuity.

TABLE 4: Complications due to treatment.

Complications	6 sectors ($n = 43$)	8 sectors ($n = 18$)	Total ($n = 61$)
Anterior chamber reaction	13	9	22
Conjunctival hyperemia	10	5	15
Keratic precipitates	9	6	15
Chemosis	8	6	14
Intraoperative pain	10	3	13
Subconjunctival hemorrhage	6	7	13
Scleral thinning	7	5	12
Foreign body sensation	4	1	5
Superficial punctate keratitis	3	1	4
Corneal edema	1	1	2
Hypotony	1	1	2
Astigmatism (>1 diopter)	1	0	1
Retinal detachment*	1	0	1

Patients with ocular signs mentioned in the table were included for analyses only if such signs occurred or aggravated after the treatment. *The causality was not confirmed due to severe cataract and no ultrasound scan of the fundus before the treatment.

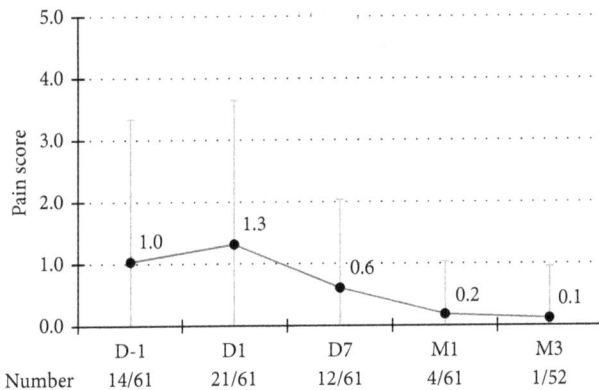

FIGURE 4: Average pain score and the number of patients suffering local pain at return visits.

4. Discussion

In this study, the efficacy and safety of HIFU-based ultrasonic cyclocoagulation was observed among end-stage glaucoma patients in China within a 3-month follow-up. The results showed that the mean IOP was decreased by 24.3%, and the success rate was 50.0% at 3 months after the treatment. There was no difference between the 6 sectors and 8 sectors groups with respect to the extent of IOP reduction at last visit. Subgroup analysis indicated that PACG had the highest success rate (80.0%) and largest percentage of IOP reduction (36.1%). However, NVG appeared to be the type that had the lowest response rate, with a success rate of 29.2% (7/24) and only 18.6% of IOP reduction at 3 months. Complications, such as scleral thinning and hypotony, were noticed in our study. The number of patients suffering from local pain and average pain score were reduced significantly at last follow-up.

At present, it is believed that the mechanism of reducing IOP by ultrasonic cyclocoagulation is mainly depending on the destruction of the nonpigmented epithelium of the ciliary body, directly influencing the production of aqueous humor. Besides, due to the shrinkage of the ciliary body after sonification, the potential space between the ciliary body and the sclera is enlarged, leading to increased outflow of aqueous humor through supraciliary and suprachoroidal space [16, 21]. In vivo study also revealed an increase of intrascleral hyporeflective spaces and conjunctival microcysts 1 month after the treatment, indicating an enhanced transscleral AH outflow [22].

The percentage of IOP reduction (24.3%) of our study remained close to the corresponding data (about 25% at 3 months) in some foreign studies [8, 9, 18, 23], and the success rate (50.0%) was only slightly lower. For failed cases with IOP reduction <20%, it is universally believed that the amount of ciliary body coagulated is insufficient, and the remaining normal epithelium will have a compensatory secretion of aqueous humor. Also, it should be taken into account that the increased transscleral outflow after insonification may decrease to some extent over time [22]. For patients with no obvious IOP reduction after treatment, some found that a secondary ultrasonic cyclocoagulation might achieve satisfactory results [23], suggesting that even if no response at the first time, repeated treatment may still be effective.

It was assumed that higher IOP reduction would be seen in the 8 sectors group, for more ciliary processes were considered to be ablated than that in the 6 sectors group. The results turned out to be a little confusing that no statistical differences in IOP reduction and success rate were present between the two groups at 3 months. Only a higher response rate of the 8 sectors group was revealed in the early follow-up. Perhaps, it is because the sample size was not big enough to demonstrate the difference.

Interestingly, we found that PACG did much better than other types of glaucoma, showing a success rate of 80% and mean IOP reduction of 36.1%. Although the mechanism is unknown, it is undoubtedly an encouraging news for Chinese glaucoma patients with a high proportion of PACG.

According to the results of multicenter clinical studies in foreign countries [9, 17, 18], minor complications were completely resolved within 1 month, and no complications such as secondary cataract, subluxation of the lens, and phthisis were observed. Denis et al. [18] (52 patients) reported one case of hypotony with choroidal detachment, one of macular edema, and six of visual acuity reduced >2 lines. Aptel et al. [9] recruited 30 patients and found that two patients developed IOP spikes (increased more than 10 mmHg within 7 days), one case had macular edema, one scleral thinning, and one astigmatism increased more than 1 diopter. In this study, minor complications basically disappeared within 1 month. 12 cases showed scleral thinning, and 2 developed hypotony (2 mmHg and 3 mmHg).

For end-stage glaucoma patients, local pain has a serious impact on the quality of life. It could be caused by uncontrolled IOP as well as corneal edema due to decompensation of corneal endothelium as a result of long-term high IOP. Although the overall success rate was only 50%, it was rather surprising that the pain score reduced massively, which, to some extent, was in line with the goal of treatment for patients with advanced glaucoma.

Compared with other cyclodestructive surgery, ultrasonic cyclocoagulation, as a relatively new method, showed no obvious advantage regarding efficacy for the moment. Taking IOP ≤ 21 mmHg as the success standard, endoscopic cyclophotocoagulation could achieve a success rate of 76.5% (mean follow-up: 10.8 months) at our center [24], which was significantly better than ultrasonic cyclocoagulation. However, cyclophotocoagulation has serious complications; for example, the incidence of phthisis was about 10% [25]. In contrast, the current HIFU-based ultrasonic cyclocoagulation has its own strengths that it is a relatively noninvasive procedure and is easy to operate, with an acceptable safety profile.

This study had some limitations. First, because of the short duration of follow-up (only 3 months), long-term efficacy need to be further evaluated. Second, the sample size (61 patients) may not be large enough for a convincing analysis of rare complications. As the individuals involved were end-stage glaucoma patients, it was difficult to effectively assess the impact of treatment on visual acuity.

In summary, HIFU-based ultrasonic cyclocoagulation is an effective treatment to reduce IOP for Chinese patients with end-stage glaucoma. It is expected to serve as a promising alternative to cyclodestructive surgery. However, long-term efficacy and safety require further investigation.

Conflicts of Interest

The authors have no conflicts of interest related to the article.

Acknowledgments

The authors were grateful for the patients who participated in this study. Staff members from the Glaucoma Department of the Zhongshan Ophthalmic Center, including Dr. Sijing Yang, Dr. Bikun Xian, Dr. Kaijing Li, Dr. Yuchun Liu, Dr. Ziming Luo, and Dr. Huifeng Rong, were also appreciated for their assistance and contribution to the research. This study was supported by the National Natural Science Foundation of China (grant no. 81371007).

References

[1] D. L. Miller, N. B. Smith, M. R. Bailey, G. J. Czarnota, K. Hynynen, and I. R. Makin, "Overview of therapeutic ultrasound applications and safety considerations," *Journal of Ultrasound in Medicine*, vol. 31, no. 4, pp. 623–634, 2012.

[2] M. Warmuth, T. Johansson, and P. Mad, "Systematic review of the efficacy and safety of high-intensity focussed ultrasound for the primary and salvage treatment of prostate cancer," *European Urology*, vol. 58, no. 6, pp. 803–815, 2010.

[3] M. C. Peek, M. Ahmed, A. Napoli et al., "Systematic review of high-intensity focused ultrasound ablation in the treatment of breast cancer," *British Journal of Surgery*, vol. 102, no. 8, pp. 873–882, 2015.

[4] T. T. Cheung, S. T. Fan, F. S. Chu et al., "Survival analysis of high-intensity focused ultrasound ablation in patients with small hepatocellular carcinoma," *HPB*, vol. 15, no. 8, pp. 567–573, 2013.

[5] F. Valtot, J. Kopel, and J. Haut, "Treatment of glaucoma with high intensity focused ultrasound," *International Ophthalmology*, vol. 13, no. 1-2, pp. 167–170, 1989.

[6] F. Aptel and C. Lafon, "Therapeutic applications of ultrasound in ophthalmology," *International Journal of Hyperthermia*, vol. 28, no. 4, pp. 405–418, 2012.

[7] T. Charrel, F. Aptel, A. Birer et al., "Development of a miniaturized HIFU device for glaucoma treatment with conformal coagulation of the ciliary bodies," *Ultrasound in Medicine & Biology*, vol. 37, no. 5, pp. 742–754, 2011.

[8] F. Aptel, C. Dupuy, and J. F. Rouland, "Treatment of refractory open-angle glaucoma using ultrasonic circular cyclocoagulation: a prospective case series," *Current Medical Research and Opinion*, vol. 30, no. 8, pp. 1599–1605, 2014.

[9] F. Aptel, P. Denis, J. F. Rouland, J. P. Renard, and A. Bron, "Multicenter clinical trial of high-intensity focused ultrasound

treatment in glaucoma patients without previous filtering surgery," *Acta Ophthalmologica*, vol. 94, no. 5, pp. e268–e277, 2016.

[10] J. W. Cheng, S. W. Cheng, X. Y. Ma, J. P. Cai, Y. Li, and R. L. Wei, "The prevalence of primary glaucoma in mainland China: a systematic review and meta-analysis," *Journal of Glaucoma*, vol. 22, no. 4, pp. 301–306, 2013.

[11] A. C. Day, G. Baio, G. Gazzard et al., "The prevalence of primary angle closure glaucoma in European derived populations: a systematic review," *British Journal of Ophthalmology*, vol. 96, no. 9, pp. 1162–1167, 2012.

[12] R. P. Mills, D. L. Budenz, P. P. Lee et al., "Categorizing the stage of glaucoma from pre-diagnosis to end-stage disease," *American Journal of Ophthalmology*, vol. 141, no. 1, pp. 24–30, 2006.

[13] M. McCaffery and A Beebe, "Pain: clinical manual for nursing practice," *Nursing Standard*, vol. 9, no. 11, p. 55, 1994.

[14] F. Aptel, T. Charrel, C. Lafon et al., "Miniaturized high-intensity focused ultrasound device in patients with glaucoma: a clinical pilot study," *Investigative Ophthalmology & Visual Science*, vol. 52, no. 12, pp. 8747–8753, 2011.

[15] J. Rouland and F. Aptel, "Treatment of refractory glaucoma using UC3 procedure with HIFU (high intensity focused ultrasound). prospective series," *Acta Ophthalmologica*, vol. 91, no. s252, 2013.

[16] F. Aptel, A. Begle, A. Razavi et al., "Short- and long-term effects on the ciliary body and the aqueous outflow pathways of high-intensity focused ultrasound cyclocoagulation," *Ultrasound in Medicine & Biology*, vol. 40, no. 9, pp. 2096–2106, 2014.

[17] F. Aptel, P. Denis, J. Rouland, J. P. Renard, and A. M. Bron, "Multicenter clinical trial of ultrasonic circular cyclo coagulation in glaucoma patients naive of filtering surgery: preliminary results at 6 months," *Acta Ophthalmologica*, vol 92, 2014.

[18] P. Denis, F. Aptel, J. F. Rouland et al., "Cyclocoagulation of the ciliary bodies by high-intensity focused ultrasound: a 12-month multicenter study," *Investigative Ophthalmology and Visual Science*, vol. 56, no. 2, pp. 1089–1096, 2015.

[19] S. Melamed, M. Goldenfeld, D. Cotlear, A. Skaat, and I. Moroz, "High-intensity focused ultrasound treatment in refractory glaucoma patients: results at 1 year of prospective clinical study," *European Journal of Ophthalmology*, vol. 25, no. 6, pp. 483–489, 2015.

[20] G. Giannaccare, A. Vagge, C. Gizzi et al., "High-intensity focused ultrasound treatment in patients with refractory glaucoma," *Graefe's Archive for Clinical and Experimental Ophthalmology*, vol. 255, no. 3, pp. 599–605, 2017.

[21] R. Mastropasqua, L. Agnifili, V. Fasanella et al., "Uveo-scleral outflow pathways after ultrasonic cyclocoagulation in refractory glaucoma: an anterior segment optical coherence tomography and in vivo confocal study," *British Journal of Ophthalmology*, vol. 100, no. 12, pp. 1668–1675, 2016.

[22] R. Mastropasqua, V. Fasanella, A. Mastropasqua, M. Ciancaglini, and L. Agnifili, "High-intensity focused ultrasound circular cyclocoagulation in glaucoma: a step forward for cyclodestruction?," *Journal of Ophthalmology*, vol. 2017, Article ID 7136275, 14 pages, 2017.

[23] S. Melamed, M. M. Goldenfeld, D. Cotlear, A. Skaat, and I. Moroz, "High-intensity focused ultrasound device in refractory Glaucoma patients. results at 1 year prospective clinical study," *European Journal of Ophthalmology*, vol. 25, no. 6, pp. 483–489, 2014.

[24] M. B. Yu, S. S. Huang, J. Ge, J. Guo, and M. Fang, "The clinical study of endoscopic cyclophotocoagulation on the management of refractory glaucoma," *Chinese Journal of Ophthalmology*, vol. 42, no. 1, pp. 27–31, 2006.

[25] F. Fankhauser, S. Kwasniewska, and E. Van der Zypen, "Cyclodestructive procedures. I. Clinical and morphological aspects: a review," *Ophthalmologica Journal International d'Ophtalmologie International Journal of Ophthalmology Zeitschrift für Augenheilkunde*, vol. 218, no. 2, pp. 77–95, 2004.

Spectral Domain Optical Coherence Tomography Assessment of Macular and Optic Nerve Alterations in Patients with Glaucoma and Correlation with Visual Field Index

Alessio Martucci ⓘ,[1] Nicola Toschi ⓘ,[2,3,4] Massimo Cesareo,[1] Clarissa Giannini,[1] Giulio Pocobelli,[1] Francesco Garaci ⓘ,[2] Raffaele Mancino,[1] and Carlo Nucci ⓘ[1]

[1]Ophthalmology Unit, Department of Experimental Medicine, University of Rome Tor Vergata, Rome, Italy
[2]Department of Biomedicine and Prevention, University of Rome Tor Vergata, Rome, Italy
[3]Department of Radiology, Athinoula A. Martinos Center for Biomedical Imaging, Boston, MA, USA
[4]Harvard Medical School, Boston, MA, USA

Correspondence should be addressed to Carlo Nucci; nucci@med.uniroma2.it

Academic Editor: Angelo Balestrazzi

Introduction. To evaluate the sectorial thickness of single retinal layers and optic nerve using spectral domain optic coherence tomography (SD-OCT) and highlight the parameters with the best diagnostic accuracy in distinguishing between normal and glaucoma subjects at different stages of the disease. *Material and Methods.* For this cross-sectional study, 25 glaucomatous (49 eyes) and 18 age-matched healthy subjects (35 eyes) underwent a complete ophthalmologic examination including visual field testing. Sectorial thickness values of each retinal layer and of the optic nerve were measured using SD-OCT Glaucoma Module Premium Edition (GMPE) software. Each parameter was compared between the groups, and the layers and sectors with the best area under the receiver operating characteristic curve (AUC) were identified. Correlation of visual field index with the most relevant structural parameters was also evaluated. *Results and Discussion.* All subjects were grouped according to stage as follows: Controls (CTRL); Early Stage Group (EG) (Stage 1 + Stage 2); Advanced Stage Group (AG) (Stage 3 + Stage 4 + Stage 5). mGCL TI, mGCL TO, mIPL TO, mean mGCL, cpRNFLt NS, and cpRNFLt TI showed the best results in terms of AUC according classification proposed by Swets ($0.9 < AUC < 1.0$). These parameters also showed significantly different values among group when CTRL vs EG, CTRL vs AG, and EG vs AG were compared. SD-OCT examination showed significant sectorial thickness differences in most of the macular layers when glaucomatous patients at different stages of the disease were compared each other and to the controls.

1. Introduction

Primary open-angle glaucoma, a leading cause of blindness in the world, is an optic neuropathy characterized by the death of ganglion cells of the retina, which is associated with the loss of axons that make up the optic nerve. These ultrastructural alterations gradually progress becoming clinically evident as an increased excavation of the optic disc and the presence of specific visual field (VF) defects [1]. Diagnosing and monitoring disease progression is therefore essential for the management of patients with glaucoma. Given that a significant structural loss usually precedes detectable function loss [2], technologies and strategies able to quantify glaucomatous changes at an early stage have the potential to impact prognosis and hence influence quality of life [3]. In this context, spectral domain-optical coherence tomography (SD-OCT) provides a tool for macular segmentation and thickness evaluation of individual retinal layers as well as retinal nerve fiber layer thickness (RNFLt) and Bruch's membrane opening (BMO)-minimum rim width (MRW) assessment. The patented Anatomic Position System (APS) creates an anatomic map of each patient's eye using the center of the fovea and the center of BMO as landmarks. In turn, this allows accurate localization and hence highly sensitive assessment of structural changes.

In this study, sectorial thickness values of each retinal layer at macular level, circumpapillary RNFLt of the optic nerve, and BMO-MRW were measured using SD-OCT Glaucoma Module Premium Edition (GMPE) software (Heidelberg Engineering, Germany) to assess the putative thickness differences between controls and initial glaucoma, controls and advanced glaucoma, and initial and advanced glaucoma.

2. Methods

In this cross-sectional study, 49 eyes of 25 glaucomatous patients and 35 age-matched healthy eyes of 18 subjects were recruited from the Glaucoma Clinic and the General Outpatients clinic (respectively) at the University Hospital "Policlinico Tor Vergata" (Rome, Italy). Patients and controls were aged 61.86 ± 6.79 and 60.58 ± 9.22 years, respectively. The study protocol was approved by the local institutional review board and adhered to the tenets of the Declaration of Helsinki. All subjects provided written informed consent.

All subjects underwent a complete ophthalmologic examination including the administration of a medical history questionnaire focused on local and systemic treatments and family history of glaucoma, determination of best-corrected visual acuity with logarithmic Early Treatment Diabetic Retinopathy Study visual acuity charts (Precision Vision, la Salle USA), slit-lamp examination of the anterior segment, intraocular pressure (IOP) evaluation using Goldmann applanation tonometry, pachymetry using an ultrasound pachymeter (Pachette DGH500; DGH Technology, Inc., Philadelphia, PA), gonioscopy, and 24-2 Swedish Interactive Threshold Algorithm (SITA) standard visual field (VF) testing. After pupillary dilation, slit-lamp fundus examination and SD-OCT were performed.

All participants met the following inclusion criteria: best-corrected visual acuity >0.1 logMAR, refractive error $< \pm 5$ spherical diopters or $< \pm 3$ cylindrical diopters, transparent ocular media, and open anterior chamber (Shaffer classification $>20°$).

The exclusion criteria comprehended previous or active optic neuropathies, retinal vascular diseases, preproliferative or proliferative diabetic retinopathy, macular degeneration, hereditary retinal dystrophy, use of medication that could affect VF, and previous or active neurological, cerebrovascular, or neurodegenerative diseases. Normal tension glaucoma (NTG) patients were also excluded.

A glaucoma diagnosis was defined, following the European Glaucoma Society criteria [4], as the presence of an elevated IOP (>21 mmHg), marked excavation of the optic nerve head with thinning of the neural rim, notching, focal or diffuse atrophy of neural rim, cup/disc ratio (CDr) in the vertical meridian >0.6, CDr asymmetry between the eyes >0.2, optic disc haemorrhages, denuded circumlinear vessels, and the presence of typical VF defects.

2.1. Visual Field Examination.
VF examination was performed using Humphrey Swedish Interactive Threshold Algorithm (SITA) standard visual fields with 24-2 test point

pattern (Carl Zeiss Meditec Inc., Dublin, CA). As reported in the literature [5], Standard Automated Perimetry (SAP) examinations were considered unreliable and discarded if fixation losses were >20%, false-positive errors >15%, and false-negative errors were >33%. The minimal glaucomatous abnormality was defined as the presence of pattern deviation probability plots with <5%, more than three of which contiguous and one of which <1%, corrected pattern standard deviation or pattern standard deviation significant at $p < 0.05$, or glaucoma hemifield test outside normal limits [5]. VFs were confirmed in at least 3 subsequent VF examinations. For this study, VFs were classified according to the glaucoma staging system based on the visual field index (VFI) [5]. VFI was found to be in excellent correlation with MD across the spectrum of glaucomatous visual loss [5]. The VFI expresses the amount of visual field loss as a percentage relative to the sensitivity of a reference group of healthy observers. To reduce the potentially confounding effects of cataract, the VFI disregards reductions in sensitivity unless they are associated with a pattern deviation probability outside normal limits. Locations at which the pattern deviations are within the 95th percentile of healthy observers are treated as normal and assigned a value of 100%. In addition, locations in the center of the visual field are more heavily weighted and therefore make a greater contribution to the VFI than do those in the periphery. This classification has been deemed easy to use, accurate, and its staging performance has been reported to be either equal or superior to other existing glaucoma staging systems [5].

All subjects were subsequently grouped according to stage as follows: Controls (CTRL); Initial Stages Group (IG) (Stage 1 + Stage 2); Advanced Stages Group (AG) (Stage 3 + Stage 4 + Stage 5).

2.2. Optical Coherence Tomography Examination.
After pupil dilation, all subjects underwent SD-OCT examination with GMPE software (Heidelberg Retinal Engineering, Dossenheim, Germany).

During the initial Anatomic Positioning System (APS) scan, the scanner performs automatic detection of landmarks and automatic alignment of scans relative to the patient's individual fovea-to-BMO center axis, hence improving accuracy and reproducibility measurements and overcoming measurement errors due to head tilt and eye rotation. Moreover, custom TruTrack™ technology actively tracks the eye during imaging with simultaneous dual-beam imaging minimizing motion artifacts. The GMPE, unlike the previous software versions, offers multi-layer segmentation for assessment of the isolated retinal layers providing a thorough assessment of the macular region via single layer thickness maps, APS, and BMO-MRW-based optic nerve head (ONH) evaluation.

To obtain perifoveal volumetric retinal scans, both eyes of all subjects were examined using the Spectralis OCT posterior pole vertical-oriented scan lines (PPoleV scan) protocols. PPoleV scan includes 19 single vertical axial scans ($30° \times 15°$ OCT volume scan), aligned to the individual fovea-to-BMO center axis with 240 microns distance between sections (Figure 1). Segmentation of the retinal layers in each

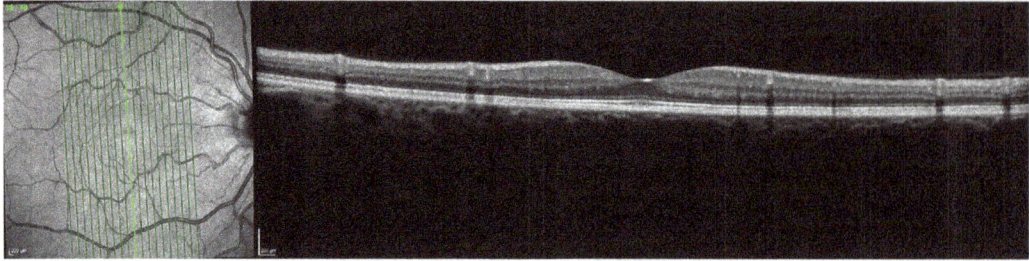

FIGURE 1: Sample Spectralis OCT posterior pole vertical-oriented scan lines (PPoleV scan) protocols.

vertical foveal scan was performed automatically using GMPE software for Spectralis OCT. For each layer provided by the new segmentation software (macular total retina (RETINA), Retinal Nerve Fiber Layer (RNFL), Ganglion Cell Layer (GCL), Inner Plexiform Layer (IPL), Inner Nuclear Layer (INL), Outer Plexiform Layer (OPL), Outer Nuclear Layer (ONL), Retinal Pigmented Epithelium (RPE), Inner Retinal Layers (IRL), and Outer Retinal Layers (ORL)), thickness measurements of all sectors, as defined by the Early Treatment Diabetic Retinopathy Study scheme (temporal inner, superior inner, nasal inner, inferior inner, temporal outer, superior outer, nasal outer, and inferior outer), were considered (Figure 2).

To perform optic nerve head (ONH) analysis, using BMO as the anatomical border of the rim, within 24 scan lines, the GMPE software automatically detects 48 BMO positions along the ONH determining the BMO-based disc margin. BMO-MRW is calculated from the BMO to the nearest point on the internal limiting membrane (ILM). In this study, for each scan, the following BMO-MRW measurements were considered: global, temporal superior, nasal superior, nasal, nasal inferior, temporal inferior, and temporal (Figure 3).

Circumpapillary RNFLt (cpRNFLt) analysis is performed acquiring three circle scans automatically centred on the individual fovea-to-BMO center axis ensuring the accurate definition of each single sector independent of head position. For each scan, the central circle has been analyzed and the following cpRNFLt measurements were considered: global, temporal superior, nasal superior, nasal, nasal inferior, temporal inferior, and temporal (Figure 4).

No manual corrections were necessary and only good quality OCT scans, with an OCT score >25, were included in the study.

2.3. Statistical Analysis.
All data were initially entered into an EXCEL database (Microsoft, Redmond, Washington, United States). Statistical analysis was performed in Statistical Package for the Social Sciences (SPSS) version 23.

Descriptive statistics consisted of the mean ± SD for parameter with Gaussian distributions (after confirmation using the Kolmogorov–Smirnov test), median and interquartile range for variables with nonGaussian distributions.

Comparisons among groups were performed using ANOVA/ANCOVA, for continuous Gaussianly distributed variables, and Mann–Whitney U test, for non-Gaussianly distributed variables. $p < 0.05$ was considered statistically significant.

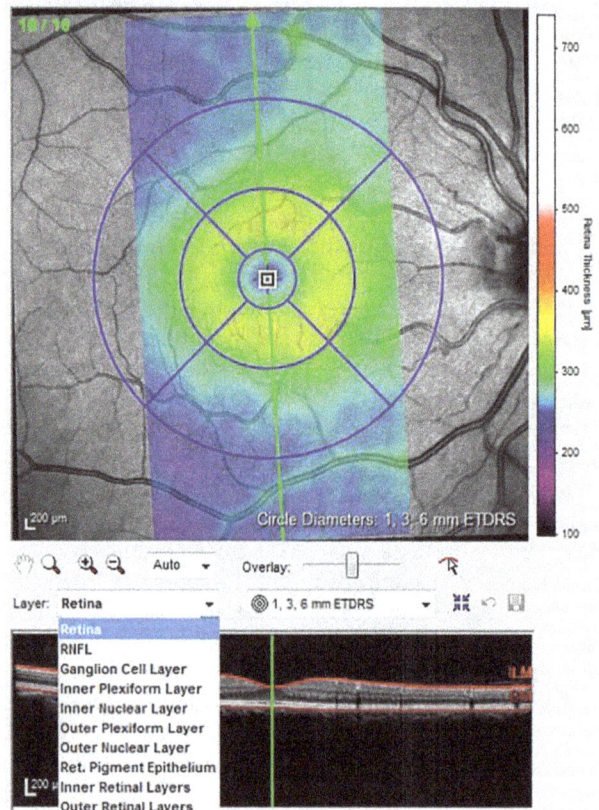

FIGURE 2: Sample of segmentation of retinal layers.

Age comparisons among groups were performed using Friedman ANOVA. A chi-square test was used to test independence among categorical variables.

For all the parameters which showed a statistically significant difference comparing controls vs. initial stages glaucoma, controls vs. advanced stages glaucoma, and initial stages glaucoma vs. advanced stages glaucoma, the diagnostic accuracy was evaluated by fitting a binary logistic regression model and examining the area under the generated receiver operating characteristics (ROC) curve (AUC).

For the interpretation of the AUC values, we referred to the classification proposed by Swets and only retained parameters with high diagnostic accuracy [6]:

(a) AUC = 0.5, the test is not informative

(b) 0.5 < AUC < 0.7, the test is not accurate

(c) 0.7 < AUC < 0.9, the test is moderately accurate

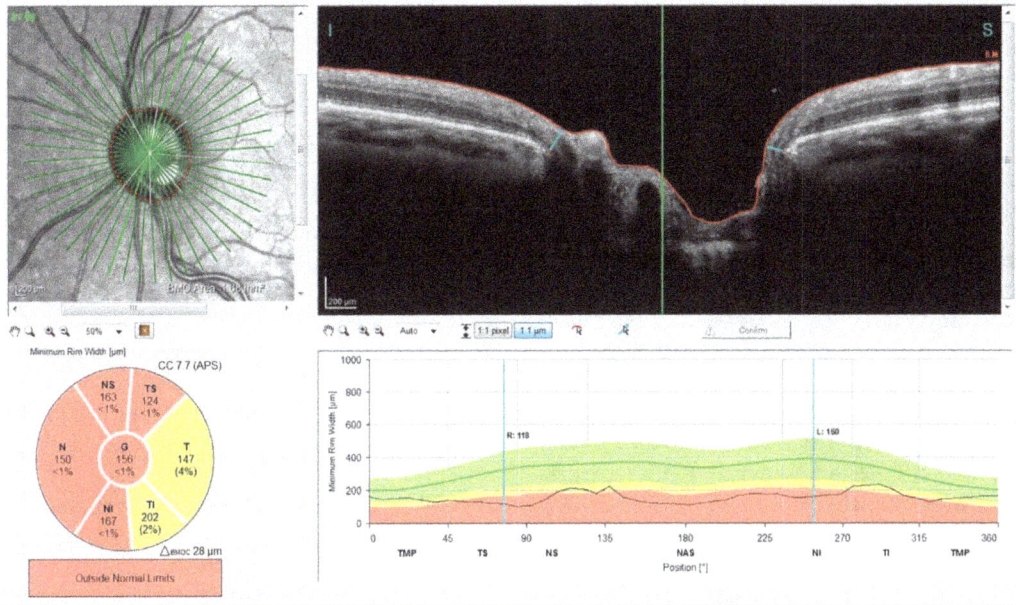

FIGURE 3: Bruch's membrane opening minimum rim width analysis.

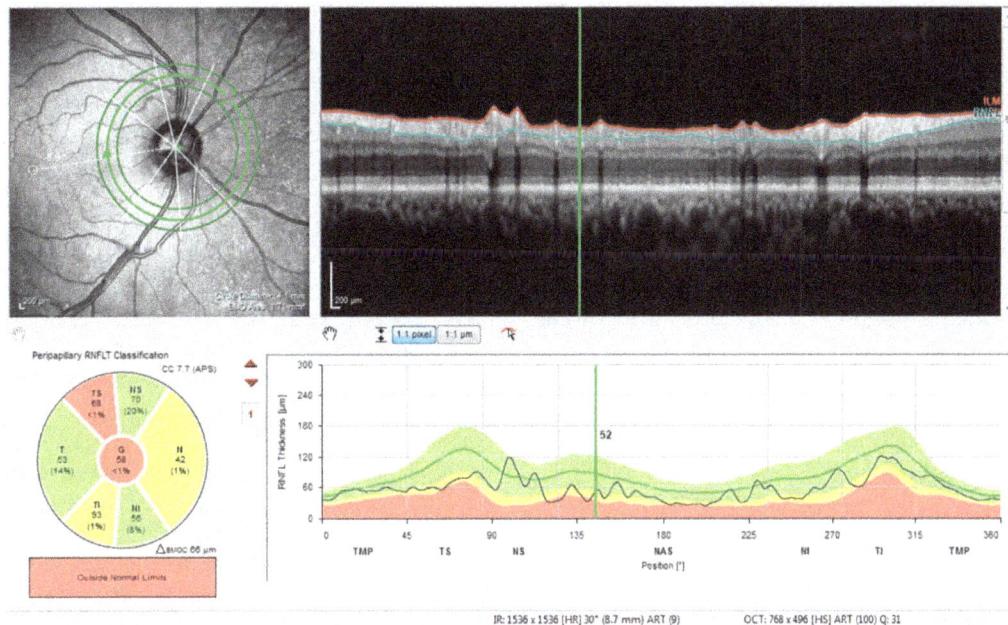

FIGURE 4: Circumpapillary retinal nerve fiber layer thickness analysis.

(d) $0.9 < AUC < 1.0$, the test is highly accurate

The correlation between functional, VFI, and structural loss, layers, and sector thicknesses was determined using Spearman's r correlation coefficient. Spearman's r correlation coefficient was classified accordingly [7]:

(a) 0.9 to 1.0 (−0.9 to −1.0): very high positive (negative) correlation

(b) 0.7 to 0.9 (−0.7 to −0.9): high positive (negative) correlation

(c) 0.5 to 0.7 (−0.5 to −0.7): moderate positive (negative) correlation

(d) 0.3 to 0.5 (−0.3 to −0.5): low positive (negative) correlation

(e) 0.0 to 0.3 (−0.0 to −0.3): negligible correlation

3. Results

A total of 84 eyes were included in the study. Control group was constituted of 35 eyes (age 60.83 ± 1.53), while initial and advanced stages glaucoma groups were constituted of 22 eyes (age 63.23 ± 1.34) and 27 eyes (age 60.52 ± 1.37), respectively.

There were no statistically significant differences in terms of age ($p = 0.58$) and gender ($p = 0.087$) among groups.

At macular level, the mean thicknesses of GCL superior, inferior, temporal, and nasal in the inner (GCL mean inner) and outer (GCL mean outer) sectors showed a highly accurate diagnostic ability in all the comparisons considered (CTRL vs. IG, AUC = 0.9; CTRL vs. AG, AUC = 1.0; IG vs. AG, AUC = 0.9). The same result was obtained when macular GCL temporal inner and outer and IPL temporal inner thicknesses were evaluated (CTRL vs. IG, AUC = 0.9; CTRL vs. AG, AUC = 1.0; IG vs. AG, AUC = 0.9). The mean of macular RNFL superior, inferior, temporal, and nasal outer sectors thickness (RNFL mean outer) also showed a highly accurate diagnostic ability in discriminating among all the groups considered for the study (CTRL vs. IG, AUC = 0.9; CTRL vs. AG, AUC = 1.0; IG vs. AG, AUC = 0.9). Moreover, at macular level, both the mean GCL and mean RNFL thickness values, given by the respective mean of superior, inferior, temporal, and nasal inner and outer sectors, resulted highly accurate in discriminating among all the groups (CTRL vs. IG, AUC = 0.9; CTRL vs. AG, AUC = 1.0; IG vs. AG, AUC = 0.9) (Table 1).

At ONH level, circumpapillary RNFL global and circumpapillary RNFL temporal superior sector thicknesses resulted highly accurate in discriminating among all the groups considered for the study (CTRL vs. IG, AUC = 0.9; CTRL vs. AG, AUC = 1.0; IG vs. AG, AUC = 0.9) (Table 1).

Table 2 reports descriptive statistics of the parameters that showed the highest diagnostic ability in all the following comparison: CTRL vs. IG, CTRL vs. AG, and IG vs. AG.

The correlation between functional, VFI, and structural loss thickness of the OCT parameters has been determined using Spearman's r correlation coefficient. Table 3 reports the OCT parameters that showed high and very high correlation coefficient with VFI (see Supplementary Material for the other parameters). Interestingly, all the parameters that showed the highest AUC also showed a positive correlation with VFI. In particular, if we consider the parameters that showed the best AUC values, at macular level, GCL mean inner ($r = 0.81$), GCL mean outer ($r = 0.75$), GCL temporal inner ($r = 0.79$), GCL temporal outer ($r = 0.72$), IPL temporal inner ($r = 0.78$), RNFL mean outer ($r = 0.71$), mean GCL ($r = 0.76$), and mean RNFL ($r = 0.73$) were highly positively correlated with VFI. On the contrary, circumpapillary RNFLt global ($r = 0.45$) and circumpapillary RNFLt temporal superior ($r = 0.52$) showed a low positive correlation with VFI.

4. Discussion

OCT technology has been proposed more than 20 years ago for noninvasive cross-sectional imaging in biological systems [8], and the first generation of time domain OCT has been superseded by the newest spectral domain instruments. Given that SD-OCT provides an accurate reconstruction of ONH and of the macular area, hence highlighting the presence of possible structural damage, it is increasingly becoming part of common clinical practice. Moreover, thanks to the faster scanning speed and the increased axial resolution, the latest OCT generation offers high resolution images which are less affected by eye movement artifacts and are more reproducible [9–11]. In this regard, local intrasession and intersession variability in OCT have been previously described as very low and uniform across eyes and layers [12, 13].

Before Zeimer et al. [14] suggested the use of macular imaging for glaucoma evaluation, the most important clinical parameter was the circumpapillary RNFL thickness [15–20]. However, due to the presence of blood vessels and the high variability of the ONH structure (even among healthy subjects), circumpapillary RNFLt measurements may not always be completely reliable in glaucoma diagnosis [21]. Instead, the macula is a relatively simple structure, constituted by multiple layers whose structure is not influenced by the presence of blood vessels. The shape of the macula, and more specifically the RGC layer, is generally less variable among healthy individuals as compared to other ocular structures such as the RNFL and ONH. Thus, in conjunction with the fact that it contains 50% of the total retinal ganglion cells (RGCs) and 35% of RNFL, macula appears to be a promising area for glaucoma evaluation [14, 21].

While previous studies with TD-OCT reported a good diagnostic ability of macular thickness, sensitivity and specificity were lower than those provided by circumpapillary RNFLt [22–28].

Using the fast-macular cube scan of a prototype software, Martinez-de-la-Martinez-de-la-Casa et al. [29] observed that with the macular segmentation software provided the Spectralis OCT, macular RNFLt measurements performed better than other algorithms in discriminating healthy subjects from glaucoma suspects. A similar result was also found considering RNFL + GCL + IPL thickness and total macular thickness [30]. Another study by Mathers et al. [31] also highlighted the usefulness of macular thickness as measured by SD-OCT in confirming the existence and extent of VF defects.

In a previous study using 3D-OCT 2000 (Topcon Corp., Tokyo, Japan), a thickness reduction of macular layers with progression of glaucoma was reported. This study showed a significantly lower ganglion cell-inner plexiform layer thickness (GCIPLT), as well as lower macular ganglion cell complex thickness (GCCT: a combination of macular RNFL thickness and GCIPLT) in POAG patients, compared to normal controls, progressing with the severity of glaucomatous damage [32].

In this study, we evaluated the ability of the parameters assessed using the GMPE software at macular and optic nerve level to discriminate among the following groups: controls versus initial glaucoma, controls versus advanced glaucoma, and initial versus advanced glaucoma. GMPE is a specific software for glaucoma diagnosis that, unlike other software, allows a layer by layer and sector by sector macular assessment. Thanks to this software, we are able to obtain, at macular level, macular total retina, retinal nerve fiber layer,

TABLE 1: Mann–Whitney and AUC of the parameters with the highest diagnostic ability in the CTRL vs. IG, CTRL vs. AG, and IG vs. AG comparisons.

CTRL vs. IG			CTRL vs. AG			IG vs. AG		
Parameter	AUC	p value	Parameter	AUC	p value	Parameter	AUC	p value
Macula GCL mean inner	0.9	$4.29449E-06$	Macula GCL mean inner	1.0	$3.94592E-10$	Macula GCL mean inner	0.9	$9.29422E-06$
Macula GCL mean outer	0.9	$2.3797E-06$	Macula GCL mean outer	1.0	$3.11259E-10$	Macula GCL mean outer	0.9	$4.87372E-07$
Macula GCL temporal inner	0.9	$6.40501E-07$	Macula GCL temporal inner	1.0	$3.59673E-10$	Macula GCL temporal inner	0.9	$3.5386E-06$
Macula GCL temporal outer	0.9	$2.26545E-07$	Macula GCL temporal outer	1.0	$1.6719E-10$	Macula GCL temporal outer	0.9	$4.12819E-06$
Macula IPL temporal inner	0.9	$4.81767E-06$	Macula IPL temporal inner	1.0	$1.67747E-10$	Macula IPL temporal inner	0.9	$1.42929E-05$
Macula RNFL mean outer	0.9	$1.6614E-05$	Macula RNFL mean outer	1.0	$4.46656E-10$	Macula RNFL mean outer	0.9	$3.41429E-06$
Macula mean GCL	0.9	$9.86195E-07$	Macula mean GCL	1.0	$1.78465E-10$	Macula mean GCL	0.9	$1.04181E-06$
Macula mean RNFL	0.9	$2.51857E-06$	Macula mean RNFL	1.0	$3.14624E-10$	Macula mean RNFL	0.9	$9.886E-07$
cpRNFL global	0.9	$3.19772E-06$	cpRNFL global	1.0	$2.68425E-10$	cpRNFL global	0.9	$7.41664E-07$
cpRNFL temporal superior	0.9	$2.83685E-06$	cpRNFL temporal superior	1.0	$2.70908E-10$	cpRNFL temporal superior	0.9	$4.33798E-06$
VFI	0.9	$2.14775E-06$	VFI	1.0	$3.81295E-11$	VFI	1.0	$6.5955E-09$

GCL: ganglion cell layer; IPL: inner plexiform layer; cpRNFL: circumpapillary retinal nerve fiber layer thickness; VFI: visual field index; CTRL: control group; IG: Early Glaucoma Group; AG: Advanced Glaucoma Group; p value Mann–Whitney <0.05.

TABLE 2: Descriptive statistics of the parameters with the highest diagnostic ability in the CTRL vs. IG, CTRL vs. AG, and IG vs. AG comparisons.

	CTRL			IG			AG		
Parameter	Median	Interquartile range low	Interquartile range high	Median	Interquartile range low	Interquartile range high	Median	Interquartile range low	Interquartile range high
Macula GCL mean inner	52.00	50.25	54.75	43.13	39.25	45.75	27.75	22.50	36.50
Macula GCL mean outer	35.50	32.75	38.50	30.13	27.75	32.25	22.50	20.75	25.75
Macula GCL temporal inner	51.00	47.00	53.00	35.00	29.00	42.00	20.00	18.00	27.00
Macula GCL temporal outer	39.00	35.00	40.00	26.50	24.00	31.00	19.00	17.00	22.00
Macula IPL temporal inner	43.00	40.00	45.00	34.00	32.00	37.00	25.00	22.00	27.00
Macula RNFL mean outer	34.75	33.50	37.00	28.88	25.25	31.50	21.00	19.00	24.50
Macula mean GCL	31.59	29.27	33.20	27.34	26.06	27.88	21.41	19.80	24.14
Macula mean RNFL	40.94	38.61	42.73	32.03	26.06	35.78	20.66	19.52	25.16
cpRNFL global	90.00	79.00	97.00	61.50	58.00	72.00	47.00	39.00	51.00
cpRNFL temporal superior	113.00	101.00	138.00	79.50	66.00	96.00	39.00	31.00	57.00
VFI	99.00	98.00	99.00	92.00	86.00	96.00	49.00	13.00	66.00

GCL: ganglion cell layer; IPL: inner plexiform layer; cpRNFL: circumpapillary retinal nerve fiber layer thickness; VFI: visual field index; CTRL: control group; IG: Early Glaucoma Group; AG: Advanced Glaucoma Group.

ganglion cell layer, inner plexiform layer, inner nuclear layer, outer plexiform layer, outer nuclear layer, retinal pigmented epithelium, inner retinal layers, and outer retinal layer thickness measurements in all sectors as defined by the Early Treatment Diabetic Retinopathy Study scheme (temporal inner, superior inner, nasal inner, inferior inner, temporal outer, superior outer, nasal outer, and inferior outer). In addition, for the purpose of the study, we calculated and evaluated the mean thickness value for each layer.

ONH was also assessed using the GMPE software and retinal nerve fiber layer thickness, and Bruch's membrane opening minimum rim width was obtained.

TABLE 3: Pearson correlation coefficient between VFI and OCT parameters.

Parameter	Correlation with VFI (r)
Macula GCL mean inner	0.81
Macula GCL temporal inner	0.79
Macula GCL superior inner	0.78
Macula IPL temporal inner	0.78
Macula IPL mean inner	0.77
Macula GCL inferior inner	0.76
Mean GCL	0.76
Macula GCL mean outer	0.75
Macula RNFL nasal outer	0.75
Mean RNFL	0.73
Macula GCL temporal outer	0.72
Macula GCL nasal outer	0.71
Macula GCL nasal inner	0.71
Macula RNFL mean outer	0.71
Macula IPL inferior inner	0.70

GCL: ganglion cell layer; IPL: inner plexiform layer; VFI: visual field index; CTRL: control group; IG: Early Glaucoma Group; AG: Advanced Glaucoma Group; r: Pearson correlation coefficient.

Of all the parameters, the presence of statistically significant differences among the groups was evaluated. Subsequently the diagnostic ability of those parameters to discriminate controls versus initial glaucoma, controls versus advanced glaucoma, and initial versus advanced glaucoma was tested using AUC. Subsequently, only the parameters with good ability to discriminate among groups in all of the three comparisons were considered. At macular level, the parameters that best performed were mean GCL, GCL mean inner and outer, GCL temporal inner and outer, IPL temporal inner, mean RNFL, and RNFL mean outer.

At ONH level, the parameters that best performed were circumpapillary RNFL global and temporal superior. None of the Bruch's membrane opening parameters had very high diagnostic accuracy in discriminating among all the groups.

Interestingly, the median of all the parameters discussed above showed reducing thickness values trend with progression of the disease.

Although many efforts have been made in the development of new technologies to diagnose and evaluate the glaucoma progression, clinicians still base their decisions on standard "white-on-white" automated VF testing, which remains the best-studied way to assess disease progression. Nevertheless, many confounding factors, such as media opacity, may affect the results. Most importantly, distraction, or other factors involving the patient's participation make VF tests unreliable. This leads to a high level of disagreement among clinicians whether or not glaucoma is progressing in their patients.

The VFI is a new global metric that represents the entire VF as a single percentage of normal. Based on an aggregate percentage of visual function with 100% being a perfect age-adjusted visual field, it assigns a number between 1% and 100%. Central VF points are more heavily weighted, and the percentage of VF loss is calculated based on pattern or total deviations depending on the depth of loss. Interestingly, the progression rates calculated by VFI are much less affected by

cataract development and cataract surgery than the traditional mean deviation index or the pattern standard deviation [33, 34].

Due to the clinical relevance of VFI, its possible correlation with the OCT parameters has been assessed in this study. Interestingly, most of the OCT parameters showed a correlation with VFI. In particular, macular parameters such as GCL mean inner, GCL temporal inner, GCL superior inner, IPL temporal inner, IPL mean inner, GCL inferior inner, mean GCL, GCL mean outer, RNFL nasal outer, mean RNFL, GCL temporal outer, GCL nasal outer, GCL nasal inner, RNFL mean outer, and IPL inferior inner showed from high to very high correlation with VFI. Thus, suggesting their possible usefulness in the objective evaluation of the progression of the disease.

Interestingly, our data go beyond those of a previous study that showed a good diagnostic ability of macular GCL temporal inner thicknesses in discriminating controls vs. initial glaucoma [35]. In fact, our results suggest that this parameter had, not only a good ability in discriminating controls from initial glaucoma, but also controls from advanced glaucoma and initial glaucoma from advanced glaucoma. Moreover, this parameter showed a very high positive correlation with VFI, showing a strong structure-function correlation, thus further supporting a possible usefulness of OCT parameters in glaucoma diagnosis and follow-up.

There is much interest in the world of scientific research regarding the use of OCT in the diagnosis and follow-up of glaucoma, which is now considered a real neurodegenerative disease [36, 37]. Many studies have focused on the analysis of the diagnostic capacity of this tool in discriminating healthy subjects from subjects with suspected glaucoma or at the initial stage of the disease. Our work has been aimed at pushing beyond searching parameters that would allow, not only an early diagnosis of the disease but also a patient evaluation during lifetime, allowing to discriminate among the patients at the initial stage of the disease and those at an advanced stage.

There are several limitations to this prospective study. The cohort included a small number of patients, and this may have affected our analysis. Moreover, while we aimed to include patients with a broad range of glaucoma severity, the group of patients affected by advanced stages of disease was smaller than all other groups, possibly affecting statistical power.

In conclusion, this study suggests a possible usefulness of macular segmentation and ONH analysis with GMPE in the evaluation of glaucoma patients. Our data suggest that OCT may be a useful tool in detecting macular microstructural changes related to the progression of glaucoma and that this tracking is possible since the early stages of the disease. Our initial results warrant further prospective longitudinal studies on a larger cohort to confirm the ability of OCT parameters, to track disease progression in glaucoma, and eventually test new neuroprotective agents in the management of glaucoma [38, 39].

Conflicts of Interest

The authors declare that they have no conflicts of interest.

References

[1] C. Cedrone, R. Mancino, A. Cerulli, M. Cesareo, and C. Nucci, "Epidemiology of primary glaucoma: prevalence, incidence, and blinding effects," *Progress in Brain Research*, vol. 173, pp. 3–14, 2008.

[2] R. Malik, W. H. Swanson, and D. F. Garway-Heath, "The "structure-function relationship" in glaucoma: past thinking and current concepts," *Clinical & Experimental Ophthalmology*, vol. 40, no. 4, pp. 369–380, 2012.

[3] M. Cesareo, E. Ciuffoletti, F. Ricci et al., "Visual disability and quality of life in glaucoma patients," *Progress in Brain Research*, vol. 221, pp. 359–374, 2015.

[4] EGS Foundation, "European glaucoma society terminology and guidelines for glaucoma, 4th edition—chapter 2: classification and terminology," *British Journal of Ophthalmology*, vol. 101, no. 5, pp. 73–127, 2017.

[5] K. Hirasawa, N. Shoji, T. Morita, and K. Shimizu, "A modified glaucoma staging system based on visual field index," *Graefe's Archive for Clinical and Experimental Ophthalmology*, vol. 251, no. 12, pp. 2747–2752, 2013.

[6] J. A. Swets, "Measuring the accuracy of diagnostic systems," *Science*, vol. 240, no. 4857, pp. 1285–1293, 1998.

[7] M. Mukaka, "A guide to appropriate use of correlation coefficient in medical research," *Malawi Medical Journal: The Journal of Medical Association of Malawi*, vol. 24, no. 3, pp. 69–71, 2012.

[8] D. Huang, E. A. Swanson, C. P. Lin et al., "Optical coherence tomography," *Science*, vol. 254, no. 5035, pp. 1178–1181, 1991.

[9] J. J. Wong, T. C. Chen, L. Q. Shen, and L. R. Pasquale, "Macular imaging for glaucoma using spectral-domain optical coherence tomography: a review," *Seminars in Ophthalmology*, vol. 27, no. 5-6, pp. 160–166, 2012.

[10] K. Mansouri, M. T. Leite, F. A. Medeiros, C. K. Leung, and R. N. Weinreb, "Assessment of rates of structural change in glaucoma using imaging technologies," *Eye*, vol. 25, no. 3, pp. 269–277, 2011.

[11] S. J. Langenegger, J. Funk, and M. Toteberg-Harms, "Reproducibility of retinal nerve fiber layer thickness measurements using the eye tracker and the retest function of spectralis SD-OCT in glaucomatous and healthy control eyes," *Investigative Opthalmology & Visual Science*, vol. 52, no. 6, pp. 3338–3344, 2011.

[12] A. Miraftabi, N. Amini, J. Gornbein et al., "Local variability of macular thickness measurements with SD-OCT and influencing factors," *Translational Vision Science & Technology*, vol. 5, no. 4, p. 5, 2016.

[13] M. Cesareo, E. Ciuffoletti, A. Martucci et al., "Automatic segmentation of posterior pole retinal layers in patients with early stage glaucoma using spectral domain optical coherence tomography," *Journal of Clinical & Experimental Ophthalmology*, vol. 7, no. 2, p. 538, 2016.

[14] R. Zeimer, S. Asrani, S. Zou, H. Quigley, and H. Jampel, "Quantitative detection of glaucomatous damage at the posterior pole by retinal thickness mapping," *A Pilot Study Ophthalmology*, vol. 105, no. 2, pp. 224–231, 1998.

[15] Z. Burgansky-Eliash, G. Wollstein, T. Chu et al., "Optical coherence tomography machine learning classifiers for glaucoma detection: a preliminary study," *Investigative Opthalmology & Visual Science*, vol. 46, no. 11, pp. 4147–4152, 2005.

[16] K. R. Sung, D. Y. Kim, S. B. Park, and M. S. Kook, "Comparison of retinal nerve fiber layer thickness measured by cirrus HD and stratus optical coherence tomography," *Ophthalmology*, vol. 116, no. 7, pp. 1264–1270, 2009.

[17] S. B. Park, K. R. Sung, S. Y. Kang, K. R. Kim, and M. S. Kook, "Comparison of glaucoma diagnostic capabilities of cirrus HD and stratus optical coherence tomography," *Archives of Ophthalmology*, vol. 127, no. 12, pp. 1603–1609, 2009.

[18] J. W. Cho, K. R. Sung, J. T. Hong, T. W. Um, S. Y. Kang, and M. S. Kook, "Detection of glaucoma by spectral domain-scanning laser ophthalmoscopy/optical coherence tomography (SD-SLO/OCT) and time domain optical coherence tomography," *Journal of Glaucoma*, vol. 20, no. 1, pp. 15–20, 2011.

[19] C. J. Shin, K. R. Sung, T. W. Um et al., "Comparison of retinal nerve fiber layer thickness measurements calculated by the optic nerve head map (NHM4) and RNFL 3.45 modes of spectral-domain optical coherence tomography (OCT) (RTVue-100)," *British Journal of Ophthalmology*, vol. 94, no. 6, pp. 763–767, 2010.

[20] H. Wu, J. F. de Boer, and T. C. Chen, "Diagnostic capability of spectral-domain optical coherence tomography for glaucoma," *American Journal of Ophthalmology*, vol. 153, no. 5, pp. 815–826.e2, 2012.

[21] K. R. Sung, G. Wollstein, N. R. Kim et al., "Macular assessment using optical coherence tomography for glaucoma diagnosis," *British Journal of Ophthalmology*, vol. 96, no. 12, pp. 1452–1455, 2012.

[22] G. Wollstein, J. S. Schuman, L. L. Price et al., "Optical coherence tomography (OCT) macular and peripapillary retinal nerve fiber layer measurements and automated visual fields," *American Journal of Ophthalmology*, vol. 138, no. 2, pp. 218–225, 2004.

[23] A. Giovannini, G. Amato, and C. Mariotti, "The macular thickness and volume in glaucoma: an analysis in normal and glaucomatous eyes using OCT," *Acta Ophthalmologica Scandinavica*, vol. 80, no. 236, pp. 34–36, 2002.

[24] D. S. Greenfield, H. Bagga, and R. W. Knighton, "Macular thickness changes in glaucomatous optic neuropathy detected using optical coherence tomography," *Archives of Ophthalmology*, vol. 121, no. 1, pp. 41–46, 2003.

[25] V. Guedes, J. S. Schuman, E. Hertzmark et al., "Optical coherence tomography measurement of macular and nerve fiber layer thickness in normal and glaucomatous human eyes," *Ophthalmology*, vol. 110, no. 1, pp. 177–189, 2003.

[26] D. E. Lederer, J. S. Schuman, E. Hertzmark et al., "Analysis of macular volume in normal and glaucomatous eyes using optical coherence tomography," *American Journal of Ophthalmology*, vol. 135, no. 6, pp. 838–843, 2003.

[27] C. K. Leung, W. M. Chan, W. H. Yung et al., "Comparison of macular and peripapillary measurements for the detection of glaucoma: an optical coherence tomography study," *Ophthalmology*, vol. 112, no. 3, pp. 391–400, 2005.

[28] F. A. Medeiros, L. M. Zangwill, C. Bowd, R. M. Vessani, R. Susanna Jr., and R. N. Weinreb, "Evaluation of retinal nerve fiber layer, optic nerve head, and macular thickness measurements for glaucoma detection using optical coherence tomography," *American Journal of Ophthalmology*, vol. 139, no. 1, pp. 44–55, 2005.

[29] J. M. Martinez-de-la-Casa, P. Cifuentes-Canorea, C. Berrozpe et al., "Diagnostic ability of macular nerve fiber layer thickness using new segmentation software in glaucoma suspects," *Investigative Ophthalmology & Visual Science*, vol. 55, no. 12, pp. 8343–8348, 2014.

[30] Y. Kotera, M. Hangai, F. Hirose, S. Mori, and N. Yoshimura, "Three-dimensional imaging of macular inner structures in glaucoma by using spectral-domain optical coherence tomography," *Investigative Ophthalmology & Visual Science*, vol. 52, no. 3, pp. 1412–1421, 2011.

[31] K. Mathers, J. A. Rosdahl, and S. Asrani, "Correlation of macular thickness with visual fields in glaucoma patients and suspects," *Journal of Glaucoma*, vol. 23, no. 2, pp. e98–e104, 2014.

[32] M. Honjo, K. Omodaka, T. Ishizaki, S. Ohkubo, M. Araie, and T. Nakazawa, "Retinal thickness and the structure/function relationship in the eyes of older adults with glaucoma," *PLoS One*, vol. 10, no. 10, Article ID e0141293, 2015.

[33] H. Bagga, G. Vizzeri, L. M. Zangwill et al., "Correlation of visual field index with optic disc topography and retinal nerve fiber layer thickness," *Investigative Ophthalmology & Visual Science*, vol. 50, no. 13, p. 3514, 2009.

[34] B. Bengtsson and A. Heijl, "A visual field index for calculation of glaucoma rate of progression," *American Journal of Ophthalmology*, vol. 145, no. 2, pp. 343–353, 2008.

[35] M. Pazos, A. A. Dyrda, M. Biarnés et al., "Diagnostic accuracy of spectralis SD OCT automated macular layers segmentation to discriminate normal from early glaucomatous eyes," *Ophthalmology*, vol. 124, no. 8, pp. 1218–1228, 2017.

[36] R. Mancino, M. Cesareo, A. Martucci et al., "Neurodegenerative process linking the eye and the brain," *Current Medicinal Chemistry*, vol. 25, 2018.

[37] R. Mancino, A. Martucci, M. Cesareo et al., "Glaucoma and alzheimer disease: a single age-related neurodegenerative disease of the brain," *Current Neuropharmacology*, vol. 16, no. 7, pp. 971–977, 2017.

[38] C. Nucci, A. Martucci, C. Giannini, L. A. Morrone, G. Bagetta, and R. Mancino, "Neuroprotective agents in the management of glaucoma," *Eye*, vol. 32, no. 5, pp. 938–945, 2018.

[39] C. Nucci, R. Russo, A Martucci et al., "New strategies for neuroprotection in glaucoma, a disease that affects the central nervous system," *European Journal of Pharmacology*, vol. 787, pp. 119–126, 2016.

10

Transpalpebral Electrical Stimulation as a Novel Therapeutic Approach to Decrease Intraocular Pressure for Open-Angle Glaucoma

Félix Gil-Carrasco,[1] **Daniel Ochoa-Contreras,**[1] **Marco A. Torres,**[1] **Jorge Santiago-Amaya,**[2]
Fidel W. Pérez-Tovar,[2] **Roberto Gonzalez-Salinas ⓘ,**[3] **and Luis Nino-de-Rivera ⓘ**[2]

[1]*Glaucoma Department, Hospital Luis Sánchez Bulnes, Asociación para Evitar la Ceguera en México I.A.P, Mexico City, Mexico*
[2]*Artificial Vision Laboratory, Instituto Politécnico Nacional, Mexico City, Mexico*
[3]*Research Department, Asociación para Evitar la Ceguera en México I.A.P, Mexico City, Mexico*

Correspondence should be addressed to Luis Nino-de-Rivera; luisninoderivera@gmail.com

Academic Editor: Enrique Mencía-Gutiérrez

Purpose. To determine the effect on intraocular pressure of transpalpebral specific exogenous voltages in a cohort of open-angle glaucoma patients. *Methods.* This is a prospective, comparative, and experimental pilot study. The electrical stimuli applied consisted of 10 Hz, biphasic, nonrectangular current pulses (100 μA) delivered from an isolated constant current stimulator. At intake, baseline IOP measurements were obtained from each eye. The measurement was repeated before and after microstimulation until the end of the treatment. *Results.* Seventy-eight eyes of 46 patients diagnosed with POAG were studied: 58 eyes with maximum tolerated medical treatment and 20 eyes without treatment (naïve). The mean baseline IOP on the treated POAG group was 19.25 mmHg ± 4.71. Baseline IOP on the naïve group was 20.38 mmHg ± 3.28. At the four-month follow-up visit, the mean IOP value on the treatment group was 14.41 mmHg ± 2.06 ($P < 0.0001$). The obtained mean IOP measurement on the treatment-naïve group was 15.29 mmHg ± 2.28 ($P < 0.0001$). *Conclusions.* The hypotensive response obtained using transpalpebral electrical stimulation on POAG patients, both on treatment-naïve patients and on patients receiving maximum tolerable treatment, was statistically significant when comparing basal IOP measurements to those obtained at the four-month follow-up visit.

1. Introduction

Primary open-angle glaucoma (POAG) is considered the world's leading cause of irreversible blindness [1]. One of the main risk factors for the occurrence and progression of this disease is an increase in intraocular pressure (IOP), primarily due to the dysfunction of the conventional drainage or trabecular pathway [2]. Oxidative stress and vascular damage play major roles in triggering apoptotic cell loss in these tissues [3, 4]. Molecular alterations occurring in the ocular anterior chamber during the early course of glaucoma trigger this cell loss [5]. Therefore, initial treatments, such as hypotensive drugs, usually aim to lower IOP. These drugs primarily focus on decreasing aqueous humor (AH) production or, alternatively, improving the outflow via nonconventional routes. Parasympathetic mimetic drugs can indirectly improve AH depletion via the trabecular route by stimulating muscular fibers contractility in the trabecular meshwork, which improves the AH outflow [5]. The trabecular meshwork is not merely a passive drainage filter but acts directly and actively on the resistance to AH passage via mechanisms that are not fully understood [6].

Several authors have described alterations in the mechanical properties of trabecular cells due to ion channel dysfunction, which affects the volume and elasticity of the cell. These changes may affect the permeability or ease of drainage of the trabecular system, and the contractile state and its induction have been recently studied in this context [7]. Stumpff et al. demonstrated that abnormal deposits of tyrosine kinase in the trabecula are related to the dysfunctional passage of the AH through the trabeculae into Schlemm's duct. These abnormal deposits cause the trabecular cell to increase in volume and lose elasticity, primarily due to the dysfunction of calcium- (Ca^{2+}-) activated potassium (maxi K) channels [8]. Moreover, tyrosine kinase inhibitors activate the maxi-KCa^{2+} ($BKCa^{2+}$) channels in the bovine trabecular veins and that hyperpolarization caused by the potassium efflux of the trabecular cells can lead to the relaxation of the trabecular meshwork to facilitate the outflow and passage of AH to Schlemm's channel [8–10]. Previous reports showed that tyrosine kinase inhibitors relax the bands of precontracted trabecular tissue. Specifically, the application of *genistein*, a tyrosine kinase inhibitor in trabecular cells previously contracted with acetylcholine, induced a dose-dependent reversible increase in the output current to 578% ± 154% ($n = 16$) of the initial current levels [1, 9]. The electrophysiology of $BKCa^{2+}$ channels observed when inhibiting tyrosine kinase demonstrates their activation and their function in the regulation of intracellular Ca^{2+}. Soto et al. showed that the concentrations of intracellular Ca^{2+} in trabecular meshwork cells (TMCs, human, and bovine) directly correlated with the magnitude of the ionic current of $BKCa^{2+}$ [11]. Furthermore, the behavior of the voltage-dependent K^+ channels in TMCs is of the current rectifier type and directly correlates with increasing concentrations of intracellular Ca to modify the membrane potential [9, 10].

Recent studies by our research group [12] and in the Andreas Schattz group [9] demonstrate that transcorneal electrical stimulation (TES) using biphasic pulses of 20 Hz and up to 1100 μA are beneficial to patients with retinitis pigmentosa (RP). Moreover, we noted that the application of TES in patients with PR decreased the IOP in several of these patients, which prompted us to study the effects of electrical stimulation as a possible alternative to control IOP.

The present pilot study aims at demonstrating a significant IOP decrease employing transpalpebral electrical stimulation (TPES) on open-angle glaucoma patients with maximum tolerated medical treatment and on those without treatment (naïve patients).

2. Materials and Methods

The Internal Review Board of the Asociación para Evitar la Ceguera en México I.A.P. approved this study. All the procedures conformed to the tenets of the Declaration of Helsinki; the good clinical practices guidelines comply with the issued regulations of the Standards for Privacy of Individually Identifiable Health Information (HIPAA). A signed written informed consent form was obtained from all of the participants after providing an explanation of the procedures to be used and possible complications.

2.1. Design. This is a prospective, comparative, and experimental study, conducted at the Glaucoma Department at

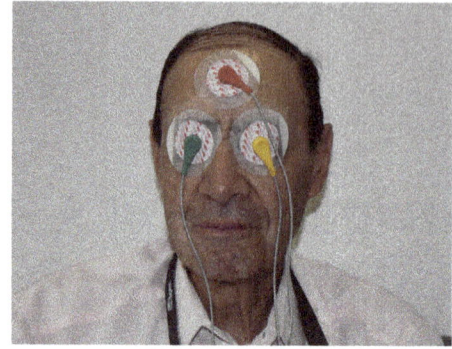

FIGURE 1: Transpalpebral electrical microstimulation procedure on a POAG patient.

the Asociación para Evitar la Ceguera en Mexico I.A.P., Luis Sánchez Bulnes Hospital in Mexico City, Mexico, in collaboration with the Vision Laboratory from the Instituto Politécnico Nacional, Mexico City, Mexico, from May 2015 to April 2017.

2.2. Patients. A total of 78 eyes from 46 patients with POAG were included in this study; 58 of these patients were receiving the maximum tolerated medical treatment and did not reach their target tensional values, whereas 20 patients were treatment naïve to drugs.

Key inclusion criteria included patients ≥40 years of age, diagnosed with POAG with or without topical treatment which required lowering the IOP to achieve their target IOP. We excluded patients with any previous ocular surgery, infectious eye disease, uveitis, or any other inflammatory ocular disorders, kwon allergies, corneal abnormalities, or previous conditions that prevent IOP measurement, as well as a history for ocular trauma.

All of the subjects had a comprehensive ocular examination including a review of the medical history, slit-lamp examination, Goldmann applanation tonometry, IOP measurement, central corneal thickness, cup to disk ratio, gonioscopy, optic nerve OCT, visual field evaluation, and dilated fundus examination.

2.3. Microstimulation Procedure. The waveform more frequently used by authors in TES is shown in Figure 1(a). However, based on the antecedents previously discussed in Introduction, the tension response to electrical stimuli delivered by a transpalpebral device was studied in patients with glaucoma. This device reproduces electric profiles analogous to those reported by Stumpff and Wiederholt [10] in the $BKCa^{2+}$ after the application of tyrosine kinase inhibitors and may be used as an adjuvant treatment to control IOP in patients with POAG. The waveform shown in Figure 1(b) fits more accurately with $BKCa^{2+}$ ionic cells in TMC.

The electrical stimuli applied in our study consisted of 10 Hz, biphasic nonrectangular current pulses (up to 100 μA) that were delivered from an isolated constant current stimulator. Every TPES application was performed at the same time of the day for all patients (between 9:00 and

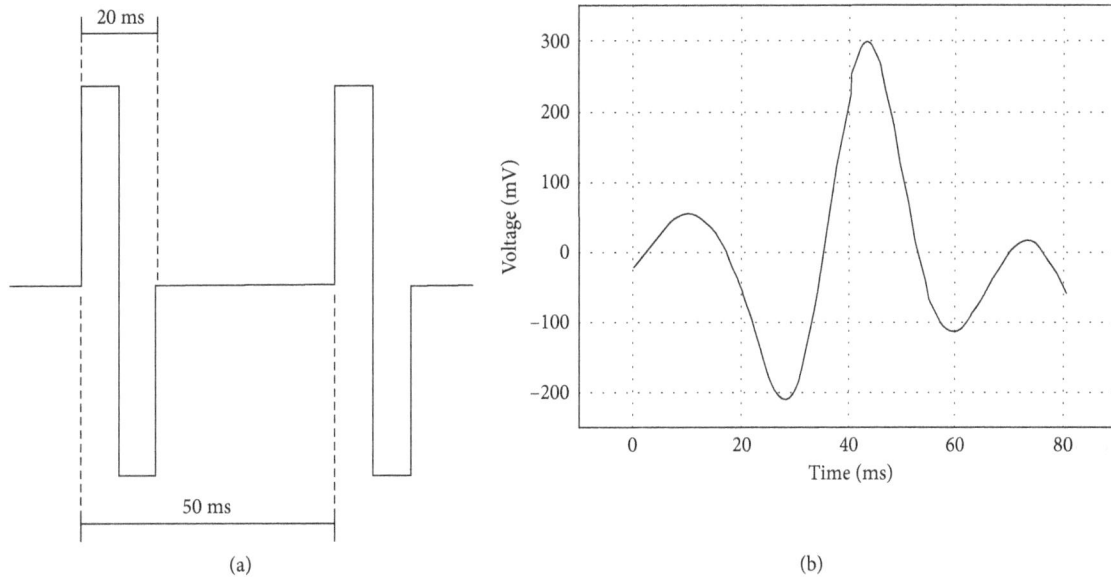

FIGURE 2: (a) Biphasic waveform applied on the most reported TES; (b) a new voltage waveform approach used in TPES.

10:00 h). The microstimulation procedure consisted of daily TPES application for 40 minutes attaching the current electrode to the eyelid employing polyurethane adhesive film fragments for a total of 10 days, divided into two 5-period days, with a rest of 2 days in between for a period of two weeks as depicted in Figure 1. Afterwards, application was continued twice per week for the remaining time until the four-month visit.

2.4. Instrumentation. The transpalpebral electronic stimulator based on a digital adaptive model delivers an electronic waveform generator specific for transpalpebral electrical stimulation. The applied waveform model is generated on a digital processor by means of an adaptive finite impulse response filter, in which the output waveform is synthesized form the original waveform registered from a multifocal electroretinograph as depicted in Figure 2.

2.5. Statistical Analysis. Statistical significance for IOP changes between groups was determined using a Student's *t*-test for normally distributed variables. Otherwise, we employed the Wilcoxon matched-pairs signed rank test. In addition, a Pearson correlation coefficient (r) and linear regression analysis were obtained between age and the fourth-month visit IOP (95% CI and a two-tailed P value). P values less than 0.05 were considered statistically significant. Normal and nonnormal distributions were determined using the Shapiro–Wilk tests for all variables.

Statistical analyses were performed using the Statistical Package for Social Sciences (SPSS) software (version 20, SPSS, Inc., Chicago, IL, USA). Graphs and layouts depicted in the Results were elaborated using the 2015 Graph Pad software Inc., Prism version 6.0.

3. Results

A total of seventy-eight eyes from 46 POAG patients were included in this study, 58 eyes with maximum tolerated medical treatment and 20 eyes without treatment (naïve). No statistically significant differences were evidenced between groups in terms of age ($P = 0.358$). All demographic data are summarized in Table 1.

The mean baseline IOP on the maximum tolerated medical treatment group was 19.25 mmHg ± 4.71. On the contrary, the mean baseline IOP on the treatment-naïve patients was 20.38 mmHg ± 3.28. At the four-month follow-up visit, the mean IOP values obtained on the maximum tolerated medical treatment group was 14.41 mmHg ± 2.06, which accounts for a 25.14% IOP reduction. The obtained mean IOP measurement on the treatment-naïve group was 15.29 mmHg ± 2.28, which represents a 25.97% IOP reduction.

In Figure 3, IOP comparison is depicted between baseline and four-month follow-up visit ($P < 0.0001$) for all POAG patients including those with maximum tolerated medical treatment (Figure 3(a)) and those without treatment ($P < 0.0001$) (Figure 3(b)).

In Figure 4, IOP comparison is described between baseline and four-month follow-up visit measurement for the right eye (Figure 4(a)) and the left eye (Figure 4(b)) on the naïve POAG patients.

The compared IOP values for POAG patients with maximum tolerated medical treatment at baseline and at the four-month follow-up visit are presented in Figure 5.

The Pearson correlation coefficient (r) and linear regression analysis (R^2) obtained between patients' years of age and the final IOP measurement at the four-month follow-up visit were as follows: $r = -0.367, R^2 = -0.134$, and $P = 0.006$, as depicted in Figure 6.

TABLE 1: Demographic data of included POAG patients.

Variable	Male	Female	Total	P value*	95% CI of the difference
Eyes (n)	37	39	76	—	—
Gender (%)	48.69	51.31	100	—	—
Age (years)					
Mean ± SD	63.24 ± 11.12	59.05 ± 15.23	68.07 ± 12.06	0.358	−4.94 to 13.31
Range	40, 79	23, 77	12, 101		

*Wilcoxon matched-pairs signed rank test.

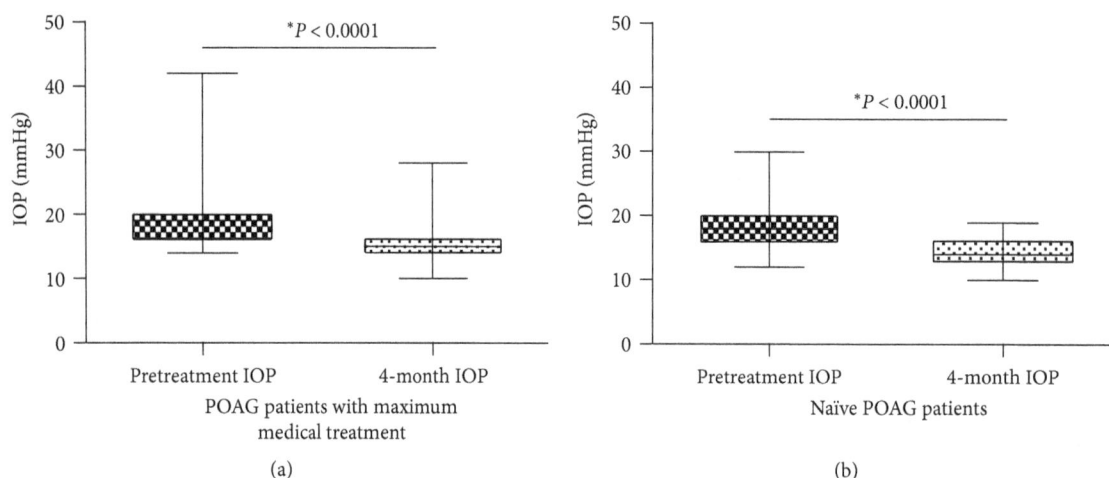

FIGURE 3: (a) Comparison between IOP values obtained before electrical stimulation to those measured at the four-month follow-up visit for POAG patients receiving the maximum tolerated medical treatment. (b) Comparison between IOP values obtained before electrical stimulation to those measured at the four-month follow-up visit from naïve patients. *Wilcoxon matched-pairs signed rank test.

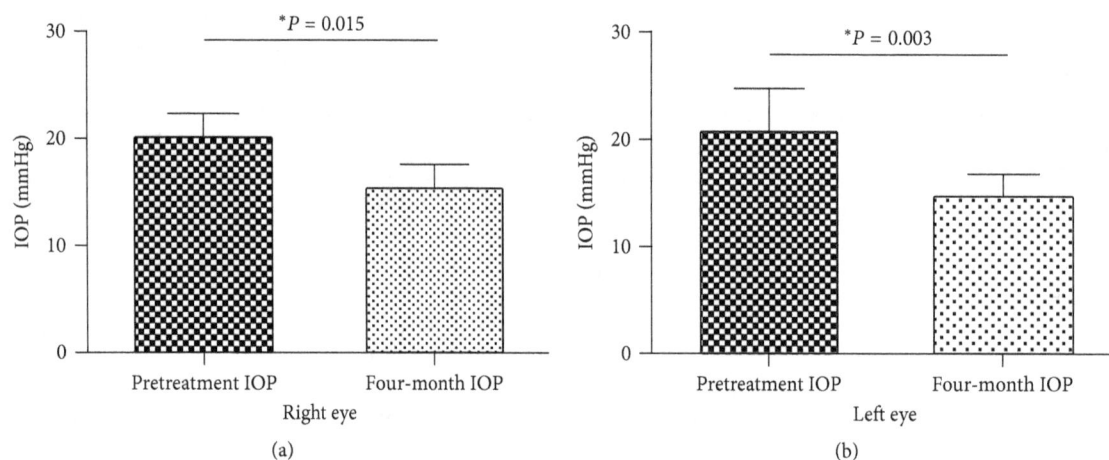

FIGURE 4: IOP measurements obtained from POAG patients without treatment (naïve): (a) comparison of IOP values before electrical stimulation to those obtained at the four-month follow-up visit for the right eye; (b) comparison of IOP values before electrical stimulation to those obtained at the four-month follow-up visit in the left eye. *Wilcoxon matched-pairs signed rank test.

4. Discussion

Understanding the physiology of the trabecular cell, the active membrane components that explain its activity, the pathophysiology of trabecular dysfunction, and the role of ion channels, primarily maxi K channels, facilitate an alternative therapeutic hypotensive ocular approach for glaucoma patients [10].

In recent years, the electrophysiology of TMCs has garnered increasing interest, and the behavior of voltage-dependent $BKCa^{2+}$ channels and their relationship to various conditions, such as POAG, has been studied [11]. There

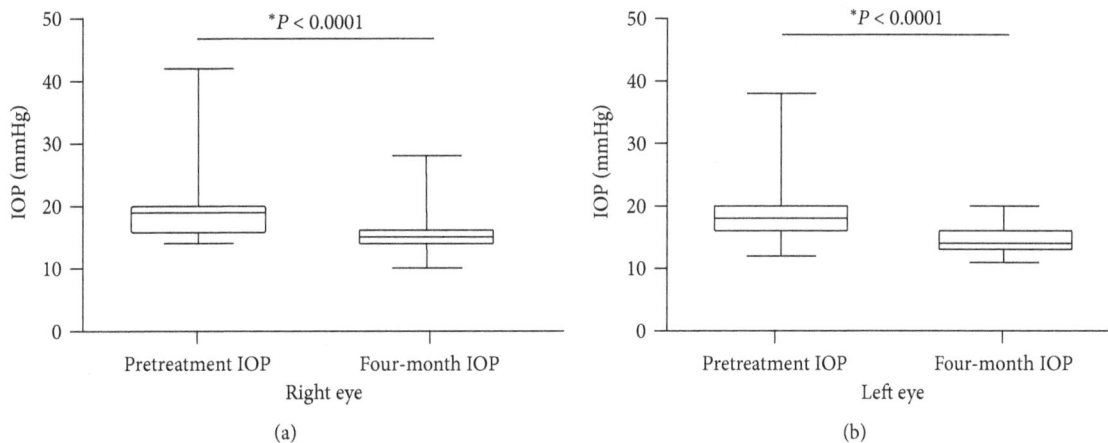

FIGURE 5: IOP measurements obtained from POAG patients receiving maximum tolerated medical treatment: (a) comparison between IOP values obtained before electrical stimulation to those obtained at the four-month follow-up visit for the right eye; (b) comparison between IOP values obtained before electrical stimulation to those obtained at the four-month follow-up visit for the left eye. *Wilcoxon matched-pairs signed rank test.

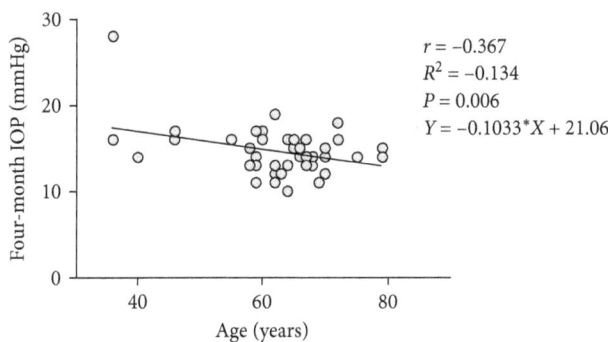

FIGURE 6: Coefficient of correlation (r) and linear regression analysis (R^2) between POAG patients' years of age and IOP measurement at the four-month follow-up visit. *Pearson correlation coefficients (r), 95% CI, and two-tailed P value.

are three types of voltage-dependent potassium channels in both healthy and glaucomatous cells. In the cases studied, the behavior of the ionic currents of 3 different K^+ channels for normal TMCs and glaucomatous TMCs (GTMCs) exhibited significant differences in membrane amplitude and voltage [11].

We propose the application of transpalpebral specific exogenous voltages to act similarly to tyrosine kinase inhibitors. Specifically, applying an electric potential from the eyelid induces membrane potentials analogous to those found by Stumpff and Wiederholt [10] and Soto et al. [11] and stimulates the reactivation of $BKCa^{2+}$ in TMCs. The application of exogenous electric fields can reactivate the $BKCa^{2+}$ sequestered by the action of kinases in patients with POAG, obtaining an analogous reaction to that reported by tyrosine kinase inhibitors, thus contributing to IOP control [10–15].

Most reported research in TES, both indirect and direct stimulation, uses simple bipolar square waveforms to target a complex neural network system at the inner retina [8, 9].

Only a few authors suggest stimulation by sinusoidal and other nonsquare waveforms [14, 15]. Square bipolar waveforms are not consistent with the typical cell ionic current patterns. However, the relationship between TES parameters and the effect on IOP and other eye structures is still unclear.

In our study, the ocular hypotensive response obtained was statistically significant for both groups, the treatment-naïve group and the group of POAG patients with previous maximum tolerable treatment. Moreover, the results of the previously treated group clinically confirm the rescue of primary trabecular function in the setting of reduced AH production and the stimulation of the uveoscleral or non-conventional drainage pathways [14].

The hypotensive response obtained in this group of patients, even in patients having received maximum tolerable treatment, was comparable to that described with prostaglandin analogues or various drug combinations [16, 17]. Therefore, this treatment could be comparable to first-line ocular hypotensive treatment but does not affect the ocular surface or exert systemic or local side effects.

The flexibility to generate any desired action potential opens fresh opportunities to brand new experiments in transpalpebral stimulation. Our stimulator system can reproduce any real biological ionic currents with 99.9% accuracy. These new approaches to stimulate TMCs open brand new opportunities to understand more precisely the neuroregulation effects of electrical stimulation in glaucoma.

Transpalpebral electrical microstimulation is not an invasive procedure. Thus, this treatment modality is advantageous to conventional medical treatment consisting of hypotensive ocular drugs, which are associated with local and possible systemic side effects. This procedure induces no changes on the ocular surface in opposition to ocular surface changes induced by the topical medication and the preservatives. No inflammatory phenomenon is generated; moreover, the immunological apparatus remains unaltered. Electrical microstimulation focuses to the true cause of ocular hypertension, that is, the treatment of the dysfunctional trabeculum, while the rest of the therapy is focused on reducing the production of the aqueous humor or the exit of it through the unconventional route. In addition, it is important to emphasize the fact that this approach is highly cost efficient, especially when compared to the gold standard antiglaucoma therapy, which can elevate the long-term overall expenditures.

Long-term follow-up of larger cohorts will allow identifying potential refractory periods in the trabecular function or functional recovery of trabecular cells. Thus, such studies are necessary to demonstrate the effectiveness of this procedure.

Conflicts of Interest

The authors declare that they have no conflicts of interest.

Acknowledgments

The present work was supported by a grant from the CONACYT, Instituto Politécnico Nacional, and Asociación para Evitar la Ceguera en México, I.A.P. (Grant no. 0261660).

References

[1] Y. C. Tham, X. Li, T. Y. Wong, H. A. Quigley, T. Aung, and C. Y. Cheng, "Global prevalence of glaucoma and projections of glaucoma burden through 2040: a systematic review and meta-analysis," *Ophthalmology*, vol. 121, no. 11, pp. 2081–2090, 2014.

[2] D. Schmidl, L. Schmetterer, G. Garhöfer, and A. Popa-Cherecheanu, "Pharmacotherapy of glaucoma," *Journal of Ocular Pharmacology and Therapeutics*, vol. 31, no. 2, pp. 63–77, 2015.

[3] G. Tezel, X. Yang, C. Luo et al., "Oxidative stress and the regulation of complement activation in human glaucoma," *Investigative Opthalmology and Visual Science*, vol. 51, no. 10, pp. 5071–5082, 2010.

[4] A. Harris, B. Siesky, and B. Wirostko, "Cerebral blood flow in glaucoma patients," *Journal of Glaucoma*, vol. 22, pp. S46–S48, 2013.

[5] S. C. Saccà, A. Pulliero, and A. Izzotti, "The dysfunction of the trabecular meshwork during glaucoma course," *Journal of Cellular Physiology*, vol. 230, no. 3, pp. 510–525, 2015.

[6] W. D. Stamer and T. S. Acott, "Current understanding of conventional outflow dysfunction in glaucoma," *Current Opinion in Ophthalmology*, vol. 23, no. 2, pp. 135–143, 2012.

[7] M. P. Fautsch and D. H. Johnson, "Aqueous humor outflow: what do we know? Where will it lead us?," *Investigative Opthalmology and Visual Science*, vol. 47, no. 10, pp. 4181–4187, 2006.

[8] F. Stumpff, Y. Que, M. Boxberger, O. Strauss, and M. Wiederholt, "Stimulation of maxi-K channels in trabecular meshwork by tyrosine kinase inhibitors," *Investigative Opthalmology and Visual Science*, vol. 40, no. 7, pp. 1404–1417, 1999.

[9] A. Schatz, J. Pach, M. Gosheva et al., "Transcorneal electrical stimulation for patients with retinitis pigmentosa: a prospective, randomized, sham-controlled follow-up study over 1 year transcorneal electrical stimulation for RP," *Investigative*

Opthalmology and Visual Science, vol. 58, no. 1, pp. 257–269, 2017.

[10] F. Stumpff and M. Wiederholt, "Regulation of trabecular meshwork contractility," *Current Opinion in Ophthalmology*, vol. 9, pp. 46–49, 1998.

[11] D. Soto, N. Comes, E. Ferrer et al., "Modulation of aqueous humor outflow by ionic mechanisms involved in trabecular meshwork cell volume regulation," *Investigative Opthalmology and Visual Science*, vol. 45, no. 10, pp. 3650–3656, 2004.

[12] J. Grant, V. Tran, S. K. Bhattacharya, and L. Bianchi, "Ionic currents of human trabecular meshwork cells from control and glaucoma subjects," *Journal of Membrane Biology*, vol. 246, no. 2, pp. 167–175, 2013.

[13] D. Robles-Camarillo, L. Niño-de-Rivera, J. López-Miranda, F. Gil-Carrasco, and H. Quiroz-Mercado, "The effect of transcorneal electrical stimulation in visual acuity: Retinitis pigmentosa," *Journal of Biomedical Science and Engineering*, vol. 6, no. 10, pp. 1–7, 2013.

[14] L. Niño-de-Rivera, F. W. Pérez-Tovar, J. S. Amaya et al., "Flexible polyimide microelectrodes array for transcorneal electrical stimulation," *Journal of Biomedical Science and Engineering*, vol. 8, no. 8, pp. 544–554, 2015.

[15] T. Morimoto, T. Miyoshi, H. Sawai, and T. Fujikado, "Optimal parameters of transcorneal electrical stimulation (TES) to be neuroprotective of axotomized RGCs in adult rats," *Experimental Eye Research*, vol. 90, no. 2, pp. 285–291, 2010.

[16] J. Xie, L. Yow, G. J. Wang et al., "Modeling and percept of transcorneal electrical stimulation in humans," *IEEE Transactions on Biomedical Engineering*, vol. 28, no. 7, pp. 1932–1939, 2011.

[17] A. G. Konstas, L. Quaranta, B. Bozkurt et al., "24-h efficacy of glaucoma treatment options," *Advances in Therapy*, vol. 33, no. 4, pp. 481–517, 2016.

11

Evaluating Eye Drop Instillation Technique and its Determinants in Glaucoma Patients

Xinbo Gao, Qiongman Yang, Wenmin Huang, Tingting Chen, Chengguo Zuo, Xinyan Li, Wuyou Gao, and Huiming Xiao ⓘ

State Key Laboratory of Ophthalmology, Zhongshan Ophthalmic Center, Sun Yat-sen University, Guangzhou 510060, China

Correspondence should be addressed to Huiming Xiao; 1250559136@qq.com

Academic Editor: Jesús Pintor

Aim. To evaluate eye drop instillation technique and to explore its determinants in glaucoma patients. *Methods.* One hundred and thirteen patients diagnosed with glaucoma and self-administering topical antiglaucoma eye drops for at least 1 month were evaluated. All patients instilled artificial tear solution in one eye as they would do at home. The whole process was evaluated by two study staff. A comprehensive score system associated with eye drop instillation techniques was used to quantify the instillation technique and explore its determinants such as demographic and clinical characteristics. *Results.* Half of the patients (48.67%) finished the administration of eye drop on first attempt.1.7 eye drops were squeezed out on average. 43 patients (37.17%) got contact with ocular surface or adnexa. Only 19.7% patients had eye drop instillation techniques being defined as well. 11 patients (9.7%) had prior instruction regarding using eye drops, while only 4 patients knew to occlude the tear duct by pressing the dacryocyst area. Older age and worse visual acuity were found to be independent risk factors for worse instillation technique. *Conclusions.* Eye drop instillation technique in glaucoma patients deserves great attention from eye care practitioners during their lifelong follow-up, especially those aged older and have worse visual acuity.

1. Introduction

Glaucoma is a chronic eye disease causing blindness in millions of people worldwide [1]. Ocular hypotensive eye drops are the most common treatment for lowering the intraocular pressure, which until now is the only proved way to slow the progression of the disease. During lifelong follow-up, a daily, correct administration by the patient is required. However, it is reported nearly half of the patients with glaucoma could not use the eye drops properly [2].

Unlike oral medicines, eye drops require patients to use proper technique for successful medication administration. This requires not only instilling a single drop accurately into the conjunctiva of the eye but also without contacting eye drop container with the ocular surface or adnexa. It is reported more than half of the patients omitted 10% of doses and 15% of patients omitted half doses [3]. Poor eye drop instillation in adherence not only leads to reduced treatment effectiveness but also increases costs in such chronic disease. Systemic side effects, infection, or trauma can also be induced

due to overdose or contacting the eye drop container with the eye [4]. Accordingly, this study aimed to explore the status of patients in busy clinical setting of a developing country and to evaluate the determinants of the drop instillation skill.

2. Methods

A cross-sectional design was used and 113 patients with glaucoma were enrolled in this study between August 1, 2016 and December 30, 2016. Nine patients who were approached to enroll in the study declined participation. All subjects were consented prior to enrollment and the protocol followed the tenets of the Declaration of Helsinki; the study was approved by the Ethic Board of Zhongshan Ophthalmic Center.

We included all consecutive subjects with diagnosis of glaucoma, aged over 18 years old, self-administrating eye drops with no compliance aids more than 6 months, having better visual acuity no less than 20/200 in either eye, using at least one topical hypotensive medications in one or both eyes. Subjects were only excluded if they had disability in

TABLE 1: Scheme used to grade eye drop instillation technique.

Description of technique	Score
Good technique, on target, and no contamination	5
Awkward technique, on target, and no contamination	4
On target but contaminates by touching the bottle tip to the lashes or lid	3
On target but contaminates by touching the bottle tip to bulbar conjunctiva or cornea*	2
Not on target, and no contamination	1
Not on target and contaminates the bottle tip by touching the eye, eyelid, or lashes	0

On target: delivered the eye drop to the eye or conjunctiva sac; *Added risk of trauma to ocular surface.

TABLE 2: Patients' demographic, clinical characteristics ($N = 113$).

Item	Result
Demographic characteristics	
Age (y), mean (SD)	56.53 (14.60)
Male sex, n (%)	62 (54.87)
Education level, n (%)	
≤middle school	60 (53.10)
>middle school	53 (46.90)
Location, n (%)	
Urban	85 (75.22)
Rural	28 (24.78)
Clinical characteristics	
UCVA, * n (%)	
Good (≥6/12)	84 (74.34)
Intermediate (<6/12 and ≥6/18)	10 (8.85)
Poor (<6/18)	19 (16.81)
Visual field stage, ** n (%)	
Early stage	42 (37.17)
Medium stage	29 (25.66)
Late stage	42 (37.17)
Number of local eye drops, n (%)	
<4	62 (54.87)
4–6	51 (45.13)
Duration of using eye drops (y), n (%)	
<1	108 (95.58)
1–5	5 (4.42)

SD: standard deviation; UCVA: uncorrected visual acuity. *Use UCVA of the eye, which had better visual acuity in this item. **Use visual field of the eye, which had better visual acuity in this item.

communication or physical impediments to eye drop use [5]. In addition, subjects were required to have had a complete ophthalmic exam within the preceding 6 months. If it was not available, the patient completed testing during study enrollment.

Subject Characteristics—we measured age as continuous variables and gender as a dichotomous variable. Levels of education was originally measured as a categorical variable and then was dichotomized for the multivariable analyses (i.e., under middle school, higher than middle school). The number of glaucoma medications being taken was measured as a continuous variable and then recoded into one versus two or more for the multivariable analyses. Length of time having using antiglaucoma eye drops was measured as a dichotomous variable: one year or more. Visual field defects were classified as mild (mean deviation ≥ −6 dB), moderate (mean deviation < −6 but > −12 dB), or severe (mean deviation ≤ −12 dB) according to Hodapp-Anderson criteria [1]. The reliability parameters of less than 20% errors were used.

Eye drop instillation technique—subjects were first escorted to an exam room and instructed to instill a 5 ml sterile artificial tear solution just as they usually did at home. They were free for a second attempt while they were not satisfied with their first attempt but no prompting was given. The right eye was assigned if the patients had prescribed eye drops for both eyes. The entire process was observed and recorded by two research staff. When there was disagreement between graders, a consensus grading was used. A comprehensive list of items associated with eye drop instillation techniques was developed, based on prior research [6]. Skill score system was based on previous studies [6, 7] which are demonstrated in Table 1. The total process patients instilled eye drops was recorded and scored on each eye drop attempt. Score of quite first drop and last drop, average score of skill of all eye drops, and total skill score were analyzed. Perfect instillation technique was defined as being to instill a single drop in the eye conjunctiva on the first attempt without touching one's eyelid or face. Participants were also asked to recall whether they had had any instruction on skills of instilling eye drops previously, and if so, from whom. Multiple linear regression was examined to explore how the demographic characteristics (gender, age, race, levels of education, number of glaucoma medications, and length of time

diagnosed with glaucoma), clinical characteristics, knowledge of using eye drops, and instruction history were associated with total skill score. Next, in a different multivariable logistic regression model, we examined the same factors whether associated with the first drop score system (whether patients had successful perfect eye drop during the first try). Variables with a $p < 0.05$ in the univariable analysis were included in the multivariable regression model.

3. Results

One hundred and thirteen subjects participated in the study and their demographic characteristics are presented in Table 2. Sixty-two of the participates were male, 85% lived in urban and 60% had education level lower than middle school and subjects aged 56.5 years on average. Percentages of subjects with early, mild, and late stage of visual field defect severity for their better eyes were, respectively, 37.2%, 25.7%, and 37.2%. More than half of the sample (54.9%) had been using less than four eye drops and most (95.6%) had a history of less than one year in this study.

As shown in Table 3, most patients (93.8%) controlled the interval between eye drops more than 5 minutes; however, only 3.5% patients knew to press the dacryocyst area

Table 3: Patients' knowledge and education experience of using eye drops ($N = 113$).

Item	Result
Knowledge of using eye drops	
Interval between each eye drops, *n* (%)	
5 minutes	7 (6.19)
10 minutes	105 (92.92)
30 minutes	1 (0.88)
Press dacryocyst area, *n* (%)	
Yes	4 (3.54)
No	109 (96.46)
Education/training experience of using eye drops	
Having training of using eye drops, *n* (%)	
Yes	11 (9.73)
No	102 (90.27)
Education method, *n* (%)	
By doctor/nurse in ZOC	8 (72.73)
By doctor/nurse in other hospital	1 (9.09)
Reading education brochure	2 (18.18)
Education time, *n* (%)	
5 minutes	4 (36.36)
10 minutes	5 (45.45)
30 minutes	2 (18.18)

SD: standard deviation; ZOC: Zhongshan Ophthalmic Center.

Table 4: Patients' skill of using eye drops.

Item	Result
Skill score system	
Score of quite first drop of eye drops (0.5), mean (SD)	0.04 (0.47)
Score of number of last drop (0–5), mean (SD)	4.35 (0.71)
Average score of skill of each eye drops (0–5), mean (SD)	2.53 (1.15)
Total skill score (0–15), mean (SD)	6.93 (1.88)
First drop score system	
Finish in first drop, *n* (%)	
Yes	55 (48.67)
No	58 (51.33)

SD: standard deviation.

after instilling the eye drops. Only a small part of patients (9.7%) have training experience of using eye drops, of which mostly (81.8%) by doctor or nurse in the hospital.

From Table 4, only half (48.67%) of the participants finish administrating eye drops on the first try. The average drops used was 1.7 ± 0.8 which transformed to 4.35 ± 0.71 in total score system. The average total skill score was 6.93 ± 1.88 and first drop skill score was 0.04 ± 0.47. Of patients regarding quite first drop, 11 (11/113, 9.7%) missed the eye and got contamination with the drop (score of 0), 46 (46/113, 40.7%) missed the eye, 7 (7/113, 6.2%) got target but touched the tip of the bottle to the bulbar conjunctiva or cornea, and 24 (24/113, 21.2%) got target but touched the eyelid or lashes with the tip of the bottle. Twenty-five subjects (25/113, 22.1%) successfully finished administration during the first try, of which eight subjects (8/113, 7.1%) had the best expertise and scored highest.

Table 5 shows the results of the linear model for predicting good drop instillation technique. Total skill score was chosen as response variable. Factors of demographic, clinical characteristics, knowledge of using eye drops, and previous education were assessed by univariable analysis. It showed that younger age, better education, better visual acuity, knowledge of pressing the dacryocyst area to occlude the punctum, and prior instruction regarding using eye drops were the factors significantly associated with a good technique ($p < 0.05$ for all). In the multivariable model, only age, visual acuity, and previous education on drop instillation technique remained significant. Table 6 shows the results of the logistic regression model for predicting whether it finished successfully in the first drop. Consistent with the total skill predicting model, same risk factors were confirmed in the univariable analysis. However, only age and visual acuity remained significant in multivariable regression. Prior instructions on using eye drops were not included in the final logistic regression model.

4. Discussion

Glaucoma is a slowly progressive eye disease, and prescribed glaucoma regimen adherence has long been an issue with glaucoma patients [5]. Improper administration of eye drops is often of a variety of unintentional noncompliance and underreported [8]. Unawareness is not only from patients but also from eye care providers especially in busy clinical practices [9]. Approximately 80% of patients instill their own eye drops by themselves and mostly, no delivery aids are adopted [10]. Our study indicates that only 19.7% patients managed to successfully instill eye drops into conjunctiva sac on first attempt.

Although volume of one drop (50 uL) dispensed from bottle far exceeds the capacity of conjunctiva sac (5 uL), our study showed it is not easy for patients to achieve the administration of medication. The mean drops squeezed by each patient per application per eye were 1.57. The mean drops instilled in the conjunctiva were 1.33. Brown et al. [11] found that 21% glaucoma patients administered 2 or more drops in their eyes by themselves. In a similar study, Dietlein et al. [12] reported that only 57% patients managed to instill eye drops in the conjunctival sac and 28.5% of patients closed their eyelids for at least 3 minutes after administration, while only 5.7% occluded the punctum. Even worse, only 3.5% (4/113) patients in our study tried to occlude the punctum after administration. A substantial amount of eye drops was wasted and increased the cost associated with treatment due to the faulty instillation technique. Unable to press the dacryocyst area again increased the bypass outflow of the medicine and systemic absorption. Unwanted adverse effects [13] includes those common side effects such as periocular

TABLE 5: Linear model of potential predictors of patients' skill score of using eye drops (skill score system) (significant items were highlighted in bold).

	Simple regression β (95% CI)	p value	Multiple regression[†] β (95% CI)	p value
Demographic characteristics				
Mean of age	**−0.05 (−0.07, −0.03)**	**<0.001**	**−0.03 (−0.05, −0.01)**	**0.002**
Male sex	−0.56 (−1.26, 0.14)	0.118		
Education level				
≤middle school	Reference			
>middle school	**0.88 (0.19, 1.56)**	**0.013**	0.51 (−0.10, 1.11)	0.100
Location				
Urban	Reference			
Rural	0.31 (−0.51, 1.13)	0.453		
Clinical characteristics				
UCVA*				
Good (≥6/12)	Reference			
Intermediate (<6/12 and ≥6/18)	0.50 (−0.71, 1.72)	0.416	0.10 (−0.94, 1.15)	0.843
Poor (<6/18)	**−1.25 (−2.18, −0.33)**	**0.008**	**−1.24 (−2.03, −0.45)**	**0.002**
Visual field stage**				
Early stage	Reference			
Medium stage	−0.61 (−1.51, 0.28)	0.179		
Late stage	0.22 (−0.59, 1.03)	0.588		
Number of local eye drops				
<4	Reference			
≥4	0.40 (−0.30, 1.11)	0.263		
Duration of using eye drops (y)				
<1	Reference			
1–5	0.70 (−1.01, 2.41)	0.421		
Knowledge of using eye drops				
Interval between each eye drops				
5 minutes	Reference			
10 minutes	−0.78 (−2.23, 0.67)	0.289		
30 minutes	−3.69 (−7.66, 0.28)	0.068		
Press dacryocyst area				
Yes	**3.70 (1.92, 5.48)**	**<0.001**	1.64 (−0.12, 3.40)	0.068
No	Reference			
Education/training experience of using eye drops				
Having training of using eye drops				
Yes	**2.54 (1.45, 3.63)**	**<0.001**	**1.71 (0.62, 2.80)**	**0.002**
No	Reference			

SD: standard deviation; UCVA: uncorrected visual acuity. *Use patient better-seeing eye's UCVA in this item. **Use patient better-seeing eye's visual field in this item. [†]All variables in the simple regression with $p < 0.05$ were included in multiple regression.

hyperpigmentation caused by prostaglandin, arrhythmias associated with b-blockers, and infrequent side effects such as airway obstruction, thrombocytopenia, and electrolyte disturbances with carbonic anhydrase inhibitors. Adverse effects may bring frustration to patients, which decreases adherence, lowers the effectiveness, and therefore facilitates the swift of treatment to surgery.

Another issue studied in this study is the potential mechanical contact with ocular surface while instilling the eye drop. Underlying complications may range from

infections of ocular surface or trauma such as corneal abrasions [14]. In developing countries, contamination to the bottle may happen due to bad living environment [15]. Dietlein et al. [12] reported that scratching of the eye drop container on the cornea or the conjunctiva was observed in 68% of the study group. Severe visual loss due to corneal ulcers caused by *Serratia marcescens*, secondary to the use of contaminated eye drop containers has been shown by Templeton et al. [16] in their study. Our study showed 37.7% patients got contamination by contacting with ocular surface or adnexa

TABLE 6: Logistic model of potential predictors of patients' skill score of using eye drops (first drop score system) (significant items were highlighted in bold).

	Simple regression		Multiple regression[†]	
	β (95% CI)	p value	β (95% CI)	p value
Demographic characteristics				
Mean of age	**−0.01 (−0.02, −0.004)**	**0.002**	**−0.01 (−0.01, −0.002)**	**0.010**
Male sex	0.14 (−0.05, 3.24)	0.151		
Education level				
≤middle school	Reference			
>middle school	0.15 (−0.04, 0.34)	0.115		
Location				
Urban	Reference			
Rural	0.07 (−0.15, 0.28)			
Clinical characteristics				
UCVA[*]				
Good (≥6/18)	Reference			
Intermediate	0.52(−0.27, 0.37)	0.747	−0.01 (−0.32, 0.30)	0.962
Poor (<6/18)	**−0.39 (−0.63, −0.15)**	**0.002**	**−0.38 (−0.61, −0.14)**	**0.002**
Visual field stage[**]				
Early stage	Reference			
Medium stage	−0.17 (−0.41, 0.07)	0.168		
Late stage	−0.05 (−0.26, 0.17)	0.665		
Number of local eye drops				
<4	Reference			
≥4	0.08 (−0.11, 0.27)	0.415		
Duration of using eye drops (y)				
<1	Reference			
1–5	−0.09 (−0.55, 0.37)	0.695		
Knowledge of using eye drops				
Interval between each eye drops				
5 minutes	Reference			
10 minutes	0.07 (−0.32, 0.46)	0.735		
30 minutes	−0.43(−1.50, 0.64)	0.428		
Press dacryocyst area				
Yes	**0.53 (0.03, 1.04)**	**0.037**	0.16 (−0.36, 0.68)	0.542
No	Reference			
Education/training experience of using eye drops				
Having training of using eye drops				
Yes	**0.37 (0.06, 0.68)**	**0.020**	0.26 (−0.06, 0.58)	0.109
No	Reference			

SD: standard deviation; UCVA: uncorrected visual acuity. [*]Use patient better-seeing eye's UCVA in this item. [**]Use patient better-seeing eye's visual field in this item. [†]All variables in the simple regression with $p < 0.05$ were included in multiple regression.

on their first attempt to instill the drops. It deserves great concern in clinical settings as the underlying devastating complications; also, the eye drops inherence such as instillation technique needs to be evaluated before changing the prescribed regime.

In this study, we investigated the associated determinants of the faulty techniques. Older age, worse visual acuity, and no instruction previously were found risk factor-associated faulty techniques. The patients in the study were aged on average 56.53 (range, 18 to 80), wherein the elderly population constitutes a major share as glaucoma mostly affected. Even though we excluded patients with physical inability for administrating eye drops, still older patients had reduced manual dexterity with age. Poor vision results in the inability of patients to visualize the tip of the bottle and erroneous judgments of the height of the tip of the bottle above the ocular plane. A lack of previous instruction obviously contributes to lack of knowledge about the correct technique, such as press the dacryocyst area and avoid the contamination of the drops. It should be an indispensable part of glaucoma care and further studies are needed to explore its positive effect on the adherence of glaucoma patients [17].

A limitation of this study should be noticed. Firstly, a confounding factor to be considered is that the eagerness of the patient to perform the task accurately when being observed by the study staff may also induce a behavioral modification. Secondly, we did not explore the difference of installation technique in either eye when patients have prescribed eye drops for both eyes. Thirdly, we only included patients with better visual acuity no less than 20/200 in either eye as those with worse visual acuity may have companions to help. However, there are still a considerable number of patients who instill eye drops by themselves, which needs more attention in further studies. Still and all, our study again confirmed the reality of poor drop technique in glaucoma patients.

Despite the ongoing challenge of poor drug adherence of patients with glaucoma, potential strategies come up day in and day out to counter the issue of poor drop adherence. Smart reminding device, ocular sprays, drug-eluting contact lenses, and other modalities of all sorts are on the way to more patients [18]. Moreover, with the advent of surgical innovations, the minimally invasive surgery may have a much smaller chance of risk. Thus, the patients have more options rather than sticking to eye drops [19].

In conclusion, this study clearly shows that a vast majority of glaucoma patients in China are not correctly instilling eye drops. This can lead to serious consequences on the quality of life of the patients. It also highlights the importance of patient education with regard to eye drop instillation whenever glaucoma topical medications are prescribed and a check on this by the eye care providers during follow-up visits.

Conflicts of Interest

None of the authors has financial or other conflicts of interest concerning this study.

Authors' Contributions

Xinbo Gao and Qiongman Yang contributed equally to this study and share the first authorship.

Acknowledgments

This work was supported in whole by the Medical Scientific Research Foundation of Guangdong Province, China (A2015370).

References

[1] R. R. A. Bourne, G. A. Stevens, R. A. White et al., "Causes of vision loss worldwide, 1990–2010: a systematic analysis," *The Lancet Global Health*, vol. 1, no. 6, pp. e339–e349, 2013.

[2] C. O. Okeke, H. A. Quigley, H. D. Jampel et al., "Adherence with topical glaucoma medication monitored electronically: the Travatan Dosing Aid study," *Ophthalmology*, vol. 116, no. 2, pp. 191–199, 2009.

[3] M. A. Kass, D. W. Meltzer, M. Gordon, D. Cooper, and J. Goldberg, "Compliance with topical pilocarpine treatment," *American Journal of Ophthalmology*, vol. 101, no. 5, pp. 515–523, 1986.

[4] T. S. Bacon, K. C. Fan, and M. A. Desai, "Electronic medical record and glaucoma medications: connecting the medication reconciliation with adherence," *Clinical Ophthalmology*, vol. 10, pp. 221–225, 2016.

[5] J. C. Tsai, "A comprehensive perspective on patient adherence to topical glaucoma therapy," *Ophthalmology*, vol. 116, no. 11, pp. S30–S36, 2009.

[6] A. J. Tatham, U. Sarodia, F. Gatrad, and A. Awan, "Eye drop instillation technique in patients with glaucoma," *Eye*, vol. 27, no. 11, pp. 1293–1298, 2013.

[7] D. M. Carpenter, R. Sayner, S. J. Blalock et al., "The effect of eye drop technique education in patients with glaucoma," *Health Communication*, vol. 31, no. 8, pp. 1036–1042, 2016.

[8] R. Gupta, B. Patil, B. M. Shah, S. J. Bali, S. K. Mishra, and T. Dada, "Evaluating eye drop instillation technique in glaucoma patients," *Journal of Glaucoma*, vol. 21, no. 3, pp. 189–192, 2012.

[9] J. C. Tsai, C. A. Mcclure, S. E. Ramos, D. G. Schlundt, and J. W. Pichert, "Compliance barriers in glaucoma: a systematic classification," *Journal of Glaucoma*, vol. 12, no. 5, pp. 393–398, 2003.

[10] M. A. Kass, E. Hodapp, M. Gordon, A. E. Kolker, and I. Goldberg, "Part I. Patient administration of eyedrops: interview," *Annals of Ophthalmology*, vol. 14, no. 8, pp. 775–779, 1982.

[11] M. M. Brown, G. C. Brown, and G. L. Spaeth, "Improper topical self-administration of ocular medication among patients with glaucoma," *Canadian Journal of Ophthalmology*, vol. 19, no. 1, pp. 2–5, 1984.

[12] T. S. Dietlein, J. F. Jordan, C. Lüke, A. Schild, S. Dinslage, and G. K. Krieglstein, "Self-application of single-use eyedrop containers in an elderly population: comparisons with standard eyedrop bottle and with younger patients," *Acta Ophthalmologica*, vol. 86, no. 8, pp. 856–859, 2008.

[13] G. Lazcano-Gomez, M. de los Angeles Ramos-Cadena, M. Torres-Tamayo, A. Hernandez de Oteyza, M. Turati-Acosta, and J. Jimenez-Román, "Cost of glaucoma treatment in a developing country over a 5-year period," *Medicine*, vol. 95, no. 47, article e5341, 2016.

[14] B. Sleath, D. M. Carpenter, S. J. Blalock et al., "Applying the resources and supports in self-management framework to examine ophthalmologist-patient communication and glaucoma medication adherence," *Health Education Research*, vol. 30, no. 5, pp. 693–705, 2015.

[15] O. Geyer, E. J. Bottone, S. M. Podos, R. A. Schumer, and P. A. Asbell, "Microbial contamination of medications used to treat glaucoma," *British Journal of Ophthalmology*, vol. 79, no. 4, pp. 376–379, 1995.

[16] W. C. Templeton III, R. A. Eiferman, J. W. Snyder, J. C. Melo, and M. J. Raff, "Serratia keratitis transmitted by contaminated eyedroppers," *American Journal of Ophthalmology*, vol. 93, no. 6, pp. 723–726, 1982.

[17] A. Feng, J. O'Neill, M. Holt, C. Georgiadis, M. M. Wright, and S. R. Montezuma, "Success of patient training in improving proficiency of eyedrop administration among various ophthalmic patient populations," *Clinical Ophthalmology*, vol. 10, pp. 1505–1511, 2016.

[18] M. V. Boland, D. S. Chang, T. Frazier, R. Plyler, J. L. Jefferys, and D. S. Friedman, "Automated telecommunication-based reminders and adherence with once-daily glaucoma medication dosing: the automated dosing reminder study," *JAMA Ophthalmology*, vol. 132, no. 7, pp. 845–850, 2014.

[19] K. W. Muir and P. P. Lee, "Glaucoma medication adherence: room for improvement in both performance and measurement," *Archives of Ophthalmology*, vol. 129, no. 2, pp. 243–245, 2011.

12

Normative Values of Peripapillary Retinal Nerve Fiber Layer Thickness in a Middle Eastern Population

Mouna M. Al-Sa'ad,[1] Amjad T. Shatarat ⓘ,[2] Justin Z. Amarin ⓘ,[3] and Darwish H. Badran[2]

[1]Department of Special Surgery, School of Medicine, The University of Jordan, Queen Rania Al-Abdullah Street, Amman 11942, Jordan
[2]Department of Anatomy and Histology, School of Medicine, The University of Jordan, Queen Rania Al-Abdullah Street, Amman 11942, Jordan
[3]School of Medicine, The University of Jordan, Queen Rania Al-Abdullah Street, Amman 11942, Jordan

Correspondence should be addressed to Amjad T. Shatarat; a.shatarat@ju.edu.jo

Academic Editor: Maurizio Uva

Purpose. Peripapillary retinal nerve fiber layer (pRNFL) thickness is subject to high variability. Normative values of pRNFL thickness remain undocumented in the Middle East. The aim of our study is to assess the normative values of pRNFL thickness in a Middle Eastern population. *Methods.* A retrospective chart review of 74 patients was conducted. Outpatients who had presented to the ophthalmology clinic at the Jordan University Hospital between January 2016 and July 2018 were consecutively sampled. Measurements had been recorded using Fourier-domain optical coherence tomography. Multivariable regression models were developed to generate predicted normative values with adjustments to candidate confounders. *Results.* The mean global pRNFL thickness was $99 \pm 11\,\mu$m. The mean quadrantic pRNFL thickness increased from the nasal quadrant ($75 \pm 16\,\mu$m) to the temporal ($82 \pm 20\,\mu$m), superior ($114 \pm 20\,\mu$m), and inferior ($125 \pm 20\,\mu$m) quadrants. Gender and eye sidedness did not contribute to the variability in pRNFL thickness. The relationship between aging and pRNFL thinning is independent of diabetes mellitus type 2 and systemic hypertension. Both systemic conditions significantly predicted pRNFL changes despite negative fundoscopic findings. *Conclusions.* Our set of predicted normative data may be used to interpret measurements of pRNFL thickness in Middle Eastern patients. Our findings suggest that systemic conditions with potential ocular manifestations may require consideration in predictive models of pRNFL thickness, even in the absence of gross fundoscopic findings. Normative data from additional Middle Eastern populations are required to appraise our models, which adjust for common clinical confounders.

1. Introduction

Glaucoma is an optic neuropathy characterized by excavation of the optic disc, thinning of the peripapillary retinal nerve fiber layer (pRNFL), and a specific pattern of visual field loss. Glaucoma, the leading cause of irreversible vision loss, affects an estimated 66.8 million people worldwide [1]. The diagnosis of glaucoma encompasses a number of clinical observations and measurement techniques [2].

Optic disc excavation and visual field defects are relatively late clinical manifestations of glaucoma. Peripapillary retinal nerve fiber layer thinning precedes these events by a considerable period of time. Therefore, quantitative assessment of pRNFL thickness is useful for the diagnosis of glaucoma in its early stages. Indeed, the measure is highly sensitive, specific, and reproducible [3, 4]. A number of techniques have been used to assess pRNFL thickness, the most notable of which is optical coherence tomography (OCT) [5].

Optical coherence tomography is a noninvasive cross-sectional imaging modality that measures internal structure in biological systems, including ocular structures [5, 6]. The ocular imaging technology is a useful tool in the inventory of the ophthalmologist. For instance, high-resolution *in vivo* imaging of retinal structure is important for the diagnosis of optic neuropathies [7]. The performance of OCT-based imaging is continually improving with further iterations of the technology [8]. Indeed, the latest iterations include Gabor-domain optical coherence microscopy, which may be used to assess the microstructures of the cornea [9]. In the clinic, Fourier-domain OCT is used in standard commercial systems and offers superior sensitivity compared to the conventional time-domain approach [8, 10].

Peripapillary retinal nerve fiber layer thickness is naturally subject to anatomic variation. Therefore, measurements are interpreted against a backdrop of normative reference values. Normative values are readily available, albeit for no more than a select number of ethnic groups [11]. The preceding fact is problematic as normative values may be highly variable between populations. Thus, their documentation in additional populations is necessary [12]. To the best of our knowledge, no study to date has documented the normative values of pRNFL thickness in a Middle Eastern population. The heterogeneity of Middle Eastern populations calls for a series of investigations to determine robust normative values of pRNFL thickness. Herein, we present a preliminary investigation of these values using Fourier-domain OCT.

2. Methods

2.1. Participants. We conducted a retrospective chart review of outpatients who had presented to the ophthalmology clinic at the Jordan University Hospital between January 2016 and July 2018. Patient data were reviewed on a workstation located in the clinic. All adult patients (≥18 years of age) who underwent complete ophthalmologic assessment and whose data were available were included. Exclusion criteria included any history of retinopathy or optic neuropathy, recent history of ocular surgery (≤1 year), family history of glaucoma, high-degree myopia, use of anti-glaucoma agents, poor scan quality, and incomplete binocular data. Institutional Review Board approval was sought and obtained (Jordan University Hospital, Amman, Jordan).

2.2. Measures. Peripapillary retinal nerve fiber layer thickness had been measured using a Fourier-domain OCT system (RTVue, Optovue, Inc., Fremont, CA). Measurements had been recorded by the same operator in all cases (MM Al-Sa'ad) using the RNFL3.45 mode. Measurements of pRNFL thickness in five areas (namely, temporal, superior, nasal, inferior, and global) were transcribed. In addition, clinical data (namely, age, gender, history of diabetes mellitus type 2, history of systemic hypertension, and refractive error) were collected.

2.3. Data Analysis. Data were entered into the IBM SPSS Statistics Data Editor (IBM Corporation, Armonk, NY). The software package was used to run descriptive statistics, bivariate statistics, and linear regression. The dataset included the complete binocular and clinical profile of each patient. To examine for intraindividual variation in pRNFL thickness,

binocular measurements were paired. Difference scores between paired measurements were computed. The scores were examined for outliers and normality using box plots and normal Q–Q plots, respectively. Paired measurements were subsequently compared using the paired-samples *t*-test. Intraindividual variation was interpreted using a significance level of 0.05.

Multivariable linear regression models were developed to predict the five measurements of pRNFL thickness (Figure 1). Candidate predictors were age, gender, eye sidedness, history of diabetes mellitus type 2, history of systemic hypertension, and refractive error. Bivariate correlations were evaluated by simple linear regression. The significance threshold for model entry was set at an uncorrected value of $P < 0.2$. Predicted normative values were generated from the calculated regression equations using the LMATRIX subcommand. The assumptions underlying linear regression were met. Briefly, plots of studentized residuals and unstandardized predicted values were examined for linearity and homoscedasticity. In addition, partial regression plots were examined for linearity. Multicollinearity was assessed using variance inflation factors. Studentized deleted residuals (>3 or <−3), Cook's D (>1), and leverage values (>0.2) were used to detect outliers, highly influential points, and high leverage points, respectively. Normality was assessed using normal P–P plots.

The Benjamini–Hochberg method was used to correct for multiple testing, unless otherwise stated. Numerical data are presented according to the recommendations of Cole [13]. Continuous data are presented as means and standard deviations (separated by a plus-minus sign). Frequencies are presented as absolute and relative values (the latter within parentheses).

3. Results

Fourteen patients were excluded for poor scan quality or incomplete binocular data. The final study population comprised 74 patients. One hundred forty-eight eyes entered statistical analysis. Thirty-five patients were male and 39 were female. The patients ranged in age from 18 to 79 years (mean age, 60 ± 12 years). The median spherical equivalent was 0.50 diopters (range, −3.50 to 2.50 diopters). Clinical characteristics of the study population are outlined in Table 1. Paired measurements of pRNFL thickness did not statistically significantly differ in any area (temporal, $P = 1$; superior, $P = 0.2$; nasal, $P = 0.6$; inferior; $P = 0.2$; global, $P = 0.2$).

The mean global pRNFL thickness in the study population was $99 \pm 11\,\mu$m. Quadrantic pRNFL thickness measurements are presented in Table 2. The mean quadrantic pRNFL thickness increased from the nasal quadrant to the temporal, superior, and inferior quadrants, in the mentioned order. In 114 eyes (77%), quadrantic measurements of pRNFL thickness did not follow the "ISNT rule" (i.e., inferior > superior > nasal > temporal). In 56 eyes (38%), quadrantic measurements of pRNFL thickness did not follow the "IST rule" (i.e., inferior > superior > temporal).

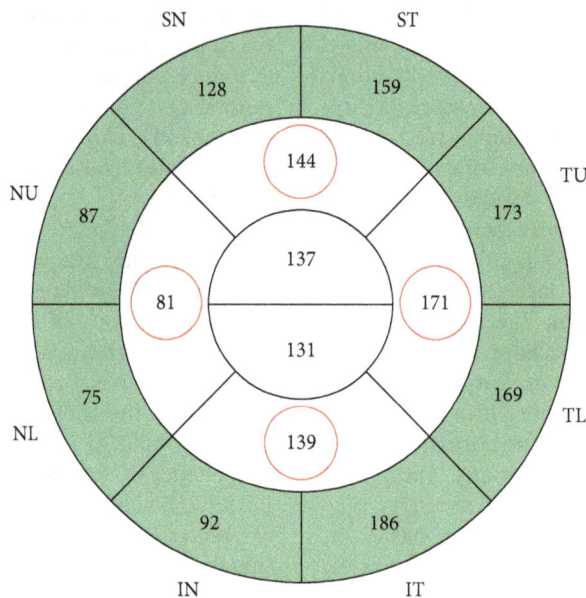

FIGURE 1: Peripapillary retinal nerve fiber layer (pRNFL) thickness analysis by the manufacturer (Optovue, Inc.). Circled in red are the four quadrantic measurements of pRNFL thickness (μm). The global RNFL thickness is the calculated mean of the four quadrantic measurements.

TABLE 1: Clinical characteristics of the study population ($N = 74$).

Characteristics	Mean or frequency
Age (years)	60 ± 12
Gender	
Male	35 (47)
Female	39 (53)
History of diabetes mellitus type 2	
Negative	39 (53)
Positive	35 (47)
History of systemic hypertension	
Negative	43 (58)
Positive	31 (42)

Continuous data are presented as means and standard deviations (separated by a plus-minus sign). Frequencies are presented as absolute and relative values (the latter within parentheses).

TABLE 2: Mean peripapillary retinal nerve fiber layer (pRNFL) thickness by area ($N = 148$ eyes).

Area	Mean pRNFL thickness (μm)
Temporal	82 ± 20
Superior	114 ± 20
Nasal	75 ± 16
Inferior	125 ± 20

Continuous data are presented as means and standard deviations (separated by a plus-minus sign).

Gender and eye sidedness did not meet the entry criterion of any model. Refractive error met the entry criterion of the model for inferior pRNFL thickness but did not statistically significantly add to the prediction. In fact, the overall model for inferior pRNFL thickness was not statistically significant ($P = 0.06$). In contrast, the remaining models were statistically significant ($P < 0.001$). Age, history

of diabetes mellitus type 2, and history of systemic hypertension contributed to the remaining models in variable patterns. Age and history of systemic hypertension generally predicted a decrease in RNFL thickness. However, history of diabetes mellitus type 2 generally predicted an increase in RNFL thickness. Full model results are shown in Table 3.

Predicted normative data are based on the regression equations calculated. The predictions assume a negative history of diabetes mellitus type 2, a negative history of systemic hypertension, and a spherical equivalent of zero. Predicted normative data are presented in Table 4 for one-decade increments in age.

4. Discussion

We developed regression models to predict the normative values of pRNFL thickness in a Middle-Eastern population. During model development, we examined pRNFL thickness measurements for sexual dimorphism, binocular asymmetry, age-related changes, and clinical association with diabetes mellitus type 2, systemic hypertension, and refractive error. In addition, we quantified deviations from the "ISNT rule" and the "IST rule" for descriptive purposes. As suggested by previous reports, neither parameter appears to be clinically useful [14, 15].

Ethnic variation in pRNFL thickness has been demonstrated in several studies [11, 12]. Though reports are incongruous, the pRNFL appears to be appreciably thinner in whites compared with Hispanics and Asians [11, 12, 16]. The mean global pRNFL thickness reported herein is highly concordant with data from previous studies on white populations and by extension, the original normative database. In addition, quadrantic measurements of pRNFL thickness in the present study are roughly consistent with

TABLE 3: Multivariable regression models of peripapillary retinal nerve fiber layer (RNFL) thickness by area in a Middle Eastern population ($N = 148$ eyes).

Variables	B value*	95% CI	P value
Temporal			<0.001
Age (years)	−0.35	−0.61 to −0.08	0.01
History of diabetes mellitus type 2	6	−1 to 12	0.09
History of systemic hypertension	11	4 to 17	0.002
Superior			<0.001
Age (years)	−0.12	−0.37 to 0.14	0.4
History of diabetes mellitus type 2	11	4 to 17	0.001
History of systemic hypertension	−14	−21 to −8	<0.001
Nasal			<0.001
History of diabetes mellitus type 2	10	5 to 15	<0.001
History of systemic hypertension	−12	−17 to −7	<0.001
Inferior			0.06
Age (years)	−0.21	−0.47 to 0.06	0.1
Refraction (spherical equivalent power)	−2.5	−5.3 to 0.2	0.07
Global			<0.001
Age (years)	−0.16	−0.31 to −0.01	0.04
History of diabetes mellitus type 2	8	4 to 11	<0.001
History of systemic hypertension	−4.2	−8.1 to −0.3	0.04

B value, regression coefficient; 95% CI, 95% confidence interval. *B values represent the change in the dependent variables (i.e., pRNFL thickness by area) for each unit of change in the independent variables (i.e., predictors).

TABLE 4: Age-adjusted normative values of peripapillary retinal nerve fiber layer thickness by area.

Age (years)	Mean predicted pRNFL thickness (95% confidence interval) in μm				
	Temporal	Superior	Nasal	Inferior	Global
20	89 (78–100)	120 (110–131)	75 (72–79)	134 (122–145)	104 (98–110)
30	85 (77–94)	119 (111–127)	75 (72–79)	132 (123–140)	102 (97–107)
40	82 (76–88)	118 (112–124)	75 (72–79)	129 (123–136)	101 (97–104)
50	79 (74–83)	117 (112–121)	75 (72–79)	127 (123–132)	99 (96–102)
60	75 (71–80)	116 (111–120)	75 (72–79)	125 (122–129)	97 (95–100)
70	72 (66–77)	114 (109–120)	75 (72–79)	123 (119–127)	96 (92–99)
80	68 (61–76)	113 (106–121)	75 (72–79)	121 (115–127)	94 (90–99)

previously reported values [12, 16]. It appears, then, that adjustments need not be made to pRNFL thickness measurements in Middle Easterners. However, the Middle Eastern population comprises a heterogeneous admixture of peoples. Therefore, normative data from additional Middle Eastern populations are required to confirm this finding.

Fundoscopic examination of all members in our study population was normal. Interestingly, a history of diabetes mellitus type 2 generally predicted a considerable increase in pRNFL thickness. In contrast, a meta-analysis of 13 studies concluded that pRNFL thickness is significantly decreased in preclinical diabetic retinopathy [17]. However, the ophthalmologic complications of diabetes mellitus type 2 include diabetic retinopathy and diabetic macular edema, and the latter entity has been shown to increase pRNFL thickness [18]. Therefore, the interpretation of pRNFL measurements in the setting of diabetes mellitus type 2 appears impractical. Indeed, Yang et al. have recently suggested a novel index to address the literary muddle [19].

In our study, gender and eye sidedness did not qualify for model entry. In support, previous studies have shown that pRNFL measurements are subject to neither sexual dimorphism nor binocular asymmetry [16, 20]. However, in our study population, age and a history of systemic hypertension generally predicted a considerable decrease in pRNFL thickness. Atherosclerosis in the setting of systemic hypertension appears to be associated with pRNFL thinning [21]. In addition, the relationship between aging and pRNFL thinning appears robust despite the presence of several confounders. In our study, age remained a significant predictor following correction for potential confounders. Indeed, a number of authors have attributed age-related thinning to senescence [12, 16, 20, 22]. The clinical significance of senescence is addressed by our set of predicted normative data.

5. Conclusions

In conclusion, our set of predicted normative data may be used to interpret measurements of pRNFL thickness in Middle Eastern patients. Our findings suggest that systemic conditions with potential ocular manifestations may require consideration in predictive models of pRNFL thickness, even in the absence of gross fundoscopic findings. Normative data from additional Middle Eastern populations are required to appraise our models.

Conflicts of Interest

The authors declare that they have no conflicts of interest.

References

[1] R. Conlon, H. Saheb, and I. I. Ahmed, "Glaucoma treatment trends: a review," *Canadian Journal of Ophthalmology*, vol. 52, no. 1, pp. 114–124, 2017.

[2] P. Azarbod, L. Crawley, F. Ahmed, M. F. Cordeiro, and P. Bloom, "Recent advances in the diagnosis and management of glaucoma," *Prescriber*, vol. 26, no. 1-2, pp. 21–25, 2015.

[3] D. L. Budenz, A. Michael, R. T. Chang, J. McSoley, and J. Katz, "Sensitivity and specificity of the StratusOCT for perimetric glaucoma," *Ophthalmology*, vol. 112, no. 1, pp. 3–9, 2005.

[4] D. L. Budenz, R. T. Chang, X. Huang, R. W. Knighton, and J. M. Tielsch, "Reproducibility of retinal nerve fiber thickness measurements using the stratus OCT in normal and glaucomatous eyes," *Investigative Opthalmology and Visual Science*, vol. 46, no. 7, pp. 2440–2443, 2005.

[5] D. Huang, E. A. Swanson, C. P. Lin et al., "Optical coherence tomography," *Science*, vol. 254, no. 5035, pp. 1178–1181, 1991.

[6] J. W. Jeoung and K. H. Park, "Comparison of cirrus OCT and stratus OCT on the ability to detect localized retinal nerve fiber layer defects in preperimetric glaucoma," *Investigative Opthalmology and Visual Science*, vol. 51, no. 2, pp. 938–945, 2010.

[7] A. Ozkok, J. C. Akkan, N. Tamcelik, M. Erdogan, D. U. Comlekoglu, and R. Yildirim, "Comparison of retinal nerve fiber layer and macular thickness measurements with Stratus OCT and OPKO/OTI OCT devices in healthy subjects," *International Journal of Ophthalmology*, vol. 8, no. 1, pp. 98–103, 2015.

[8] A. G. Podoleanu and R. B. Rosen, "Combinations of techniques in imaging the retina with high resolution," *Progress in Retinal and Eye Research*, vol. 27, no. 4, pp. 464–499, 2008.

[9] P. Tankam, Z. He, Y. J. Chu et al., "Assessing microstructures of the cornea with Gabor-domain optical coherence microscopy: pathway for corneal physiology and diseases," *Optics Letters*, vol. 40, no. 6, pp. 1113–1116, 2015.

[10] M. Choma, M. Sarunic, C. Yang, and J. Izatt, "Sensitivity advantage of swept source and Fourier domain optical coherence tomography," *Optics Express*, vol. 11, no. 18, pp. 2183–2189, 2003.

[11] A. Manassakorn, W. Chaidaroon, S. Ausayakhun, S. Aupapong, and S. Wattananikorn, "Normative database of retinal nerve fiber layer and macular retinal thickness in a Thai population," *Japanese Journal of Ophthalmology*, vol. 52, no. 6, pp. 450–456, 2008.

[12] D. L. Budenz, D. R. Anderson, R. Varma et al., "Determinants of normal retinal nerve fiber layer thickness measured by stratus OCT," *Ophthalmology*, vol. 114, no. 6, pp. 1046–1052, 2007.

[13] T. J. Cole, "Too many digits: the presentation of numerical data," *Archives of Disease in Childhood*, vol. 100, no. 7, pp. 608-609, 2015.

[14] Y. M. Tariq, H. Li, G. Burlutsky, and P. Mitchell, "Retinal nerve fiber layer and optic disc measurements by spectral domain OCT: normative values and associations in young adults," *Eye*, vol. 26, no. 12, pp. 1563–1570, 2012.

[15] Z. S. Pradhan, A. Braganza, and L. M. Abraham, "Does the ISNT rule apply to the retinal nerve fiber layer?," *Journal of Glaucoma*, vol. 25, no. 1, pp. e1-e4, 2016.

[16] P. Dave and J. Shah, "Applicability of ISNT and IST rules to the retinal nerve fibre layer using spectral domain optical coherence tomography in early glaucoma," *British Journal of Ophthalmology*, vol. 99, no. 12, pp. 1713–1717, 2015.

[17] D. J. Hwang, E. J. Lee, S. Y. Lee, K. H. Park, and S. J. Woo, "Effect of diabetic macular edema on peripapillary retinal nerve fiber layer thickness profiles," *Investigative Opthalmology and Visual Science*, vol. 55, no. 7, pp. 4213–4219, 2014.

[18] X. Chen, C. Nie, Y. Gong et al., "Peripapillary retinal nerve fiber layer changes in preclinical diabetic retinopathy: a meta-analysis," *PLoS One*, vol. 10, no. 5, Article ID e0125919, 2015.

[19] H. S. Yang, J. E. Woo, M. H. Kim, D. Y. Kim, and Y. H. Yoon, "Co-evaluation of peripapillary RNFL thickness and retinal thickness in patients with diabetic macular edema: RNFL misinterpretation and its adjustment," *PLoS One*, vol. 12, no. 1, Article ID e0170341, 2017.

[20] X. Zhang, B. A. Francis, A. Dastiridou et al., "Longitudinal and cross-sectional analyses of age effects on retinal nerve fiber layer and ganglion cell complex thickness by fourier-domain OCT," *Translational Vision Science and Technology*, vol. 5, no. 2, p. 1, 2016.

[21] O. Z. Sahin, S. B. Sahin, T. Ayaz et al., "The impact of hypertension on retinal nerve fiber layer thickness and its association with carotid intima media thickness," *Blood Pressure*, vol. 24, no. 3, pp. 178–184, 2015.

[22] A. R. Celebi and G. E. Mirza, "Age-related change in retinal nerve fiber layer thickness measured with spectral domain optical coherence tomography," *Investigative Opthalmology and Visual Science*, vol. 54, no. 13, pp. 8095–8103, 2013.

13

When is Evidence Enough Evidence? A Systematic Review and Meta-Analysis of the Trabectome as a Solo Procedure in Patients with Primary Open-Angle Glaucoma

Jeffrey T. Y. Chow,[1] Cindy M. L. Hutnik,[2] Karla Solo,[1] and Monali S. Malvankar-Mehta[1,2]

[1]Department of Epidemiology and Biostatistics, Schulich School of Medicine and Dentistry, Western University, London, ON, Canada
[2]Department of Ophthalmology, Schulich School of Medicine and Dentistry, Western University, London, ON, Canada

Correspondence should be addressed to Monali S. Malvankar-Mehta; monali.malvankar@sjhc.london.on.ca

Academic Editor: Van C. Lansingh

The purpose of this systematic review and meta-analysis was to examine the availability of evidence for one of the earliest available minimally invasive glaucoma surgery (MIGS) procedures, the Trabectome. Various databases were searched up to December 20, 2016, for any published studies assessing the use of the Trabectome as a solo procedure in patients with primary open-angle glaucoma (POAG). The standardized mean differences (SMD) were calculated for the change in intraocular pressure (IOP) and number of glaucoma mediations used at 1-month, 6-month, and 12-month follow-up. After screening, three studies and one abstract with analyzable data were included. The meta-analysis showed statistically significant reductions in IOP and number of glaucoma medications used at all time points. Though the Trabectome as a solo procedure appears to lower IOP and reduces the number of glaucoma medications, more high-quality studies are required to make definitive conclusions. The difficulty of obtaining evidence may be one of the many obstacles that limit a full understanding of the potential safety and/or efficacy benefits compared to standard treatments. The time has come for a thoughtful and integrated approach with stakeholders to determine optimal access to care strategies for our patients.

1. Introduction

As the second leading cause of blindness in the world, [1] glaucoma is an important disease that affects millions of people. In 2010, there were 60.5 million people in the world living with glaucoma and this number is predicted to rise to 80 million by 2020 [2]. Glaucoma costs the United States economy over 2.9 billion dollars every year from direct costs and productivity losses [3]. The most common type of glaucoma, primary open-angle glaucoma (POAG), occurs when the angle between the cornea and the iris is anatomically open, but functionally impaired, leading to increased pressure in the eye and potential optic nerve damage [4]. There is no cure for POAG. Current treatments are aimed at lowering intraocular pressure (IOP) with the goal of slowing or halting the progression of POAG.

Surgery is typically required when medication and laser treatments fail to deliver the necessary reduction in IOP. Minimally invasive glaucoma surgeries (MIGS) have become more popular due to their perceived safety and lack of complications [5]. One of these MIGS is the Trabectome surgical system developed by NeoMedix Inc. in Tustin, CA.

The Trabectome allows trained ophthalmologists to perform an ab interno partial trabeculectomy, a procedure that uses high-frequency electrocautery to selectively ablate the trabecular meshwork and inner wall of Schlemm's canal. The procedure results in IOP reduction by creating a more direct communication between the anterior chamber and the collector channels [6]. The Trabectome procedure has been reported to reduce the IOP to the midteens and has low complication rates [7]. Potential benefits associated with the Trabectome include being less invasive as an ab interno approach is used and increased compliance as fewer glaucoma medications are needed afterwards [7]. When performed in conjunction with cataract surgery, the benefit to the patient is a single incision that can be used for the combined procedure. Recently, the Trabectome has been used more as a solo procedure, without concurrent cataract surgery. Under the Ontario Health Insurance Plan, the Trabectome is projected to offer a moderate cost savings compared to glaucoma medications over time [8].

In a 2011 review, Vold suggested that more long-term data and randomized controlled trials were required to adequately assess the efficacy of Trabectome [7]. However, no systematic reviews focused on using Trabectome to treat POAG were found in the literature. A recent systematic review of patients with all types of glaucoma found that overall, Trabectome on average reduces the IOP by approximately 31% to a final IOP near 15 mmHg [9]. Because of the multitude and growing number of potential surgical glaucoma treatments available, there is a need to synthesize the literature available for Trabectome to ensure a full understanding of its position in the glaucoma treatment paradigm. While the original objective of the current systematic review was to analyze all data available for the Trabectome and determine its performance as a solo procedure in patients with POAG, a lack of high-quality evidence (despite years of use) resulted in a new objective to discuss the difficulty with obtaining enough evidence to fully understand the benefits of an intervention compared to potential alternatives.

2. Methods

2.1. Literature Search Strategy. A systematic review was conducted by searching several databases and pertinent grey literature for all relevant articles. PubMed, MEDLINE, EMBASE, Web of Science Core Collection, and CINAHL were searched until December 20, 2016, using a keyword string (see Appendix 1A available online at https://doi.org/10.1155/2017/2965725). Since, there were no MeSH terms or subject headings available for the Trabectome, only keyword searching was used. The search strategy was designed to reflect naming variations for the Trabectome surgical system and the associated surgical procedure. Since the number of results from database searching was low (see Appendix 1B), the concept of POAG was not included in the keywords. Instead, screening questions were used to ensure that only studies with POAG patients were included.

Grey literature was identified by searching ClinicalTrials.gov, the International Clinical Trials Registry Platform, ProQuest Dissertations and Theses, the Networked Digital Library of Theses and Dissertations, the Electronic Thesis Online Service, the Theses Canada Portal, the Canadian Health Research Collection, the Agency for Healthcare Research and Quality, and the Canadian Agency for Drugs and Technologies in Health for all relevant studies. BIOSIS Previews (using the Web of Science platform), the Association for Research in Vision and Ophthalmology (ARVO), the American Academy of Ophthalmology (AAO), and the Canadian Ophthalmological Society (COS) were searched for meeting abstracts that met the criteria described in the database search. Since the Trabectome is manufactured by NeoMedix Inc., its website was also searched for any publications not identified from previous searches. The PRISMA flow diagram for the literature search is presented in Figure 1.

2.2. Inclusion and Exclusion Criteria. Primary research studies were included in this systematic review. Secondary research studies such as review articles, case reports, systematic reviews, opinions, and editorials were excluded. Studies presenting outcomes for the Trabectome as a solo procedure in humans with POAG were included. Studies that measured the effect of the Trabectome with concurrent cataract surgery were excluded unless the study also presented the effect of the Trabectome performed alone. No restrictions were made on study location or year of publication. Studies were included if they were published in English and had a sample size over 20. EPPI Reviewer [10] was used to gather data from various published and unpublished sources as well as for duplicate removal. Covidence [11] software was used for the three screening stages, with the titles screened in level 1, the abstracts screened in level 2, and the full texts screened in level 3 (see Appendix 2). Two reviewers (JC and KS) independently screened each study with any disagreements resolved by consensus.

2.3. Quality Assessment and Data Extraction. All included studies except for the abstract-only study [12] were assessed for quality using the Downs and Black checklist [13]. All three included full-text studies [14–16] were determined to be of moderate quality with scores of 14, 16, and 15, respectively. Due to limited evidence, none of the studies were excluded from the analysis based on quality. For each of the included studies, the following data was extracted: author name, year of publication, study design, study location, sample size, demographic characteristics of subjects, baseline intraocular pressure, and baseline number of glaucoma medications. Postoperative characteristics such as intraocular pressure and number of glaucoma medications were also extracted for all time points provided in the study.

2.4. Statistical Analyses. Meta-analysis was completed using STATA versus 13.0 (STATA Corporation, College Station, TX). Percentage of IOP reduction (IOPR%) and standard error of percentage of IOP reduction ($SE_{IOPR\%}$) were calculated using the extracted IOP and standard deviation at each time point according to equations described in similar studies [17, 18]. The outcomes of interest were the standardized mean differences (SMD) for change in intraocular pressure and change in glaucoma medications at 6-month and 12-month follow-up. To calculate the SMD for each study, the difference between the mean pre- and postoperative values for each outcome measure was divided by the SD for that outcomes measure. Each SMD then had weights assigned according to the inverse of its variance in order to compute the average. Based on I^2 statistics and p values (>0.01) observed, heterogeneity was determined and fixed-effect or random-effect models were used accordingly. Forest plots were generated for each outcome of interest, and funnel plots were generated to check for publication bias.

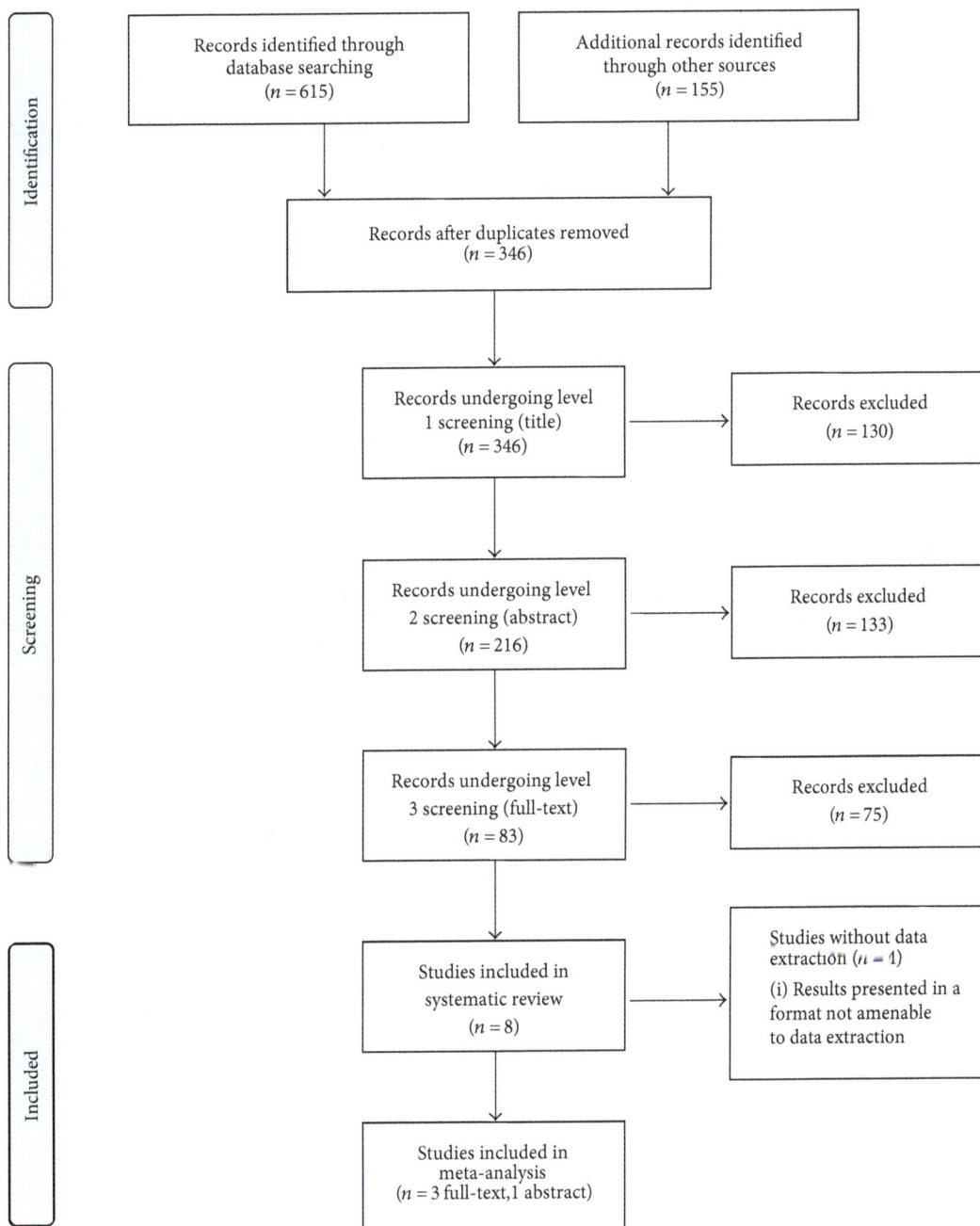

FIGURE 1: PRISMA flow diagram.

3. Results

3.1. Search Results. Figure 1 describes the flow diagram for the literature search and screening process. The database search located 615 studies (see Appendix 1B), and the grey literature search located a further 155 studies (see Appendix 1C). After removing duplicates, 346 studies were included for screening, with 8 studies remaining after three levels of screening. Four studies had results that were in a format that was not amenable to data extraction (data presented in a graph format or full text not in English) [19–21]. As a result, three studies and one abstract were included in the final meta-analysis. (see Figure 1) [12, 14–16]. Though the full text

was in German, the abstract was included since there was sufficient information provided in the abstract [12].

3.2. Study Characteristics. All included studies [12, 14–16] measured IOP and glaucoma medications used at baseline and postoperative time points with subgroups for POAG and pseudoexfoliation glaucoma (XFG) patients. The Pahlitzsch et al. study was available as an abstract since the full text was in German [12].

In the Ting et al. study, there were 450 cases of POAG from Canada, Japan, Mexico, and the United States that underwent the Trabectome alone, with an average age of 68 (SD = 15) years, consisting of 40% male [14]. In comparison,

Table 1: Reported pre- and postoperative IOP and number of glaucoma medications for POAG cases undergoing Trabectome as a solo procedure.

Author, year	Time point	N	Mean IOP (mmHg (SD))	IOPR%	SE$_{IOPR\%}$	N	Mean number of medications (mean (SD))	Mean reduction in number of medications
Ting et al. [14]	Baseline	450	25.5 (7.9)	—	—	450	2.73 (1.33)	—
	1 day	450	16.5 (7.9)	35%	44%	450	2.21 (1.73)	0.52
	1 month	420	18.1 (5.8)	29%	38%	420	2.50 (1.45)	0.23
	3 months	384	17.6 (5.3)	31%	37%	384	2.34 (1.42)	0.39
	6 months	327	17.3 (4.0)	32%	35%	327	2.14 (1.34)	0.59
	12 months	293	16.8 (3.9)	34%	35%	293	2.16 (1.29)	0.57
Mizoguchi et al. [15]	Baseline	82	23.5 (7.2)	—	—	43	2.8 (0.8)	—
	6 months	74	16.2 (3.4)	31%	34%	37	2.5 (0.9)	0.3
	12 months	60	15.7 (3.0)	33%	33%	29	2.4 (0.8)	0.4
	18 months	43	15.3 (2.4)	35%	32%	23	2.5 (0.7)	0.3
	24 months	22	14.1 (2.2)	40%	32%	8	1.8 (1.0)	1
Pahlitzsch et al. [12]	Baseline	—	19.8 (5.9)	—	—	—	Not available	—
	12 months	—	14.8 (3.2)	25%	34%	—	2.1 (1.2)	—
Akil et al. [16]	Baseline	18	24.2 (4.7)	—	—	18	2.6 (1.2)	—
	1 month	18	14.6 (3.2)	40%	23%	18	1.7 (1.2)	0.9

IOP: intraocular pressure; IOPR%: percentage reduction in intraocular pressure; SE$_{IOPR\%}$: standard error of percentage reduction in intraocular pressure. IOP refers to intraocular pressure and SD refers to standard deviation.

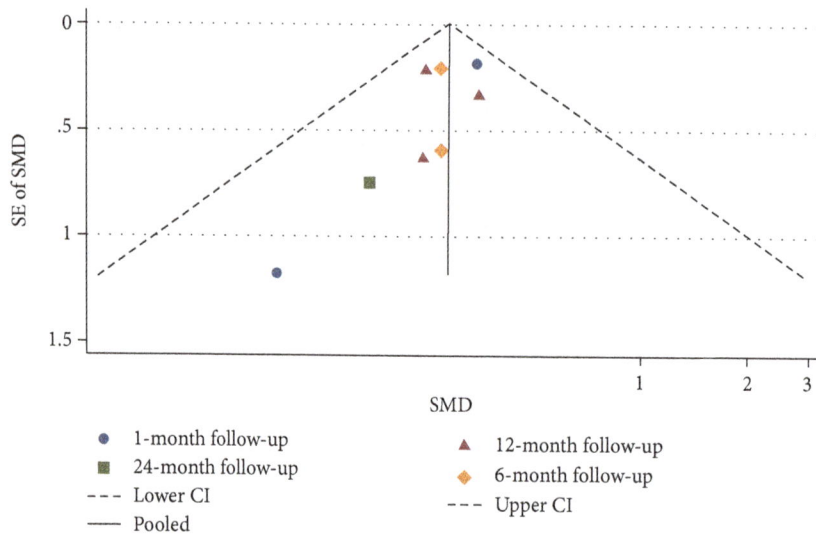

Figure 2: Funnel plot for studies examining change in intraocular pressure (mmHg) by follow-up (months). The dashed line represents the confidence interval (CI).

the Mizoguchi et al. study included 43 cases of POAG that underwent the Trabectome alone, with an average age of 67.4 (SD = 14.1) years and consisting of 37% male [15]. Akil et al. included 18 cases of POAG from the United States that underwent the Trabectome alone with an average of 72.5 (SD = 7) years and consisting of 44% male [16]. In all four studies where the results were not amenable to replication, Trabectome as a solo procedure reduced the IOP and glaucoma medications used [19–22]. The results for the other four studies are summarized in Table 1 for the POAG cases undergoing the Trabectome surgery.

3.3. Publication Bias. Visual inspection of the funnel plots presented in Figures 2 and 3 does not show any asymmetry, suggesting a lack of publication bias for the average change in IOP and topical glaucoma medications used, stratified by the length of follow-up.

3.4. Effect on Intraocular Pressure. Figure 4 summarizes the results for the change in IOP at 6-month and 12-month follow-up. There were 2 studies with 1 month follow-up, 2 studies with 6 months follow-up, and 3 studies with 12 months follow-up. There was significant heterogeneity

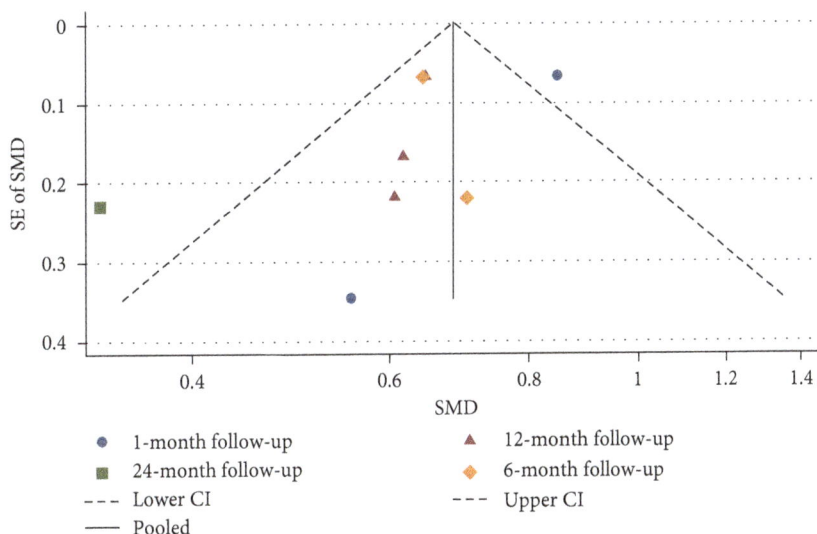

FIGURE 3: Funnel plot for studies examining change in number of glaucoma medications used by follow-up (months). The dashed line represents the confidence interval (CI).

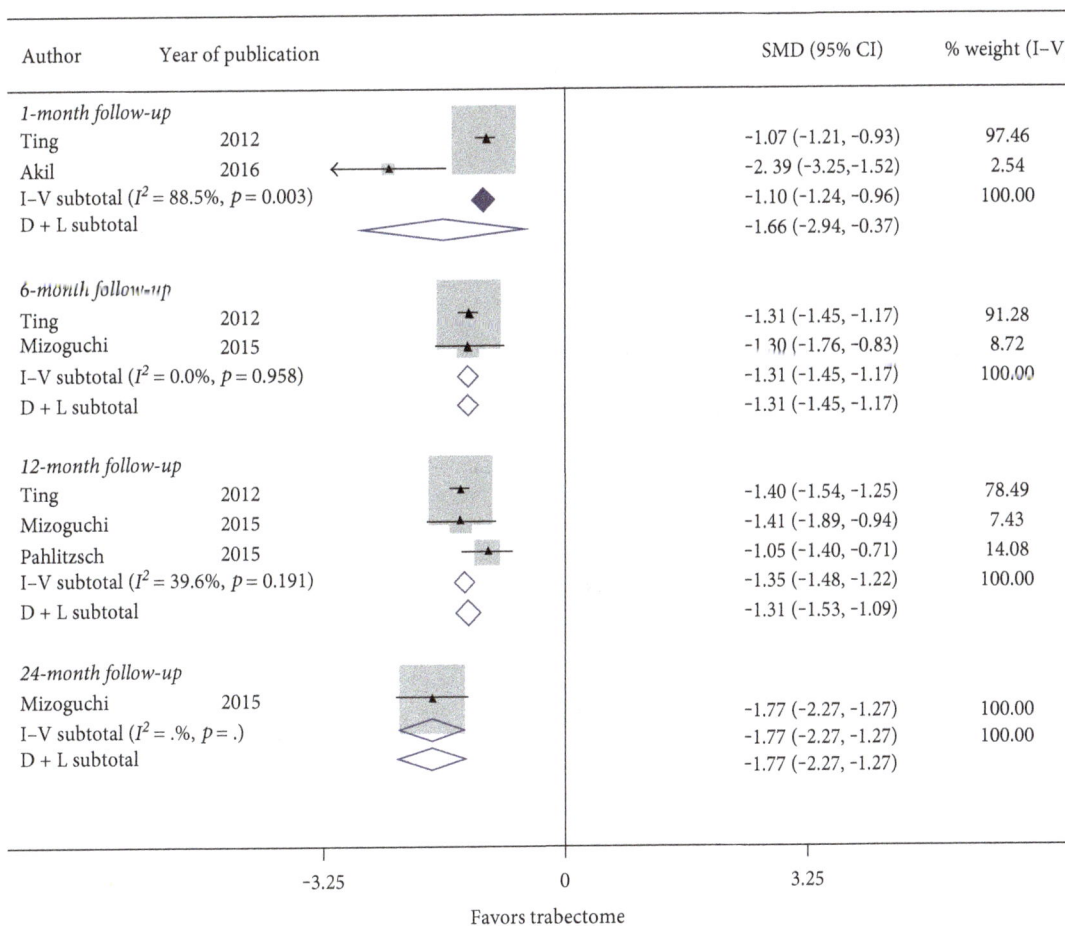

FIGURE 4: Forest plot for studies examining change in intraocular pressure (mmHg) by follow-up (months).

between studies examining 1 month follow-up ($I^2 = 88.5\%$, p value = 0.03), but nonsignificant heterogeneity between studies examining 6 months follow-up ($I^2 = 0.0\%$, p value = 0.958) and 12 months follow-up ($I^2 = 39.6\%$, p value = 0.191).

Figure 4 showed a nonstatistically significant reduction in IOP with a SMD of −1.66 (CI: [−2.94, −0.37]) at 1 month and a statistically significant reduction in IOP with a SMD of −1.31 (CI: [−1.45, −1.17]) at 6 months and −1.35

Author	Year of publication		SMD (95% CI)	% weight (I–V)
1-month follow-up				
Ting	2012		−0.17 (−0.30, −0.03)	96.30
Akil	2016		−0.59 (−1.26, 0.08)	3.70
I–V subtotal ($I^2 = 32.8\%$, $p = 0.223$)			−0.18 (−0.31, −0.05)	100.00
D + L subtotal			−0.25 (−0.57, 0.08)	
6-month follow-up				
Ting	2012		−0.44 (−0.57, −0.31)	91.21
Mizoguchi	2015		−0.35 (−0.78, 0.07)	8.79
I–V subtotal ($I^2 = 0.0\%$, $p = 0.694$)			−0.43 (−0.56, −0.31)	100.00
D + L subtotal			−0.43 (−0.56, −0.31)	
12-month follow-up				
Ting	2012		−0.44 (−0.57, −0.30)	79.47
Mizoguchi	2015		−0.50 (−93, −0.07)	7.53
Pahlitzsch	2015		−0.48 (−0.81, −0.16)	12.99
I–V subtotal ($I^2 = 0.0\%$, $p = 0.934$)			−0.45 (−0.56, −0.33)	100.00
D + L subtotal			−0.45 (−0.56, −0.33)	
24-month follow-up				
Mizoguchi	2015		−1.10 (−1.56, −0.65)	100.00
I–V subtotal ($I^2 = .\%$, $p = .$)			−1.10 (−1.56, −0.65)	100.00
D + L subtotal			−1.10 (−1.56, −0.65)	

−1.56   0   1.56

Favors trabectome

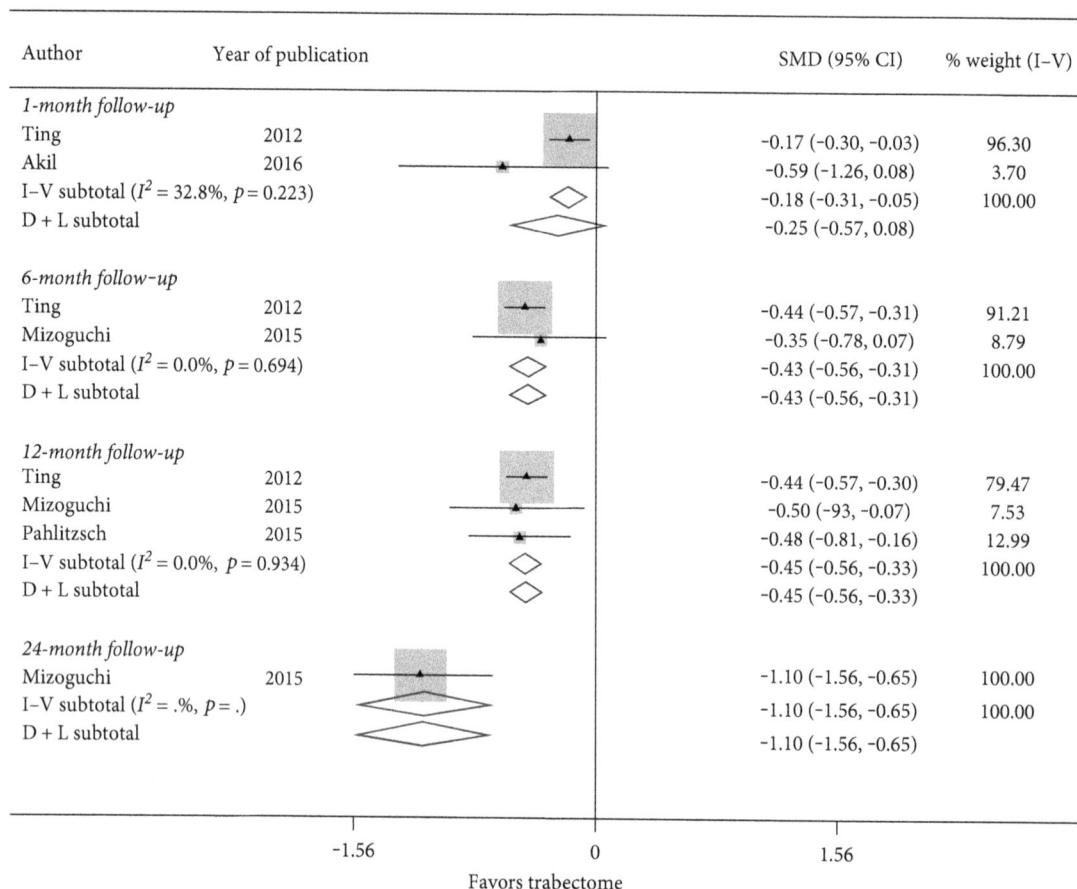

FIGURE 5: Forest plot for studies examining change in number of glaucoma medications used by follow-up (months).

(CI: [−1.48, −1.22]) at 12 months follow-up. This suggests that the significant reduction in IOP from the Trabectome procedure persists even after 12 months.

3.5. Effect on Glaucoma Medication Use. Figure 5 summarizes the results for the change in glaucoma medications used at 6 months and 12 months follow-up. There were 2 studies considering follow-up of 6 months and 3 studies inspecting 12 months follow-up. Nonsignificant heterogeneity between studies examining follow-up at 1 month ($I^2 = 32.8\%$, p value = 0.223), 6 months ($I^2 = 0.0\%$, p value = 0.694), and 12 months ($I^2 = 0.0\%$, p value = 0.934) was used to determine the fixed-effect computations. In Figure 5, there was a statistically significant reduction in postoperative glaucoma medications used with a SMD of −0.18 (CI: [−0.31, −0.05]) at 1 month, SMD of −0.43 (CI: [−0.56, −0.31]) at 6 months, and a SMD of −0.45 (CI: [−0.56, −0.33]) at 12 months follow-up. Thus, Trabectome surgery may significantly reduce dependence on glaucoma medications at 12 months follow-up.

4. Discussion

A systematic review of the literature was conducted to determine the performance of the Trabectome as a solo procedure in patients with POAG. The primary outcomes measured were IOP and glaucoma medications used. Various bibliographic databases and grey literature were searched resulting

in inclusion of three relevant full-text studies and one abstract after three levels of screening, indicating a lack of published evidence available for this topic. Thus, it would be ideal if more studies could be conducted to better understand the optimal role of Trabectome in IOP management and topical glaucoma medication management.

In all included studies, the results suggested that the Trabectome surgery resulted in significant reduction in IOP and glaucoma medications in POAG patients [12, 14–16]. While the included studies showed a 25–34% reduction in IOP at 12 months follow-up and the $SE_{IOPR\%}$ ranged from 33–35%—large standard errors suggest that the Trabectome may have differing levels of efficacy between patients. In addition, the Trabectome was not compared to a placebo (or standard of care/alternative treatment) as the key objective of this study was to determine whether the primary diagnosis of the patients had an effect on the Trabectome's success. Without an adequate control group, a strong conclusion cannot be made for the efficacy of the Trabectome as a solo procedure in POAG patients.

A recent systematic review that included all glaucoma subjects, regardless of type, also found that IOP and glaucoma medications used decreased significantly from baseline [9]. A significant strength of this analysis stems from the fact that all the included studies had coherent results of reduction in IOP as well topical glaucoma medications due to Trabectome surgery.

The study limitations for meta-analyses such as this are necessary to ponder before inferences may be considered. The primary limitation of this systematic review was the narrow inclusion criteria and the resulting low number of included studies. One reason for the low number of included studies was the lack of availability of studies that specifically examined the effect of the Trabectome in patients with POAG. In two of the included studies, the XFG group had a higher mean reduction in IOP than the POAG group, which could be due to the higher preoperative IOP levels in XFG patients [14, 19]. The Mizoguchi et al. study also showed that the XFG had a higher percent mean reduction in IOP than the POAG group, but the preoperative IOP levels were higher in the POAG patients [15]. This difference between primary and secondary glaucoma reinforces the decision to exclude studies where the POAG results are not presented separately from the secondary open-angle glaucoma such as XFG. Many studies located in the literature search were excluded because they presented the results for all types of glaucoma and pooled patients with differing glaucoma diagnoses. The lack of evidence stratified by glaucoma subgroup makes clinical decision-making difficult since physicians will be unable to determine whether the intervention is suitable for their specific patients. Further, complication and failure rates may have more to do with the type of glaucoma rather than the procedure.

Secondly, it is necessary to consider the quality of the included studies. In this meta-analysis, the Downs and Black checklist [13] was employed and none of the included studies were found to be of high quality. The included studies lacked elements such as randomization, blinding, and a control group. Nevertheless, due to limited number of studies available for the analysis, all were included, irrespective of their quality. This is a recognized, but necessary, limitation due to the few clinical studies currently available.

Thirdly, meta-analysis of observational studies is influenced by inherent biases in the included articles [23]. For example, a multitude of other factors such as level of education, ethnicity, income status, socioeconomic status, previous ocular and nonocular surgeries, family history, other ocular and nonocular diseases, preoperative and postoperative medications, number of medications, and comorbidities (e.g., high blood pressure, diabetes, stroke, and heart conditions) could influence the estimates in the original studies. Potential bias related to industry sponsorship of a study also exists, as well as methods of patient selection. Variations in surgical technique may be a major factor as well.

The results of this meta-analysis showed reduction in IOP and topical glaucoma medications after Trabectome surgery. However, the current literature suggests that additional research is warranted to best understand how to maximize the utility of Trabectome in the management of glaucoma patients. Even though the Trabectome has been available for over ten years, no randomized controlled trials have been published comparing the Trabectome with other potential glaucoma treatments [24]. As a result, it is challenging for hospitals, physicians, and other decision-makers to determine if the available evidence is sufficient to warrant publicly funded access to innovations in technology such as the Trabectome. A notable lack of published research on rates of early and late postoperative complications suggests that more research is also needed in this area.

5. Conclusions

In conclusion, this systematic review suggests that the Trabectome may be helpful in reducing the IOP and the number of glaucoma medications used in POAG patients. However, there is a need for sufficient evidence to determine Trabectome's effectiveness as a solo procedure in treating POAG due to the low number and quality of available studies. These results are concerning as the Trabectome has been used to treat open-angle glaucoma since 2006 in the United States without sufficient evidence to support anecdotal experience. The Trabectome is just one example of a technological innovation in which funding challenges have impeded access to the evidence that would allow a more definitive understanding of its role in the glaucoma treatment paradigm. There is a strong need for more studies to be conducted on the Trabectome to show effectiveness, especially randomized controlled trials and trials comparing the Trabectome to control treatments. As the Trabectome is not the only intervention in which there is a paucity of relevant research to allow evidence-based decision-making, it may be time for all stakeholders (physicians, hospitals, government, and industry) to come together to determine collective strategies that will ensure access to optimal care for patients with glaucoma.

Disclosure

The authors alone are responsible for the content and writing of the paper.

Conflicts of Interest

The authors report no conflicts of interest.

Acknowledgments

The authors wish to acknowledge John Costella for the assistance in designing the search strategy and Rohin Krishnan for the additional comments.

References

[1] S. Resnikoff, D. Pascolini, D. Etya'ale et al., "Policy and practice," *Bulletin of the World Health Organization*, vol. 82, no. 11, pp. 844–851, 2004.

[2] H. A. Quigley and A. T. Broman, "The number of people with glaucoma worldwide in 2010 and 2020," *The British Journal of Ophthalmology*, vol. 90, no. 3, pp. 262–267, 2006.

[3] D. B. Rein, P. Zhang, K. E. Wirth et al., "The economic burden of major adult visual disorders in the United States," *Archives of Ophthalmology*, vol. 124, no. 12, pp. 1754–1760, 2006.

[4] Glaucoma Research Foundation, "Types of glaucoma gleams [Internet]," May 2010, http://www.glaucoma.org/glaucoma/types-of-glaucoma.php.

[5] L. M. Brandão and M. C. Grieshaber, "Update on minimally invasive glaucoma surgery (MIGS) and new implants," *Journal of Ophthalmology*, vol. 2013, Article ID 705915, 12 pages, 2013.

[6] B. a. Francis, "Ab interno trabeculectomy: development of a novel device (Trabectome) and surgery for open-angle glaucoma," *Journal of Glaucoma*, vol. 15, no. 1, pp. 68–73, 2006.

[7] S. D. Vold, "Ab interno trabeculotomy with the trabectome system: what does the data tell us?" *International Ophthalmology Clinics*, vol. 51, no. 3, pp. 65–81, 2011.

[8] Y. Iordanous, J. S. Kent, C. M. L. Hutnik, and M. S. Malvankar-Mehta, "Projected cost comparison of Trabectome, iStent, and endoscopic cyclophotocoagulation versus glaucoma medication in the Ontario Health Insurance Plan," *Journal of Glaucoma*, vol. 23, no. 2, pp. e112–e118, 2014.

[9] K. Kaplowitz, I. I. Bussel, R. Honkanen, J. S. Schuman, and N. A. Loewen, "Review and meta-analysis of ab-interno trabeculectomy outcomes," *The British Journal of Ophthalmology*, vol. 100, no. 5, pp. 594–600, 2016.

[10] J. Thomas, J. Brunton, and S. Graziosi, *EPPI-Reviewer 4: Software for Research Synthesis [Internet]*, EPPI-Centre Software, London, 2010, http://eppi.ioe.ac.uk/cms/Default.aspx?alias=eppi.ioe.ac.uk/cms/er4.

[11] Veritas Health Innovation, "Covidence systematic review software [Internet]," Cochrane, Melbourne, 2016, http://www.covidence.org.

[12] M. Pahlitzsch, J. Gonnermann, A. K. Maier et al., "Trabekulotomie ab interno (Trabectome) – Kumulierte klinische Ergebnisse eines großen Glaukomkollektivs," *Klinische Monatsblätter für Augenheilkunde*, vol. 232, no. 10, pp. 1198–1207, 2015.

[13] S. H. Downs and N. Black, "The feasibility of creating a checklist for the assessment of the methodological quality both of randomised and non-randomised studies of health care interventions," *Journal of Epidemiology and Community Health*, vol. 52, no. 6, pp. 377–384, 1998.

[14] J. L. M. Ting, K. F. Damji, and M. C. Stiles, "Ab interno trabeculectomy: outcomes in exfoliation versus primary open-angle glaucoma," *Journal of Cataract & Refractive Surgery*, vol. 38, no. 2, pp. 315–323, 2012, ASCRS and ESCRS.

[15] T. Mizoguchi, S. Nishigaki, T. Sato, H. Wakiyama, and N. Ogino, "Clinical results of Trabectome surgery for open-angle glaucoma," *Clinical Ophthalmology*, vol. 9, pp. 1889–1894, 2015.

[16] H. Akil, P. Huang, V. Chopra, and B. Francis, "Assessment of anterior segment measurements with swept source optical coherence tomography before and after ab interno trabeculotomy (Trabectome) surgery," *Journal of Ophthalmology*, vol. 2016, pp. 1–7, 2016.

[17] M. S. Malvankar-Mehta, Y. N. Chen, Y. Iordanous, W. W. Wang, J. Costella, and C. M. L. Hutnik, "iStent as a solo procedure for glaucoma patients: a systematic review and meta-analysis," *PloS One*, vol. 10, no. article e0128146, 2015.

[18] W. Y. Zhang, A. L. Po, H. S. Dua, and A. Azuara-Blanco, "Meta-analysis of randomised controlled trials comparing latanoprost with timolol in the treatment of patients with open angle glaucoma or ocular hypertension," *The British Journal of Ophthalmology*, vol. 85, no. 8, pp. 983–990, 2001.

[19] J. F. Jordan, T. Wecker, C. van Oterendorp et al., "Trabectome surgery for primary and secondary open angle glaucomas," *Graefe's Archive for Clinical and Experimental Ophthalmology*, vol. 251, no. 12, pp. 2753–2760, 2013.

[20] H. Akil, V. Chopra, A. Huang, N. Loewen, J. Noguchi, and B. A. Francis, "Clinical results of ab interno trabeculotomy using the Trabectome in patients with pigmentary glaucoma compared to primary open angle glaucoma," *Clinical & Experimental Ophthalmology*, vol. 44, no. 7, pp. 563–569, 2016.

[21] R. T. Loewen, P. Roy, H. A. Parikh, Y. Dang, J. S. Schuman, and N. A. Loewen, "Impact of a glaucoma severity index on results of Trabectome surgery: larger pressure reduction in more severe glaucoma," *PloS One*, T. S. Acott, Ed., vol. 11, no. article e0151926, 2016.

[22] J. Werth, C. Gesser, and M. Klemm, "Unterschiedliche Effekte der Trabektomoperation auf unterschiedliche Glaukomformen," *Klinische Monatsblätter für Augenheilkunde*, vol. 232, no. 01, pp. 72–78, 2015.

[23] M. Egger, G. D. Smith, M. Schneider, and C. Minder, "Bias in meta-analysis detected by a simple, graphical test," *BMJ*, vol. 315, no. 7109, pp. 629–634, 1997.

[24] K. Hu, G. Gazzard, C. Bunce, and R. Wormald, *Ab Interno Trabecular Bypass Surgery with Trabectome for Open Angle Glaucoma. In: Hu K, Editor. Cochrane Database Syst. Rev*, Chichester, UK, John Wiley & Sons, Ltd, 2016.

14

Phenotypic Description of the Spanish Multicentre Genetic Glaucoma Group Cohort

Elena Milla,[1,2] **Maria José Gamundi,**[3] **Susana Duch,**[2] **Jose Rios,**[4] **Miguel Carballo,**[3] **and EMEIGG Study Group**[5]

[1]*Unidad de Glaucoma, Institut Clínic d'Oftalmologia (ICOF), Hospital Clínic, Barcelona, Spain*
[2]*Unidad de Glaucoma y Genética, Institut Comtal d'Oftalmologia, Barcelona, Spain*
[3]*Servicio de Laboratorio, Hospital de Terrassa, Barcelona, Spain*
[4]*Servicio de Estadística, Hospital Clinic, Barcelona, Spain*
[5]*EMEIGG, Spanish Multicentre Glaucoma Group (Estudio Multicéntrico Español de Investigaciones Genéticas en Glaucoma), Spain*

Correspondence should be addressed to Elena Milla; emilla@clinic.cat

Academic Editor: Carlo Nucci

Introduction. The aim of the study was to make a phenotypic description of the Spanish multicentre glaucoma group cohort of patients. *Design.* Retrospective, observational, multicentre, cohort study. *Material and Methods.* The clinical charts of 152 patients with hereditary glaucoma from18 Spanish eye centres were reviewed in order to make an epidemiologic description of the type of glaucoma and associated factors. True hereditary cases were compared with familiar cases according to the Gong et al. criteria. *Results.* 61% were true hereditary cases and 39% familiar cases. Ocular comorbidity, optic disc damage, and visual field mean defect were significantly more severe in hereditary patients, who required significantly more first-line hypotensive drugs and surgical interventions to control intraocular pressure than familiar patients. *Conclusions.* The strength of the hereditary component of glaucoma seems to worsen the clinical course, causing more structural and functional damage and requiring more intense glaucoma treatment. The family history of glaucoma should be carefully investigated and taken into consideration when making treatment decisions or intensifying previous treatment.

1. Introduction

By 2020, 79.6 million people will have glaucoma or ocular hypertension (OHT) and, of these, 74% will have primary open angle glaucoma (POAG). Glaucoma will continue to be the second leading cause of blindness worldwide [1]. In POAG, early detection and treatment is effective in reducing disease progression [2]. However, 50% of cases are known to be undiagnosed. The two main reasons for underdetection of glaucoma are poor uptake of community eye care services and cases missed by primary eye care services [3]. Due to the public health importance of glaucoma, it has been suggested as a condition that might merit population-based screening programs.

However, as Lander and Shork stated, glaucoma is a complex trait and, in the majority of cases, does not follow a clear-cut inheritance pattern, has a variable penetrance transmission and an insidious progression, and usually has a late onset [4].

Paradoxically, other hereditable ophthalmic pathologies, such as retinitis pigmentosa (RP), are far less common but their genetic profile has been much better characterized [5]. The difference between RP and glaucoma is that the latter is treatable if detected early [6–9]. Therefore, the development of an accurate test to detect presymptomatic carriers at risk is important for the management of glaucomatous optic neuropathy (GON).

Despite considerable research efforts, the aetiology of POAG remains unknown, probably due to the heterogeneous and complex clinical and molecular nature of the disease. In the last decade, much effort has gone into elucidating the genetic causes and risk factors of POAG. The application of advanced genetic technology, such as Genome-Wide

Association Studies (GWAS), large-scale gene expression studies, and proteomics, has yielded a wealth of information. A large amount of candidate POAG disease genes have been identified, and there is increasing insight into the molecular mechanisms underlying POAG [10]. Unfortunately, the underlying molecular mechanisms cannot be elucidated in the majority of glaucoma cases, although a familiar component is clearly present in a large number.

In 2009, our research group initiated a prospective multi-centre study which collected blood samples from patients with familial and hereditary glaucoma throughout Spain in order to carry out genetic characterization with the aim of describing the mutational profile of glaucoma in Spain. After the results were published [11], we assessed the phenotypic data of the study population to characterize the clinical profile of this sample of Spanish glaucoma patients. This is the first description of the phenotypic mapping of glaucoma in Spain.

Therefore, the objective of this study was to describe the epidemiologic features of patients included in our database.

2. Patients and Methods

Before study inclusion, all participants were informed of the study objectives. All gave informed consent to participate in the study, which adhered to the tenets of the Declaration of Helsinki. All were asked to complete a questionnaire that included personal, biographic, demographic, family, and clinical data.

This study was approved by the Ethics Committee of the Hospital Clinic of Barcelona.

Patients from 18 Spanish hospitals were enrolled by their treating ophthalmologists in a collaborative study named Estudio Multicéntrico Español de Investigación Genética del Glaucoma (EMEIGG). We did not include the total EMEIGG population in the present study. An equitable proportion of patients from each eye centre were included in order to homogenize the results between the different Spanish regions.

Patients were enrolled consecutively by their glaucoma specialist if they accomplished the inclusion criteria described below.

Inclusion criteria were POAG patients diagnosed with familiar or hereditary glaucoma and sporadic single patients (without affected relatives) with congenital, juvenile, or any kind of syndromic glaucoma. Glaucoma was diagnosed on the basis of intraocular pressure over 21 mmHg and/or the presence of glaucomatous optic neuropathy and/or glaucomatous changes in perimetry.

Exclusion criteria were other types of glaucoma (closed angle, phacomorphic, augmented episcleral venous pressure, inflammatory, and uveitic glaucoma), a history of ocular hypertension after retinal detachment, intraocular tumour, haemorrhage, postsurgical patients, and trauma.

Hereditary glaucoma/OHT was determined according to the Gong et al. criteria (index case and two affected first degree relatives from consecutive generations) [12]; the remaining cases that did not comply with this definition were classified as familial glaucoma/OHT.

All participating ophthalmologists completed a standardized Excel questionnaire in order to homogenize the collection of epidemiological and clinical data. All patients underwent a full history including systemic and ophthalmologic pathologies, other family members affected by glaucoma (number and type of relative), a family history of consanguinity, and whether they were born in a municipality with <500 inhabitants (to check for masked consanguinity).

Patients were also asked about the places of naissance of their parents and relatives in order to confirm that they were all from Spanish origin.

Patients also underwent a complete ophthalmologic examination including LOG-MAR best-corrected visual acuity, refractive status, slit lamp examination, Goldmann applanation tonometry, and funduscopy. Ancillary tests included computerized perimetry, ultrasound pachymetry, gonioscopy, optic disc photography, and optical coherence tomography (OCT).

Each referring ophthalmologist graded the disease stage, taking into account the ophthalmologic exams, the aspect of the optic disc, and visual field testing results and classified each case as ocular hypertension, initial, moderate, or severe glaucoma. Visual field damage was quantified according to Hodapp-Parrish-Anderson grading scale according to mean defect MD (initial if $MD < -6\,dB$, moderate if MD between -6 and $-12\,dB$, and advanced if $MD > -12\,dB$). Data on the number and type of ocular surgeries (including phacoemulsification) were recorded, as were current ocular hypotensive medicines.

2.1. Statistical Analysis. Quantitative variables were described using medians and interquartile ranges [P25, P75] and absolute ranges (minimum and maximum) and qualitative variables using relative frequencies. Groups were compared using the Mann–Whitney U test for quantitative variables and Fisher's exact test for qualitative variables. The analysis was made using the SPSS statistical program v20. A type I bilateral error of 5% was applied.

3. Results

The results are summarized in Tables 1 and 2. We collected data from 152 index patients included in the EMEIGG study database of unrelated glaucoma families throughout Spain [11]. Of these, 92 (61%) were true hereditary cases and 60 (39%) were familiar cases.

The median age was 64 (46; 75) years, and 83 (54.6%) were female (52 [56.5%] in hereditary patients and 31 [51.7%] in familiar patients). POAG was the most frequent type of glaucoma in both hereditary and familial patients, followed by secondary open angle glaucoma (pseudoexfoliative and pigmentary), congenital glaucoma, and juvenile glaucoma. No significant differences were found between hereditary and familial patients with respect to disease type.

Hereditary cases had a significantly older mean age and more ophthalmologic comorbidity and presented with a lower spherical equivalent but had more surgeries.

There were no significant differences in LogMAR visual acuity values in hereditary and familial patients,

TABLE 1: Demographic, clinical, and treatment variables in hereditary and familiar glaucoma patients. Spain, 2015.

Group	Hereditary	Familiar	p value
Number of cases	92 (61%)	60 (39%)	
Age (Yrs)	66 (46;75)	59 (39;68)	0.007
Sex (female)	52 (56.5%)	31 (51.7%)	0.618
Glaucoma Subtype			
POAG	72 (78.3%)	40 (66.7%)	0.335
Secondary	6 (6.5%)	4 (6.7%)	
Juvenile	7 (7.6%)	8 (13.3%)	
Congenital	6 (6.5%)	8 (13.3%)	
Syndromic	1 (1.1%)	0 (0%)	
Severity of glaucoma			
OHT	4 (4.3%)	5 (8.3%)	0.319
Initial glaucoma	19 (20.7%)	22 (36.7%)	0.039
Moderate glaucoma	29 (31.5%)	12 (20%)	0.137
Severe glaucoma	40 (43.5%)	19 (31.7%)	0.174
Ophthalmic Variables			
Ophthalmic comorbidities	20 (32.8%)	4 (10%)	0.09
VA (LOGMAR)	0.22 [0.05; 0.4]	0.1 [0; 0.3]	0.067
Spherical equivalent	−0.75 (−2;1)	−1.25 (−3.5; −0.25)	0.046
Optic disk lesions (Splinter Hemorrhages)	15 (16.5%)	3 (5%)	0.04
VF MD	−10.42 [−18; −4.39]	−5.475 [−13.51; −2.78]	0.046
Surgeries	63 (68.5%)	28 (46.7%)	0.01
Medical treatments			
Prostaglandin analogs	45 (48.9%)	18 (30%)	0.028
Alpha adrenerics	7 (7.6%)	11 (18.3%)	0.07

YRS: years; OHT: ocular hypertension; VA: visual acuity; VF MD: visual field mean defect; median and range values are provided.

TABLE 2: Reported relatives with glaucoma in hereditary and familiar glaucoma patients. Spain, 2015.

	Hereditary	Familiar	p value
Median number of reported relatives with glaucoma (P25; P75)	2 (1; 4)	1 (1; 3)	0.003
Father	29 (31.5%)	7 (11.7%)	0.006
Mother	32 (34.8%)	11 (18.3%)	0.029
Brothers	30 (32.6%)	19 (31.7%)	1
Sisters	29 (31.5%)	15 (25%)	0.465
Sons	24 (26.1%)	8 (13.3%)	0.069
Daughters	19 (20.7%)	0 (0%)	<0.001
Paternal uncles	2 (2.2%)	2 (3.3%)	0.647
Paternal aunts	0 (0%)	2 (3.3%)	0.154
Maternal uncles	3 (3.3%)	0 (0%)	0.278
Maternal aunts	5 (5.4%)	1 (1.7%)	0.404
Paternal grandfather	5 (5.4%)	0 (0%)	0.157
Paternal grandmother	1 (1.1%)	0 (0%)	1
Maternal grandfather	2 (2.2%)	1 (1.7%)	1
Maternal grandmother	2 (2.2%	0 (0%)	0.519
Others	8 (8.7%)	6 (10%)	0.782

although hereditary patients had more advanced perimetry damage (greater negative mean defect values), more severe structural damage to the optic disc (significantly higher proportion of splinter haemorrhages among the other GON factors), and a lower proportion of initial glaucoma cases.

No significant differences were found between familial and hereditary patients in other parameters studied, including intraocular pressure, gonioscopy, anterior segment anomalies, or pachymetry.

Medically, hereditary patients more frequently used first-line drugs, and familial patients second-line drugs. Hereditary patients had a greater frequency of surgical interventions (including phacoemulsification).

The median number of affected relatives was 2 [1; 4] in hereditary patients and 1 [1; 3] in familiar patients ($p = 0.003$). Affected relatives were most frequently parents and offspring, although the only significant relationship was for daughters ($p = < 0.001$) (Table 2).

No differences were found between patients born in municipalities with <500 inhabitants or >500 inhabitants.

4. Discussion

Familial clustering has been a known risk factor for glaucoma for decades and has gradually gained more weight as a decisive factor for the initiation or not of glaucoma treatment. Initial reports suggested a 30% risk of developing glaucoma in relatives of an index case, but later reports have suggested the risk could be 56% or even 75% [12]. This suggests that POAG has a strong genetic component. The family history is clinically important because the risk of POAG among first-degree relatives of a POAG patient is 7–10 times higher than that of the general population, and surveillance targeting these individuals is indicated for the early detection and treatment of POAG [13].

In the Thessaloniki Eye Study (TES), the prevalence of undiagnosed glaucoma in POAG patients was 57.1%, which was significantly higher than the 34.9% found in pseudoexfoliative glaucoma patients. Other population-based studies throughout the world have reported higher estimated prevalences of undiagnosed glaucoma (60% to 93.3%). The natural history of the disease shows that glaucoma is a silent, asymptomatic disease before advanced damage with significant visual impairment occurs. The TES showed a trend to reduce odds of undiagnosed glaucoma in POAG patients who reported a family history of glaucoma [14].

Weih et al. found that, other than age, the strongest risk factor for glaucoma was a family history of glaucoma and that, in definite glaucoma cases, a family history of glaucoma was the only significant risk factor other than age. However, the authors concluded that reporting of a family history of glaucoma is likely to be underestimated, resulting in an underestimate of the strength of the association between family history and the risk of glaucoma. As in the Baltimore Eye Survey, they found a substantial bias in the reported family history between patients who were diagnosed or undiagnosed at the time of the study. Although not statistically significant, 29% of patients who were already diagnosed reported a family history of glaucoma compared with 15%

who were undiagnosed [13, 15]. The study was carried out in urban and rural zones of Australia and found an unexplained higher concentration of glaucoma cases in rural areas [15]. This might possibly be explained by the hypothesis that there were higher rates of masked consanguinity in smaller rural locations. We found no evidence of this in Spain today, but it may have been more plausible in rural Victoria 15 years ago.

In our study, hereditary glaucoma cases were significantly more severe than familial cases and tended to appear in older patients who presented with optic nerves with greater structural and functional damage and required more aggressive medical treatments and more surgeries to control the disease. The median of affected relatives was significantly higher, as expected due to the definitions used.

Potential biases of our study could include the presence of real hereditary cases hidden among familial cases due to the patient's lack of knowledge of affected relatives and the higher rates of ocular surgeries, including phacoemulsification, in hereditary patients. Cataract surgery could have modified other ocular parameters (central visual acuity, pachymetry, etc.) and caused bias (no significant differences in visual acuity between hereditary and familial patients and a lower spherical equivalent in hereditary patients).

A family history of glaucoma is a risk factor that all ophthalmologists should bear in mind when taking decisions on treatment, especially when there is low concordance between the myriad of structural and functional glaucoma tests or progression algorithms currently in use or when there is a borderline result [16]. However, a negative family history of glaucoma does not always imply that it does not exist, as it may be caused by patients' unawareness or confusion with other ocular conditions. The Ocular Hypertension Treatment Study (OHTS) data on family history were collected by patient recall with no verification by chart review or contact with the relatives; thus, this information is likely to be incomplete and incorrect. A family history of glaucoma was not significant in the 2002 OHTS multivariate analysis of risk factors, and this information was not collected in the European Glaucoma Prevention Study (EGPS) Group [17–19].

Screening for glaucoma is difficult, and it has repeatedly been shown that half the patients with glaucoma are undiagnosed and, in at least one study, half of these patients have had an eye examination in the preceding twelve months and had still been missed. One study showed that 97% of patients with undiagnosed glaucoma had a visual field defect, 66% had a vertical-cup-disc ratio of ≥0.7, and 12% had cup asymmetry of ≥0.3 [20]. To date, no single test has been shown to be satisfactory for glaucoma screening, and thus an appropriate strategy would require a combination of several tests. However, the single biggest risk factor for glaucoma is a positive family history. Most people are unaware of whether they have a first-degree relative with a history of glaucoma, and this reflects a breakdown in our responsibility to inform our patients with glaucoma of the importance of the family history. The single biggest impact physicians may have in the detection of undiagnosed glaucoma is to ask all glaucoma patients to inform their first-degree relatives of their substantially increased risk and encourage relatives to inform the specialist at the next eye examination [21].

It is known that glaucoma cases with a positive mutational diagnosis are frequently more severe [22]. In our study, only 5% of POAG cases presented with a detectable mutation, in line with other reports [11, 23]. However, the remaining true hereditary cases are also consistent with the presence of more advanced glaucoma. These cases presented significantly worse structural and functional optic nerve characteristics, more ocular comorbidities, and needed greater amount of medical and surgical treatment to control intraocular pressure with respect to the familiar cases. Therefore, it may be suggested that the more patent the genetic component in a glaucoma case, the worse the prognosis irrespectively of other factors such as age of diagnosis, level of intraocular pressure, and treatment required.

In light of these results, ophthalmologists should first be encouraged to specifically search for a family history of glaucoma when examining a patient and, secondly, to consider more aggressive treatment when there is greater suspicion of a hereditary component.

Conflicts of Interest

The authors declare that they have no conflicts of interest.

Acknowledgments

The authors would like to thank the EMEIGG group components for their contribution to the study: EMEIGG: Spanish Multicentre Glaucoma Group (Estudio Multicéntrico Español de Investigación Genética del Glaucoma): Mahtab Djavanmardi (Institut Comtal d'Oftalmologia, Barcelona); Esperanza Gutiérrez and Marta Montero (Hosp. Doce de Octubre, Madrid); José Abreu (Hosp. Universitario Canarias); Carmen Cabarga (Hosp. Ramón y Cajal, Madrid); Cristina Vendrell (Hosp. Viladecans, Barcelona); Soledad Jiménez (Hosp. Universitario Puerta del Mar, Cádiz); Miguel Angel Almela (Hosp. Lluis Alcanyís, Xàtiva); Jordi Loscos (Hosp. Can Ruti, Barcelona); Carlos Martínez Bello (Hosp. Dos de Maig, Barcelona); Ignacio Vinuesa (Hosp. Punta de Europa, Cádiz); Rosa Martínez (Hosp. Infanta Leonor, Madrid); Tiburcio Ibáñez (Hosp. San Agustín, Linares); Lourdes Iglesias (Hosp. Universitario La Princesa, Madrid); Pere Viñallonga (Institut Oftalmològic, Menorca); Lluis Soler (Hosp. de Manresa, Barcelona); and Carmen Carrasco (Hosp. de Alcorcón, Madrid).

References

[1] H. A. Quigley and A. T. Broman, "The number of people with glaucoma worldwide in 2010 and 2020," *The British Journal of Ophthalmology*, vol. 90, pp. 262–267, 2006.

[2] B. RRA, P. Sukudom, P. J. Foster et al., "Prevalence of glaucoma in Thailand: a population based survey in Rom Klao District, Bangkok," *The British Journal of Ophthalmology*, vol. 87, pp. 1069–1074, 2003.

[3] P. Mitchell, W. Smith, K. Attebo, and P. R. Healey, "Prevalence of open-angle glaucoma in Australia. The Blue Mountains Eye Study," *Ophthalmology*, vol. 103, pp. 1661–1669, 1996.

[4] E. S. Lander and N. J. Shork, "Genetic dissection of complex traits," *Science*, vol. 265, pp. 2037–2048, 1994.

[5] C. Kim, K. J. Kim, J. Bok et al., "Microarray-based mutation detection and phenotypic characterization in Korean patients with retinitis pigmentosa," *Molecular Vision*, vol. 18, pp. 2398–2410, 2012.

[6] M. C. Leskea, A. Heijl, L. Hyman, B. Bengtsson, and E. Komaroff, "Factors for progression and glaucoma treatment: the early manifest glaucoma trial," *Current Opinion in Ophthalmology*, vol. 15, pp. 102–106, 2004.

[7] R. Shaffer, ""Glaucoma suspect" or "ocular hypertension"?" *Archives of Ophthalmology*, vol. 95, p. 588, 1977.

[8] C. Migdal, "Which therapy to use in glaucoma?" in *Ophthalmology*, M. Yanoff and J. S. Duker, Eds., vol. 12, pp. 23–25, Mosby, London, 1999.

[9] J. A. Lusthaus and I. Goldberg, "Investigational and experimental drugs for intraocular pressure reduction in ocular hypertension and glaucoma," *Expert Opinion on Investigational Drugs*, vol. 25, pp. 1201–1208, 2016.

[10] S. F. Janssen, T. G. Gorgels, W. D. Ramdas et al., "The vast complexity of primary open angle glaucoma: disease genes, risks, molecular mechanisms and pathobiology," *Progress in Retinal and Eye Research*, vol. 37, pp. 31–67, 2013.

[11] E. Millá, B. Mañé, S. Duch et al., "Survey of familial glaucoma shows a high incidence of cytochrome P450, family1, subfamily B, polypeptide 1 (CYP1B1) mutations in nonconsanguineous congenital forms in a Spanish population," *Molecular Vision*, vol. 19, pp. 1707–1722, 2013.

[12] G. Gong, S. Kosoko-Lasaki, G. Haynatzki, H. T. Lynch, J. A. Lynch, and M. R. Wilson, "Inherited, familial and sporadic primary open-angle glaucoma," *Journal of the National Medical Association*, vol. 99, pp. 559–563, 2007.

[13] J. M. Tielsch, J. Katz, A. Sommer, H. A. Quigley, and J. C. Javitt, "Family history and risk of primary open angle glaucoma: The Baltimore Eye Survey," *Archives of Ophthalmology*, vol. 112, pp. 69–73, 1994.

[14] F. Topouzis, A. L. Coleman, A. Harris et al., "Factors associated with undiagnosed open-angle glaucoma: the Thessaloniki eye study," *American Journal of Ophthalmology*, vol. 145, pp. 327–335, 2008.

[15] L. M. Weih, M. Nanjan, C. A. McCarty, and H. R. Taylor, "Prevalence and predictors of open-angle glaucoma: results from the visual impairment project," *Ophthalmology*, vol. 108, pp. 1966–1972, 2001.

[16] J. Sherman, S. Slotnick, and J. Boneta, "Discordance between structure and function in glaucoma: possible anatomical explanations," *Optometry*, vol. 80, pp. 487–501, 2009.

[17] M. O. Gordon, J. A. Beiser, J. D. Brandt et al., "The ocular hypertension treatment study: baseline factors that predict the onset of primary open-angle glaucoma," *Archives of Ophthalmology*, vol. 120, pp. 714–720, 2002.

[18] European Glaucoma Prevention Study (EGPS) Group, "Results of the European glaucoma prevention study," *Ophthalmology*, vol. 112, pp. 366–375, 2005.

[19] Ocular Hypertension Treatment Study Group, European Glaucoma Prevention Study Group, M. O. Gordon et al., "Validated prediction model for the development of primary open-angle glaucoma in individuals with ocular hypertension," *Ophthalmology*, vol. 114, pp. 10–19, 2007.

[20] E. A. Maul and H. D. Jampel, "Glaucoma screening in the real world," *Ophthalmology*, vol. 117, pp. 1665-1666, 2010.

[21] H. Taylor, "Glaucoma screening in the real world. Letter to the Editor," *Ophthalmology*, vol. 118, p. 100, 2011.

[22] E. I. Souzeau, K. P. Burdon, A. Dubowsky et al., "Higher prevalence of myocilin mutations in advanced glaucoma in comparison with less advanced disease in an Australasian disease registry," *Ophthalmology*, vol. 120, pp. 1135–1143, 2013.

[23] S. Kumar, M. A. Malik, S. Goswami, R. Sihota, and J. Kaur, "Candidate genes involved in the susceptibility of primary open angle glaucoma," *Gene*, vol. 577, pp. 119–131, 2016.

15

The Pattern of Retinal Nerve Fiber Layer and Macular Ganglion Cell-Inner Plexiform Layer Thickness Changes in Glaucoma

Jin A Choi,[1] Hye-Young Shin,[2] Hae-Young Lopilly Park,[3] and Chan Kee Park[3]

[1]*Department of Ophthalmology, College of Medicine, St. Vincent's Hospital, Catholic University of Korea, Suwon, Republic of Korea*
[2]*Department of Ophthalmology, College of Medicine, Uijeongbu St. Mary's Hospital, Catholic University of Korea, Uijeongbu, Republic of Korea*
[3]*Department of Ophthalmology, College of Medicine, Seoul St. Mary's Hospital, Catholic University of Korea, Seoul, Republic of Korea*

Correspondence should be addressed to Chan Kee Park; ckpark@catholic.ac.kr

Academic Editor: Tomomi Higashide

Background/Aims. To investigate the patterns of retinal ganglion cell damage at different stages of glaucoma, using the circumpapillary retinal nerve fiber layer (RNFL) and macula ganglion cell-inner plexiform layer (GCIPL) thicknesses. *Methods.* In 296 eyes of 296 glaucoma patients and 55 eyes of 55 healthy controls, the correlations of mean deviation (MD) with the superior and inferior quadrant RNFL/GCIPL thickness (defined as the average of three superior and inferior sectors, resp.) were analyzed. *Results.* In early to moderate glaucoma, most of the RNFL/GCIPL thicknesses had significant positive correlations with the MD. In advanced glaucoma, the superior GCIPL thickness showed the highest correlation with MD ($r = 0.495$), followed by the superior RNFL ($r = 0.452$) (all; $P < 0.05$). The correlation coefficient of the inferior RNFL thickness with MD ($r < 0.471$) was significantly stronger in early to moderate glaucoma compared to that in advanced glaucoma ($r = 0.192$; $P < 0.001$). In contrast, the correlations of the superior GCIPL thickness with MD ($r = 0.452$) in advanced glaucoma was significantly stronger compared to that in early to moderate glaucoma ($r = 0.159$; $P < 0.001$). *Conclusions.* The most preserved region in advanced glaucoma appears to be the superior macular GCIPL, whereas the most vulnerable region for initial glaucoma is the inferior RNFL around the optic disc.

1. Introduction

Glaucomatous damage usually spares the horizontal meridian in the early stage and occurs asymmetrically across the horizontal meridian [1]. In the early stages of glaucoma, the inferior retina, corresponding to superior hemifield, is involved more frequently [2, 3], with faster progression, compared with the superior retina, corresponding to the inferior hemifield [4]. In terms of progression, the retinal nerve fiber layer (RNFL) on the inferotemporal side (324–336°) is the most common location of progressive changes detected by optical coherence tomography (OCT) [5]. Studies of the disparity in glaucomatous damage between the superior and inferior retina have focused on the relatively early stages of glaucoma [4–6]. By

contrast, in advanced glaucoma, few studies have addressed the pattern of structural loss because, in this stage, extensive RNFL loss in both the superior and inferior retina has already occurred, and the assessment of the severity of disease is based largely on visual field (VF) parameters.

It has been well known that the selective retinal ganglion cell loss is a pathological hallmark of the glaucoma optic neuropathy. That begins at optic disc lamina as it is compressed and deformed by intraocular pressure (IOP) and makes the axonal damage as a consequence [7]. In practical field, we can observe them as a cupping enlargement in the disc and an RNFL defect. The next sequence might be a soma change, and that would be a natural history of the retinal ganglion cell loss in the glaucomatous optic neuropathy [8–10]. But unfortunately, this sequence is hardly recognizable by the clinical observations.

Cirrus high-definition- (HD-) OCT (Carl Zeiss Meditec, Dublin, CA), a commercial OCT device, can measure the macular ganglion cell-inner plexiform layer (GCIPL) thickness using a ganglion cell analysis (GCA) algorithm [11–13]. With an aid of this recent advancement of OCT technology, we can now figure out the structure of the whole retinal ganglion cell from the dendrite/soma (GCIPL) to the axon (cpRNFL). So we hope, in this study, we can evaluate the whole sequence of the retinal ganglion cell damage by observing the cpRNFL and GCIPL thickness changes in different stages of glaucoma from the beginning to the end. This would help us clinically to know the sensitive sites and the parameters for glaucoma severity in different stages and, in addition, help us academically to understand the natural history of the retinal ganglion cell death in glaucoma.

2. Patients and Methods

2.1. Study Samples. The medical records of all consecutive patients with open-angle glaucoma and healthy controls examined by a glaucoma specialist (CKP) between April 2012 and May 2013 at the glaucoma clinic of Seoul St. Mary's Hospital (Seoul, Korea) were reviewed retrospectively. This study was performed according to the tenets of the Declaration of Helsinki after approval by our institutional review board. When both eyes met the inclusion criteria, one eye was chosen randomly for the study.

All subjects underwent a medical history review, measurement of the best-corrected visual acuity, refraction, slit-lamp biomicroscopy, gonioscopy, Goldmann applanation tonometry, dilated stereoscopic examination of the optic disc, disc and red-free fundus photography (Canon, Tokyo, Japan), standard perimetry (24-2 Swedish Interactive Threshold Algorithm SAP, Humphrey Field Analyzer II; Carl Zeiss Meditec, Dublin, CA), and spectral-domain OCT (Cirrus HD-OCT; Carl Zeiss Meditec). All included subjects had a best-corrected visual acuity $\geq 20/40$, spherical refraction within ± 6.0 diopters, cylinder correction within ± 3.0 diopters, and normal and open anterior chamber angle by gonioscopy, and no history or evidence of retinal disease or nonglaucomatous optic nerve diseases. Patients with neurological or intraocular diseases that could cause VF defects and eyes with consistently unreliable VF results (defined as >25% false-negative results, >25% false-positive results, or >20% fixation losses) were excluded from the study.

Glaucoma was diagnosed when patient had a glaucomatous VF defect on two consecutive, reliable VF examinations and by the presence of typical glaucomatous optic disc damage (diffuse or localized rim thinning on stereoscopic color fundus photographs), irrespective of the level of IOP. A glaucomatous VF change was defined as the consistent presence of a cluster of three or more points on the pattern deviation plot with a probability of occurrence of <5% in the normal population, having one point with a

probability of occurrence in <1% of the normal population, glaucoma hemifield test results outside the normal limits, or a pattern standard deviation (PSD) with $P < 5\%$.

The severity of the glaucomatous damage was classified into early, moderate, and advanced stages according to the Hodapp-Parrish-Anderson criteria [14]. Healthy control eyes had an IOP ≤ 21 mmHg, no glaucomatous disc appearance, no visible RNFL defect on red-free RNFL photography, and a reliable normal VF test (an MD or PSD within the 95% confidence interval (CI) and a normal glaucoma hemifield test).

2.2. OCT Imaging. All subjects underwent imaging using spectral-domain OCT (Cirrus high-definition-OCT; Carl Zeiss Meditec) to acquire one optic disc (Optic Disc Cube 200×200 protocol) scan and one macular (Macular Cube 514×128 protocol) by the same operator on the same day. The circumpapillary scan allowed measurement of the RNFL thickness, whereas the macular scan allowed determination of the macular GCIPL thickness using the GCA algorithm [11–13, 15]. The circumpapillary scan measures on the 6 mm $\times 6$ mm data and the GCA algorithm detect and measure macular GCIPL thickness within an annulus with inner vertical and horizontal diameters of 1 and 1.2 mm, respectively, and outer vertical and horizontal diameters of 4 and 4.8 mm, respectively. Image quality was assessed by an experienced examiner blinded to the patient's identity and other test results. Only well-focused, well-centered images without eye movement with signal strengths of 6/10 or greater were used.

For the cpRNFL thickness measurements, the average, superior, and inferior quadrant and clock-hour thicknesses were used. The following GCIPL thickness measurements were analyzed: average, sectoral (superior (S), superonasal (SN), inferonasal (IN), inferior (I), inferotemporal (IT), superotemporal (ST)), the superior GCIPL thickness (defined as the average of the measurements in the S, SN, and ST sectors), and the inferior GCIPL thickness (defined as the average of the measurements in the I, IN, and IT sectors). Right eye orientation was used for the documentation of measurements in left eye.

2.3. Cross-Sectional Analysis of VF Progression Patterns in Advanced Stage Glaucoma. To visualize the average maps at different disease stage in advanced glaucoma, eyes with advanced stage glaucoma were further classified into 5 subgroups according to MD (I: -12 dB $\geq$ MD > -15 dB, II: MD > -18 dB, III: MD > -21 dB, IV: MD > -24 dB, V: MD ≤ -24 dB). Within each subgroup, threshold sensitivity map numeric values of the 24-2 VF tests were averaged for each VF test point, generating 1 average map for each subgroup. Based on the maximum and minimum threshold sensitivity values of all average maps, a linear grayscale was generated and applied to all maps [16].

2.4. Data Analysis. Multiple comparisons among the groups were conducted using one-way analysis of variance (ANOVA) and Tukey's test. The independent Student's t-test was used to compare the superior and inferior cpRNFL/

TABLE 1: Demographic and clinical characteristics of the total studied populations.

	Normal controls ($n = 55$)	Early glaucoma ($n = 190$)	Moderate glaucoma ($n = 58$)	Advanced glaucoma ($n = 48$)	P	Post hoc
Age (years)	48 ± 12	53 ± 12	53 ± 10	60 ± 13	<0.001	N = E = M < A
Gender (% of female)	41.8	46.3	43.1	62.5	0.399	
Spherical equivalent (diopter)	-1.00 ± 1.62	-1.65 ± 2.31	-1.53 ± 2.61	-2.07 ± 3.18	0.232	
Axial length (mm)	24.0 ± 0.75	24.4 ± 1.2	24.3 ± 1.3	24.3 ± 1.3	0.348	
CCT (μm)	552.0 ± 26.1	538.6 ± 35.9	529.2 ± 30.1	528.9 ± 32.5	0.004	N > E = M = A
MD (dB)	-0.38 ± 1.39	-2.43 ± 1.70	-8.55 ± 1.92	-19.24 ± 5.63	0.000	N > E > M > A
PSD (dB)	1.43 ± 0.29	4.41 ± 2.41	11.13 ± 2.92	11.80 ± 3.02	0.000	N < E < M < A
VFI	100 ± 1	94 ± 5	76 ± 8	45 ± 18	0.000	N > E > M > A
Average cpRNFL thickness (μm)	100.0 ± 7.7	80.3 ± 9.5	70.5 ± 8.9	62.5 ± 8.9	0.000	N > E > M > A
Average macular GCIPL thickness (μm)	85.9 ± 4.3	74.0 ± 6.3	69.1 ± 5.4	59.8 ± 14.0	0.000	N > E > M > A
ONH parameters						
Rim area (mm^2)	1.31 ± 0.19	0.94 ± 0.20	0.76 ± 0.15	0.63 ± 0.19	0.000	N > E > M > A
Cup area (mm^2)	0.19 ± 0.16	0.46 ± 0.30	0.51 ± 0.30	0.56 ± 0.31	0.102	N > E = M = A
VCD	0.50 ± 0.11	0.72 ± 0.11	0.77 ± 0.08	0.81 ± 0.07	0.000	N < E < M = A

CCT: central corneal thickness; MD: mean deviation of perimetry; PSD: pattern standard deviation of perimetry; VFI: visual field index; dB: decibels; cpRNFL: circumpapillary retinal nerve fiber layer; GCIPL: ganglion cell-inner plexiform layer; VCD: vertical cup to disc ratio. The severity of the glaucomatous damage was classified into early (MD ≥ -6.00 dB), moderate (-12.00 dB $\leq$ MD < -6.00 dB), and advanced glaucoma (MD < -12.00 dB). Values are mean $\pm$ standard deviation. Comparison among study groups was done by analysis of variance (Tukey multiple comparison).

GCIPL thicknesses in each group. The associations of MD and cpRNFL/GCIPL thicknesses were evaluated using Pearson's correlation coefficient. To compare the associations between the VF MD and sectoral OCT measurements obtained using ONH scan and macular GCIPL modes, the bootstrap method (1000 replicates) using the R means from 1000 samples reported for each relationship was used to assess the significance of differences between any two correlation coefficients. And a t-test was done to test the null hypothesis that the R value between two models is equal. To evaluate the goodness of fit of the prediction curve to our dataset, we plotted locally weighted scatterplot smoothing (LOWESS) curves. All statistical analyses were performed using SPSS software ver. 17.0 (SPSS, Chicago, IL). Values of $P < 0.05$ (two-tailed) were considered to be significant.

3. Results

The study included 296 eyes of 296 patients with open-angle glaucoma and 55 eyes of 55 healthy controls. According to the glaucoma classification criteria, 190, 58, and 48 eyes had early, moderate, and advanced glaucoma, respectively.

Among the demographic and ocular parameters, age and central corneal thickness (CCT) differed significantly between the healthy control and glaucomatous eyes ($P < 0.001$ and 0.004, resp.) (Table 1).

Figure 1 shows the overall patterns of the average, superior, and inferior cpRNFL/GCIPL thicknesses according to disease severity assessed by the MD in the study population. The LOWESS plot suggests a curvilinear relationship of the MD with the average, superior, and inferior cpRNFL/GCIPL thicknesses. In advanced disease, the relationship between

the MD and the superior versus inferior cpRNFL/GCIPL thicknesses differed. The relationship with the MD was stronger for the superior cpRNFL/GCIPL (Figures 1(e) and 1(h)) than that for the inferior cpRNFL/GCIPL thicknesses (Figures 1(f) and 1(i)). Particularly, the superior GCIPL thickness had a strong relationship with the MD in advanced disease (Figure 1(h)).

In the healthy controls, the inferior cpRNFL ($130.07 \pm 11.6 \mu$m) tended to be thicker than the superior cpRNFL ($126.96 \pm 14.6 \mu$m), but with marginal significance ($P = 0.079$; Figure 2(a)), whereas the superior GCIPL ($86.71 \pm 4.53 \mu$m) was significantly thicker than the inferior GCIPL ($85.25 \pm 4.40 \mu$m; $P < 0.001$; Figure 2(b)). In early, moderate, and advanced glaucoma, the inferior cpRNFL/GCIPL thicknesses were persistently and significantly thinner than the superior cpRNFL/GCIPL thicknesses (all $P < 0.05$; Figures 2(a) and 2(b)).

In early to moderate glaucoma, most of the cpRNFL/GCIPL thicknesses had significant positive correlations with the MD; particularly, the average ($r = 0.477$) and inferior cpRNFL ($r = 0.471$) thickness showed relatively high correlations with the MD (Table 2). In advanced glaucoma, the superior GCIPL thickness ($r = 0.495$) was most strongly correlated with the MD, followed by the superior cpRNFL thickness ($r = 0.452$) and inferior GCIPL ($r = 0.342$) thickness (all $P < 0.05$). The correlation coefficient of the inferior RNFL thickness with MD ($r = 0.471$) was significantly stronger in early to moderate glaucoma compared to that in advanced glaucoma ($r = 0.192$; $P < 0.001$). In contrast, in advanced glaucoma, the correlations of the superior GCIPL thickness with MD ($r = 0.495$) were significantly stronger compared to those in early to moderate glaucoma ($r = 0.159$; $P < 0.001$).

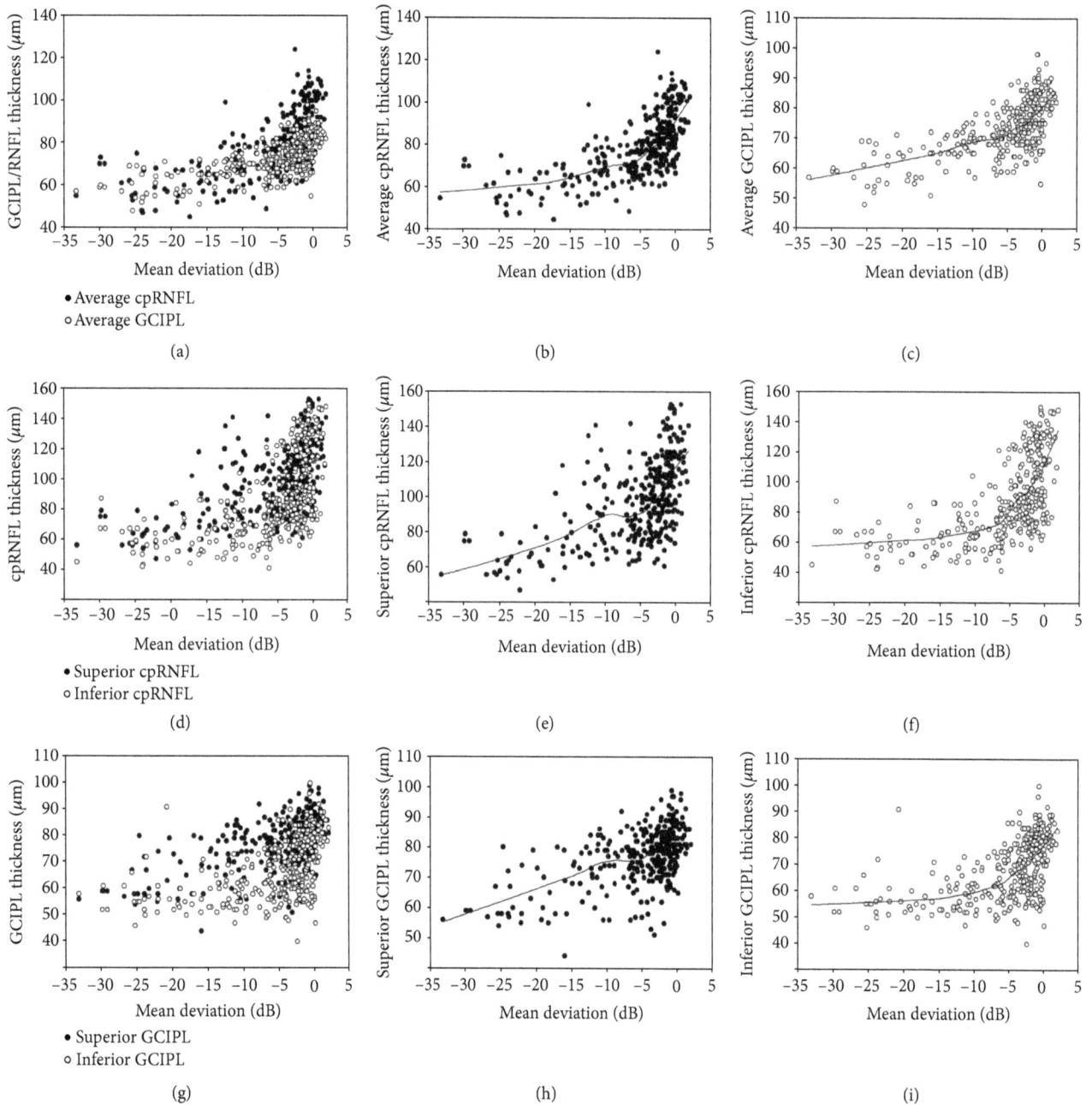

FIGURE 1: Scatterplot showing the average, superior, and inferior cpRNFL/GCIPL thicknesses according to glaucoma severity assessed using mean deviation (MD) in the study population.

Figure 3 shows the correlation coefficients of the MD with the cpRNFL and GCIPL sectoral parameters in early to moderate and advanced glaucoma. In early to moderate glaucoma, the inferior cpRNFL clock-hour thickness (clock hours 6–8) and inferior GCIPL sectors (IN, I, and IT) showed relatively high correlations with the MD. However, in advanced glaucoma, the superior cpRNFL clock-hour thicknesses (clock hours 10–12) and superior GCIPL sectors (ST, S, and IT) and IN sector showed relatively high correlations with the MD.

Figure 4(a) shows the average threshold sensitivity maps of the 24-2 VF tests for subgroups by disease severity assessed

by MD in advanced glaucoma. With increasing disease severity, the deepening and enlargement of scotomas occurred more frequently in superior hemifield. The scotomas in both hemifields spread toward the physiologic blind spot and toward the nasal periphery in an arcuate pattern. The scotomas in superior hemifield occurred very closely to the area corresponding to the papillomacular bundle, whereas the parafoveal area of inferior hemifield was relatively spared. With the disease severity, superior cpRNFL thickness became significantly thinner ($P = 0.003$) with disease severity, whereas changes of inferior cpRNFL was not significant ($P = 0.505$; Figure 4(b)). Superior GCIPL thickness became

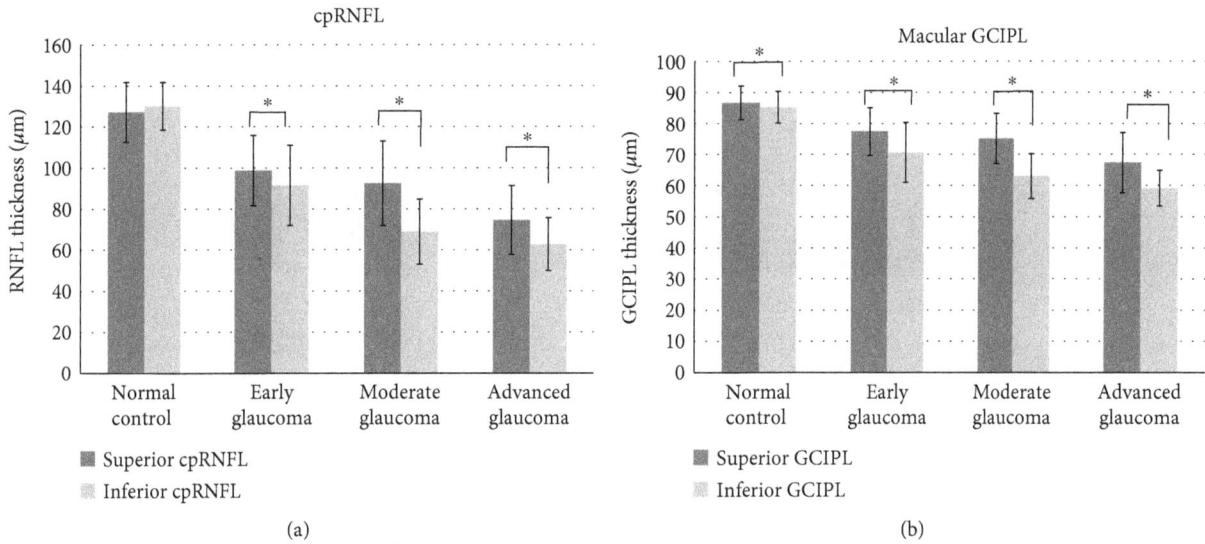

(a)   (b)

FIGURE 2: Comparisons of the superior and inferior cpRNFL/GCIPL thickness in healthy controls, in early, moderate, and advanced glaucomatous eyes. $^*P < 0.05$.

TABLE 2: Correlation coefficient for MD on Humphrey visual field analysis with circumpapillary RNFL and GCIPL parameters on OCT in different stages of glaucomatous eyes.

	Early to moderate glaucoma*			Advanced glaucoma*		
	R	R^2	P	R	R^2	P
cpRNFL						
Average	0.477	0.227	<0.001	0.198	0.039	0.177
Superior (quadrant)	0.252	0.063	<0.001	0.452	0.204	0.001
Inferior (quadrant)	0.471	0.221	<0.001	0.192	0.037	0.191
GCIPL thickness						
Average	0.345	0.119	<0.001	0.093	0.009	0.528
Superior	0.159	0.025	0.012	0.495	0.245	<0.001
Inferior	0.397	0.157	<0.001	0.342	0.117	0.020

*The severity of the glaucomatous damage was classified into early (MD $\geq$ −6.00 dB), moderate, (−12.00 dB $\leq$ MD < −6.00 dB), and advanced glaucoma (MD < −12.00 dB).

significantly thinner ($P = 0.005$) with disease severity, whereas changes of inferior GCIPL was not significant ($P = 0.109$; Figure 4(c)).

4. Discussion

Our study was designed with the purpose of investigating the patterns of retinal ganglion cell damage at different stages of glaucoma, using the cpRNFL and macula GCIPL thicknesses. We observed that the inferior cpRNFL change had the highest correlation with the MD in early stage glaucoma as well as the superior GCIPL change in advanced glaucoma (Table 2).

Through the patterns of structural loss observed in the present study, the natural history of retinal ganglion cell degeneration may be inferred. At initial stage, the glaucomatous damage remains localized involving the inferior (mainly) or superior temporal RNFL. With the progression of disease, lesions are expanded and deepened and new lesion

is developed [5, 17]. Finally, at the far advanced stage, extensive glaucomatous damage occurs, with the relative preservation of retinal ganglion cell bodies at superior macula area. This is further supported by the finding that the VF in far advanced glaucoma is gradually reduced to small central VF area, called the "central isle," which involves mainly the inferior temporal parafoveal VF area next to the blind scotoma [18]. In accordance with this, we found that superior cpRNFL/GCIPL thickness corresponding to inferior hemifield became significantly thinner, whereas changes of inferior cpRNFL/GCIPL corresponding to superior hemifield were not significant (Figures 4(b) and 4(c)). It is well known that OCT is less clinically useful due to a "floor effect" of RNFL thickness. At this stage of disease, sequential VF tests are more reliable to detect progression. Our study results suggest that the detection of progressive thinning of the superior cpRNFL/GCIPL may be useful in determining the progression of the disease in advanced glaucomatous eyes before reaching a "floor effect."

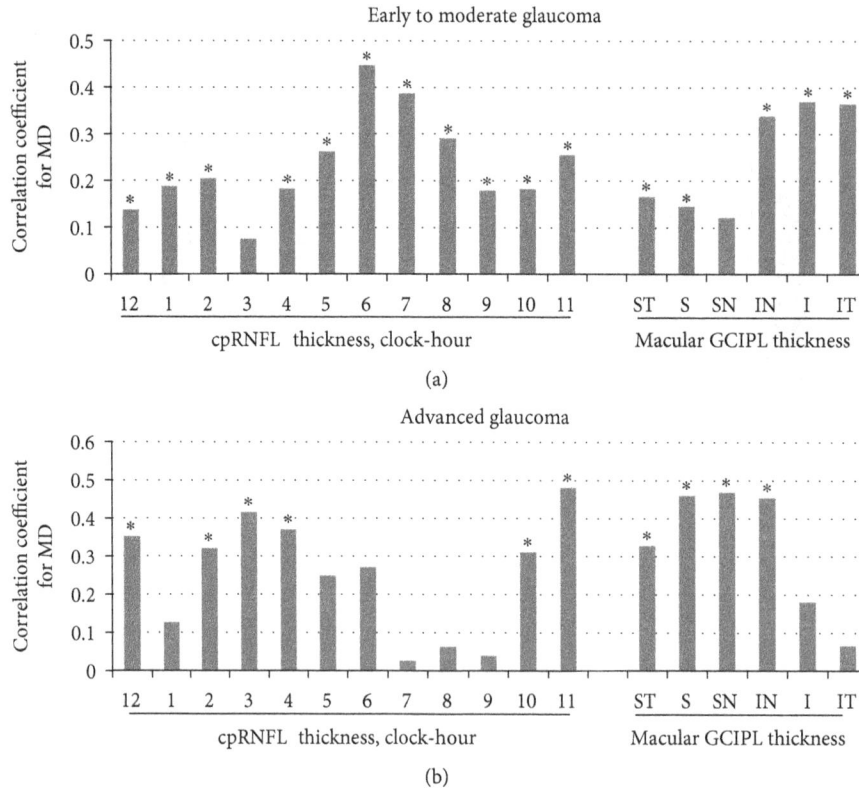

FIGURE 3: Correlation coefficients for the MD from the Humphrey visual field analysis with the cpRNFL and GCIPL sectoral parameters by OCT in glaucomatous eyes at different stages. $^*P < 0.05$.

The reason for the relative sparing of the retinal ganglion cells in the superior macula at advanced stage remains obscure. First, the inferior temporal lamina cribrosa has larger single pores and the least supporting connective tissue [3, 19], which might render the region more susceptible to glaucomatous damage. In addition, the superior GCIPL is reported to be thicker than the inferior GCIPL in normal populations [20]. In this study, the superior GCIPL was also significantly thicker on average than the inferior GCIPL in healthy controls (Figure 2(b)). These findings suggest that relatively more ganglion cells exist in the superior macula compared to the inferior macula.

In glaucoma, structural loss precedes functional changes [21, 22]. Accordingly, most of the RNFL/GCIPL thicknesses, particularly the average and inferior cpRNFL/ GCIPL thicknesses, had significant correlations with disease severity assessed by the MD in early to moderate glaucoma (Table 2 and Figure 3). This observation is in agreement with previous reports that the RNFL loss was most evident at the inferotemporal meridian in the frequency distribution and progression analysis [5, 22]. The inferior quadrant RNFL has also been considered to be the best RNFL parameters discriminating glaucoma from normal control [11, 23]. Regarding the GCIPL parameters, the inferotemporal GCIPL sectors also showed the high diagnostic accuracy in early glaucoma, regardless of the initial location (superior versus inferior) of the glaucomatous damage [11, 13, 24]. These results suggest that the

inferior temporal RNFL is particularly susceptible to the glaucomatous damage and tends to be involved frequently in the initial stage of disease.

Conversely, in advanced glaucoma, the superior GCIPL thickness had the highest correlation with the MD, followed by the superior cpRNFL thickness, whereas the inferior cpRNFL and inferior GCIPL thicknesses had relatively low correlations with the MD (Table 2). In the sectoral analysis in advanced glaucoma, the superior (ST, S, and SN) and some of inferior (IN) GCIPL sectors were also found to have relatively higher correlations with the MD compared to the inferior (I and IT) GCIPL sectors (Figure 3). At advanced stages of glaucoma, it is often difficult for clinicians to detect progression of the disease because extensive structural damage has been occurring. The evaluation of VF parameters constitutes an important part of progression detection. However, due to low reliability and low reproducibility of the VF results in the advanced stage [25], there has been a need for an objective method for assessing glaucomatous damage in the advanced stage. In this regard, the superior GCIPL thickness parameter may represent a complementary tool to the VF assessment for the monitoring of advanced glaucomatous eyes.

Our study had limitations to be acknowledged. First, this study had a cross-sectional study design; to confirm our study finding, longitudinal studies are necessary. Next, the mean age of the advanced glaucoma group is older than that

I (−15 dB < MD ≤ −12 dB) II (−18 dB < MD ≤ −15 dB) III (−21 dB < MD ≤ −18 dB) IV (−24 dB < MD ≤ −21 dB) V (MD ≤ −24 dB)

≥ 30 dB	< 15 dB
< 30 dB	< 10 dB
< 25 dB	< 5 dB
< 20 dB	0 dB

(a)

— Superior cpRNFL
⋯ Inferior cpRNFL

(b)

— Superior GCIPL
⋯ Inferior GCIPL

(c)

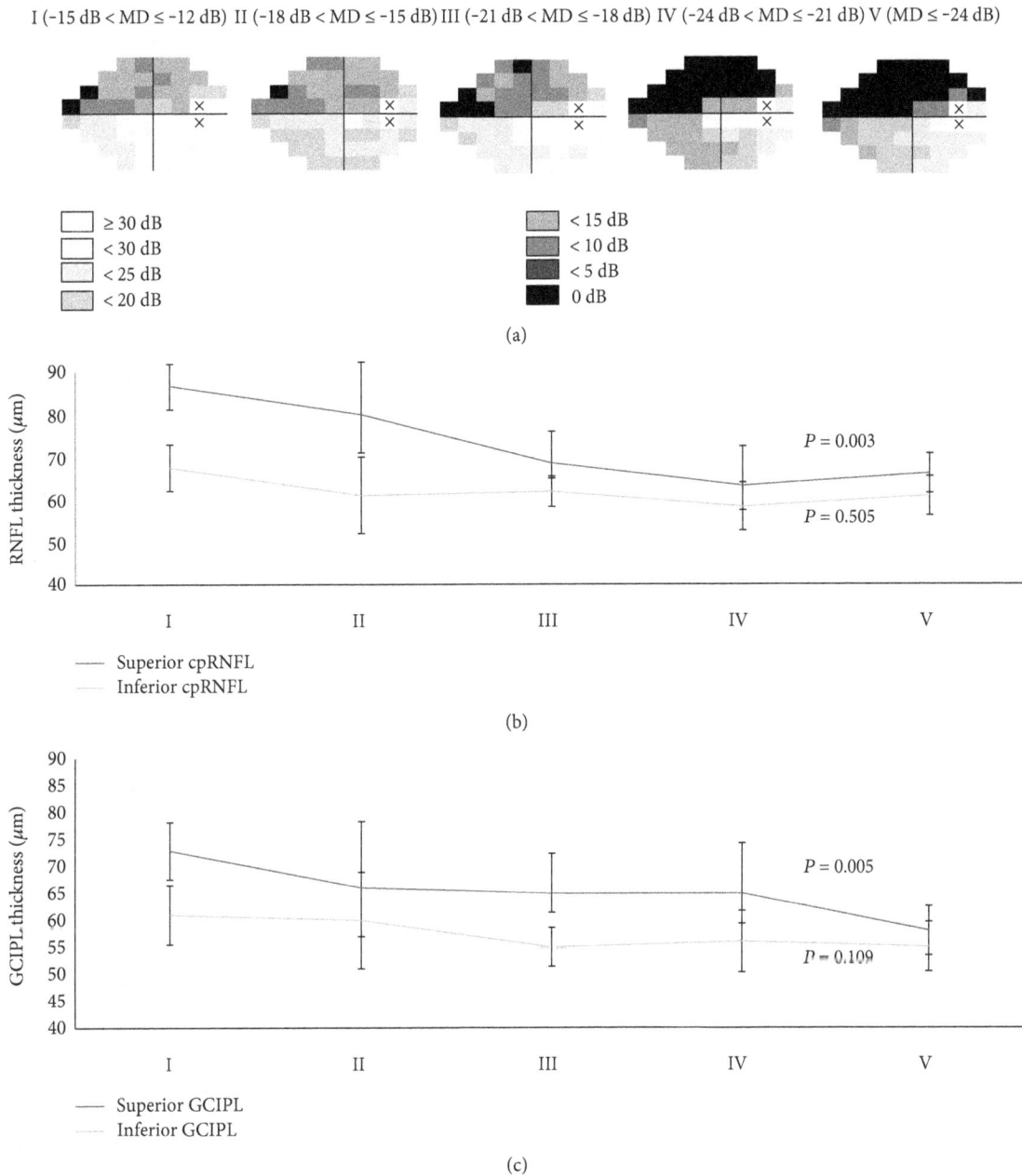

Figure 4: Average threshold sensitivity maps of the advance glaucoma subgroups (I to V) in cross-sectional analysis. The grayscale applied is shown on the top left. With increasing disease severity, the deepening and enlargement of scotomas occurred more frequently in superior hemifield. The scotomas in both hemifields spread toward the physiologic blind spot and toward the nasal periphery in an arcuate pattern. The scotomas in superior hemifield occurred very closely to the area corresponding to the papillomacular bundle, whereas the parafoveal area of inferior hemifield was relatively spared (a). With the disease severity (I to V), superior RNFL and superior GCIPL thickness became significantly thinner ($P = 0.003$ and 0.005, resp.), whereas changes of inferior RNFL and inferior GCIPL were not significant ($P = 0.505$ and 0.109, resp.) (b and c). "X" indicates blind spot; dB = decibel.

of the other group. As aging could be a potential factor that alters the RNFL and GCIPL, the correlation coefficient and changes of RNFL and GCIPL thicknesses were separately analyzed in early to moderate glaucoma and advanced glaucoma. Finally, potential misclassification of the study groups and inaccurate assessment of disease severity, based on the MD of perimetry, are possible, due to the high test-retest variability of the VF test.

In conclusion, we observed that the distinct patterns of the cpRNFL and GCIPL change in different stages of glaucoma. The findings in this study suggest that the most vulnerable region for initial glaucoma is the inferior RNFL around the optic disc, whereas the most preserved region in advanced glaucoma is the superior macular GCIPL. This information may provide important insights into understanding the natural history of retinal ganglion cell death in glaucoma.

Conflicts of Interest

No conflicting relationship exists for any author.

References

[1] C. Boden, P. A. Sample, A. G. Boehm, C. Vasile, R. Akinepalli, and R. N. Weinreb, "The structure-function relationship in eyes with glaucomatous visual field loss that crosses the horizontal meridian," *Archives of Ophthalmology*, vol. 120, pp. 907–912, 2002.

[2] A. Heijl and L. Lundqvist, "The frequency distribution of earliest glaucomatous visual field defects documented by automatic perimetry," *Acta Ophthalmologica*, vol. 62, pp. 658–664, 1984.

[3] H. A. Quigley, E. M. Addicks, W. R. Green, and A. E. Maumenee, "Optic nerve damage in human glaucoma. II. The site of injury and susceptibility to damage," *Archives of Ophthalmology*, vol. 99, pp. 635–649, 1981.

[4] H. K. Cho and C. Kee, "Comparison of the progression rates of the superior, inferior, and both hemifield defects in normal-tension glaucoma patients," *American Journal of Ophthalmology*, vol. 154, no. 6, pp. 958.e1–968.e1, 2012.

[5] C. K. Leung, M. Yu, R. N. Weinreb, G. Lai, G. Xu, and D. S. Lam, "Retinal nerve fiber layer imaging with spectral-domain optical coherence tomography: patterns of retinal nerve fiber layer progression," *Ophthalmology*, vol. 119, pp. 1858–1866, 2012.

[6] J. A. Choi, H. Y. Park, K. I. Jung, K. H. Hong, and C. K. Park, "Difference in the properties of retinal nerve fiber layer defect between superior and inferior visual field loss in glaucoma," *Investigative Ophthalmology & Visual Science*, vol. 54, pp. 6982–6990, 2013.

[7] H. A. Quigley, "Glaucoma," *Lancet*, vol. 377, pp. 1367–1377, 2011.

[8] D. R. Anderson and A. Hendrickson, "Effect of intraocular pressure on rapid axoplasmic transport in monkey optic nerve," *Investigative Ophthalmology*, vol. 13, pp. 771–783, 1974.

[9] B. P. Buckingham, D. M. Inman, W. Lambert et al., "Progressive ganglion cell degeneration precedes neuronal loss in a mouse model of glaucoma," *The Journal of Neuroscience*, vol. 28, pp. 2735–2744, 2008.

[10] Y. Munemasa and Y. Kitaoka, "Molecular mechanisms of retinal ganglion cell degeneration in glaucoma and future prospects for cell body and axonal protection," *Frontiers in Cellular Neuroscience*, vol. 6, p. 60, 2012.

[11] J. C. Mwanza, D. L. Budenz, D. G. Godfrey et al., "Diagnostic performance of optical coherence tomography ganglion cell-inner plexiform layer thickness measurements in early glaucoma," *Ophthalmology*, vol. 121, pp. 849–854, 2014.

[12] J. C. Mwanza, J. L. Warren, and D. L. Budenz, "Combining spectral domain optical coherence tomography structural parameters for the diagnosis of glaucoma with early visual field loss," *Investigative Ophthalmology & Visual Science*, vol. 54, pp. 8393–8400, 2013.

[13] J. C. Mwanza, M. K. Durbin, D. L. Budenz et al., "Glaucoma diagnostic accuracy of ganglion cell-inner plexiform layer thickness: comparison with nerve fiber layer and optic nerve head," *Ophthalmology*, vol. 119, pp. 1151–1158, 2012.

[14] E. Hodapp, R. K. Parrish, and D. R. Anderson, *Clinical Decisions in Glaucoma*, Mosby, St. Louis, Mo, 1993.

[15] J. C. Mwanza, J. D. Oakley, D. L. Budenz, R. T. Chang, O. J. Knight, and W. J. Feuer, "Macular ganglion cell-inner plexiform layer: automated detection and thickness reproducibility with spectral domain-optical coherence tomography in glaucoma," *Investigative Ophthalmology & Visual Science*, vol. 52, pp. 8323–8329, 2011.

[16] D. Su, S. C. Park, J. L. Simonson, J. M. Liebmann, and R. Ritch, "Progression pattern of initial parafoveal scotomas in glaucoma," *Ophthalmology*, vol. 120, pp. 520–527, 2013.

[17] M. H. Suh, D. M. Kim, Y. K. Kim, T. W. Kim, and K. H. Park, "Patterns of progression of localized retinal nerve fibre layer defect on red-free fundus photographs in normal-tension glaucoma," *Eye (London, England)*, vol. 24, pp. 857–863, 2010.

[18] J. Weber, T. Schultze, and H. Ulrich, "The visual field in advanced glaucoma," *International Ophthalmology*, vol. 13, pp. 47–50, 1989.

[19] H. A. Quigley and W. R. Green, "The histology of human glaucoma cupping and optic nerve damage: clinicopathologic correlation in 21 eyes," *Ophthalmology*, vol. 86, pp. 1803–1827, 1979.

[20] J. C. Mwanza, M. K. Durbin, D. L. Budenz et al., "Profile and predictors of normal ganglion cell-inner plexiform layer thickness measured with frequency-domain optical coherence tomography," *Investigative Ophthalmology & Visual Science*, vol. 52, pp. 7872–7879, 2011.

[21] A. Sommer, J. Katz, H. A. Quigley et al., "Clinically detectable nerve fiber atrophy precedes the onset of glaucomatous field loss," *Archives of Ophthalmology*, vol. 109, pp. 77–83, 1991.

[22] H. A. Quigley, E. M. Addicks, and W. R. Green, "Optic nerve damage in human glaucoma. III. Quantitative correlation of nerve fiber loss and visual field defect in glaucoma, ischemic neuropathy, papilledema, and toxic neuropathy," *Archives of Ophthalmology*, vol. 100, pp. 135–146, 1982.

[23] R. Sihota, P. Sony, V. Gupta, T. Dada, and R. Singh, "Diagnostic capability of optical coherence tomography in evaluating the degree of glaucomatous retinal nerve fiber damage," *Investigative Ophthalmology & Visual Science*, vol. 47, pp. 2006–2010, 2006.

[24] J. W. Jeoung, Y. J. Choi, K. H. Park, and D. M. Kim, "Macular ganglion cell imaging study: glaucoma diagnostic accuracy of spectral-domain optical coherence tomography," *Investigative Ophthalmology & Visual Science*, vol. 54, pp. 4422–4429, 2013.

[25] E. Z. Blumenthal and R. Sapir-Pichhadze, "Misleading statistical calculations in far-advanced glaucomatous visual field loss," *Ophthalmology*, vol. 110, pp. 196–200, 2003.

16

Nanophthalmos: A Review of the Clinical Spectrum and Genetics

Pedro C. Carricondo [ID],[1] Thais Andrade,[1] Lev Prasov,[2] Bernadete M. Ayres,[2] and Sayoko E. Moroi[2]

[1]Department of Ophthalmology, Hospital das Clínicas HCFMUSP, Faculdade de Medicina, Universidade de São Paulo, São Paulo, SP, Brazil
[2]Department of Ophthalmology and Visual Sciences, Kellogg Eye Center, University of Michigan, 1000 Wall St., Ann Arbor, MI 48105, USA

Correspondence should be addressed to Pedro C. Carricondo; pedro.carricondo@gmail.com

Academic Editor: Lisa Toto

Nanophthalmos is a clinical spectrum of disorders with a phenotypically small but structurally normal eye. These disorders present significant clinical challenges to ophthalmologists due to a high rate of secondary angle-closure glaucoma, spontaneous choroidal effusions, and perioperative complications with cataract and retinal surgeries. Nanophthalmos may present as a sporadic or familial disorder, with autosomal-dominant or recessive inheritance. To date, five genes (i.e., *MFRP*, *TMEM98*, *PRSS56*, *BEST1*, and *CRB1*) and two loci have been implicated in familial forms of nanophthalmos. Here, we review the definition of nanophthalmos, the clinical and pathogenic features of the condition, and the genetics of this disorder.

1. Introduction

The clinical spectrum of the small eye phenotype comprises conditions in which there is a global ocular reduction in size (e.g., microphthalmos and nanophthalmos) or shortening of either the anterior or posterior segments of the eye (e.g., relative anterior and posterior microphthalmos, resp.) (Table 1) [1–3]. The axial length and anterior chamber structures present a continuum of sizes (Table 2), where microphthalmos and nanophthalmos comprise the smallest or shortest eyes. Nanophthalmos derives from Greek "dwarf eye." In this ocular condition, the anterior and posterior segments have no other congenital malformations, but are both reduced in size, with secondary thickening of choroid and sclera.

The management of the small eye phenotype represents a major challenge for all ophthalmologists, from cataract surgeons to glaucoma and retina specialists. Small eyes may be associated with ophthalmic or systemic comorbidities. These eyes represent significant surgical challenges with a very high rate of intraoperative complications [4] and require a surgical approach that involves precision and care.

Recognizing and correctly diagnosing the diverse presentations of this condition is of great importance for appropriate clinical and surgical management. Understanding the genetic mechanisms involved in the pathogenesis of nanophthalmos will ultimately help us to provide potential markers for genetic diagnosis and development of innovative therapies for this condition. The goal of this review is to define nanophthalmos and provide a brief summary of the advances in the clinical characterization and genetic basis for nanophthalmos.

2. Methods

A Medline/PubMed search was performed using the terms "nanophthalmos," "ocular development," and "genetics" and their combinations. All studies published in English, Portuguese, or Spanish up to December 2017 were reviewed, and relevant publications were included in this review. The pertinent references of the selected articles were also included. All patient images were obtained with the permission of participating individuals or from parents of minor patients, as part of a study on nanophthalmos. This study

Table 1: The clinical spectrum of the small eye phenotype.

Anophthalmia	Absence of the eye
Simple microphthalmos	Short axial length due to global eye reduction with no other findings
Complex microphthalmos	Short axial length due to global eye reduction and associated ocular malformations (e.g., colobomas, persistent fetal vasculature, retinal dysplasia)
Relative anterior microphthalmos	Short axial length due to reduced anterior chamber dimension only, with normal posterior segment dimension and normal scleral thickness
Posterior microphthalmos	Short axial length due to reduced posterior segment dimension with normal anterior chamber dimensions
Nanophthalmos	Short axial length due to small anterior and posterior segments with thickened choroid and sclera and normal lens volume

was approved by the University of Michigan Institutional Review Board and complied with the US Health Insurance Portability and Accountability Act of 1996 and the Declaration of Helsinki.

3. Nanophthalmos: Definition and Clinical Features

Microphthalmos is a developmental disorder of the eye characterized by an axial length of at least 2 standard deviations below the mean for age [1]. This condition is classified as simple, when presented as an isolated finding, or complex, when accompanied by other malformations such as colobomas, anterior segment dysgenesis, lens abnormalities, and posterior segment anomalies [1]. It may also appear as a syndrome with other systemic features. These malformations result from a variety of genetic defects that induce abnormalities in early ocular embryogenesis [9–13].

Nanophthalmos is a special subtype of microphthalmia, in which the eye, although small, has preserved functionality and organization (Figure 1) [13, 14]. It usually presents as a small hyperopic eye set into a deep orbit, with narrow palpebral fissures [15, 16]. A high hypermetropic refractive error is an invariable feature, ranging from +8.00 D sphere to +25.00 or higher [2, 17]. However, the diagnostic criteria vary widely across the literature and considering only one parameter is simplistic. Wu et al. considered shallow anterior chamber, high hyperopia, axial length up to 21 mm, and posterior wall thickness greater than 1.7 mm as conditions to define nanophthalmic eyes [18]. Similarly, Yalvac et al. considered the same characteristics (with axial length defined as less than 20.5 mm) as diagnostic criteria but also added the high lens/eye volume ratio [19].

Another diagnostic issue that has been debated in the literature is the distinction between nanophthalmos and posterior microphthalmos. Posterior microphthalmos is described as a subtype of microphthalmia, in which the axial length is shortened in the posterior segment only. In this condition, the anterior segment of the eye has normal depth and angle configuration. Some investigators consider that nanophthalmos and posterior microphthalmos are synonymous [20]. The report that the reduction of the corneal diameter in high hyperopia is proportional to the axial shortening of the eye supports the hypothesis that these entities represent manifestations of the spectrum of hyperopia, rather than two completely different conditions. In addition, the fact that mutations in the same genes may cause both posterior microphthalmos and nanophthalmos reinforces this idea [20, 21].

However, other groups point to the clinical and structural differences between these conditions, such as the cornea size and curvature, anterior chamber depth, lens thickness, angle characteristics, and propensity for complications [2, 3, 20]. Relhan et al. [2] biometrically analyzed eyes of 38 patients with high hyperopia (defined in the study as greater than +7.00 D spherical equivalent on refraction), all of them with an axial length equal or less than 20.5 mm. In this study, they defined the patients with corneal diameters below 11.0 mm as nanophthalmic and those with corneal diameters greater than or equal to 11.0 mm as posterior microphthalmos. They found that nanophthalmic eyes have shallow anterior chamber depth, thicker lens, and steeper cornea, in comparison with posterior microphthalmic eyes [2]. They also reported different tendencies to complications: the incidence of angle-closure glaucoma was 69.23% in the nanophthalmos group versus 0% in the posterior microphthalmos group, while the incidence of macular folds was 0% versus 24%, respectively [2].

In addition to these clinical features, nanophthalmic eyes have abnormal collagen fibrils in each of the three layers of the sclera [22]. These abnormal fibers are thought to be the cause for the increase scleral thickness as mentioned above (Figure 1). In addition, the combination of increased scleral thickness and abnormal collagen also contributes to its inelasticity, which impairs vortex venous drainage and reduces transcleral flow of proteins [22]. These histopathologic features and anatomy described above are thought to be the mechanism by which nanophthalmic eyes develop complications of angle-closure glaucoma, uveal effusion syndrome, and retinal detachment [19, 22–28]. However, it is unclear whether the abnormal scleral structure is a primary or secondary effect of the genetic changes that induce nanophthalmos as many of the genes implicated in this condition are expressed in retina and retinal pigment epithelium [14, 29–32].

Other ocular findings include topographic corneal steepening and irregular astigmatism [33], absent or rudimentary foveal avascular zone [34], optic disc drusen, retinoschisis and foveoschisis and retinitis pigmentosa (RP) [35, 36], crowded optic disk, chorioretinal folds, and retinal cysts [37], central retinal vein occlusion [38], increased subfoveal choroidal thickness [39], and abnormalities in the retinal layers' thickness and distribution [40, 41] (Figure 1).

In summary, the described anatomical features and histopathology of the nanophthalmic eye explain the severe visual consequences in individuals with nanophthalmos. If the axial hyperopia is not corrected in early childhood,

TABLE 2: Clinical spectrum of eye size phenotypes based on axial length [5] and anterior segment features by anterior chamber depth and white-to-white corneal diameter [6–8].

| | | Axial length | | |
		Short (<21 mm)	Average (24 mm)	Long (>27 mm)
Anterior segment	Small (WTW < 11 mm; ACD < 3.0 mm)	Microphthalmos and nanophthalmos	Relative anterior microphthalmos	Complex dysgenesis
	Average (WTW~11–12.5 mm; ACD~3.3 mm)	Hyperopia posterior microphthalmos	Normal	Myopia
	Large (WTW > 12.5 mm ACD > 3.3 mm)	Complex dysgenesis	Megalocornea	Infantile or congenital glaucoma myopia

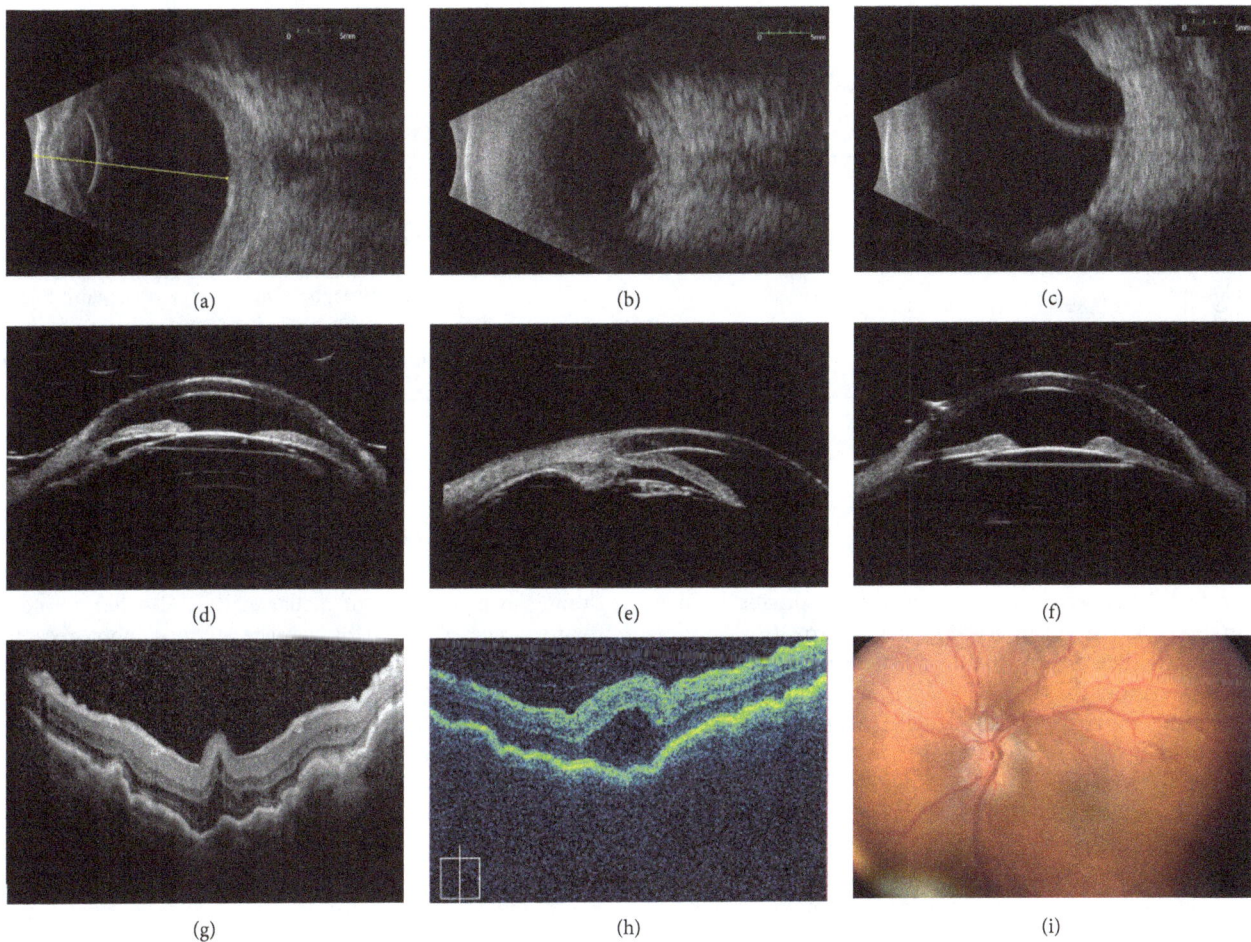

(a)   (b)   (c)

(d)   (e)   (f)

(g)   (h)   (i)

FIGURE 1: Typical ultrasonographic and retinal features of nanophthalmos. (a–c) B-scan ultrasounds showing features of nanophthalmos including short axial length, thickened sclera, and choroid (a), serous retinal detachment (b), and choroidal effusion (c). (d–f) Ultrasound biomicroscopy in a nanophthalmic eyes showing shallow anterior chamber (d), angle closure (e), and anterior rotation of the lens-iris diaphragm (f). (g) Heidelberg Spectralis OCT showing prominent choroidal and retinal folds in a small eye. (h) Zeiss Cirrus OCT showing foveoschisis and choroidal folds in a nanophthalmic eye. (i) Fundus photos in a patient with nanophthalmos and optic disc drusen, showing chorioretinal folds and crowded disc with mild vascular tortuousity.

then this results in irreversible amblyopia. The unrecognized and untreated angle-closure glaucoma can lead to progressive optic nerve damage and blindness [26]. Furthermore, intraocular surgeries in nanophthalmic eyes have significant risks and complications, both intraoperatively and postoperatively [3, 25, 42, 43]. Proper preoperative planning and anatomic understanding can lead to good outcomes and improved quality of life in these patients [18],

despite a nearly 40–60% rate of intraoperative complications [4, 22, 44, 45].

4. Genetic Aspects of Nanophthalmos

Nanophthalmos occurs due to arrested development of the eye in the early stages of embryogenesis. It is thought to have a strong genetic basis. There are many reported familial cases

TABLE 3: Genes and phenotypes in nanophthalmos.

Gene (locus)	OMIM	Location	Inheritance	Gene expression (localization)	Gene function	Phenotypic characteristics of mutations
MFRP (NNO2)	606227	11q23.3	AR	RPE/CB (transmembrane)	Wnt signalling pathway effector	(i) Nanopthalmos, high hyperopia, and angle-closure glaucoma (ii) Retinitis pigmentosa, foveoschisis, and optic disc drusen syndrome
TMEM98 (NNO4)	615949	17q11.2	AD	RPE/CB/sclera (transmembrane)	Unknown	(i) High hyperopia, angle-closure glaucoma, and increased optic disc drusen
PRSS56 (MCOP6)	613858	2q37.1	AR	Retina/sclera (cytoplasmic)	Serine protease	(i) Nanophthalmos, angle-closure glaucoma, and high hyperopia (ii) Posterior microphthalmia
CRB1	604210	1q31.3	AR	Retina (transmembrane)	Controls cell polarity	(i) Nanophthalmos and retinitis pigmentosa (ii) Leber congenital amaurosis 8 (iii) Pigmented paravenous chorioretinal atrophy (iv) Retinitis pigmentosa
Best1/VMD2	607854	11q12	AD or AR	RPE/CB (transmembrane)	Chloride channel	(i) ADVIRC: autosomal-dominant vitreoretinochoroidopathy with nanophthalmos (ii) ARB: autosomal-recessive bestrophinopathy (iii) BVMD: best vitelliform macular dystrophy
Unknown (NNO3)	611897	2q11-q14	AD			(i) Microphthalmia, microcornea, and high hyperopia
Unknown (NNO1)	600165	11p12-11q13	AD			(i) High hyperopia, high lens/eye volume ratio, and angle-closure glaucoma

RPE: retinal pigment epithelium; CB: ciliary body.

with autosomal-dominant and recessive forms of inheritance [26, 30, 46, 47]. However, nanophthalmos can also occur as a sporadic condition [23, 28, 48, 49], which may represent either environmental effects or somatic or new mutations that result in arrest of ocular growth.

To date, five genetic loci (Table 3) were reported to be linked to nanophthalmos: NNOS 2 is related to mutations in membrane frizzled-related protein (*MFRP*); NNOS 4 is related to mutations in *TMEM98*; MCOP6 is related to mutations in serine protease 56 (*PRSS56*) [50, 51]; and NNOS 1 and 3 were localized to chromosomal regions only (11p12-11q13 and 2q11-q14) [26, 29, 30]. Two additional genes, *CRB1* and *BEST1* (*VMD2*), have been implicated in nanophthalmos (Table 3) and have profound roles in photoreceptor and retinal pigment epithelial (RPE) function, respectively.

4.1. Membrane-Type Frizzled-Related Protein Gene (MFRP). A significant number of cases of recessive nanophthalmos have been assigned to mutations in the membrane-type frizzled-related protein gene (*MFRP*, OMIM 606227) [29]. This gene is located in chromosome 11q23 and encodes a glycosylated transmembrane protein that has an extracellular frizzled-related cysteine-rich domain. Frizzled proteins are receptors involved in the regulation of growth, differentiation, and cell polarity during development through the Wnt signaling pathway [52, 53].

In humans, the *MFRP* gene is expressed in the retinal pigment epithelium and in the ciliary body [14, 29]. Outside of the eye, it can only be found at very low levels in the brain,

likely accounting for the localized ocular phenotype in MFRP deficiency [29]. This gene seems to play an important role in both the ocular growth during childhood, functioning as a regulator of ocular size. It also has a role in maintenance of the RPE, which supports photoreceptor function [14, 54–56]. Mouse models of MFRP deficiency, such as rd6 (Mfrp^{rd6}) and rdx (Mfrp^{174delG}) mice, have flecked retina disorders and photoreceptor degeneration, supporting the importance of this gene for retinal and RPE physiology [57–60].

The link between eye size and RPE/ciliary body function has yet to be elucidated. It has been proposed that MFRP affects the physiologic mechanism of emmetropization, in which the refractive error is corrected by postnatal axial growth during the first six years of life [14]. Soundrarajan suggested that a complex regulatory network may influence the postnatal eye development and indicated the participation of another gene (*PRSS56*) in the same pathway [61]. Besides these, other proposed mechanisms for the role of the RPE/ciliary body in eye size include the mechanical stress effects and the inflammatory response observed in the retina [14, 62, 63]. Most recently, Velez et al. [64] found that introducing a normal copy of *Mfrp* gene through adenoviral-based gene therapy may reverse some of these pathogenic changes in Mfrp rd6/rd6 mice. Specifically, subretinal injection of this vector resulted in rescue of photoreceptor death, normalization of retinal function, and regulation of eye length in adult mice. These findings suggest that gene therapy may be a viable option for this disease.

Mouse models of *Mfrp* loss-of-function have failed to demonstrate the full nanophthalmic phenotype observed in humans and instead present with predominant retinal degeneration [57–60]. This may be in part due to the differences in the lens size and ocular anatomy in mice and humans. Collery et al. proposed a new model using zebrafish (*Danio rerio*) that better mimics the human phenotype and may be useful in studying and better understanding this condition [62].

To date, several cases of MFRP mutations leading to reduced eye axial length have been reported. According to Wasmann et al. [65], by the time of the publication in 2014, there were 14 different described *MFRP* mutations: two of them were single amino acid substitutions at extremely conserved sites and 12 caused severe truncation of the protein. Since that time, three new mutations have been described [55], and additional known mutations have been reported in other populations [36, 66]. All of these cases presented with high hyperopia, but the effect of the mutation on retinal rod photoreceptor function was different between individuals, and the clinical spectrum of age of onset and severity of disease was quite variable [65]. The reason for this clinical variability may be a combination of the spectrum of genetic mutations in *MFRP* and other genetic or environmental modifiers that remain to be determined [67].

Wasmann et al. reported a case of two sisters with confirmed *MFRP* mutations. They both presented low visual acuity, high hyperopia, macular retinal folds, with the older sibling also having thickened sclera, and optic nerve head drusen [65]. The mutations in the *MFRP* gene have also been linked to the autosomal-recessive syndrome of posterior microphthalmos, retinitis pigmentosa, foveoschisis, and optic disc drusen [29, 35, 66–68]. These results represent the broad clinical spectrum of *MFRP* mutations, which occurs likely due to differences in early gene expression and environmental factors that shape the development of the eye.

4.2. Transmembrane Protein 98 Gene (TMEM98).

The transmembrane protein 98 (*TMEM98*, OMIM 615949) gene encodes a transmembrane protein that is universally expressed in the human body, including in the ocular tissues, such as iris, choroid, retinal pigment epithelium, and sclera. Its specific function still remains unclear, but it is hypothesized to lead to pathologic scleral pathologic thickening and secondary glaucoma development in nanophthalmic eyes or play a role in the development of the RPE [30, 31].

In a large pedigree, Awadalla and coworkers found a missense mutation in the *TMEM98* (A193P) that could be associated with autosomal-dominant nanophthalmos [30]. Although its pathogenic relationship with the disease was not clear, this association has been greatly strengthened by Khorram and colleagues' recent report of two novel *TMEM98* mutations (His196Pro and c.694_721delAG AAT-GAAGACTGGATCGAAGATGCCTCgtaagg) in autosomal-dominant nanophthalmic patients [31]. Additional studies are still needed to identify the specific role of this gene in the pathogenesis of nanophthalmos.

4.3. Protease Serine 56 (PRSS56).

PRSS56, also known as LOC646960, is located in the chromosome 2q37.1 and encodes a protein of 603 amino acids, which functions as a serine protease. It is suggested that it is expressed in the embryonic tissue, brain, testis, and eye [50]. There are reports of its association with nanophthalmos and posterior microphthalmos cases [21, 50, 69] although its physiologic and pathogenic mechanisms remain to be fully determined [21].

It has been reported that *PRSS56* is highly expressed in retinal ganglion cells of adult animals [50], and its presence in this tissue and in the brain cells suggest its relevance in the regulation of ocular development [69]. Nair et al. [51] demonstrated this role in the homozygous mutant mice Prss56^{Grm4}, which showed shortened axial length and higher susceptibility to angle closure. Furthermore, they found that the differences in ocular size between mutant mice and wild-type controls were progressively greater after birth, with no significant difference prior to that time [51]. They found that the genetic background had a strong influence of magnitude of eye size differences between wild-type and mutant mice, suggesting the existence of genetic modifiers that influence eye growth in concert with *Prss56*. Soundararajan et al. also suggested that PRSS56 and MFRP may function through a common biological pathway that affects the emmetropization process, but nature of this interaction is still unclear [61].

4.4. Crumbs Homologue 1 Gene (CRB1).

Human *CRB1* is a 1406 amino acids transmembrane protein that localizes to photoreceptor inner segments and is vital for the neuronal development of the retina [70, 71]. The *CRB1* gene is located in chromosome 1, in the interval 1q31.2-1q32.1, and its mutations are classically associated with various heritable retinal dystrophies, including Leber Congenital Amaurosis [70, 72, 73]. Furthermore, some recent reports showed association of mutation in *CRB1* with nanophthalmos and retinitis pigmentosa [74, 75].

4.5. Bestrophin 1 (BEST1/VMD2).

The *BEST1* (*VMD2*) gene is located on chromosome 11q12 and is primarily expressed in the RPE [32]. It encodes an integral membrane protein, bestrophin 1, localized predominantly in the basolateral plasma membrane of the RPE and most prominently near the macula [76, 77]. *BEST1* mutations are classically associated with Best vitelliform macular dystrophy (BVMD), a disease restricted to the macula. However, it has been reported to be in association with other widespread ocular abnormalities, such as autosomal-dominant vitreoretinochoroidopathy (ADVIRC) and autosomal-recessive bestrophinopathy (ARB), which are both associated with nanophthalmos [76]. Other studies also strongly suggest an association between *BEST1* mutations and angle-closure glaucoma [77, 78].

ADVIRC is a rare condition characterized by a peripheral circumferential hyperpigmented band with punctate white opacities in the retina, chorioretinal atrophy in the midperipheral or peripapillary retina, and vitreous fibrillary condensations [76, 79]. There are reports of association of this condition with nanophthalmos and a higher incidence of angle-closure glaucoma [79, 80].

ARB is also a rare condition characterized by macular and midperipheral subretinal whitish to yellowish deposits that may become scars and lead to decrease in visual acuity [81–83]. Patients are usually hyperopic and have a shallow anterior chamber and a higher propensity to angle-closure glaucoma [81–85].

4.6. Other Loci for Nanophthalmos. The autosomal-dominant nanophthalmos NNO1 (OMIM 600165) is caused by a defect on chromosome 11, between D11S905 and D11S987. This region may also be associated with severity of angle-closure glaucoma manifestations [26]. The precise genetic change at this locus has yet to be confirmed, though coding and regulatory mutations in BEST1 have been excluded as a cause (data not shown). Another form of autosomal-dominant disease, NNO3 (OMIM 611897), was described in a family with simple microphthalmia, microcornea, and high hyperopia, and it was reported to be linked to chromosome 2q11-14 [86].

5. Conclusion

With the progress of the imaging and surgical technologies, there have been significant advances in the diagnosis and management of the nanophthalmic eye. These have improved outcomes for individuals with such challenging eyes. Furthermore, substantial new discoveries in the genetics of nanophthalmos have led to the discovery of many new genes and pathways in the pathogenesis of this condition. These advances will ultimately improve early detection of this condition and provide novel avenues for treatment, including the possibility for gene therapy. Genetic diagnoses will facilitate genetic counseling for familial forms of this condition and may help to decrease amblyopia from uncorrected hyperopia, prevent vision loss from complications, and improve monitoring to minimize glaucoma and retinal complications from nanophthalmos.

Conflicts of Interest

The authors declare that they have no conflicts of interest.

Acknowledgments

This work was supported in part by a Career Starter Award from the Knights Templar Eye Foundation to Lev Prasov. The authors thank the clinicians and the photographers who participated in the care of these patients at the Kellogg Eye Center at the University of Michigan.

References

[1] M. J. Elder, "Aetiology of severe visual impairment and blindness in microphthalmos," *British Journal of Ophthalmology*, vol. 78, no. 5, pp. 332–334, 1994.

[2] N. Relhan, S. Jalali, N. Pehre, H. L. Rao, U. Manusani, and L. Bodduluri, "High-hyperopia database, part I: clinical characterisation including morphometric (biometric) differentiation of posterior microphthalmos from nanophthalmos," *Eye*, vol. 30, no. 1, pp. 120–126, 2016.

[3] R. S. Hoffman, A. R. Vasavada, Q. B. Allen et al., "Cataract surgery in the small eye," *Journal of Cataract and Refractive Surgery*, vol. 41, no. 11, pp. 2565–2575, 2015.

[4] S. Rajendrababu, N. Babu, S. Sinha et al., "A randomized controlled trial comparing outcomes of cataract surgery in nanophthalmos with and without prophylactic sclerostomy," *American Journal of Ophthalmology*, vol. 183, pp. 125–133, 2017.

[5] M. De Bernardo, L. Zeppa, R. Forte et al., "Can we use the fellow eye biometric data to predict IOL power?," *Seminars in Ophthalmology*, vol. 32, no. 3, pp. 363–370, 2017.

[6] G. U. Auffarth, M. Blum, U. Faller, M. R. Tetz, and H. E. Volcker, "Relative anterior microphthalmos: morphometric analysis and its implications for cataract surgery," *Ophthalmology*, vol. 107, no. 8, pp. 1555–1560, 2000.

[7] M. Khairallah, R. Messaoud, S. Zaouali, S. Ben Yahia, A. Ladjimi, and S. Jenzri, "Posterior segment changes associated with posterior microphthalmos," *Ophthalmology*, vol. 109, no. 3, pp. 569–574, 2002.

[8] I. Guber, C. Bergin, S. Perritaz, and F. Majo, "Correcting interdevice bias of horizontal white-to-white and sulcus-to-sulcus measures used for implantable collamer lens sizing," *American Journal of Ophthalmology*, vol. 161, pp. 116–125 e1, 2016.

[9] A. M. Slavotinek, "Eye development genes and known syndromes," *Molecular Genetics and Metabolism*, vol. 104, no. 4, pp. 448–456, 2011.

[10] T. M. Bardakjian and A. Schneider, "The genetics of anophthalmia and microphthalmia," *Current Opinion in Ophthalmology*, vol. 22, no. 5, pp. 309–313, 2011.

[11] D. R. Fitzpatrick and V. van Heyningen, "Developmental eye disorders," *Current Opinion in Genetics and Development*, vol. 15, no. 3, pp. 348–353, 2005.

[12] M. Warburg, "Classification of microphthalmos and coloboma," *Journal of Medical Genetics*, vol. 30, no. 8, pp. 664–669, 1993.

[13] A. S. Verma and D. R. Fitzpatrick, "Anophthalmia and microphthalmia," *Orphanet Journal of Rare Diseases*, vol. 2, p. 47, 2007.

[14] O. H. Sundin, S. Dharmaraj, I. A. Bhutto et al., "Developmental basis of nanophthalmos: MFRP is required for both prenatal ocular growth and postnatal emmetropization," *Ophthalmic Genetics*, vol. 29, no. 1, pp. 1–9, 2008.

[15] O. S. Singh, R. J. Simmons, R. J. Brockhurst, and C. L. Trempe, "Nanophthalmos: a perspective on identification and therapy," *Ophthalmology*, vol. 89, no. 9, pp. 1006–1012, 1982.

[16] A. K. Altintaş, M. A. Acar, I. S. Yalvaç, I. Koçak, A. Nurözler, and S. Duman, "Autosomal recessive nanophthalmos," *Acta Ophthalmologica Scandinavica*, vol. 75, no. 3, pp. 325–328, 1997.

[17] A. O. Khan, "Posterior microphthalmos versus nanophthalmos," *Ophthalmic Genetics*, vol. 29, no. 4, p. 189, 2008.

[18] W. Wu, D. G. Dawson, A. Sugar et al., "Cataract surgery in patients with nanophthalmos: results and complications," *Journal of Cataract and Refractive Surgery*, vol. 30, no. 3, pp. 584–590, 2004.

[19] I. S. Yalvac, B. Satana, G. Ozkan, U. Eksioglu, and S. Duman, "Management of glaucoma in patients with nanophthalmos," *Eye*, vol. 22, no. 6, pp. 838–843, 2008.

[20] S. R. Nowilaty, A. O. Khan, M. A. Aldahmesh, K. F. Tabbara, A. Al-Amri, and F. S. Alkuraya, "Biometric and molecular characterization of clinically diagnosed posterior microphthalmos," *American Journal of Ophthalmology*, vol. 155, no. 2, pp. 361–372.e7, 2013.

[21] M. B. Said, E. Chouchène, S. B. Salem et al., "Posterior microphthalmia and nanophthalmia in Tunisia caused by a founder c.1059_1066insC mutation of the PRSS56 gene," *Gene*, vol. 528, no. 2, pp. 288–294, 2013.

[22] A. Yamani, I. Wood, I. Sugino, M. Wanner, and M. A. Zarbin, "Abnormal collagen fibrils in nanophthalmos: a clinical and histologic study," *American Journal of Ophthalmology*, vol. 127, no. 1, pp. 106–108, 1999.

[23] Y. M. Buys and C. J. Pavlin, "Retinitis pigmentosa, nanophthalmos, and optic disc drusen: a case report," *Ophthalmology*, vol. 106, no. 3, pp. 619–622, 1999.

[24] A. Neelakantan, P. Venkataramakrishnan, B. S. Rao et al., "Familial nanophthalmos: management and complications," *Indian Journal of Ophthalmology*, vol. 42, no. 3, pp. 139–143, 1994.

[25] E. Areiter, M. Neale, and S. M. Johnson, "Spectrum of angle closure, uveal effusion syndrome, and nanophthalmos," *Journal of Current Glaucoma Practice*, vol. 10, no. 3, pp. 113–117, 2016.

[26] M. I. Othman, S. A. Sullivan, G. L. Skuta et al., "Autosomal dominant nanophthalmos (NNO1) with high hyperopia and angle-closure glaucoma maps to chromosome 11," *American Journal of Human Genetics*, vol. 63, no. 5, pp. 1411–1418, 1998.

[27] N. Kara, O. Baz, H. Altinkaynak, C. Altan, and A. Demirok, "Assessment of the anterior chamber angle in patients with nanophthalmos: an anterior segment optical coherence tomography study," *Current Eye Research*, vol. 38, no. 5, pp. 563–568, 2013.

[28] A. K. Mandal, T. Das, and V. K. Gothwal, "Angle closure glaucoma in nanophthalmos and pigmentary retinal dystrophy: a rare syndrome," *Indian Journal of Ophthalmology*, vol. 49, no. 4, pp. 271–272, 2001.

[29] O. H. Sundin, G. S. Leppert, E. D. Silva et al., "Extreme hyperopia is the result of null mutations in MFRP, which encodes a frizzled-related protein," *Proceedings of the National Academy of Sciences of the United States of America*, vol. 102, no. 27, pp. 9553–9558, 2005.

[30] M. S. Awadalla, K. P. Burdon, E. Souzeau et al., "Mutation in TMEM98 in a large white kindred with autosomal dominant nanophthalmos linked to 17p12-q12," *JAMA Ophthalmology*, vol. 132, no. 8, pp. 970–977, 2014.

[31] D. Khorram, M. Choi, B. R. Roos et al., "Novel TMEM98 mutations in pedigrees with autosomal dominant nanophthalmos," *Molecular Vision*, vol. 21, pp. 1017–1023, 2015.

[32] K. Petrukhin, M. J. Koisti, B. Bakall et al., "Identification of the gene responsible for Best macular dystrophy," *Nature Genetics*, vol. 19, no. 3, pp. 241–247, 1998.

[33] S. Srinivasan, M. Batterbury, I. B. Marsh, A. C. Fisher, C. Willoughby, and S. B. Kaye, "Corneal topographic features in a family with nanophthalmos," *Cornea*, vol. 25, no. 6, pp. 750–756, 2006.

[34] M. K. Walsh and M. F. Goldberg, "Abnormal foveal avascular zone in nanophthalmos," *American Journal of Ophthalmology*, vol. 143, no. 6, pp. 1067-1068, 2007.

[35] J. Crespí, J. A. Buil, F. Bassaganyas et al., "A novel mutation confirms MFRP as the gene causing the syndrome of nanophthalmos–renititis pigmentosa–foveoschisis–optic disk drusen," *American Journal of Ophthalmology*, vol. 146, no. 2, pp. 323–328, 2008.

[36] L. C. Zacharias, R. Susanna, O. Sundin, S. Finzi, B. N. Susanna, and W. Y. Takahashi, "Efficacy of topical dorzolamide therapy for cystoid macular edema in a patient with MFRP-related nanophthalmos–retinitis pigmentosa–foveoschisis–optic disk drusen syndrome," *Retinal Cases and Brief Reports*, vol. 9, no. 1, pp. 61–63, 2015.

[37] C. J. MacKay, M. S. Shek, R. E. Carr, L. A. Yanuzzi, and P. Gouras, "Retinal degeneration with nanophthalmos, cystic macular degeneration, and angle closure glaucoma. A new recessive syndrome," *Archives of Ophthalmology*, vol. 105, no. 3, pp. 366–371, 1987.

[38] A. A. Albar, S. R. Nowilaty, and N. G. Ghazi, "Nanophthalmos and hemiretinal vein occlusion: a case report," *Saudi Journal of Ophthalmology*, vol. 29, no. 1, pp. 89–91, 2015.

[39] A. Demircan, C. Altan, O. A. Osmanbasoglu, U. Celik, N. Kara, and A. Demirok, "Subfoveal choroidal thickness measurements with enhanced depth imaging optical coherence tomography in patients with nanophthalmos," *British Journal of Ophthalmology*, vol. 98, no. 3, pp. 345–349, 2014.

[40] H. Xiao, X. Guo, Y. Zhong, and X. Liu, "Retinal and choroidal changes of nanophthalmic eyes with and without secondary glaucoma," *Retina*, vol. 35, no. 10, pp. 2121–2129, 2015.

[41] F. Helvacioglu, Z. Kapran, S. Sencan, M. Uyar, and O. Cam, "Optical coherence tomography of bilateral nanophthalmos with macular folds and high hyperopia," *Case Reports in Ophthalmological Medicine*, vol. 2014, Article ID 173853, 3 pages, 2014.

[42] J. S. Chang, J. C. Ng, V. K. Chan, and A. K. Law, "Cataract surgery with a new fluidics control phacoemulsification system in nanophthalmic eyes," *Case Reports in Ophthalmology*, vol. 7, no. 3, pp. 218–226, 2016.

[43] S. Srinivasan, "Small eyes-big problems," *Journal of Cataract and Refractive Surgery*, vol. 41, no. 11, pp. 2345-2346, 2015.

[44] G. Carifi, F. Safa, F. Aiello, C. Baumann, and V. Maurino, "Cataract surgery in small adult eyes," *British Journal of Ophthalmology*, vol. 98, no. 9, pp. 1261–1265, 2014.

[45] H. Singh, J. C. Wang, D. C. Desjardins, K. Baig, S. Gagné, and I. I. Ahmed, "Refractive outcomes in nanophthalmic eyes after phacoemulsification and implantation of a high-refractive-power foldable intraocular lens," *Journal of Cataract and Refractive Surgery*, vol. 41, no. 11, pp. 2394–2402, 2015.

[46] S. Moradian, A. Kanani, and H. Esfandiari, "Nanophthalmos," *Journal of Ophthalmic and Vision Research*, vol. 6, no. 2, pp. 145-146, 2011.

[47] M. Martorina, "Familial nanophthalmos," *Journal Français D'Ophtalmologie*, vol. 11, no. 4, pp. 357–361, 1988.

[48] S. Ghose, M. S. Sachdev, and H. Kumar, "Bilateral nanophthalmos, pigmentary retinal dystrophy, and angle closure glaucoma—a new syndrome?," *British Journal of Ophthalmology*, vol. 69, no. 8, pp. 624–628, 1985.

[49] H. Proença, A. Castanheira-Dinis, and M. Monteiro-Grillo, "Bilateral nanophthalmos and pigmentary retinal dystrophy–an unusual syndrome," *Graefe's Archive for Clinical and Experimental Ophthalmology*, vol. 244, no. 9, pp. 1203–1205, 2006.

[50] A. Gal, I. Rau, L. El Matri et al., "Autosomal-recessive posterior microphthalmos is caused by mutations in PRSS56, a gene encoding a trypsin-like serine protease," *American Journal of Human Genetics*, vol. 88, no. 3, pp. 382–390, 2011.

[51] K. S. Nair, M. Hmani-Aifa, Z. Ali et al., "Alteration of the serine protease PRSS56 causes angle-closure glaucoma in mice and posterior microphthalmia in humans and mice," *Nature Genetics*, vol. 43, no. 6, pp. 579–584, 2011.

[52] P. Bhanot, M. Brink, C. H. Samos et al., "A new member of the frizzled family from drosophila functions as a wingless receptor," *Nature*, vol. 382, no. 6588, pp. 225–230, 1996.

[53] M. Katoh, "Molecular cloning and characterization of MFRP, a novel gene encoding a membrane-type frizzled-related protein," *Biochemical and Biophysical Research Communications*, vol. 282, no. 1, pp. 116–123, 2001.

[54] M. Mameesh, A. Ganesh, B. Harikrishna et al., "Co-inheritance of the membrane frizzled-related protein ocular phenotype and glycogen storage disease type Ib," *Ophthalmic Genetics*, vol. 38, no. 6, pp. 1–5, 2017.

[55] R. Mukhopadhyay, P. I. Sergouniotis, D. S. Mackay et al., "A detailed phenotypic assessment of individuals affected by MFRP-related oculopathy," *Molecular Vision*, vol. 16, pp. 540–548, 2010.

[56] M. N. Mandal, V. Vasireddy, M. M. Jablonski et al., "Spatial and temporal expression of MFRP and its interaction with CTRP5," *Investigative Ophthalmology and Visual Science*, vol. 47, no. 12, pp. 5514–5521, 2006.

[57] S. Kameya, N. L. Hawes, B. Chang, J. R. Heckenlively, J. K. Naggert, and P. M. Nishina, "Mfrp, a gene encoding a frizzled related protein, is mutated in the mouse retinal degeneration 6," *Human Molecular Genetics*, vol. 11, no. 16, pp. 1879–1886, 2002.

[58] J. Fogerty and J. C. Besharse, "174delG mutation in mouse MFRP causes photoreceptor degeneration and RPE atrophy," *Investigative Ophthalmology and Visual Science*, vol. 52, no. 10, pp. 7256–7266, 2011.

[59] N. L. Hawes, B. Chang, G. S. Hageman et al., "Retinal degeneration 6 (rd6): a new mouse model for human retinitis punctata albescens," *Investigative Ophthalmology and Visual Science*, vol. 41, no. 10, pp. 3149–3157, 2000.

[60] O. H. Sundin, "The mouse's eye and Mfrp: not quite human," *Ophthalmic Genetics*, vol. 26, no. 4, pp. 153–155, 2005.

[61] R. Soundararajan, J. Won, T. M. Stearns et al., "Gene profiling of postnatal Mfrprd6 mutant eyes reveals differential accumulation of Prss56, visual cycle and phototransduction mRNAs," *PLoS One*, vol. 9, no. 10, article e110299, 2014.

[62] R. F. Collery, P. J. Volberding, J. R. Bostrom, B. A. Link, and J. C. Besharse, "Loss of zebrafish Mfrp causes nanophthalmia, hyperopia, and accumulation of subretinal macrophages," *Investigative Ophthalmology and Visual Science*, vol. 57, no. 15, pp. 6805–6814, 2016.

[63] P. Wang, Z. Yang, S. Li, X. Xiao, X. Guo, and Q. Zhang, "Evaluation of MFRP as a candidate gene for high hyperopia," *Molecular Vision*, vol. 15, pp. 181–186, 2009.

[64] G. Velez, S. H. Tsang, Y. T. Tsai et al., "Gene therapy restores Mfrp and corrects axial eye length," *Scientific Reports*, vol. 7, no. 1, p. 16151, 2017.

[65] R. A. Wasmann, J. S. Wassink-Ruiter, O. H. Sundin, E. Morales, J. B. Verheij, and J. W. Pott, "Novel membrane frizzled-related protein gene mutation as cause of posterior microphthalmia resulting in high hyperopia with macular folds," *Acta Ophthalmologica*, vol. 92, no. 3, pp. 276–281, 2014.

[66] A. Neri, R. Leaci, J. C. Zenteno, C. Casubolo, E. Delfini, and C. Macaluso, "Membrane frizzled-related protein gene-related ophthalmological syndrome: 30-month follow-up of a sporadic case and review of genotype-phenotype correlation in the literature," *Molecular Vision*, vol. 18, pp. 2623–2632, 2012.

[67] R. Ayala-Ramirez, F. Graue-Wiechers, V. Robredo, M. Amato-Almanza, I. Horta-Diez, and J. C. Zenteno, "A new autosomal recessive syndrome consisting of posterior microphthalmos, retinitis pigmentosa, foveoschisis, and optic disc drusen is caused by a MFRP gene mutation," *Molecular Vision*, vol. 12, pp. 1483–1489, 2006.

[68] J. C. Zenteno, B. Buentello-Volante, M. A. Quiroz-González, and M. A. Quiroz-Reyes, "Compound heterozygosity for a novel and a recurrent MFRP gene mutation in a family with the nanophthalmos-retinitis pigmentosa complex," *Molecular Vision*, vol. 15, pp. 1794–1798, 2009.

[69] A. Orr, M. P. Dubé, J. C. Zenteno et al., "Mutations in a novel serine protease PRSS56 in families with nanophthalmos," *Molecular Vision*, vol. 17, pp. 1850–1861, 2011.

[70] A. J. Lotery, S. G. Jacobson, G. A. Fishman et al., "Mutations in the CRB1 gene cause Leber congenital amaurosis," *Archives of Ophthalmology*, vol. 119, no. 3, pp. 415–420, 2001.

[71] S. G. Jacobson, A. V. Cideciyan, T. S. Aleman et al., "Crumbs homolog 1 (CRB1) mutations result in a thick human retina with abnormal lamination," *Human Molecular Genetics*, vol. 12, no. 9, pp. 1073–1078, 2003.

[72] A. I. den Hollander, J. R. Heckenlively, L. I. van den Born et al., "Leber congenital amaurosis and retinitis pigmentosa with Coats-like exudative vasculopathy are associated with mutations in the crumbs homologue 1 (CRB1) gene," *American Journal of Human Genetics*, vol. 69, no. 1, pp. 198–203, 2001.

[73] H. Abouzeid, Y. Li, I. H. Maumenee, S. Dharmaraj, and O. Sundin, "A G1103R mutation in CRB1 is co-inherited with high hyperopia and Leber congenital amaurosis," *Ophthalmic Genetics*, vol. 27, no. 1, pp. 15–20, 2006.

[74] C. C. Paun, B. J. Pijl, A. M. Siemiatkowska et al., "A novel crumbs homolog 1 mutation in a family with retinitis pigmentosa, nanophthalmos, and optic disc drusen," *Molecular Vision*, vol. 18, pp. 2447–2453, 2012.

[75] J. C. Zenteno, B. Buentello-Volante, R. Ayala-Ramirez, and C. Villanueva-Mendoza, "Homozygosity mapping identifies the Crumbs homologue 1 (Crb1) gene as responsible for a recessive syndrome of retinitis pigmentosa and nanophthalmos," *American Journal of Medical Genetics Part A*, vol. 155A, no. 5, pp. 1001–1006, 2011.

[76] C. J. Boon, B. J. Klevering, B. P. Leroy, C. B. Hoyng, J. E. Keunen, and A. I. den Hollander, "The spectrum of ocular phenotypes caused by mutations in the BEST1 gene," *Progress in Retinal and Eye Research*, vol. 28, no. 3, pp. 187–205, 2009.

[77] L. Toto, C. J. Boon, L. Di Antonio et al., "Bestrophinopathy: a spectrum of ocular abnormalities caused by the c.614T>C mutation in the BEST1 gene," *Retina*, vol. 36, no. 8, pp. 1586–1595, 2016.

[78] E. Wittström, V. Ponjavic, M. L. Bondeson, and S. Andréasson, "Anterior segment abnormalities and angle-closure glaucoma in a family with a mutation in the BEST1 gene and Best vitelliform macular dystrophy," *Ophthalmic Genetics*, vol. 32, no. 4, pp. 217–227, 2011.

[79] J. Yardley, B. P. Leroy, N. Hart-Holden et al., "Mutations of VMD2 splicing regulators cause nanophthalmos and autosomal dominant vitreoretinochoroidopathy (ADVIRC)," *Investigative Ophthalmology and Visual Science*, vol. 45, no. 10, pp. 3683–3689, 2004.

[80] B. A. Lafaut, B. Loeys, B. P. Leroy, W. Spileers, J. J. De Laey, and P. Kestelyn, "Clinical and electrophysiological findings in autosomal dominant vitreoretinochoroidopathy: report of a new pedigree," *Graefe's Archive for Clinical and Experimental Ophthalmology*, vol. 239, no. 8, pp. 575–582, 2001.

[81] R. Burgess, I. D. Millar, B. P. Leroy et al., "Biallelic mutation of BEST1 causes a distinct retinopathy in humans," *American Journal of Human Genetics*, vol. 82, no. 1, pp. 19–31, 2008.

[82] R. Burgess, R. E. MacLaren, A. E. Davidson et al., "ADVIRC is caused by distinct mutations in BEST1 that alter pre-mRNA splicing," *Journal of Medical Genetics*, vol. 46, no. 9, pp. 620–625, 2009.

[83] C. J. Boon, L. I. van den Born, L. Visser et al., "Autosomal recessive bestrophinopathy: differential diagnosis and treatment options," *Ophthalmology*, vol. 120, no. 4, pp. 809–820, 2013.

[84] A. E. Davidson, P. I. Sergouniotis, R. Burgess-Mullan et al., "A synonymous codon variant in two patients with autosomal recessive bestrophinopathy alters in vitro splicing of BEST1," *Molecular Vision*, vol. 16, pp. 2916–2922, 2010.

[85] C. Crowley, R. Paterson, T. Lamey et al., "Autosomal recessive bestrophinopathy associated with angle-closure glaucoma," *Documenta Ophthalmologica*, vol. 129, no. 1, pp. 57–63, 2014.

[86] H. Li, J. X. Wang, C. Y. Wang et al., "Localization of a novel gene for congenital nonsyndromic simple microphthalmia to chromosome 2q11-14," *Human Genetics*, vol. 122, no. 6, pp. 589–593, 2008.

17

Changes in Glaucoma Medication during the Past Eight Years and Future Directions in Japan based on an Insurance Medical Claim Database

Masako Sakamoto, Kazuyoshi Kitamura, and Kenji Kashiwagi

Department of Ophthalmology, University of Yamanashi Faculty of Medicine, Chuo, Yamanashi, Japan

Correspondence should be addressed to Kenji Kashiwagi; kenjik@yamanashi.ac.jp

Academic Editor: Ciro Costagliola

Purpose. To investigate changes in the status of glaucoma care between 2006 and 2013 and to predict future directions of glaucoma care in Japan. *Subjects and Methods*. Japanese subjects registered in the largest national insurance claim database in Japan from 2006 to 2013 were analyzed. Estimations of the number of glaucoma patients during the past eight years and of the number of future patients were calculated. Changes in prescription trends among the same patients in the three-year period after initiating antiglaucoma medication were also investigated. *Results*. There was a total of 3,016,000 subjects in the database. The proportion of glaucoma patients increased consistently from 2.5% in 2006 to 4.5% in 2013. This trend was predicted to continue until 2025, followed by a constant decrease with age. The most frequently prescribed antiglaucoma medications were prostaglandin analogues (PGs); however, in recent years, fixed combination therapy has emerged as a major treatment. Among 2856 newly diagnosed glaucoma patients; 94.7% of the patients initially received a single medication, but 25% of the patients received additional medications within 3 years. *Conclusions*. The prevalence of glaucoma patients has significantly increased during the past eight years. The number of antiglaucoma medications continuously increased during the treatment period.

1. Introduction

Glaucoma is one of the major ocular diseases that results in acquired blindness. The prevalence of glaucoma among subjects 40 years of age or older is 5%, and there are estimated four million glaucoma patients in Japan [1]. Aging is one of the major risk factors for glaucoma [1, 2], and it is predicted that the prevalence of glaucoma will increase in an aging society [3].

Reduction of intraocular pressure is the only proven treatment for glaucoma [4]. Glaucoma treatments consist of ophthalmic solutions, laser treatments, and surgical procedures. We have described the changes in antiglaucoma ophthalmic solutions prescribed in Japan in 2010 [5]. The glaucoma treatment regimen has markedly improved, as exemplified by new antiglaucoma ophthalmic solutions and minimally invasive glaucoma surgeries becoming available during the past years [6, 7]. Unfortunately, few studies have investigated the current status of glaucoma care, including changes in the number of glaucoma patients and large-scale treatment regimens in Japan.

It is important to investigate changes in glaucoma treatment from medical and surgical viewpoints to elucidate the current tasks of glaucoma care and to assist with future predictions of the glaucoma burden; we accomplished this aim by analyzing national insurance claim data in the present study.

2. Subjects and Methods

This study adhered to the tenets of the Declaration of Helsinki and was approved by the University of Yamanashi Ethical Review Board. Because the data used in this study do not contain any personal information, the Ethical Review Board agreed to permit this study without requiring written informed consent from all patients.

Changes in Glaucoma Medication during the Past Eight Years and Future Directions in Japan...

125

2.1. Database. In this study, we used the claim database of the Japan Medical Data Center (JMDC), established in 2003, to accumulate receipt data and perform epidemiological and health service research [8]. The JMDC is the largest medical database in Japan, and the details of this database have been described elsewhere [5, 8, 9]. In brief, the database employs an anonymous linkage system using an encryption code and combines individual medical claim information from different health insurance societies through a computer-aided, post-entry standardization method. This database covers employees and their dependents who belong to Japan Health Insurance Society, one of two major Health Insurance systems in Japan. The data include the patients' encrypted personal identifiers, age, sex, and International Classification of Diseases version 10 (ICD-10) diagnosis codes, the names of dispensed drugs, and the size of medical institutions. The encrypted personal identifiers could be used to link claim data from different hospitals, clinics, and pharmacies.

2.2. Subjects. The total number of subjects registered in the database from January 2006 to December 2013 was 3,016,666.

2.3. Definition of Glaucoma. Glaucoma was defined as having any of glaucoma diagnosis according to the ICD-10 diagnosis codes (Supplemental Table 1 available online at https://doi.org/10.1155/2017/7642049), having a history of antiglaucoma medication use and/or glaucoma surgery (including laser treatment) and having a three-month or longer history of any glaucoma treatment, including an antiglaucoma prescription, laser procedures, and glaucoma surgeries. Patients who met the following criteria were excluded from the analysis. patients who changed insurance systems, those who had no records in the Japan Health Insurance Society database, and those whose glaucoma diagnosis were retracted. The details of data extraction have been shown elsewhere [8, 9].

2.4. Data Adjustment. The estimated number of glaucoma patients in each study year was adjusted based on the 2010 Japanese census to compare proportions among years during the study period. Future trends in the estimated number of glaucoma patients were evaluated based on a combination of data from the 2013 database and official prediction data from the National Institute of Population and Social Security Research based on birth and mortality rates in January 2012.

2.5. Changes in Antiglaucoma Ophthalmic Solutions during a Three-Year Period among Newly Diagnosed and Prescribed Glaucoma Patients. Subjects with newly diagnosed glaucoma were defined as having belonged to the Japan Health Insurance Society union for more than one year before entry, having no history of any type of glaucoma, having been prescribed antiglaucoma ophthalmic solutions, and having no laser and/or surgical treatments recorded in the JMDC database. Among glaucoma patients who were newly diagnosed, those who had been registered in the database were evaluated to determine changes made to their medical treatment regimen during a three-year period. Glaucoma subjects with a history of any laser or surgical treatments

over the three-year period were excluded from this study because of investigating changing in medication precisely.

2.6. Statistical Analysis. For the statistical analysis, all commercially available ophthalmic solutions in Japan were classified into the following categories: prostaglandin analogues (PGs), beta-blocker (BB), carbonic anhydrase inhibitor (CAI), and others (Supplemental Table 2).

The data were analyzed with JMP 11.0 software (SAS Institute Inc., Cary, NC, USA), and values are presented as the means ± standard deviations. Correlations between the proportion of glaucoma patients, frequency of glaucoma medication, and glaucoma surgery and the changes in the number of antiglaucoma ophthalmic solutions per patient were evaluated using Pearson's correlation coefficient or the Wilcoxon signed-rank test. P values less than 0.05 were considered statistically significant.

3. Results

3.1. Changes in the Estimated Number of Glaucoma Patients. The estimated number of glaucoma patients in 2006 was 3,140,000. This number significantly ($P < 0.0001$) increased by year, reaching 5,750,000 in 2013 (Figure 1a). When comparing age groups, the estimated number of glaucoma patients did not significantly change among patients younger than 50 years old, but the number of patients the same or older than 50 years of age significantly increased each year over the 7-year period between 2006 and 2016 ($P < 0.0001$); the magnitude of the increase was greater with age (Figure 1(b)).

3.2. Future Prediction of the Estimated Number of Glaucoma Patients. The number of glaucoma patients was predicted to increase to approximately 5,890,000 by 2025, and thereafter, it was predicted to decrease due to a reduction of the population. Changes in profiles were not the same among age groups. The number of patients aged 60 or older was expected to increase by 2035, whereas the profile of those under 50 years of age showed a consistent reduction during the study period (Figure 2).

3.3. Comparison of Ratios of Medicated Patients among Age Groups. The ratio of glaucoma patients using any medications significantly increased with age ($P < 0.001$). The rates of glaucoma patients using any medications among less than 40 years old, 40–49 years old, 50–59 years old, 60–69 years old, and 70 years old or older were 19.3%, 37.1%, 48.1%, 53.4%, and 58.0%, respectively.

3.4. Changes in the Number of Prescribed Antiglaucoma Ophthalmic Solutions per Patient. The number of antiglaucoma agents significantly increased during the study period. The introduction of fixed combination therapy drastically changed the trend in the prescription of antiglaucoma ophthalmic solutions. The number of prescribed ophthalmic solutions per patient was 1.49 agents in 2006, which was relatively constant by 2009; however, after 2010, when fixed combination ophthalmic solutions became available in Japan, the number of antiglaucoma agents was increased, reaching 1.71 in 2013.

(a)

(b)

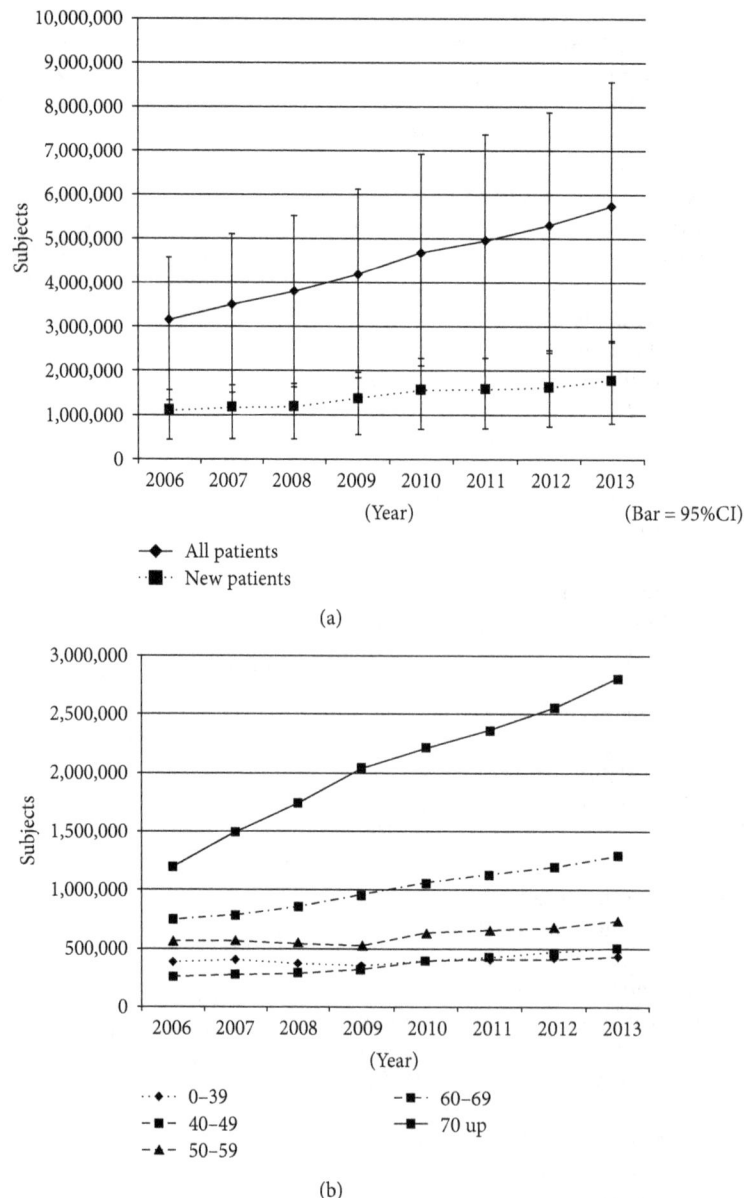

FIGURE 1: Changes in the estimated number of glaucoma patients. (a) Changes in the estimated number of all glaucoma patients and of newly diagnosed glaucoma patients. (b) Changes in the estimated number of glaucoma patients among generations. Bar = SD.

3.5. Trends in Antiglaucoma Ophthalmic Solutions. Figure 3 shows the yearly change in the contents of antiglaucoma ophthalmic solutions. PGs, BBs, and CAIs were the major antiglaucoma ophthalmic solutions used throughout the study period. The proportion of PGs was similar, while those of BBs and CAIs gradually decreased during the study period. The proportion of fixed combination therapy significantly increased after its introduction in 2010. An analysis based on antiglaucoma agents showed that PGs and PG-containing fixed combination therapy accounted for 51.8% of all antiglaucoma agents in 2013.

3.6. Frequency of Glaucoma Surgery. Because the number of glaucoma surgeries was limited for each year, the total number of glaucoma surgeries during the study period was included in the analysis. The mean frequency of glaucoma

surgery was 0.57%, but the frequency of glaucoma surgery significantly increased with age, with a peak at 0.70% in patients in their 60s.

3.7. Changes in Antiglaucoma Ophthalmic Solutions during a Three-Year Period among Newly Diagnosed and Prescribed Glaucoma Patients. A total of 2856 glaucoma patients were eligible for the analysis. Almost all newly medicated glaucoma patients (96.6%) received a single antiglaucoma ophthalmic solution. In the three-year follow up, 14.1% of these patients were administered the same or more than two antiglaucoma ophthalmic solutions (Figure 4(a)). There were 1.03 ± 0.20 bottles of antiglaucoma ophthalmic solutions and 1.06 ± 0.26 types of agents during the first year. By contrast, after three years of follow-up, the numbers were 1.21 ± 0.48 bottles and 1.35 ± 0.68 types, respectively. The

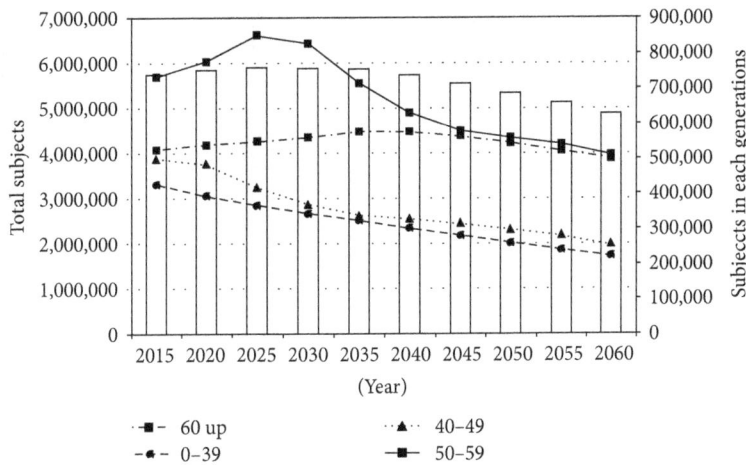

FIGURE 2: Future prediction of the number of glaucoma patients.

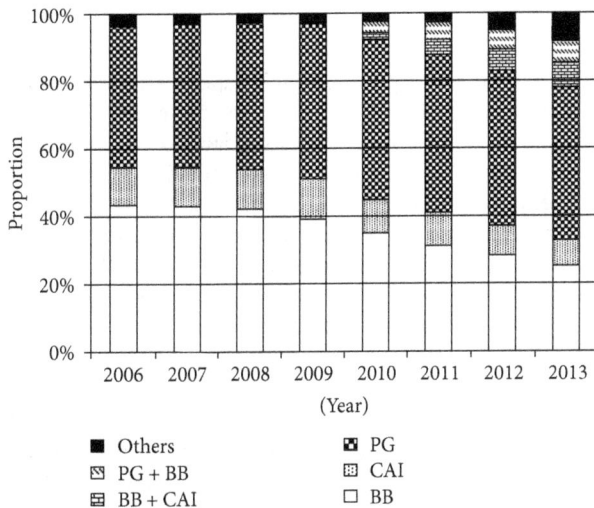

FIGURE 3: Trends in antiglaucoma ophthalmic solutions. PG: prostaglandin analogue; BB: beta blocker; CAI: carbonic anhydrase inhibitor.

numbers of antiglaucoma ophthalmic solutions and agents significantly increased during the first three years ($P < 0.0001$, Wilcoxon signed-rank test). PGs were the most popular type of antiglaucoma ophthalmic solution, followed by BBs, but the treatment regimens became complicated during the three-year period (Figure 4(b)).

4. Discussion

The current study revealed the number of Japanese glaucoma patients in recent years and the frequencies of medications, and surgeries among these patients. The proportion of glaucoma patients significantly increased during the eight years of the study, especially among elderly subjects. The total number of patients of glaucoma patients increased with age. It is expected to increase until 2025 and decrease thereafter due to the aging and reduction of birthrate of Japanese society.

In recent years, many antiglaucoma ophthalmic solutions have become available, resulting in diversification of antiglaucoma ophthalmic solutions. The frequency of glaucoma medication significantly increased with age, and the total number of antiglaucoma agents increased. Therefore, medical expenses for glaucoma treatment will likely increase, and the development of less expensive and more effective therapies for glaucoma is needed.

The frequency of glaucoma surgery increased with age as expected, but the frequency of glaucoma surgery did not significantly change during the study period. Several new surgeries had been introduced recently, which may drastically change glaucoma care. Therefore, it is important to investigate changes in glaucoma surgery. However, the number of glaucoma surgery was not sufficient to investigate this in the present study. Further investigations should be necessary. The introduction of new antiglaucoma ophthalmic solutions may have contributed to this finding. New surgical approaches have been developed recently, including minimally invasive glaucoma surgery, which has been reported to be effective for IOP reduction without severe complications [6, 10, 11]. Although new glaucoma surgeries have not been widely applied in Japan, this trend may change glaucoma care in the near future.

The current study revealed that PGs occupied a major position among antiglaucoma ophthalmic solutions. BBs and CAIs were second and third, respectively, at the beginning of the study period, but their use was gradually reduced over time.

Recently, new categories of antiglaucoma ophthalmic solutions have become available, such as an alpha 2 agonist and fixed combinations. It has been reported that the alpha 2 agonist brimonidine exerts an IOP-independent neuroprotective effect [12]. It is well known that normal tension glaucoma is the most common glaucoma subtype, especially in Asian countries, including Japan [1, 13-17]. Antiglaucoma medications with an IOP-independent neuroprotective effect are highly preferred for glaucoma treatment. The ROCK inhibitor, which is an ophthalmic solution that reduces the IOP by enhancing conventional outflow, became available

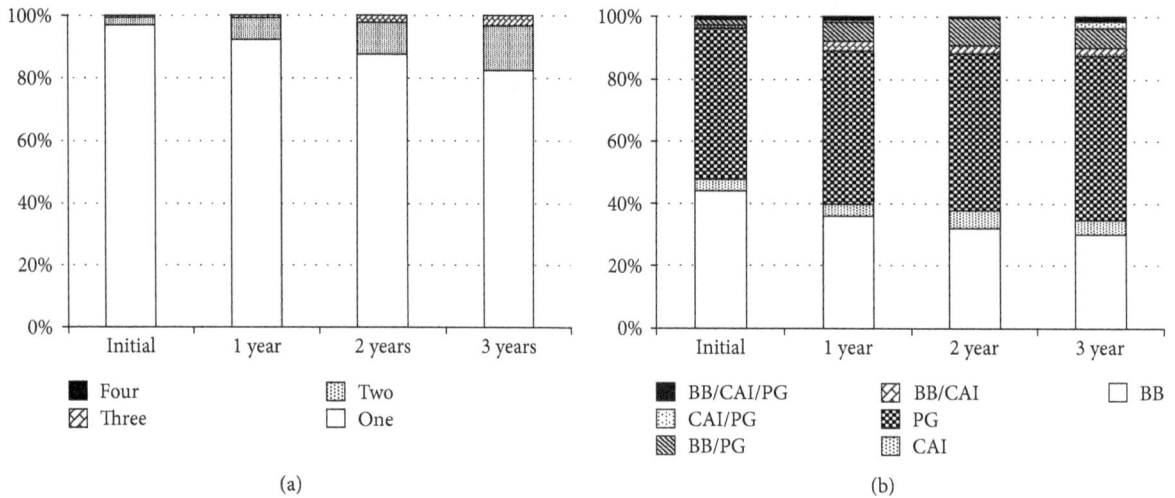

FIGURE 4: Change in antiglaucoma ophthalmic solutions in three years among newly medicated patients. (a) Change in bottles of antiglaucoma ophthalmic solution. (b) Change in the number of antiglaucoma ophthalmic agents. PG: prostaglandin analogue; BB: beta blocker; CAI: carbonic anhydrase inhibitor.

in Japan very recently and has been reported to show an additional IOP reduction in combination with other antiglaucoma ophthalmic solutions [18-21]. Thus, the prescription trend for antiglaucoma ophthalmic solutions may change in the future.

The number of antiglaucoma agents of newly-medicated glaucoma patients increased significantly during a three-year period; 20.4% of glaucoma patients treated by one antiglaucoma agent required two or more agents during this period. It has been noted that increasing the number of ophthalmic solutions results in deterioration of adherence and/or continuity, as well as increasing the risk of side effects [22, 23]. It will be important to develop better treatments that control the IOP using fewer antiglaucoma ophthalmic solutions.

The results of this study demonstrate that the number of glaucoma patients increased during the study period, which also indicates that the medical expenses may accelerate in the future. Comprehensive new glaucoma treatments involving medical, surgical, and laser approaches should be investigated from a socioeconomic perspective.

The results of this study cannot be directly compared to data from epidemiological studies because the current study employed claim data. The accuracy of diagnosis in the current study may be lower than that of an epidemiological study. We could not obtain some important data from the currently employed database including severity of glaucomatous optic neuropathy, visual filed defect, visual acuity, IOP, and other glaucoma-related parameters, which could result in some limitations in the current study. The claim data in the current study were limited to patients in the Social Health Insurance Database. Therefore, we cannot eliminate some possibility of bias in terms of both subject selection and future prediction completely. All Japanese citizens are obligated to register for public insurance systems. Two main types of public insurance systems are available in Japan: National Health Insurance for retired persons and the self-employed and their dependents and Employee Health

Insurance for employees and their dependents. It is difficult to collect combined data from subjects registered in the National Insurance System because data are managed independently by local autonomies. No clear evidence is available that demonstrates the differences between the two insurance systems regarding subject characteristics, including socioeconomic status and disease prevalence. Therefore, the status of glaucoma care between two insurance systems could be similar. Ratios of medicated or operated patients seem to be fewer than expected. Possible explanations could be considered. Firstly, prevalence of patients with normal tension glaucoma (NTG) is higher in Japan compared to other countries [1]. The rate of progress of glaucomatous optic neuropathy among patients with NTG is generally slower than that among those with other types of glaucoma. Secondly, advancement of apparatus such as optical coherence tomography may result in much frequent discovery of very early stage of glaucoma named preperimetric glaucoma which is sometimes subject to observation Thirdly, there were some patients who had been simply followed up after well-performed glaucoma surgery. It is impossible to judge if patients had a history of glaucoma surgery before 2006. Lastly, physicians may not terminate glaucoma diagnosis due to some reasons.

5. Conclusion

This study revealed the current status of glaucoma care in Japan. The proportion of glaucoma patients has significantly increased during the past eight years, but it may begin to decrease after 2025. PGs were the most frequently prescribed antiglaucoma medications, and the number of antiglaucoma medications continuously increased during the treatment period. These data may be adapted to other countries. It is necessary to pursue a more effective and less expensive glaucoma care system by developing new treatment methods and a better screening system.

Conflicts of Interest

All authors have no conflict of interest in this study.

Acknowledgments

The authors appreciate the kind cooperation of Ms. Makiko Kaneko and Ms. Rie Nishikino in providing and analyzing the data. This study was performed with the assistance of JMDC.

References

[1] A. Iwase, Y. Suzuki, M. Araie et al., "The prevalence of primary open-angle glaucoma in Japanese: the Tajimi study," *Ophthalmology*, vol. 111, no. 9, pp. 1641–1648, 2004.

[2] A. L. Coleman and S. Miglior, "Risk factors for glaucoma onset and progression," *Survey of Ophthalmology*, vol. 53, Supplement 1, pp. S3–S10, 2008.

[3] Y. C. Tham, X. Li, T. Y. Wong, H. A. Quigley, T. Aung, and C. Y. Cheng, "Global prevalence of glaucoma and projections of glaucoma burden through 2040: a systematic review and meta-analysis," *Ophthalmology*, vol. 121, no. 11, pp. 2081–2090, 2014.

[4] D. F. Garway-Heath, D. P. Crabb, C. Bunce et al., "Latanoprost for open-angle glaucoma (UKGTS): a randomised, multicentre, placebo-controlled trial," *Lancet*, vol. 385, no. 9975, pp. 1295–1304, 2015.

[5] K. Kashiwagi, "Changes in trend of newly prescribed antiglaucoma medications in recent nine years in a Japanese local community," *Open Journal of Ophthalmology*, vol. 4, pp. 7–11, 2010.

[6] G. M. Richter and A. L. Coleman, "Minimally invasive glaucoma surgery: current status and future prospects," *Clinical Ophthalmology*, vol. 10, pp. 189–206, 2016.

[7] M. Nardi, G. Casini, G. Guidi, and M. Figus, "Emerging surgical therapy in the treatment of glaucoma," *Progress in Brain Research*, vol. 221, pp. 341–357, 2015.

[8] S. Kimura, T. Sato, S. Ikeda, and M. Noda, "Nakayama T development of a database of health insurance claims: standardization of disease classifications and anonymous record linkage," *Journal of Epidemiology*, vol. 20, no. 5, pp. 413–419, 2010.

[9] K. Kashiwagi and T. Furuya, "Persistence with topical glaucoma therapy among newly diagnosed Japanese patients," *Japanese Journal of Ophthalmology*, vol. 58, no. 1, pp. 68–74, 2014.

[10] C. E. Bovee and L. R. Pasquale, "Evolving surgical interventions in the treatment of glaucoma," *Seminars in Ophthalmology*, vol. 32, no. 1, pp. 91–95, 2017.

[11] D. Z. Chen and C. C. A. Sng, "Safety and efficacy of microinvasive glaucoma surgery," *Journal of Ophthalmology*, vol. 2017, Article ID 3182935, 13 pages, 2017.

[12] T. Krupin, J. M. Liebmann, D. S. Greenfield, R. Ritch, S. Gardiner, and Low-Pressure Glaucoma Study Group, "A randomized trial of brimonidine versus timolol in preserving visual function: results from the Low Pressure Glaucoma Treatment Study," *American Journal of Ophthalmology*, vol. 151, no. 4, pp. 671–681, 2011.

[13] C. S. Kim, G. J. Seong, N. H. Lee, K. C. Song, and Namil Study Group, Korean Glaucoma Society, "Prevalence of primary open-angle glaucoma in central South Korea the Namil study," *Ophthalmology*, vol. 118, no. 6, pp. 1024–1030, 2011.

[14] L. Dandona, R. Dandona, M. Srinivas et al., "Open-angle glaucoma in an urban population in southern India: the Andhra Pradesh eye disease study," *Ophthalmology*, vol. 107, no. 9, pp. 1702–1709, 2000.

[15] Y. B. Liang, D. S. Friedman, Q. Zhou et al., "Prevalence of primary open angle glaucoma in a rural adult Chinese population: the Handan eye study," *Investigative Ophthalmology & Visual Science*, vol. 52, no. 11, pp. 8250–8257, 2011.

[16] S. Y. Shen, T. Y. Wong, P. J. Foster et al., "The prevalence and types of glaucoma in Malay people: the Singapore Malay eye study," *Investigative Ophthalmology & Visual Science*, vol. 49, no. 9, pp. 3846–3851, 2008.

[17] L. Vijaya, R. George, H. Arvind et al., "Prevalence of primary angle-closure disease in an urban south Indian population and comparison with a rural population. The Chennai Glaucoma Study," *Ophthalmology*, vol. 115, no. 4, pp. 655–660.e1, 2008.

[18] H. Tanihara, T. Inoue, T. Yamamoto et al., "One-year clinical evaluation of 0.4% ripasudil (K-115) in patients with open-angle glaucoma and ocular hypertension," *Acta Ophthalmologica*, vol. 94, no. 1, pp. e26–e34, 2016.

[19] H. Tanihara, T. Inoue, T. Yamamoto et al., "Additive intraocular pressure-lowering effects of the rho kinase inhibitor ripasudil (K-115) combined with timolol or latanoprost: a report of 2 randomized clinical trials," *JAMA Ophthalmology*, vol. 133, no. 7, pp. 755–761, 2015.

[20] H. Tanihara, T. Inoue, T. Yamamoto et al., "Intra-ocular pressure-lowering effects of a Rho kinase inhibitor, ripasudil (K-115), over 24 hours in primary open-angle glaucoma and ocular hypertension: a randomized, open-label, crossover study," *Acta Ophthalmologica*, vol. 93, no. 4, pp. e254–e260, 2015.

[21] K. Yamamoto, K. Maruyama, N. Himori et al., "The novel rho kinase (ROCK) inhibitor K-115. a new candidate drug for neuroprotective treatment in glaucoma," *Investigative Ophthalmology & Visual Science*, vol. 55, no. 11, pp. 7126–7136, 2014.

[22] F. Djafari, M. R. Lesk, P. J. Harasymowycz, D. Desjardins, and J. Lachaine, "Determinants of adherence to glaucoma medical therapy in a long-term patient population," *Journal of Glaucoma*, vol. 18, no. 3, pp. 238–243, 2009.

[23] J. H. Gurwitz, R. J. Glynn, M. Monane et al., "Treatment for glaucoma: adherence by the elderly," *American Journal of Public Health*, vol. 83, no. 5, pp. 711–716, 1993.

18

Combined Application of Bevacizumab and Mitomycin C or Bevacizumab and 5-Fluorouracil in Experimental Glaucoma Filtration Surgery

Lei Zuo,[1] **Jianhong Zhang,**[1] **and Xun Xu** ⓘ[2]

[1]*Department of Ophthalmology, Shanghai Fourth People's Hospital, Shanghai 200081, China*
[2]*Department of Ophthalmology, Shanghai General Hospital, Shanghai Jiao Tong University School of Medicine, Shanghai 200080, China*

Correspondence should be addressed to Xun Xu; drxuxun@sjtu.edu.cn

Academic Editor: Ozlem G. Koz

The present study aimed at observing the effect of a single subconjunctival injection of bevacizumab (BVZ) combined with 5-fluorouracil (5-Fu) or mitomycin C (MMC) on the antiscarring effect of glaucoma filtration surgery (GFS). The inhibitory effect of combined BVZ and 5-Fu in retinal pigment epithelial cells on vascular endothelial growth factor (VEGF) levels was demonstrated through *in vitro* experiments. Combined BVZ and 5-Fu and combined BVZ and MMC inhibited cell cycle, induced apoptosis, and inhibited human umbilical vein endothelial cell migration. Also, the cytotoxicity of combined BVZ and 5-Fu was lower. In animal experiments, the observation of filtering bleb survival, hematoxylin and eosin and Masson staining of filtering bleb scars, and mRNA expression levels of fibrosis markers in filtering blebs showed that combined BVZ and 5-Fu had a better antiscarring effect compared with single drugs; however, the antiscarring effect of combined BVZ and MMC was not significantly different from MMC. Therefore, the findings of this study provided more reference for the clinical use of adjuncts to inhibit scarring after GFS and helped understand the regulatory effect of combined anti-VEGF antibody BVZ and antimetabolites on wound healing more comprehensively.

1. Introduction

Glaucoma is a serious irreversible optic neuropathy that ultimately causes blindness. When maximum drug therapy cannot control intraocular pressure in patients with glaucoma, laser therapy or surgery must be performed. Glaucoma filtration surgery (GFS) is currently one of the most effective methods for treating glaucoma [1, 2]. Unlike with most operations, the success of GFS is achieved by inhibiting wound healing [3]. In the 1990s, antimetabolic drugs, such as fluorouracil (5-Fu) and mitomycin (MMC), were used to reduce scar formation after a trabeculectomy and to maintain continuous unobstructed filtering, thereby improving the success rate of surgery [4]. However, despite their effectiveness, these drugs were related to several types of life-threatening visual acuity complications [5, 6].

Vascular endothelial growth factor (VEGF) is a signaling protein that promotes vascular endothelial growth and permeability [7]. Also, it has a key role in angiogenesis and embryonic angiogenesis. Further, it participates in pathological angiogenesis, such as tumor growth [8, 9] and ocular diseases. VEGF concentration increases in all ocular diseases involving neovascularization and/or inflammation, such as proliferative diabetic retinopathy [10], neovascular glaucoma [11], uveitis [12], and age-related macular degeneration [13]. In addition, VEGF is related to fibrosis and inflammation [14, 15].

Bevacizumab (BVZ) is a synthetic anti-VEGF monoclonal antibody [16, 17]. Recent studies found that VEGF concentration increased and VEGF levels in the aqueous humor were upregulated in patients after glaucoma surgery. This postsurgery upregulation could be suppressed by the anti-VEGF antibody, BVZ, administered during the surgery [18]. BVZ reduces the migration of VEGF into injured vessels and significantly inhibits scar formation during wound healing [18, 19]. Furthermore, the watertight suture in the conjunctiva can antagonize BVZ-induced delayed healing of the conjunctival wound [20]. Subconjunctival injection of BVZ could reach an effective level in the intraocular tissues in the treated eyes [21]. On the basis of these findings, doses of BVZ were injected to inhibit scar formation after trabeculectomy.

Kahook et al. first reported and used the anti-VEGF antibody as a potential wound-healing regulator; 1 mg BVZ was injected around a filtering bleb using a fine needle after MMC application failed [22]. In other cases, Grewal reported that a subconjunctival injection of BVZ helped save the failed filtering blebs [23]. Some animal studies also demonstrated the effectiveness of BVZ combined with 5-Fu (BVZ + 5-Fu) in preventing scarring after GFS [24]. Some animal studies used a sustained-release device carrying MMC in trabeculectomy, suggesting that BVZ combined with MMC (BVZ + MMC) had synergistic effects [25]. Although reports on the antiproliferative effect and toxicity of BVZ on ocular cells have been reported [26], the role of BVZ + 5-Fu and BVZ + MMC in human ocular cells has rarely been investigated, and the comparison of the application of BVZ + 5-Fu or BVZ + MMC in experimental GFS surgery and their effectiveness remains unclear.

This study evaluated the safety and effect of a single subconjunctival injection of BVZ combined with 5-Fu or MMC on the antiscarring effect of GFS and compared them with the use of uncombined agents in *in vitro* and animal experiments. Cytotoxicity, the survival time of filtering blebs, and mRNA expression levels of fibrosis markers were observed. These findings provided a reference for glaucoma treatment in clinical surgeries.

2. Materials and Methods

2.1. In Vitro Experiment

2.1.1. Drugs and Reagents. Medium, antibiotics, trypsin (1 : 250), recombinant human VEGF, 3-(4,5-dimethylthiazol-2-yl)-2,5-diphenyltetrazolium bromide (MTT), and heat-inactivated fetal bovine serum (FBS) were purchased from Invitrogen (CA, USA). Endothelial cell culture medium was purchased from PromoCell GmbH (Heidelberg, Germany). Bevacizumab (Avastin), PhosSTOP, and protease inhibitors were purchased from Roche (Basel, Switzerland). The enzyme-linked immunosorbent assay (ELISA) kit was purchased from R&D Systems (MN, USA). The Bradford protein assay was purchased from Bio-Rad (Hercules, CA, USA). Fluorouracil (25 mg/mL) was purchased from Shanghai Xudong Haipu Pharmaceutical Co. Ltd. (China), and mitomycin was purchased from Zhejiang Hisun Pharmaceutical Co., Ltd. (China). Phosphate-buffered saline (PBS) and 0.9% sodium chloride were purchased from Baxter Healthcare Ltd. Human retinal pigment epithelial cells (ARPE-19) and human umbilical vein endothelial cells (HUVECs) were cultured in DMEM/F12 culture medium

containing 10% FBS and antibiotics, respectively. ARPE-19 and HUVEC lines were purchased from American Type Culture Collection (VA, USA).

2.1.2. Detection of Cytotoxicity/Proliferation. A single-cell suspension within the logarithmic growth period cultured under normal conditions was inoculated into a six-well culture plate at a cell density of 5×10^4 cells per well. After synchronization using serum-free RPMI 1640 culture medium, ARPE-19 cells were incubated with 0.05, 0.5, or 5 mg/mL 5-Fu; 0.0002, 0.002, or 0.02 mg/mL MMC; 0.025, 0.25, or 2.5 mg/mL BVZ; 0.05, 0.5, or 5 mg/mL 5-Fu + 2.5 mg/mL BVZ; 0.0002, 0.002, or 0.02 mg/mL MMC + 2.5 mg/mL BVZ; or PBS as the control for 24 h, after which they were washed with PBS. Fresh serum-free medium with or without 0.5 mg/mL MTT was added to the cells. After incubating for 2 h, the colorimetric analysis was conducted to determine formazan extraction and ELISA (Emax, Molecular Devices Corporation, CA, USA) was conducted to measure the absorbance of each well at 570 nm [27].

2.1.3. VEGF Level Determination. ARPE-19 cells were treated with 5 mg/mL 5-Fu, 0.02 mg/mL MMC, 2.5 mg/mL BVZ, 5 mg/mL 5-Fu + 2.5 mg/mL BVZ, 0.02 mg/mL MMC + 2.5 mg/mL BVZ, or PBS as the control. After 24 h, 200 μL of the supernatant per well was collected and analyzed using a VEGF ELISA Kit (R&D Systems) according to the manufacturer's protocol [28].

2.1.4. Assessment of Cell Cycle Changes Using Flow Cytometry with Propidium Iodide Staining. A single-cell suspension during the logarithmic growth period and cultured under normal conditions was inoculated into a six-well culture plate at a cell density of 5×10^4 cells per well. After synchronization using serum-free RPMI 1640 culture medium, ARPE-19 cells were incubated with 5 mg/mL 5-Fu, 0.02 mg/mL MMC, 2.5 mg/mL BVZ, 5 mg/mL 5-Fu + 2.5 mg/mL BVZ, 0.02 mg/mL MMC + 2.5 mg/mL BVZ, or PBS as the control for 48 h. Each application was done in triplicate. The cells were collected, washed with PBS, counted, adjusted into a single-cell suspension at 1×10^6/mL, fixed with 70% ethanol, preserved at 4°C, and washed with PBS to remove the fixative before staining. RNase A (100 μL) was added to the cell suspension. The cells were incubated in a 37°C water bath for 30 min, and 400 μL of propidium iodide (PI) was added and mixed for staining. The suspension was then incubated again in the dark at 4°C for 30 min, and the cells were detected using flow cytometry. The percentage of cells in each cycle was fitted according to the cell distribution diagram of relative DNA content [29].

2.1.5. Detection of Cell Apoptosis by Annexin V-FITC Staining. ARPE-19 cells were treated with 5 mg/mL 5-Fu, 0.02 mg/mL MMC, 2.5 mg/mL BVZ 5 mg/mL 5-Fu + 2.5 mg/mL BVZ, 0.02 mg/mL MMC + 2.5 mg/mL BVZ, or PBS as the control and incubated at 37°C in 50 mL/LCO$_2$ for 48 h. Each application was done in triplicate. The cells were collected and washed with PBS. A binding buffer (500 μL) was added to suspend the cells. Then, 5 μL of Annexin V-FITC was added to the suspension and mixed, after which 5 μL of PI was added and mixed. The cells were incubated in the dark at room temperature for 15 min, and the apoptotic cells were detected using flow cytometry [30].

2.1.6. Migration Analysis of Endothelial Cells. HUVECs were cultured *in vitro* to 80% density. A 1 mm pipette tip was used to make three equidistant scratches perpendicular to the bottom of the cell culture dish. PBS was used to remove the cells floating on the scratches, and images using six different fields of vision were taken using the Leica DM IRB microscope (40×). The time point was set at 0 h and the cells were treated with 0.05 mg/mL 5-Fu, 0.0002 mg/mL MMC, 2.5 mg/mL BVZ, 0.05 mg/mL 5-Fu + 2.5 mg/mL BVZ, or 0.0002 mg/mL MMC + 2.5 mg/mL BVZ. The treatments were combined with 40 ng/mL VEGF; 40 ng/mL VEGF alone was added into 0.2% FBS culture medium as the control. The control group without drug intervention was set. Images using the Leica DM IRB microscope were taken after culturing for 24 h. Each treatment culture was duplicated, and the same area of each duplicate was selected for photographing. The scratch area at each time point was analyzed using the ImageJ software. The wound closure rate = (area of the wound at 0 h − area of the wound at 24 h)/area of the wound at 0 h [31].

2.7. Animal Experiment

2.7.1. Animal Model. Sixty healthy male New Zealand white rabbits (aged 12–14 weeks and weighing 2.0–2.5 kg each) were used in this study. All animal experiments were approved by the Shanghai Science and Technology Committee (permit number: SYXK[hu]2015-0014) and were in accordance with the Association for Research in Vision and Ophthalmology declaration of animal use. The experimental animals were kept under a 12/12 h light/dark cycle with random feeding. They were domesticated for 1 week before the experiment.

Trabeculectomy surgery was performed according to the standard protocol. An intramuscular injection of 50 mg/kg ketamine hydrochloride (Gutian Pharmaceutical Company, Fujian, China) and 25 mg/kg chlorpromazine hydrochloride (Gutian Pharmaceutical Company) was administered for general anesthesia. Proparacaine hydrochloride eyedrops (Alcon USA, TX, USA) were applied as local anesthesia. The conjunctiva was separated along the corneal limbus, and then a scleral flap of 3×4 mm^2 with the corneal limbus as the base and a thickness of one-half of the sclera was made. The iris root was excised after a trabecular meshwork of 1.5×2 mm^2 was removed. The scleral flap was sutured with a 10-0 nylon thread, and the conjunctiva was sutured to a watertight seal [32]. The surgery was performed by an experienced physician.

All New Zealand white rabbits received GFS in their right eye and were randomly divided into the following six groups ($n = 10$):

Group 1. The control group: GFS, no ancillary drugs;

Group 2. 5-Fu treatment group: at the end of GFS, 0.1 mL (50 mg/mL) of 5-Fu was injected under the conjunctiva next to the filtering bleb; attention was paid to avoid 5-Fu from entering the eye.

Group 3. MMC group: before resection of the sclera and trabecular tissue, an absorbent cotton pad of 1×4 mm^2 (0.2 mg/mL) was placed between the scleral bed and the scleral flap and covered with the conjunctiva and Tenon's capsule. Attention was paid to avoid the contact between the conjunctival flap and the cotton pad. After 3 min, the area was washed with 30 mL of balanced salt solution. The sclera was then resected, and the peripheral iridectomy was performed. The conjunctival incision was tightly sutured [33].

Group 4. BVZ treatment group: at the end of GFS, 0.1 mL (25 mg/mL) of BVZ was injected under the conjunctiva next to the filtering bleb.

Group 5. 5-Fu + BVZ treatment group: at the end of GFS, 0.1 mL of 5-Fu and 0.1 mL of BVZ were injected under the conjunctiva into one side of the filtering bleb.

Group 6. MMC + BVZ treatment group: an MMC cotton pad (0.2 mg/mL) was placed for 3 min; after the surgery, 0.1 mL of BVZ was injected under the contralateral conjunctiva of the filtering blebs.

2.7.2. Clinical Observation. A Kaplan–Meier survival curve (56 days of observation time) was drawn according to the survival time of the filtering blebs in each group [34]. The failure of a filtering bleb was defined as a flat, neovascularized, and scared filtering bleb with a deep anterior chamber [35]. The incidence of complications, such as wound leakage and corneal opacity, was observed.

2.7.3. Polymerase Chain Reaction Analysis. Pentobarbital sodium (60–150 mg/kg) was injected intravenously 28 and 56 days after the surgery, and the filtering bleb tissue was removed. A polymerase chain reaction (PCR) analysis ($n = 3$) was conducted to quantitatively analyze the expression of collagen I and fibronectin [24]. Total mRNA of the filtering bleb tissue was extracted and separated using TRIzol reagents (Invitrogen), and cDNA was synthesized using the Tetro cDNA Synthesis Kit (Bioline, London, UK). The mRNA expression level was detected by real-time (RT) PCR using the SensiFAST SYBR Hi-ROX Kit (Bioline) and analyzed with ABI Prism 7500 (SDS Software, USA). Table 1 lists the primer sequences. The primers and probes for RT-PCR were designed by Shanghai Generay Biotech Co., Ltd. The expression levels of type I collagen and fibronectin mRNA were normalized using mRNA of glyceraldehyde-3-phosphate dehydrogenase (GAPDH).

2.7.4. Tissue Sections. Pentobarbital sodium (60–150 mg/kg) was injected intravenously to remove the eyeball 56 days after the surgery. After denucleation, all eyeballs were fixed in the formalin acetate alcohol solution for 24 h, preserved in

TABLE 1: Primers used in real-time polymerase chain reaction.

Gene name	Primer sequences
Collagen I	Forward: 5′-CAGCCGCTTCACCTACAGC-3′ Reverse: 5′-TTTTGTATTCAATCACTGTCTTGCC-3′
Fibronectin	Forward: 5′-ACC AAC CTT AAT CCG GGC AC-3′ Reverse: 5′-TCA GAA ACT GTG GCT TGC TGG-3′
GAPDH	Forward: 5′-AGACAGCCGCATCTTCTTGT-3′ Reverse: 5′-CTTGCCGTGGGTAGAGTCAT-3′

70% ethanol, and fixed with paraffin. Sequential 5 μm sections were prepared and stained with hematoxylin and eosin (H&E) for histological observation and Masson for detection of collagen deposition [36] ($n = 4$).

2.7.5. Statistical Analyses. The mean ± standard deviation was used to describe the variables. When the variance was homogeneous, the LSD and SNK tests of the analysis of variance were used. When the difference was inhomogeneous, the differences between experimental groups were analyzed using the rank-sum test. The Kaplan–Meier survival analysis and Mantel–Cox log-rank test were used to analyze the differences in survival time of the filtering blebs. All statistical analyses were carried out using SPSS 13.0 (SPSS Inc., IL, USA). A $P < 0.05$ was considered to be statistically significant.

3. Results

3.1. In Vitro Experiments

3.1.1. Cytotoxicity Analyses. After adding 0.025, 0.25, and 2.5 mg/mL BVZ to the cultured ARPE-19 cells, no significant cytotoxicity was observed compared with that in the PBS group. After 0.0002, 0.002, and 0.02 mg/mL MMC were added, the viability of the ARPE-19 cells was significantly lower than that in the PBS group, with no significance difference between the MMC and MMC + BVZ groups. When 0.05, 0.5, and 5 mg/mL 5-Fu were added, the number of apoptotic ARPE-19 cells significantly increased. However, when 0.5 and 5 mg/mL 5-Fu + BVZ were added, the survival of ARPE-19 cells significantly increased (Figure 1).

3.1.2. Detection of VEGF Level in Retinal Pigment Endothelium Cells. The ELISA method was used to analyze the VEGF levels in the medium to be able to detect VEGF expression in retinal pigment endothelium (RPE) cells after drug intervention. After culturing for 24 h, the VEGF levels in RPE cells in the BVZ and BVZ + 5-Fu groups were significantly lower than that in the control group, while the VEGF levels in the 5-Fu and MMC groups significantly increased (Figure 2).

3.1.3. Cell Cycle and Apoptosis. The effects of 5-Fu, MMC, BVZ, BVZ + 5-Fu, and BVZ + MMC on the cell cycle and apoptosis of RPE cells were evaluated using flow cytometry.

The results showed that the proliferation of RPE cells was significantly inhibited after 5-Fu, MMC, BVZ + 5-Fu, or BVZ + MMC was added to RPE cells and incubated for 48 h compared to with those in the control group (Figure 3(a)). Treatment with 5-Fu, MMC, BVZ, BVZ + 5-Fu, or BVZ + MMC could significantly induce RPE cell apoptosis, and the inhibitory effect of the combined drugs was higher than that of the single drugs (Figure 3(b)).

3.1.4. Cell Migration. The scratch-wound assay was used to evaluate the inhibitory effects of 5-Fu, MMC, BVZ, BVZ + 5-Fu, and BVZ + MMC on the migration of HUVECs. Figure 4 shows the changes in the migration of HUVECs after 24 h under the action of VEGF and 5-Fu, MMC, BVZ, BVZ + 5-Fu, or BVZ + MMC. The wound closure rate of cells in the VEGF control group was 0.2215 ± 0.0117 after 24 h, and that of cells in the negative control group without drug intervention was 0.0454 ± 0.0216. The rate in the 5-Fu/VEGF, 5-Fu/BVZ/VEGF, BVZ/VEGF, MMC/VEGF, and MMC/BVZ/VEGF groups was 0.1402 ± 0.0183, 0.1811 ± 0.0147, 0.1438 ± 0.0194, 0.1086 ± 0.0132, and 0.0695 ± 0.0191, respectively. 5-Fu, MMC, BVZ, 5-Fu + BVZ, and MMC + BVZ could significantly inhibit the migration of HUVECs under the action of VEGF, and the inhibitory effect of MMC + BVZ was higher than that of MMC or BVZ alone (Figure 4).

3.2. Animal Experiments

3.2.1. Survival of Filtering Blebs. The average survival time of filtering blebs in groups 1 (control), 2 (5-Fu), 3 (MMC), 4 (BVZ), 5 (BVZ + 5-Fu), and 6 (BVZ + MMC) was 6.3 ± 0.7, 22.4 ± 2.7, 35.5 ± 5.0, 23.8 ± 2.9, 36.0 ± 5.2, and 35.2 ± 5.6 days, respectively (Figure 5). The Kaplan–Meier analysis showed significant differences among the six groups (log-rank = 46.18; $P < 0.001$). The survival time of filtering blebs in the BVZ + 5-Fu group was significantly longer than that in the BVZ, control, and 5-Fu groups, with no significant difference compared with the MMC group. The survival time of filtering blebs was significantly longer in the BVZ + MMC group than in the control, 5-Fu, and BVZ groups, with no significant difference compared with that in the MMC or BVZ + 5-Fu group (Table 2).

3.2.2. Bleb Vascularity. Figure 6 shows the bleb vascularity in the six groups of filtering blebs. No complications, such as wound leakage, encysted bleb, or corneal opacity, were observed during the study.

3.2.3. Histopathological Features. H&E and Masson staining of the tissue sections of the 56-day filtering blebs showed histological features and subconjunctival collagen deposition in the control (Figures 7(a) and 7(g)), BVZ (Figures 7(b) and 7(h)), 5-Fu (Figures 7(c) and 7(i)), MMC (Figures 7(d) and 7(j)), 5-FU + BVZ (Figures 7(e) and 7(k)), and MMC + BVZ (Figures 7(f) and 7(l)) treatment groups.

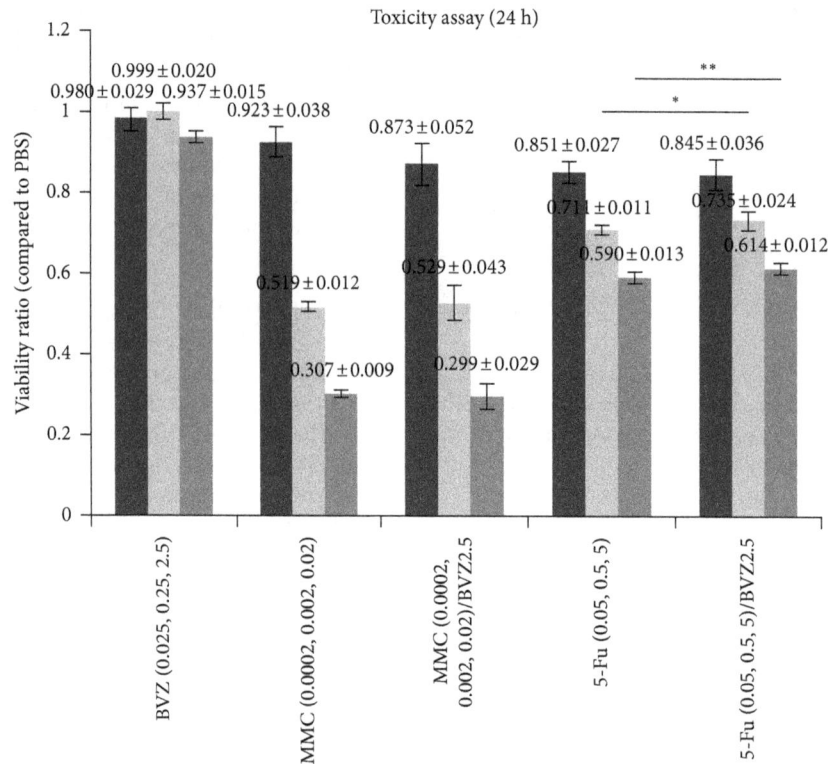

FIGURE 1: Cell viability of ARPE-19 after treatment with bevacizumab (BVZ), mitomycin C (MMC), 5-fluorouracil (5-Fu), MMC + BVZ, and 5-Fu + BVZ. The cell viability of the control group was set at 100%. Unit: mg/mL. $^{*}P < 0.05$, $^{**}P < 0.01$.

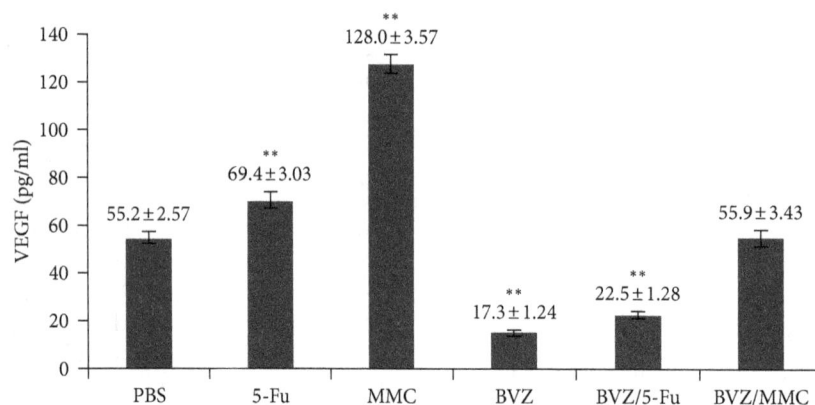

FIGURE 2: Effects of bevacizumab (BVZ), mitomycin C (MMC), 5-fluorouracil (5-Fu), MMC + BVZ, and 5-Fu + BVZ on vascular endothelial growth factor (VEGF) levels in retinal pigment endothelium (RPE) cells. $^{**}P < 0.001$.

3.2.4. mRNA Quantitation of Type I Collagen Fiber and Fibronectin in Filtering Blebs. In the BVZ, 5-Fu + BVZ, and MMC + BVZ groups, the mRNA expression levels of type I collagen fiber (Figures 8(a)) and fibronectin (Figure 8(b)) in the filtering blebs after 1 and 2 months were significantly lower than those in the control group.

4. Discussion

This study observed the safety and the antiscarring effects of the use of BVZ + 5-Fu and BVZ + MMC in *in vitro* experiments and experimental GFS. The results showed that the use of BVZ + 5-Fu had better antiscarring effects and provided better cell safety. However, BVZ + MMC showed no significant advantage over MMC alone. The findings provided more reference for the clinical use of adjuncts to inhibit wound healing of the bleb after GFS, contributing to the overall knowledge on wound modulation by the combined use of BVZ and antimetabolic drugs.

The purpose of the GFS surgery was to relieve elevated intraocular pressure by creating an incision to bypass the trabecular meshwork and drain the aqueous humor outward through subconjunctival filtering blebs [37]. The neovascularization of the conjunctiva and migration of the

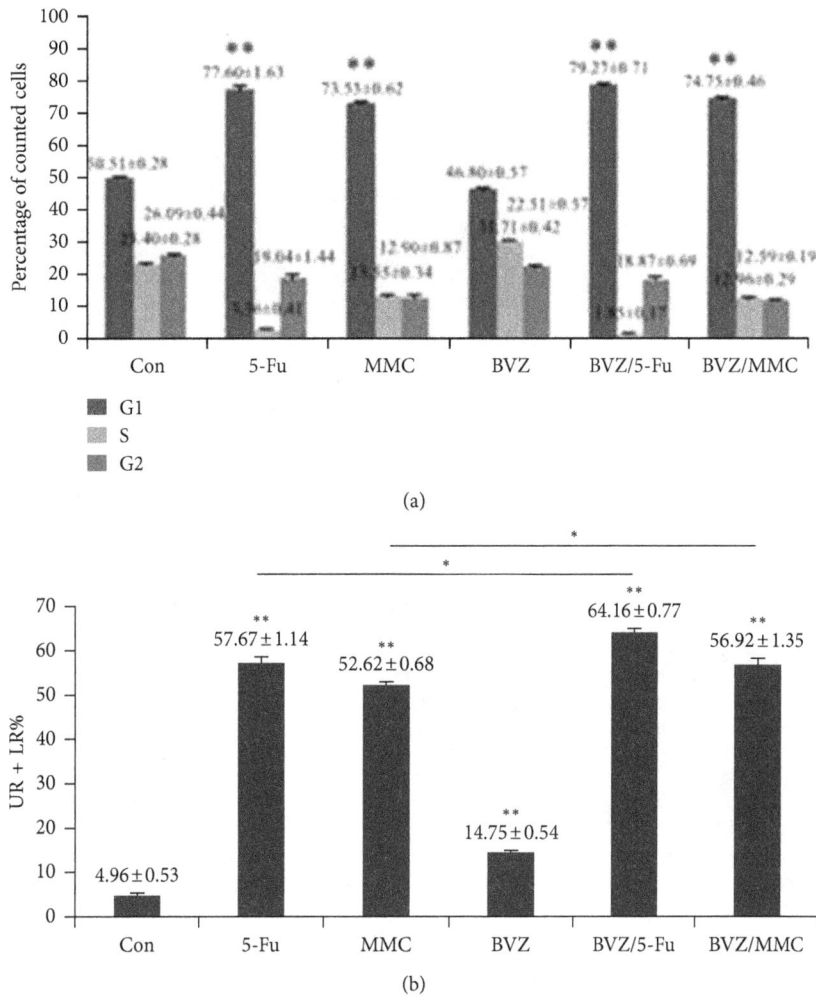

Figure 3: Analysis of the cell cycle and apoptosis of retinal pigment endothelium (RPE) cells. (a) Percentage of RPE cells in G1/G0, G2/M, and S phases after 48 h of incubation in PBS control, 5 mg/mL 5-fluorouracil (5-Fu), 0.02 mg/mL mitomycin C (MMC), 2.5 mg/mL bevacizumab (BVZ), 2.5 mg/mL BVZ + 5 mg/mL 5-Fu, and 2.5 mg/mL BVZ + 0.02 mg/mL MMC. $^{**}P < 0.001$. (b) Effects of 48 h of incubation in the same concentrations of drugs on RPE cell apoptosis. $^{*}P < 0.01$.

fibroblasts resulted in the proliferation of fibroblasts accompanied by collagen deposits, which directly caused the failure of filtering bleb drainage [38]. Angiogenesis is a process of growing new blood vessels from existing blood vessels. This important process occurs naturally during growth, reproduction, and wound healing to supply nutrients and oxygen to the tissues. VEGF is the most common stimulator for endothelial growth and vascular permeability [39, 40]. It not only regulates fibrosis through angiogenesis but also acts as a mediator in signaling pathways that promote fibroblast migration, proliferation, and collagen production [41, 42].

Seet et al. [43] used mouse models to analyze the time and space of the reaction stages during wound healing after GFS. They found that the tissue reaction after surgery could be divided into two stages: early "acute inflammation" and late "fibrosis" stages. The early acute inflammation stage is characterized by significantly elevated transcriptional expressions of VEGF, chemokines (C-X-C motif), ligand (CXCL), and matrix metalloproteinase (MMP), besides

increased infiltration by inflammatory cells. The late fibrosis stage is characterized by the significantly elevated expression of transforming growth factor (TGF)-$\beta 2$ and extracellular matrix genes, whereas the infiltration of inflammatory cells reduced. VEGF-A is the only VEGF subtype significantly elevated during the late stage of wound healing [43], suggesting that it might be involved in the transition of the early to late stage [44]. VEGF signaling is involved in both angiogenesis and fibrosis, two critical processes in scar formation [43, 45]. This has led to studies investigating the ability of anti-VEGF therapy to improve the outcomes of GFS. However, the treatment for one target might not offer adequate benefit for GFS because of the complex wound-healing process. Therefore, this study was concerned not only with the use of BVZ in GFS but also whether the use of BVZ + 5-Fu or BVZ + MMC could better inhibit wound scar formation after GFS. Also, the safety and possible mechanism of action of the aforementioned drugs were investigated.

The present study tested the cytotoxicities of BVZ + 5Fu and BVZ + MMC in vitro. Previous studies have used the

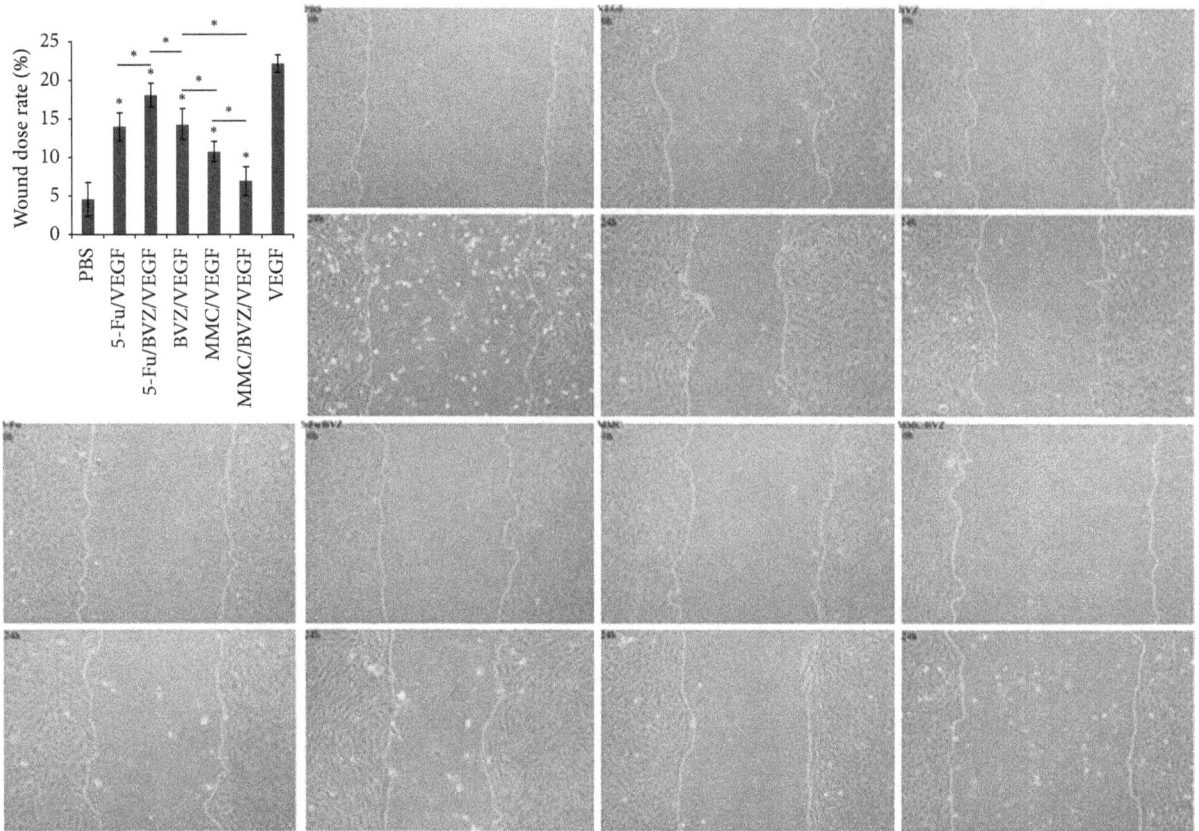

FIGURE 4: Cell migration analysis. The scratch-wound assay of human umbilical vein endothelial cells (HUVECs) after treatment with bevacizumab (BVZ), mitomycin C (MMC), 5-fluorouracil (5-Fu), MMC + BVZ, and 5-Fu + BVZ on the migration of endothelial cells under the action of vascular endothelial growth factor (VEGF). ($P < 0.05$).

MTT assay to observe the cytotoxicity of BVZ to ARPE19 cell lines [26]. The cytotoxicity of selected herbal chemicals with potent antiangiogenic therapeutic properties was studied by performing the MTT cell viability/proliferation assay on ARPE19 cells [27]. Therefore, the same method was used in the present study to observe the cytotoxicity of BVZ combined with antimetabolites. The study found that the toxicity of treatment with 0.5 and 5 mg/mL 5-Fu + 2.5 mg/mL BVZ was lower than that of 5-Fu alone. However, the treatment with MMC + 2.5 mg/mL BVZ had toxicity equivalent to that of MMC alone.

Since RPE and endothelial cells are known to express VEGF [46, 47], the impact of combination drugs on RPE cells at the level of VEGF was tested to observe the comprehensive effect of these combinations on wound healing. Further, the study attempted to explore the mechanism of action of combined drugs and examined the cell cycle and apoptosis of RPE cells. The treatment with BVZ + 5-Fu was found to have a significant inhibitory effect on VEGF levels in RPE cells, but BVZ + MMC had no such effect. Both BVZ + 5-Fu and BVZ + MMC blocked the proliferation of RPE cells in the G1/G0 phase and significantly induced RPE cell apoptosis.

Tenon's fibroblast cells are the important mediators in the formation of filtering blebs scar after GFS [48]. *In vitro* studies have reported the inhibitory effect of BVZ on the proliferation and migration of Tenon's fibroblast cells

[18, 49]. VEGF signaling is involved in both angiogenesis and fibrosis, two critical processes in scar formation [43, 45]. The present study paid attention to the effect of combined drugs on vascular endothelial cells, which were involved in angiogenesis [50]. The scratch-wound assay is a classic method for studying the spread, proliferation, and migration of vascular endothelial cells, which are typical events in the wound-healing process [27]. Therefore, scratch-wound assay and HUVECs were chosen to observe the effects of BVZ combined with antimetabolites on the migration of vascular endothelial cells. Both BVZ + 5-Fu and BVZ + MMC inhibited the migration of HUVECs.

Animal experiments and small clinical trials showed that BVZ treatment delayed the healing process of filtering blebs after GFS [18, 23, 51]. How et al. [24] performed the subconjunctival injection of BVZ + 5-Fu in an experimental rabbit eye GFS model and observed that the antiproliferative effect of the combined treatment was better than that of each drug alone. In clinical trials, Suh and Kee [52] and Chua et al. [53] also administered BVZ + 5-Fu in GFS. Compared with 5-Fu alone, no significant difference was found in vision, postoperative intraocular pressure, or antiglaucoma drug use. Kahook et al. [54] randomly divided patients with primary open-angle glaucoma into an MMC group and a group treated with MMC and an intravitreal injection of ranibizumab (RBZ). They found that the bleb morphology, such as filtering bleb dispersion and neovascularization, in

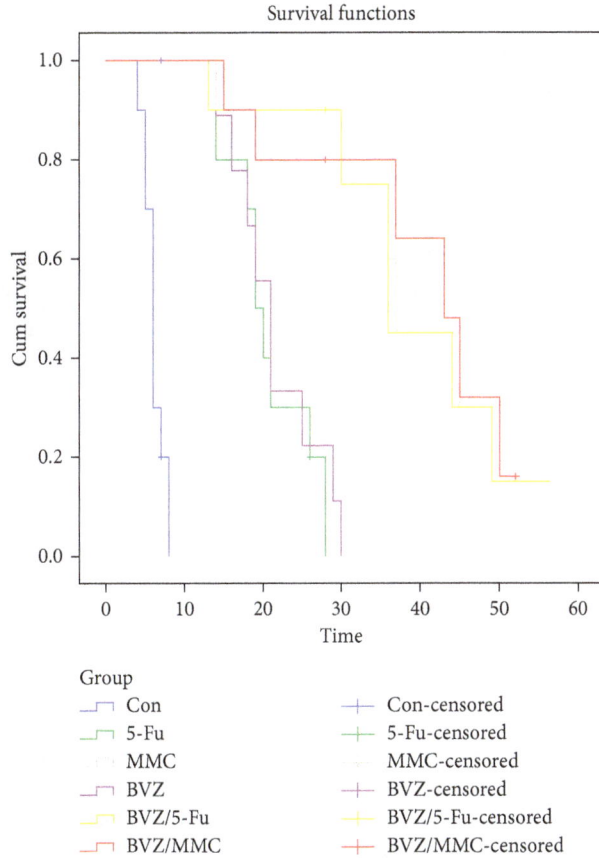

FIGURE 5: Kaplan–Meier analysis of the survival time of filtering blebs in each group.

TABLE 2: Kaplan–Meier analysis and Mantel–Cox log-rank test of the survival time of filtering blebs in each group.

Group	Con P value	5-Fu P value	MMC P value	BVZ P value	BVZ + 5-Fu P value	BVZ + MMC P value
Con	—	<0.0001	<0.0001	<0.0001	<0.0001	<0.0001
5-Fu	<0.0001	—	<0.0001	0.588	<0.0001	0.002
MMC	<0.0001	<0.0001	—	<0.0001	0.851	0.920
BVZ	<0.0001	0.588	<0.0001	—	<0.0001	0.002
BVZ + 5-Fu	<0.0001	<0.0001	0.851	<0.0001	—	0.794
BVZ + MMC	<0.0001	0.002	0.920	0.002	0.794	—

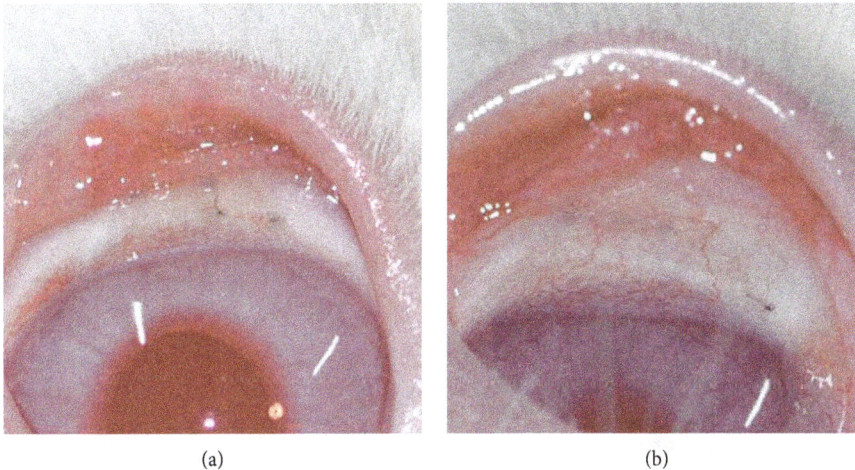

(a)

(b)

FIGURE 6: Continued.

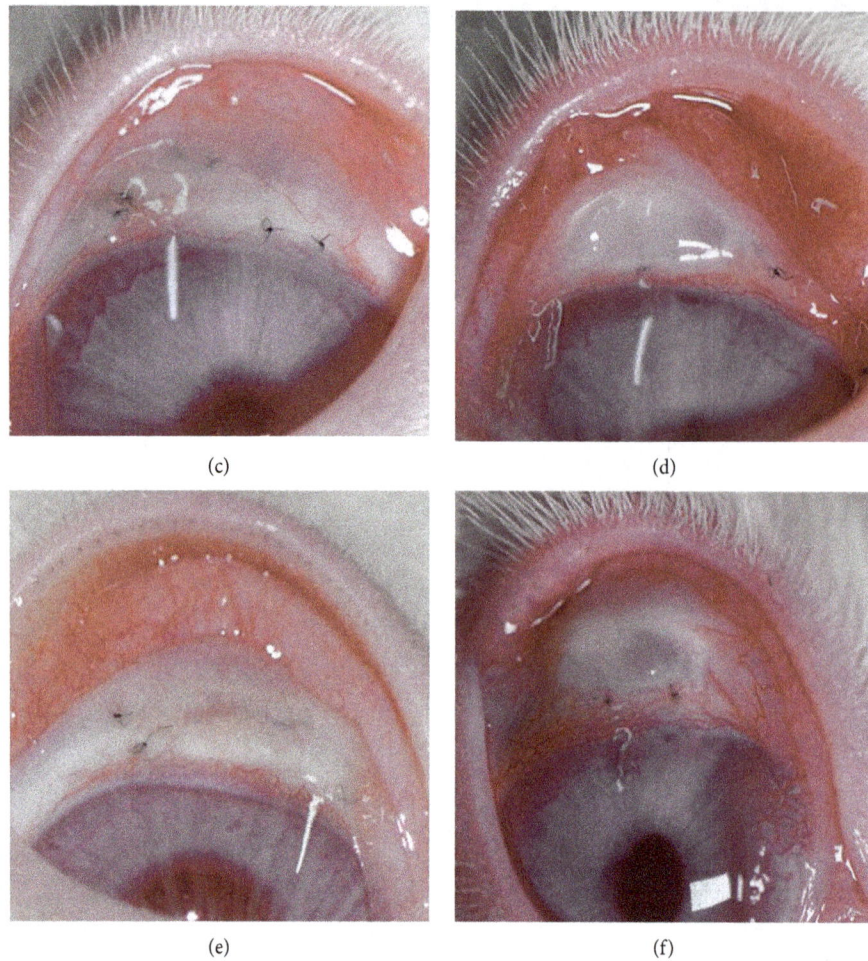

Figure 6: Bleb photograph examples in rabbit subconjunctival scar models 20 days after the surgery. Compared with the control group (a), 5-fluorouracil (5-Fu) treatment group (b) had a nearly normal distribution of blood vessels with filtering blebs low and flat. Compared with the control group (a), bevacizumab (BVZ) treatment (c) and 5-Fu + BVZ groups (e) showed slightly higher and diffused filtering blebs, and the distribution of blood vessels was not obvious. Compared with the control group (a), mitomycin C (MMC) (d) and MMC + BVZ groups (f) showed more conjunctival blood vessels with obviously bulged filtering blebs.

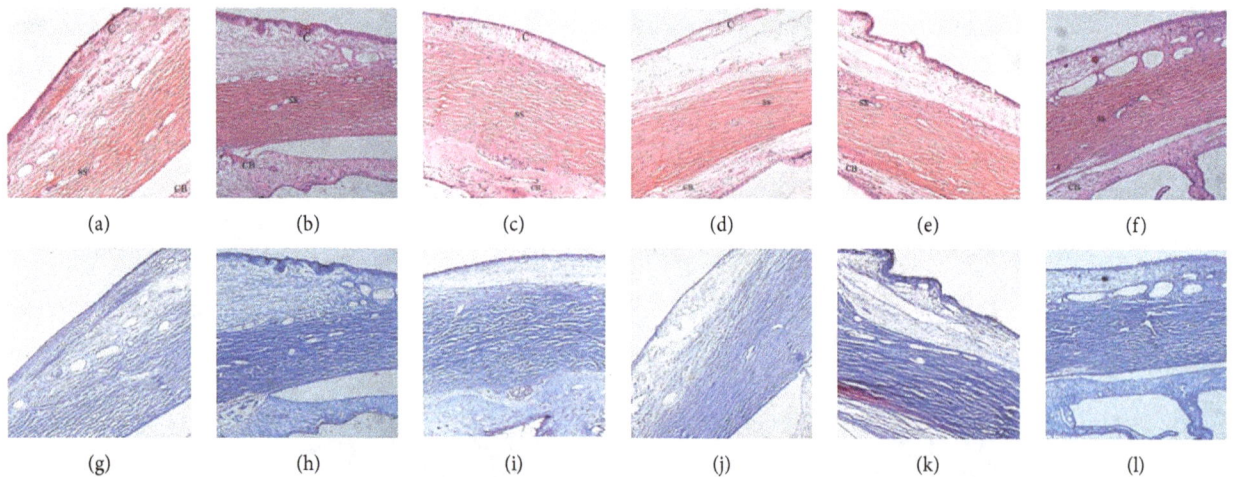

Figure 7: Histological features of filtering positions after 56 days (magnification ratio ×100). (a–f) Hematoxylin and eosin (H&E) staining, (g–l) Masson staining of the tissue sections. In the control (a and g) and 5-fluorouracil (5-Fu) treatment groups (c and i), the subconjunctival fibrous scar tissues were dense. The collagen deposition was relatively loose in the bevacizumab (BVZ) treatment group (b and h), and the structures of filtering blebs could not be distinguished in the three groups. In the mitomycin C (MMC) (d and j), 5-FU + BVZ (e and k), and MMC + BVZ (f and l) treatment groups, the subconjunctival collagen deposition was spare, and the residual filtering bleb structure was observed in all these groups. CB, ciliary body; C, conjunctiva; SS, scleral excision position.

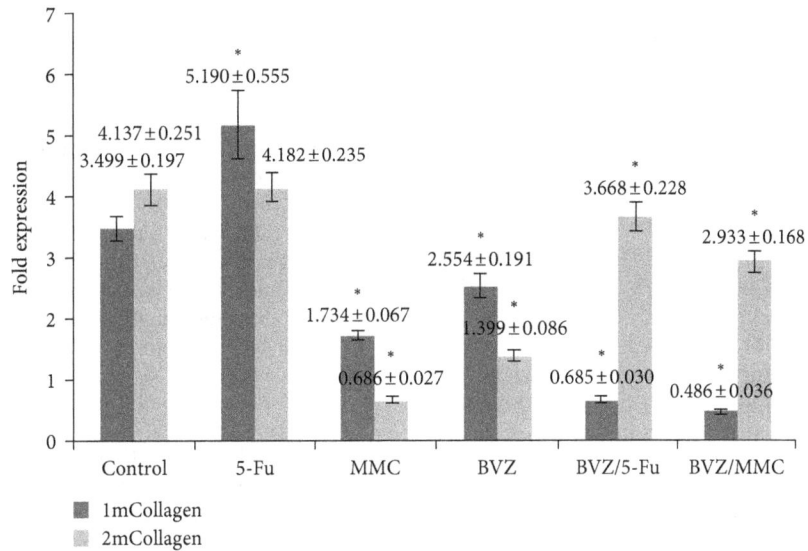

(a)

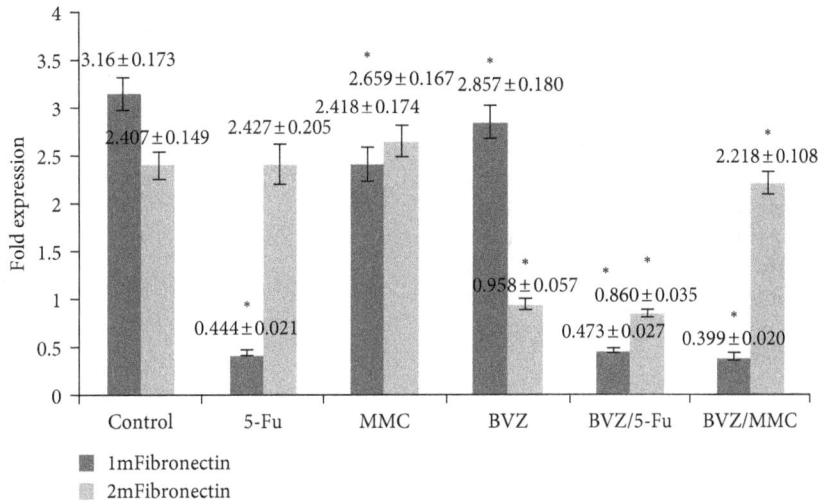

(b)

FIGURE 8: mRNA expression levels of fibrotic markers in the tissues of filtering blebs. In the bevacizumab (BVZ), 5-fluorouracil (5-Fu) + BVZ, and mitomycin C (MMC) + BVZ groups, the mRNA expression levels of type I collagen (a) and fibronectin (b) in filtering blebs were significantly lower than those in the control group. The data in the MMC and 5-Fu treatment groups were not significantly different from those in the control group after both 1 and 2 months ($^*P < 0.05$).

the combined treatment group was better than that in the single treatment group; however, the intraocular pressure was not different between the groups.

The results of this study showed that BVZ + 5-Fu had a better antiscarring effect, whereas the effect of a single drug was similar to that in the control group. The use of BVZ in combination with antimetabolic drug 5-Fu reduced the VEGF level significantly, which not only inhibited both early and late stages of scar formation but also enhanced the potential anti-inflammatory effects. Therefore, BVZ and 5-Fu might work synergistically [24] and the antiscarring effect was greater than that of the use of the single drug. However, it should be clearly understood that experimental study or clinical outcomes in animal studies may not predict outcomes in human clinical use (such as the CAT-152 trials [55]).

The shortcoming of this study was the lack of the measurement of intraocular pressure. However, the reduction of subconjunctival scars should have a positive effect on the function of filtering blebs.

Since Tenon's fibroblast cells are important mediators in the formation of filtering blebs scar after GFS [48], further studies should include observing the cytotoxicity of combined drugs on human Tenon's fibroblasts (HTF) and the effect of combined drugs on the migration of HTF.

In the present study, the mRNA expression levels on the two fibrotic markers in the BVZ + 5-Fu and BVZ + MMC groups were significantly reduced in the first month, but increased by varying degrees in the second month. This finding suggested that a subsequent study could repeat the BVZ injection in the second month to verify whether it could persistently inhibit the formation of type 1 collagen fibers and fibrin and prolong the survival of filtering blebs [45].

The general and local effects of the subconjunctival injection of BVZ should be further considered. A pharmacokinetic study showed that both subconjunctival and intravitreal injections of BVZ could achieve effective intraocular concentration [21]. Wang and Harasymowycz [56] reported that 3 of 28 patients who received a subconjunctival injection of BVZ during GFS had retinal vein branch occlusion. The combined results of clinical trials showed that patients receiving high doses of RBZ (e.g., 0.5 mg) had a higher incidence of stroke compared with patients receiving a low dose (e.g., 0.3 mg) of intravitreal injection [57]. The safety of anti-VEGF antibodies, including the potential side effects on the eye and entire body, must be more clearly defined.

5. Conclusion

The experimental results showed that a single subconjunctival injection of BVZ combined with 5-Fu in experimental GFS has a better antiscarring effect compared with a single drug. BVZ + 5-Fu could significantly prolong the survival time of the filtering bleb with lower cytotoxicity. However, no significant difference was observed between the MMC + BVZ and single MMC groups. The present study provided a more comprehensive reference for clinical improvement in GFS prognosis. The subsequent studies should focus on establishing the mode and frequency of administration of BVZ + 5-Fu and also on further investigating the mechanism of action of BVZ + 5-Fu.

Conflicts of Interest

The authors declare that there are no conflicts of interest regarding the publication of this manuscript.

Acknowledgments

This study was supported by the Key Project Funds for Scientific Research of the Shanghai Municipal Committee of Health and Family Planning (Grant no. 201640027).

References

[1] J. Burr, A. Azuara-Blanco, and A. Avenell, "Medical versus surgical interventions for open angle glaucoma," *Cochrane Database of Systematic Reviews*, vol. 18, no. 2, article CD004399, 2005.

[2] R. Hitchings, "Initial treatment for open-angle glaucoma-medical, laser, or surgical? Surgery is the treatment of choice for open-angle glaucoma," *Archives of Ophthalmology*, vol. 116, no. 2, pp. 241-242, 1998.

[3] G. L. Skuta and R. K. Parrish II, "Wound healing in glaucoma filtering surgery," *Survey of Ophthalmology*, vol. 32, no. 3, pp. 149-170, 1987.

[4] G. L. Skuta, C. C. Beeson, E. J. Higginbotham et al., "Intraoperative mitomycin versus postoperative 5-fluorouracil in high-risk glaucoma filtering surgery," *Ophthalmology*, vol. 99, no. 3, pp. 438-444, 1992.

[5] S. Smith, P. A. D'Amore, and E. B. Dreyer, "Comparative toxicity of mitomycin C and 5-fluorouracil in vitro," *American Journal of Ophthalmology*, vol. 118, no. 3, pp. 332-337, 1994.

[6] K. Schwartz and D. Budenz, "Current management of glaucoma," *Current Opinion in Ophthalmology*, vol. 15, no. 2, pp. 119-126, 2004.

[7] P. Carmeliet, V. Ferreira, G. Breier et al., "Abnormal blood vessel development and lethality in embryos lacking a single VEGF allele," *Nature*, vol. 380, no. 6573, pp. 435-439, 1996.

[8] T. E. 1 Fitzpatrick, G. E. Lash, A. Yanaihara et al., "Inhibition of breast carcinoma and trophoblast cell invasiveness by vascular endothelial growth factor," *Experimental Cell Research*, vol. 283, no. 2, pp. 247-255, 2003.

[9] M. Kowanetz and N. Ferrara, "Vascular endothelial growth factor signaling pathways: therapeutic perspective," *Clinical Cancer Research*, vol. 12, no. 17, pp. 5018-5022, 2006.

[10] A. Kakehashi, S. Inoda, C. Mameuda et al., "Relationship among VEGF, VEGF receptor, AGEs, and macrophages in proliferative diabetic retinopathy," *Diabetes Research and Clinical Practice*, vol. 79, no. 3, pp. 438-445, 2008.

[11] R. C. Tripathi, J. Li, B. Tripathi et al., "Increased level of vascular endothelial growth factor in aqueous humor of patients with neovascular glaucoma," *Ophthalmology*, vol. 105, no. 2, pp. 232-237, 1998.

[12] S. A. Vinores, C. C. Chan, M. A. Vinores et al., "Increased vascular endothelial growth factor (VEGF) and transforming growth factor beta (TGFbeta) in experimental autoimmune uveoretinitis: upregulation of VEGF without neovascularization," *Journal of Neuroimmunology*, vol. 89, no. 12, pp. 43-50, 1998.

[13] R. N. Frank, "Growth factors in age-related macular degeneration: pathogenic and therapeutic implications," *Ophthalmic Research*, vol. 29, no. 5, pp. 341-353, 1997.

[14] M. Murakami, S. Iwai, S Hiratsuka et al., "Signaling of vascular endothelial growth factor receptor-1 tyrosine kinase promotes rheumatoid arthritis through activation of monocytes/macrophages," *Blood*, vol. 108, no. 6, pp. 1849-1856, 2006.

[15] D. Beddy, R. W. Watson, J. M. Fitzpatrick et al., "Increased vascular endothelial growth factor production in fibroblasts isolated from strictures in patients with Crohn's disease," *British Journal of Surgery*, vol. 91, no. 1, pp. 72-77, 2004.

[16] L. G. Presta, H. Chen, S. J. O'Connor et al., "Humanization of an anti-vascular endothelial growth factor monoclonal antibody for the therapy of solid tumors and other disorders," *Cancer Research*, vol. 57, no. 20, pp. 4593-4599, 1997.

[17] H. Hurwitz, L. Fehrenbacher, W. Novotny et al., "Bevacizumab plus irinotecan, fluorouracil, and leucovorin for metastatic colorectal cancer," *New England Journal of Medicine*, vol. 350, no. 23, pp. 2335-2342, 2004.

[18] Z. Li, T. Van Bergen, S. Van de Veire et al., "Inhibition of vascular endothelial growth factor reduces scar formation after glaucoma filtration surgery," *Investigative Opthalmology and Visual Science*, vol. 50, no. 11, pp. 5217-5225, 2009.

[19] J. B. Jonas, U. H. Spandau, and F. Schlichtenbrede, "Intravitreal bevacizumab for filtering surgery," *Ophthalmic Research*, vol. 39, no. 2, pp. 121-122, 2007.

[20] N. Nilforushan, M. Yadgari, S. K. Kish et al., "Subconjunctival bevacizumab versus mitomycin C adjunctive to trabeculectomy," *American Journal of Ophthalmology*, vol. 153, no. 2, pp. 352-357, 2012.

[21] H. Nomoto, F. Shiraga, N. Kuno et al., "Pharmacokinetics of bevacizumab after topical, subconjunctival, and intravitreal administration in rabbits," *Investigative Opthalmology and Visual Science*, vol. 50, no. 10, pp. 4807–4813, 2009.

[22] M. Y. Kahook, J. S. Schuman, and R. J. Noecker, "Intravitreal bevacizumab in a patient with neovascular glaucoma," *Ophthalmic Surgery, Lasers, and Imaging*, vol. 37, no. 2, pp. 144–146, 2006.

[23] D. S. Grewal, R. Jain, H. Kumar et al., "Evaluation of subconjunctival bevacizumab as an adjunct to trabeculectomy: a pilot study," *Ophthalmology*, vol. 115, no. 12, pp. 2141–2145, 2008.

[24] A. How, J. L. L. Chua, A. Charlton et al., "Combined treatment with bevacizumab and 5-fluorouracil attenuates the postoperative scarring response after experimental glaucoma filtration surgery," *Investigative Opthalmology and Visual Science*, vol. 51, pp. 928–932, 2010.

[25] R A. Ignacio, V. Sandra Clarissa, R. Ricardo et al., "The PLGA implant as an antimitotic delivery system after experimental trabeculectomy," *Investigative Opthalmology and Visual Science*, vol. 54, no. 8, pp. 5227–5235, 2013.

[26] M. S. Spitzer, B. Wallenfels-Thilo, A. Sierra et al., "Antiproliferative and cytotoxic properties of bevacizumab on different ocular cells," *British Journal of Ophthalmology*, vol. 90, pp. 1316–1321, 2006.

[27] L. Cao, H. Liu, D. S. Lam et al., "In vitro screening for angiostatic potential of herbal chemicals," *Investigative Opthalmology and Visual Science*, vol. 51, no. 12, pp. 6658–6664, 2010.

[28] J. Tong, D. Lam, W. Chan et al., "Effects of triamcinolone on the expression of VEGF and PEDF in human retinal pigment epithelial and human umbilical vein endothelial cells," *Molecular Vision*, vol. 12, pp. 1490–1495, 2006.

[29] K. Steindl-Kuscher, W. Krugluger, M. E. Boulton et al., "Activation of the β-catenin signaling pathway and its impact on RPE cell cycle," *Investigative Opthalmology and Visual Science*, vol. 50, pp. 4471–4476, 2009.

[30] Y. Bai, W. Yu, N. Han et al., "Effects of semaphorin 3A on retinal pigment epithelial cell activity," *Investigative Opthalmology and Visual Science*, vol. 54, no. 10, pp. 6628–6637, 2013.

[31] A. Wang, N. X. Landén, F. Meisgen et al., "MicroRNA-31 is overexpressed in cutaneous squamous cell carcinoma and regulates cell motility and colony formation ability of tumor cells," *PLoS One*, vol. 9, no. 7, Article ID e103206, 2014.

[32] H. Zhong, G. Sun, X. Lin et al., "Evaluation of pirfenidone as a new postoperative antiscarring agent in experimental glaucoma surgery," *Investigative Opthalmology and Visual Science*, vol. 52, no. 6, pp. 3136–3142, 2011.

[33] M. F. Cordeiro, P. H. Constable, R. A. Alexander et al., "Effect of varying the mitomycin-C treatment area in glaucoma filtration surgery in the rabbit," *Investigative Opthalmology and Visual Science*, vol. 38, no. 8, pp. 1639–1646, 1997.

[34] T. T. I. Wong, A. L. Mead, and P. T. Khaw, "Prolonged antiscarring effects of ilomastat and MMC after experimental glaucoma filtration surgery," *Investigative Opthalmology and Visual Science*, vol. 46, pp. 2018–2022, 2005.

[35] A. P. Wells, J. G. Crowston, J. Marks et al., "A pilot study of a system for grading of drainage blebs after glaucoma surgery," *Journal of Glaucoma*, vol. 13, no. 6, pp. 454–460, 2004.

[36] Z. Yan, Y. Bai, Z. Tian et al., "Anti-proliferation effects of Sirolimus sustained delivery film in rabbit glaucoma filtration surgery," *Molecular Vision*, vol. 17, pp. 2495–2506, 2011.

[37] E. M. Addicks, H. A. Quigley, W. R. Green et al., "Histologic characteristics of filtering blebs in glaucomatous eyes," *Archives of Ophthalmology*, vol. 101, no. 5, pp. 795–798, 1983.

[38] L. K. Seibold, M. B. Sherwood, and M. Y. Kahook, "Wound modulation after filtration surgery," *Survey of Ophthalmology*, vol. 57, no. 6, pp. 530–550, 2012.

[39] P. Bao, A. Kodra, M. Tomic-Canic et al., "The role of vascular endothelial growth factor in wound healing," *Journal of Surgical Research*, vol. 153, no. 2, pp. 347–358, 2009.

[40] T. H. Adair and J. P. Montani, "Angiogenesis," *Colloquium Series on Integrated Systems Physiology: From Molecule to Function*, vol. 2, no. 1, pp. 1–84, 2010.

[41] D. T. Azar, "Corneal angiogenic privilege: angiogenic and antiangiogenic factors in corneal avascularity, vasculogenesis, and wound healing (an American Ophthalmological Society thesis)," *Transactions of the American Ophthalmological Society*, vol. 104, pp. 264–302, 2006.

[42] W. W. Li, K. E. Talcott, A. W. Zhai et al., "The role of therapeutic angiogenesis in tissue repair and regeneration," *Advances in Skin and Wound Care*, vol. 18, no. 9, pp. 491–500, 2005.

[43] L. F. Seet, S. N. Finger, S. W. Chu et al., "Novel insight into the inflammatory and cellular responses following experimental glaucoma surgery: a roadmap for inhibiting fibrosis," *Current Molecular Medicine*, vol. 13, no. 6, pp. 911–928, 2013.

[44] T. A. Wilgus, A. M. Ferreira, T. M. Oberyszyn et al., "Regulation of scar formation by vascular endothelial growth factor," *Laboratory Investigation*, vol. 88, no. 6, pp. 579–590, 2008.

[45] M. Kim, C. Lee, R. Payne et al., "Angiogenesis in glaucoma filtration surgery and neovascular glaucoma: a review," *Survey of Ophthalmology*, vol. 60, no. 6, pp. 524–535, 2015.

[46] I. Kim, A. M. Ryan, R. Rohan et al., "Constitutive expression of VEGF, VEGFR-1, and VEGFR-2 in normal eyes," *Investigative Opthalmology and Visual Science*, vol. 40, pp. 2115–2121, 1999.

[47] P. A. Campochiaro and First ARVO/Pfizer Institute Working Group, "Ocular versus extraocular neovascularization: mirror images or vague resemblances," *Investigative Opthalmology and Visual Science*, vol. 47, no. 2, p. 462, 2006.

[48] P. J. Lama and R. D. Fechtner, "Antifibrotic and wound healing in glaucoma surgery," *Survey of Ophthalmology*, vol. 48, no. 3, pp. 314–346, 2003.

[49] E. C. O'Neill, Q. Qin, N. J. Van Bergen et al., "Antifibrotic activity of bevacizumab on human Tenon's fibroblasts in vitro," *Investigative Opthalmology and Visual Science*, vol. 51, no. 12, pp. 6524–6532, 2010.

[50] A. F. Karamysheva, "Mechanisms of angiogenesis," *Biochemistry*, vol. 73, no. 7, pp. 751–762, 2008.

[51] E. Vandewalle, L. Abegao Pinto, T. Van Bergen et al., "Intracameral bevacizumab as an adjunct to trabeculectomy: a 1-year prospective, randomised study," *British Journal of Ophthalmology*, vol. 98, no. 1, pp. 73–78, 2014.

[52] W. Suh and C. Kee, "The effect of bevacizumab on the outcome of trabeculectomy with 5-Fluorouracil," *Journal of Ocular Pharmacology and Therapeutics*, vol. 29, no. 7, pp. 646–651, 2013.

[53] B. E. Chua, D. Q. Nguyen, Q. Qin et al., "Bleb vascularity following post-trabeculectomy subconjunctival bevacizumab: a pilot study," *Clinical and Experimental Ophthalmology*, vol. 40, no. 8, pp. 773–779, 2012.

[54] M. Y. Kahook, "Bleb morphology and vascularity after trabeculectomy with intravitreal ranibizumab: a pilot study,"

American Journal of Ophthalmology, vol. 150, no. 3, pp. 399–403, 2010.

[55] F. Grehn, G. Hollo, CAT-152 Trabeculectomy Study Group et al., "Factors affecting the outcome of trabeculectomy: an analysis based on combined data from two phase III studies of an antibody to transforming growth factor beta2, CAT-152," *Ophthalmology*, vol. 114, no. 10, pp. 1831–1838, 2007.

[56] J. Wang and P. Harasymowycz, "Subconjunctival bevacizumab injection in glaucoma filtering surgery: a case control series," *ISRN Ophthalmology*, vol. 2013, pp. 1–6, 2013.

[57] N. M. Bressler, D. S. Boyer, D. F. Williams et al., "Cerebrovascular accidents in patients treated for choroidal neovascularization with ranibizumab in randomized controlled trials," *Retina*, vol. 32, no. 9, pp. 1821–1828, 2012.

19

Short-Term Clinical Results of Ab Interno Trabeculotomy using the Trabectome with or without Cataract Surgery for Open-Angle Glaucoma Patients of High Intraocular Pressure

Handan Akil,[1,2] Vikas Chopra,[1,2] Alex S. Huang,[1,2] Ramya Swamy,[1,2] and Brian A. Francis[1,2]

[1]Doheny Image Reading Center, Doheny Eye Institute, Los Angeles, CA, USA
[2]Department of Ophthalmology, David Geffen School of Medicine, Los Angeles, CA, USA

Correspondence should be addressed to Brian A. Francis; bfrancis@doheny.org

Academic Editor: Chelvin Sng

Purpose. To assess the safety and efficacy of Trabectome procedure in patients with preoperative intraocular pressure (IOP) of 30 mmHg or higher. *Methods.* All patients who had underwent Trabectome stand-alone or Trabectome combined with phacoemulsification were included. Survival analysis was performed by using Kaplan-Meier, and success was defined as IOP ≤ 21 mmHg, 20% or more IOP reduction from baseline for any two consecutive visits after 3 months, and no secondary glaucoma surgery. *Results.* A total of 49 cases were included with an average age of 66 (range: 13–91). 28 cases had Trabectome stand-alone and 21 cases had Trabectome combined with phacoemulsification. Mean IOP was reduced from a baseline of 35.6 ± 6.3 mmHg to 16.8 ± 3.8 mmHg at 12 months ($p < 0.01^*$), while the number of medications was reduced from 3.1 ± 1.3 to 1.8 ± 1.4 ($p < 0.01^*$). Survival rate at 12 months was 80%. 9 cases required secondary glaucoma surgery, and 1 case was reported with hypotony at day one, but resolved within one week. *Conclusion.* Trabectome seems to be safe and effective in patients with preoperative IOP of 30 mmHg or greater. Even in this cohort with high preoperative IOP, the end result is a mean IOP in the physiologic range.

1. Introduction

Glaucoma is a progressive disease which causes irreversible damage to the optic nerve [1]. The main goal of treatment is to lower intraocular pressure (IOP) to a level which is safe for the optic nerve head. Although trabeculectomy or episcleral aqueous drainage implants demonstrated a permanent IOP reduction, they may have a high risk profile regarding the intraoperative and postoperative complications [2]. This has influenced the development of a less invasive surgical technique, trabeculotomy by internal approach with the Trabectome (NeoMedix Corp., Tustin, CA), which works on the trabecular meshwork and inner wall of Schlemm's canal to reduce

outflow resistance [3, 4]. This surgical approach provides a postoperatively stable eye without damaging the conjunctiva and can be further combined with cataract surgery easily with low incidence of intraoperative and postoperative complications.

Results of Trabectome in various types of open-angle glaucoma patients with preoperative IOP of less than 30 mmHg have been shown to be favorable with fewer rates of complication compared to those of traditional trabeculectomy, giving the surgeons hope of an effective and safe treatment option for patients with higher preoperative IOPs [2–4].

The study was conducted to report the success rate of ab interno trabeculotomy within a single-surgeon, single-

TABLE 1: Demographics and descriptive statistics of all the patients with IOP ≥ 30 mmHg.

	$n = 49$
Age	
Mean ± SD	66 ± 18
Range	18–91
Gender	
Female	19 (39%)
Male	30 (61%)
Race	
African American	2 (4%)
Asian	5 (10%)
Caucasian	31 (63%)
Hispanics	7 (14%)
Others	4 (8%)
Diagnosis	
POAG	24 (49%)
Pseudoexfoliation glaucoma	12 (24%)
ACG	2 (4%)
Pigment dispersion	5 (10%)
Ocular hypertension	2 (4%)
Secondary glaucoma	2 (4%)
Others	2 (4%)
Preop Snellen acuity	
20/20–20/40	22 (45%)
20/50–20/70	9 (18%)
20/80–20/100	4 (8%)
20/200–20/400	8 (16%)
<20/400	1 (2%)
NR	5 (10%)
VF	
Mild	4 (8%)
Moderate	12 (24%)
Advanced	3 (6%)
MD/others	30 (61%)
Disc C/D	
<0.7	13 (27%)
0.7 to 0.8	17 (35%)
>0.8	11 (22%)
NR	8 (16%)
Lens status	
Phakic	39 (80%)
Pseudophakic	8 (16%)
Aphakic	0 (0%)
NR	2 (4%)
Shaffer grade	
I	0 (0%)
II	2 (4%)
III	11 (22%)
IV	5 (10%)
NR	31 (63%)

TABLE 1: Continued.

	$n = 49$
Prior surgeries	
SLT	17 (35%)
ALT	4 (8%)
Trabeculectomy	1 (2%)
Trabectome	2 (4%)
YAG	1 (2%)
Combined surgeries	
Trabectome + Phaco	21 (43%)
Trabectome only	28 (57%)

center cohort of patients with a preoperative IOP of 30 mmHg or higher.

2. Patient and Methods

This is a nonrandomized prospective analysis of patients treated by a single experienced surgeon (BAF). The study followed the tenets of the Declaration of Helsinki and the Health Insurance Portability and Accountability Act and had the Institutional Review Board approval. Cohort comparison was studied between patients with open-angle glaucoma-receiving Trabectome combined with phacoemulsification cataract extraction and intraocular lens (IOL) and patients receiving Trabectome alone.

The inclusion criteria for both the combined Trabectome group and Trabectome-alone group were as follows: open-angle glaucoma (as defined by glaucomatous optic nerve appearance with or without glaucomatous visual field damage)—an unobstructed view of the angle, age greater than or equal to 18, a visually significant cataract, and follow-up of at least 2 years. The severity of visual fields was graded according to the Hodapp-Anderson-Parrish (HAP) classification and visual field index (VFI) score [5]. Exclusion criteria were as follows: angle closure, uveitic or neovascular glaucoma, previous glaucoma surgery, and no clear view of the nasal angle.

A total number of 49 eyes of 49 patients were included in the study. Twenty-one eyes underwent combined Trabectome surgery and 28 eyes underwent Trabectome-alone surgery. In each group, patient demographics, preoperative cup-to-disc ratio, preoperative and postoperative visual acuity, IOP, and medications were recorded. Postoperative data at day one and months 1, 3, 6, and 12 were collected.

The surgical procedure has been described in detail elsewhere [2–4]. Briefly, the surgery was performed with the Trabectome® system, including the single-use handpiece with an irrigation-aspiration (I/A) system (Neomedix Inc., Tustin, USA). In combined surgery, the Trabectome surgery was performed prior to phacoemulsification. The head and microscope were tilted to give a gonioscopic view of the angle. The goniosurgical lens (a modified Swann-Jacobs lens)

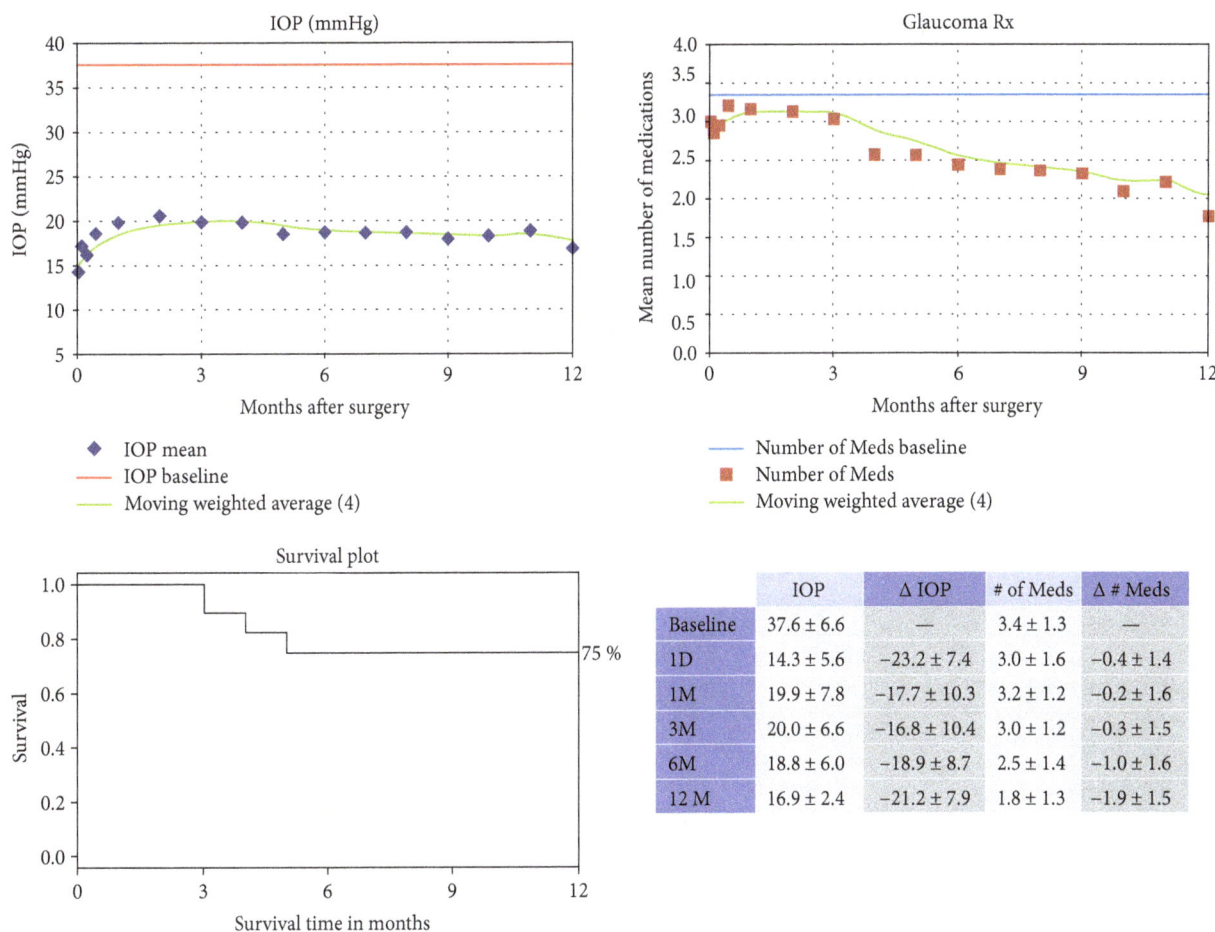

FIGURE 1: Intraocular pressure (IOP) and number of glaucoma medications data with survival rate over time from all the eyes with IOP > 30 mmHg and having undergone Trabectome surgery with or without cataract extraction. Kaplan-Meier survival curve of the success of the procedure defined as decrease in IOP of 20% or more or a decrease in glaucoma medications with no need for additional medications or glaucoma procedures.

was placed on the cornea to visualize the angle structures. A 1.7 mm keratome was used to create a temporal corneal incision. An ophthalmic viscosurgical device (OVD) was injected to form the anterior chamber. The Trabectome handpiece was inserted and advanced along the meshwork, ablating and removing between 90 and 150 degrees of the nasal trabecular meshwork and inner wall of Schlemm's canal. The power was adjusted up or down depending on the desire to ablate a wider strip of trabecular meshwork or to minimize burning of tissue, respectively. Irrigation and aspiration were then used to remove any remaining blood, viscoelastic, or cellular material.

Postoperative care is varied according to clinical presentation but routinely includes topical steroids four times per day tapered over 8 weeks, topical antibiotics four times per day for 7 days, and pilocarpine 1% three to four times per day tapering over two to eight weeks. Typically, the patients were advised to continue preoperative glaucoma medications after surgery if needed.

The estimated cumulative success rate was obtained by Kaplan-Meier life-table analyses using the following criteria: Kaplan-Meier survival curve of the success of the procedure

defined as a decrease in IOP of 20% or more or a decrease in glaucoma medications with no need for additional medications or glaucoma procedures.

3. Statistical Analysis

One-way repeated-measures analysis of variance (ANOVA) test was used for the baseline and postoperative values for each group. The difference in IOP and number of antiglaucoma medications between groups were assessed by an unpaired t-test. Pearson's χ^2 test was used for subgroup comparison of sex and lens status before surgery. We estimated the cumulative percentages of success as well as the failure rates over time with the Kaplan-Meier method. Statistical significance was assumed for $p \leq 0.05$.

4. Results

Demographic data and descriptive statistics of 49 cases were included into the study (Table 1). The mean age of the study population was 66 ± 18 and 39% were females. The proportion of Caucasians was higher (63%) and the proportion of

TABLE 2: Demographics and descriptive statistics of the patients with IOP ≥ 30 mmHg and having undergone combined Trabectome surgery.

	$n = 21$
Age	
Mean ± SD	72 ± 17
Range	23–88
Gender	
Female	12 (57%)
Male	9 (43%)
Race	
African American	1 (5%)
Asian	3 (14%)
Caucasian	12 (57%)
Hispanics	5 (24%)
Diagnosis	
POAG	6 (29%)
Pseudoexfoliation glaucoma	9 (43%)
ACG	2 (10%)
Ocular hypertension	1 (5%)
Secondary glaucoma	1 (5%)
Others	2 (10%)
Preop Snellen acuity	
20/20–20/40	5 (24%)
20/50–20/70	6 (29%)
20/80–20/100	3 (14%)
20/200–20/400	6 (29%)
<20/400	0 (0%)
NR	1 (5%)
VF	
Mild	1 (5%)
Moderate	4 (19%)
Advanced	0 (0%)
MD/others	16 (76%)
Disc C/D	
<0.7	5 (24%)
0.7 to 0.8	9 (43%)
>0.8	5 (24%)
NR	2 (10%)
Lens status	
Phakic	20 (95%)
Pseudophakic	0 (0%)
Aphakic	0 (0%)
NR	1 (5%)
Shaffer grade	
I	0 (0%)
II	1 (5%)
III	4 (19%)
IV	1 (5%)
NR	15 (71%)

TABLE 2: Continued.

	$n = 21$
Prior surgeries	
SLT	9 (43%)
ALT	1 (5%)
Trabeculectomy	1 (5%)

African American patients was lower (4%) in the study group. The mean preoperative IOP was 35.6 ± 6.3 mmHg. By postoperative month 12, the average IOP was 16.8 ± 3.8 (55.3% decrease) ($p < 0.01$). The average number of glaucoma medication use was significantly decreased from 3.1 ± 1.3 to 1.8 ± 1.3 at month 12 ($p < 0.01$). Primary open-angle glaucoma (POAG) was the major diagnosis (49%) in the study group and it was followed by pseudoexfoliation glaucoma (24%). Nine patients (18%) needed secondary surgery one year after the surgery and 1 case was reported with hypotony at postoperative 1st day but resolved within one week. The overall survival rate was 80% by postoperative month 12. Figure 1 shows the IOP and glaucoma medication trend with the survival rate of the procedure during the postoperative follow-up.

Twenty-eight cases had Trabectome-alone surgery and 21 cases had combined Trabectome phacoemulsification surgery. There were some statistically significant differences found between the two groups. The preoperative IOP was significantly lower in the combined Trabectome group (33.0 ± 4.9 mmHg) compared to that in the Trabectome-alone group (37.6 ± 6.6 mmHg) ($p = 0.01$). The Trabectome only group had a better preoperative visual acuity, which reflects the presence of the cataract in the combined Trabectome group. The mean age of the combined Trabectome group was 72 ± 17 and 57% were female. However, the mean age of the Trabectome-alone group was 62 ± 18 and 75% were male ($p = 0.06$). The study reported a higher proportion of Caucasians and lower proportion of Asian patients in both groups. The Trabectome-alone group showed a higher proportion of severe visual field defects compared to the combined Trabectome group. Tables 2 and 3 give the demographic data of each group.

5. Combined Trabectome Group

The mean preoperative IOP was 33.0 ± 4.9 mmHg (Figure 2) and by postoperative month 1, it has dropped to 18.5 ± 6.4 (44.2% decrease). By postoperative month 12, the average IOP was even lower at 16.6 ± 4.8 (51.8% decrease) ($p < 0.01$). Figure 2 shows the IOP and glaucoma medication trend with the survival rate during the postoperative follow-up. The average number of glaucoma medications use in the group was 2.7 ± 1.1. By postoperative month 12, it has significantly decreased to 1.8 ± 1.5 ($p < 0.01$). Survival rate at 12 months of follow-up was 86%. One eye (5%) needed secondary surgery to control IOP one year after the surgery. Hypotony, aqueous misdirection, wound leak, and postoperative infection were not reported in any of the patients. There was no clinically significant bleeding which may require intervention.

TABLE 3: Demographics and descriptive statistics of the patients with IOP $\geq$ 30 mmHg and having undergone Trabectome-alone surgery.

	$n = 28$
Age	
Mean $\pm$ SD	62 ± 18
Range	30–91
Gender	
Female	7 (25%)
Male	21 (75%)
Race	
African American	1 (4%)
Asian	2 (7%)
Caucasian	19 (68%)
Hispanics	2 (7%)
Other	4 (14%)
Diagnosis	
POAG	18 (64%)
Pseudoexfoliation glaucoma	3 (11%)
Pigment dispersion	5 (18%)
Ocular hypertension	1 (4%)
Secondary glaucoma	1 (4%)
Preop Snellen acuity	
20/20–20/40	17 (61%)
20/50–20/70	3 (11%)
20/80–20/100	1 (4%)
20/200–20/400	2 (7%)
<20/400	1 (4%)
NR	4 (14%)
VF	
Mild	3 (11%)
Moderate	8 (29%)
Advanced	3 (11%)
MD/others	14 (50%)
Disc C/D	
<0.7	8 (29%)
0.7 to 0.8	8 (29%)
>0.8	6 (21%)
NR	6 (21%)
Lens status	
Phakic	19 (68%)
Pseudophakic	8 (29%)
NR	1 (4%)
Shaffer grade	
I	0 (0%)
II	1 (4%)
III	7 (25%)
IV	4 (14%)
NR	16 (57%)

TABLE 3: Continued.

	$n = 28$
Prior surgeries	
SLT	8 (29%)
ALT	3 (11%)
Trabectome	2 (7%)
YAG	1 (4%)

6. Trabectome-Alone Group

The mean preoperative IOP was 37.6 ± 6.6 mmHg (Figure 3) and on postoperative day 1, it has decreased to 14.3 ± 5.6 mmHg (61.7% decrease). But by postoperative month 1, IOP increased to 19.9 ± 7.8 (47.1% decrease). By postoperative month 12, the IOP was stable at 16.9 ± 2.4 (56.9% decrease). The average number of glaucoma medications used in the group was 3.4 ± 1.3. By postoperative month 12, it has significantly decreased to 1.8 ± 1.3 ($p < 0.01$). Figure 3 shows the IOP and glaucoma medication trend with the survival rate during the postoperative follow-up. Eight cases required secondary surgery. Hypotony (IOP < 5 mmHg) at postoperative day one was observed in one patient (4%) and resolved later.

7. Discussion

The Trabectome seems to be a favorable method of minimal invasive glaucoma surgery with or without cataract surgery in patients with preoperative IOP of 30 mmHg or greater. The current data also suggests the effectiveness of Trabectome-alone surgery in reducing IOP and postoperative number of medications compared to combined Trabectome surgery.

The baseline IOP in our study was 33.0 ± 4.9 mmHg in the combined Trabectome group and 37.6 ± 6.6 in the Trabectome-alone group which is higher than the values in the studies by Francis [3] (22 mmHg). Minckler et al. [4] (25.7 mmHg), Jea et al. [6] (28.1 mmHg), or Trabectome-alone surgery significantly reduced the postoperative IOP in our study patients as well as combined Trabectome surgery. The IOPs at 1 year after surgery were significantly reduced from baseline to mid teens (16.9 ± 2.4 mmHg and 16.6 ± 4.8 mmHg, resp.) which is similar to those previously reported [2–6]. These results suggest that Trabectome surgery with or without cataract extraction may offer a clinically useful control on IOP levels. Some studies reported IOPs as 16.1 mmHg [4], 17.4 mmHg [6], and 16.6 mmHg [7] after 1 year of Trabectome surgery. Moreover, in this study, the number of medications were significantly reduced after both surgeries similar to other studies [3, 4, 8]. The success rate after Trabectome surgery has been reported to be about 30%–50% in the literature [2–4, 6–8]. In our study, the success rate for IOP decrease was 55% in the overall study population, 51.8% in the combined group, and 56.8% in the Trabectome-alone group. Mizoguchi et al. [9] reported that their Trabectome failure rate was higher in the eyes with a preoperative IOP <18 mmHg and lower in those with a preoperative IOP of 18–22 mmHg, and they concluded that the

IOP (mmHg)

- ◆ IOP mean
- — IOP baseline
- — Moving weighted average (4)

Glaucoma Rx

- — Number of Meds baseline
- ■ Number of Meds
- — Moving weighted average (4)

Survival plot

75 %

	IOP	Δ IOP	# of Meds	Δ # Meds
Baseline	33.0 ± 4.9	—	2.7 ± 1.1	—
1D	19.7 ± 10.0	−13.4 ± 9.6	2.0 ± 1.2	−0.8 ± 1.5
1M	18.5 ± 6.4	−14.6 ± 8.0	2.4 ± 1.6	−0.3 ± 1.4
3M	15.1 ± 4.5	−18.1 ± 7.6	2.2 ± 1.3	−0.4 ± 1.0
6M	18.1 ± 6.5	−15.1 ± 9.0	1.8 ± 1.2	−0.8 ± 1.2
12 M	16.6 ± 4.8	−17.1 ± 7.7	1.8 ± 1.5	−1.0 ± 1.7

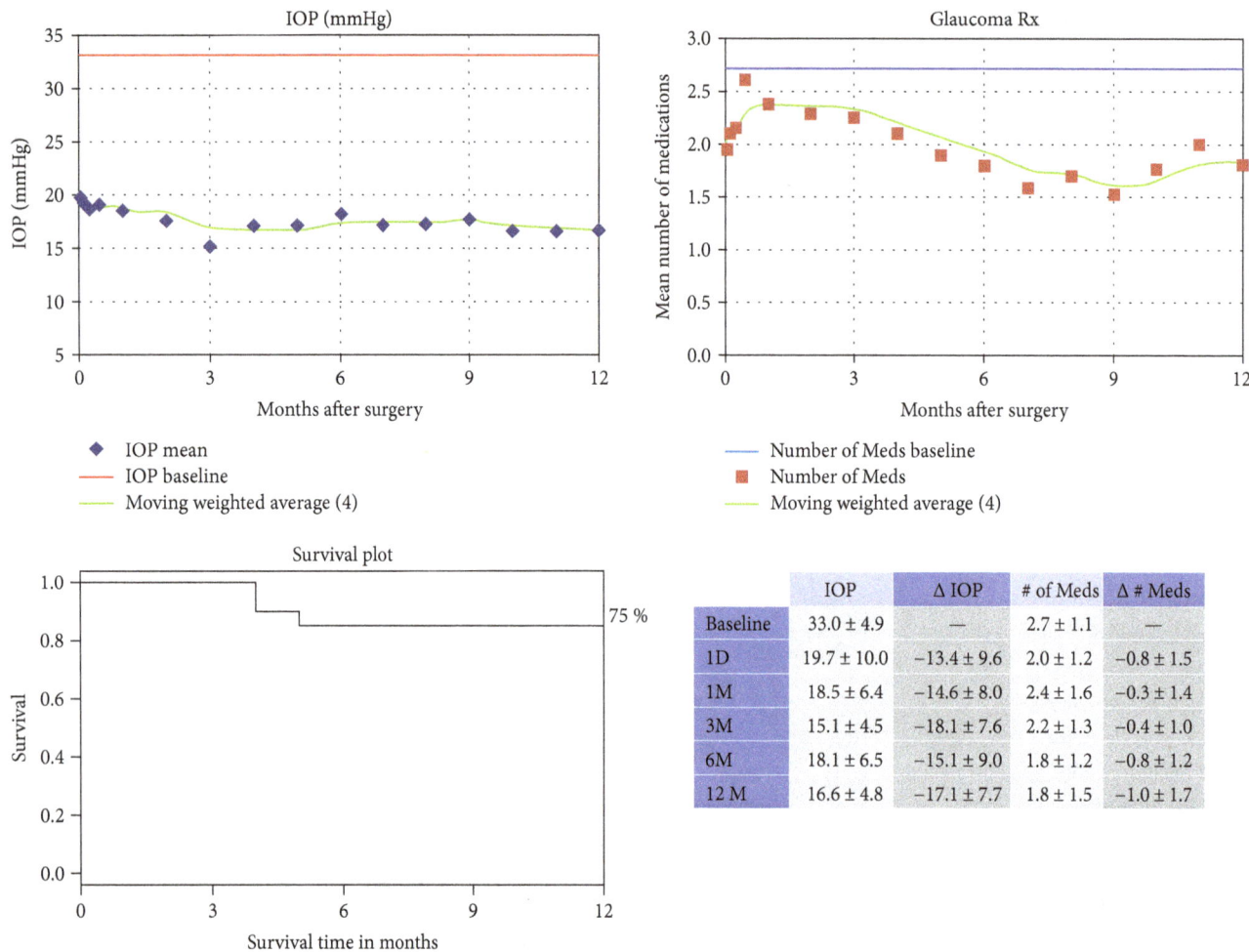

FIGURE 2: Intraocular pressure (IOP) and number of glaucoma medications data with survival rate over time from the eyes with IOP > 30 mmHg and having undergone combined Trabectome surgery. Kaplan-Meier survival curve of the success of the procedure defined as decrease in IOP of 20% or more or a decrease in glaucoma medications with no need for additional medications or glaucoma procedures.

results of Trabectome surgery may differ according to baseline IOP. Although the relationship of the surgical success and preoperative IOP level has not been established yet, our study showed that Trabectome surgery can be effective and safe at baseline IOP levels around 35.6 (±6.3) mmHg. Markedly high and low baseline IOPs have been reported as risk factors for poor surgical outcomes [6, 7].

The current study had a control group of glaucoma patients having Trabectome surgery alone; therefore, it was possible to determine to what extent Trabectome trabeculotomy or cataract extraction contributed to the lowering of IOP and medications. The IOP was lowered by 17.7 ± 7.7 mmHg (51.8% decrease) in the combined Trabectome group and 21.2 ± 7.9 mmHg (56.9% decrease) in the Trabectome-alone group by postoperative month 12. It has been generally suggested that phacoemulsification cataract extraction alone may lower IOP in glaucoma patients as well as in nonglaucomatous individuals, with the amount of 2–4 mmHg [10, 11]. Our study showed that there is a decrease to the normal physiologic level in IOP after a Trabectome procedure. Although a higher proportion of IOP decrease was reported

in the Trabectome-alone group, it may be caused by higher baseline IOP levels compared to that in the combined Trabectome group.

In a prospective interventional study [12], patients with open-angle glaucoma underwent combined Trabectome surgery. Mean preoperative IOP was 20.0 ± 6.3 mmHg, and mean postoperative IOP was 15.5 ± 2.9 mmHg, with a 1.4 ± 1.3 mean number of glaucoma medications after one year of follow-up. Nine patients needed additional glaucoma procedures.

Another study with a large number of case series evaluated the outcomes of Trabectome-alone versus combined procedures with phacoemulsification [4]. At 24 months, IOP decreased by 40% from 25.7 ± 7.7 mmHg preoperatively to 16.6 ± 4.0 mmHg in the Trabectome-alone group compared to 30% from 20.0 ± 6.2 mmHg to 14.9 ± 3.1 mmHg in the combined Trabectome group. Mean number of medications decreased from 2.9 to 1.2 in the Trabectome group and from 2.6 to 1.5 in the combined group. A total of 14% of patients were considered failure cases from the Trabectome-alone group.

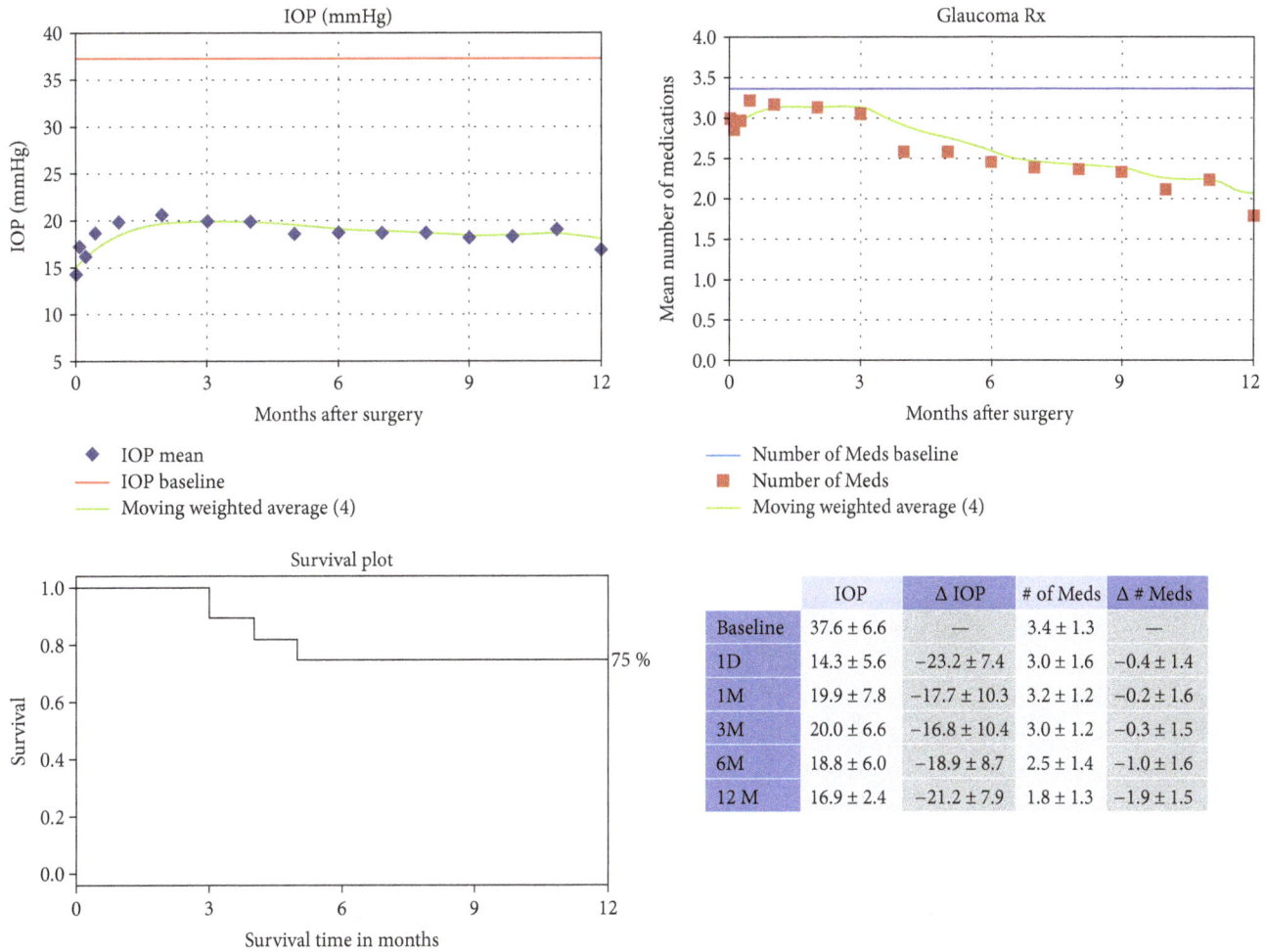

IOP (mmHg) chart

- ◆ IOP mean
- — IOP baseline
- — Moving weighted average (4)

Glaucoma Rx chart

- — Number of Meds baseline
- ■ Number of Meds
- — Moving weighted average (4)

Survival plot — 75 %

	IOP	Δ IOP	# of Meds	Δ # Meds
Baseline	37.6 ± 6.6	—	3.4 ± 1.3	—
1D	14.3 ± 5.6	−23.2 ± 7.4	3.0 ± 1.6	−0.4 ± 1.4
1M	19.9 ± 7.8	−17.7 ± 10.3	3.2 ± 1.2	−0.2 ± 1.6
3M	20.0 ± 6.6	−16.8 ± 10.4	3.0 ± 1.2	−0.3 ± 1.5
6M	18.8 ± 6.0	−18.9 ± 8.7	2.5 ± 1.4	−1.0 ± 1.6
12 M	16.9 ± 2.4	−21.2 ± 7.9	1.8 ± 1.3	−1.9 ± 1.5

FIGURE 3: Intraocular pressure (IOP) and number of glaucoma medications data over time from the eyes with IOP> 30 mmHg and having undergone Trabectome-alone surgery. Kaplan-Meier survival curve of the success of the procedure defined as decrease in IOP of 20% or more or a decrease in glaucoma medications with no need for additional medications or glaucoma procedures.

A prospective nonrandomized study grouped open-angle glaucoma patients who underwent Trabectome procedures according to baseline IOP levels [13]. In the group with preoperative IOP levels ≤17 mmHg, the IOP mean reduction was 7% mmHg with a 35% reduction in IOP-lowering medications. However, patients having IOP ≥ 30 mmHg showed IOP reduction as 48% with a 25% reduction in IOP-lowering medications.

Maeda et al. [14] also reported a decrease from mean preoperative IOP of 26.6 ± 8.1 mmHg to 17.4 ± 3.4 mmHg after surgery. The number of IOP-lowering medications decreased from 4.0 ± 1.4 to 2.3 ± 1.2 at 6 months.

In our study, Trabectome surgery with or without cataract surgery achieved fairly good IOP levels from the values of 30 mmHg or higher to mid teens (16.8 ± 3.8). The number of IOP-lowering medications also decreased from 3.1 ± 1.3 to 1.8 ± 1.4 at 12 months.

The strengths of our study include having the Trabectome-alone group as controls to determine the IOP-lowering effect of procedures accurately and close monitoring of IOP, medications, and complications in a prospective fashion. Results are presented by differences in mean IOP and glaucoma medications as well as by a Kaplan-Meier survival curve. Our study covers high IOP cases with short-term follow-up; so, it might be valuable to compare the results with the long-term follow-up studies (Figure 4) [4, 6–8, 12, 14–16]. Severe complications like expulsive hemorrhage which may be caused by sudden drop of IOP after the surgery have not been reported yet; therefore, ab interno trabeculotomy using Trabectome might be safer compared to filtration procedures regarding the pressure changes. One of the major limitations of this study is the inclusion of the patients with a high initial IOP (presumably above the mean baseline of all patients undergoing Trabectome). One would anticipate that repeated IOP measurements in this group (even without Trabectome) would be closer to the mean (i.e., lower) on subsequent readings. The other limitations include the nonrandomized design of the study, with the inherent selection bias and dropout issues. Although IOP and a number of medications were found to be lower during follow-up after the surgery, it cannot be claimed that the surgery itself lowered the pressure without a comparison group. Additionally, the patients who maintained a one-year follow-up may have a selection bias. In our study, we did not have a wash-out time interval for

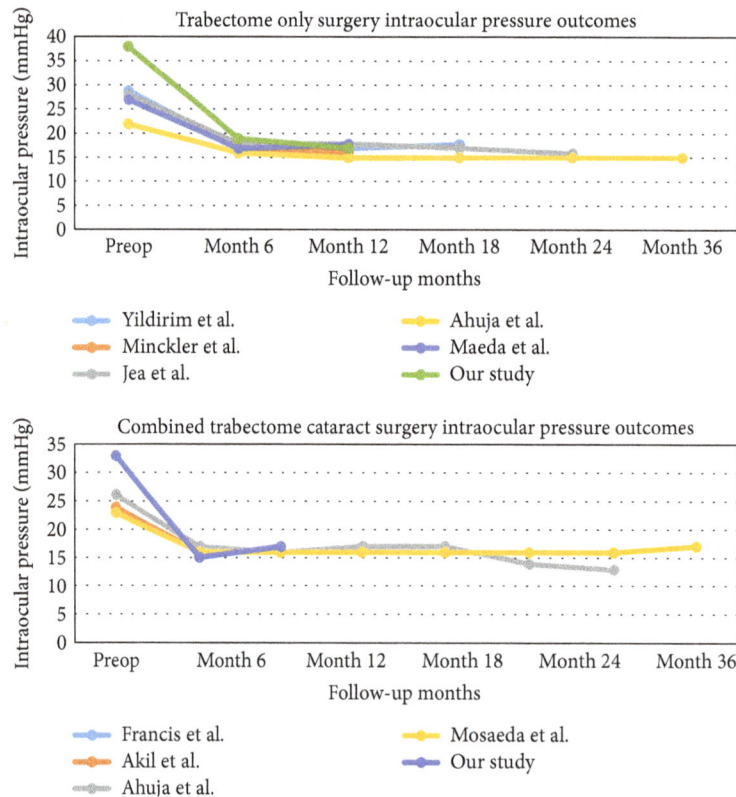

FIGURE 4: Intraocular pressure (IOP) changes over time after the Trabectome surgery with or without cataract extraction in different studies.

glaucoma medications before or after surgery; so, we cannot be certain as to the efficacy or necessity of the number of medications either pre- or posttreatment. We included a comparison group of glaucoma patients who had Trabectome-alone surgery. We encountered some differences between the groups in ethnicity, type of glaucoma, amount of visual field loss, prior surgeries, and degree of angle opening. However, these differences can be expected given the pathogenesis and epidemiology of cataract and glaucoma. The next step would be the establishment of randomized trials to determine the efficacy of Trabectome surgery compared with newer IOP-lowering surgeries for OAG, with one another, and with phacoemulsification alone (in the case of combined procedures).

In conclusion, the risk-to-benefit profile of trabeculotomy by internal approach in patients with high IOP levels has not been studied yet. The results of our study showed that the Trabectome, as a minimally invasive glaucoma surgery, might be considered as an alternative to standard filtration surgery in the surgical treatment of the open-angle glaucoma patients with higher IOP levels because of its internal approach, giving a good option for the combined cataract-glaucoma surgery, the low-risk profile, and the remaining of the future option for filtration surgery.

Disclosure

An earlier version of this work was presented as a poster at the 25th Annual Meeting of the American Glaucoma Society, 2015.

Conflicts of Interest

Dr. Brian A. Francis reports consulting agreements with Neomedix company (Trabectome). No other author has a financial or proprietary interest in any material or method mentioned.

References

[1] H. A. Quigley and A. T. Broman, "The number of people with glaucoma worldwide in 2010 and 2020," *The British Journal of Ophthalmology*, vol. 90, no. 3, pp. 262–267, 2006.

[2] J. F. Jordan, T. Wecker, C. van Oterendorp et al., "Trabectome surgery for primary and secondary open angle glaucomas," *Graefe's Archive for Clinical and Experimental Ophthalmology*, vol. 251, no. 12, pp. 2753–2760, 2013.

[3] B. A. Francis, "Trabectome combined with phacoemulsification versus phacoemulsification alone: a prospective, non-randomized controlled surgical trial," *Clinical Surgery Journal Ophthalmology*, vol. 28, pp. 1–7, 2010.

[4] D. Minckler, S. Mosaed, L. Dustin, B. Francis, and the Trabectome Study Group, "Trabectome (trabeculectomy-internal approach): additional experience and extended follow-up," *Transactions of the American Ophthalmological Society*, vol. 106, pp. 149–159, 2008.

[5] E. Hodapp, R. K. Parrish II, and D. R. Anderson, *Clinical Decisions in Glaucoma*, Mosby–Year Book, St Louis, Mo, 1993.

[6] S. Y. Jea, S. Mosaed, S. D. Vold, and D. J. Rhee, "Effect of a failed Trabectome on subsequent trabeculectomy," *Journal of Glaucoma*, vol. 21, no. 2, pp. 71–75, 2012.

[7] Y. Ahuja, S. Ma Khin Pyi, M. Malihi, D. O. Hodge, and A. J. Sit, "Clinical results of ab interno trabeculotomy using the Trabectome for open-angle glaucoma: the Mayo Clinic series in Rochester, Minnesota," *American Journal of Ophthalmology*, vol. 156, no. 5, pp. 927–935, 2013.

[8] H. Akil, V. Chopra, A. Huang, N. Loewen, J. Noguchi, and B. Francis, "Clinical results of ab interno trabeculotomy using the Trabectome in patients with pigmentary glaucoma compared to primary open angle glaucoma," *Clinical & Experimental Ophthalmology*, vol. 44, no. 7, pp. 563–569, 2016.

[9] T. Mizoguchi, S. Nishigaki, T. Sato, H. Wakiyama, and N. Ogino, "Clinical results of Trabectome surgery for open-angle glaucoma," *Clinical Ophthalmology (Auckland, NZ)*, vol. 9, pp. 1889–1894, 2015.

[10] N. Mathalone, M. Hyams, S. Neiman, G. Buckman, Y. Hod, and O. Geyer, "Long-term intraocular pressure control after clear corneal phacoemulsification in glaucoma patients," *Journal of Cataract and Refractive Surgery*, vol. 31, no. 3, pp. 479–483, 2005.

[11] B. J. Shingleton, J. J. Pasternack, J. W. Hung, and M. W. O'Donoghue, "Three and five year changes in intraocular pressures after clear corneal phacoemulsification in open angle glaucoma patients, glaucoma suspects, and normal patients," *Journal of Glaucoma*, vol. 15, no. 6, pp. 494–498, 2006.

[12] B. A. Francis, D. Minckler, L. Dustin et al., "Combined cataract extraction and trabeculotomy by the internal approach for coexisting cataract and open-angle glaucoma: initial results," *Journal of Cataract and Refractive Surgery*, vol. 34, no. 7, pp. 1096–1103, 2008.

[13] S. D. Vold, "Ab interno trabeculotomy with the Trabectome system: what does the data tell us?" *International Ophthalmology Clinics*, vol. 51, no. 3, pp. 65–81, 2011.

[14] M. Maeda, M. Watanabe, and K. Ichikawa, "Evaluation of Trabectome in open-angle glaucoma," *Journal of Glaucoma*, vol. 22, no. 3, pp. 205–220, 2013.

[15] Y. Yildirim, T. Kar, E. Duzgun, S. K. Sagdic, A. Ayata, and M. H. Unal, "Evaluation of the long-term results of Trabectome surgery," *International Ophthalmology*, vol. 36, no. 5, pp. 719–726, 2016.

[16] S. Mosaed, "The first decade of global Trabectome outcomes," *European Ophthalmic Review*, vol. 8, pp. 113–119, 2014.

20

Ahmed Glaucoma Valves versus EX-PRESS Devices in Glaucoma Secondary to Silicone Oil Emulsification

Zhuyun Qian,[1] **Kai Xu,**[1] **Xiangmei Kong** (ID),[1,2,3] **and Huan Xu**[1]

[1]*Department of Ophthalmology and Visual Science, Eye, Ear, Nose, and Throat Hospital, Shanghai Medical College, Fudan University, Shanghai, China*
[2]*Key Laboratory of Myopia, Ministry of Health, Fudan University, Shanghai, China*
[3]*Shanghai Key Laboratory of Visual Impairment and Restoration, Fudan University, Shanghai, China*

Correspondence should be addressed to Xiangmei Kong; kongxm95@163.com

Academic Editor: Lisa Toto

Objective. To evaluate and compare the clinical effects of Ahmed glaucoma valves (AGVs) and EX-PRESS implants on glaucoma secondary to silicone oil (SO) emulsification. *Methods.* A retrospective case-series study was designed. A total of 23 eyes with late intraocular pressure (IOP) elevation secondary to SO emulsification were included in the study. Antiglaucoma surgery with implantation of AGVs or EX-PRESS devices was performed. Pre- and postoperative ocular parameters were recorded at each visit during a 1-year follow-up period. The rates of complete success (IOP < 21 mmHg without medication) and qualified success (IOP < 21 mmHg with ≤3 glaucoma medications) were analyzed. *Results.* A total of 14 eyes underwent AGV implantation, and 9 underwent EX-PRESS implantation. The mean IOP and number of medications used at the last follow-up decreased significantly compared with that before surgery ($P < 0.001$). The total success rate for all eyes including complete success (7/23) and qualified success (7/23) was 60.9% (14/23) at 1 year. The total success rate in the AGV group was 78.6% (11/14), whereas it was 33.3% (3/9) in the EX-PRESS group; the difference between the 2 groups was significant ($P < 0.05$). *Conclusion.* For glaucoma secondary to SO emulsification, glaucoma implants could be effective at lowering IOP, and AGVs might produce better outcomes than EX-PRESS devices.

1. Introduction

Silicone oil (SO) is widely used in the management of complicated retinal detachment. However, a series of complications can be caused by intraocular SO tamponade, including transient or permanent intraocular pressure (IOP) elevation [1–3]. A major reason for the occurrence of glaucoma secondary to SO tamponade is SO emulsification. The incidence of open-angle glaucoma (OAG) after SO emulsification varies from 11% to 56% [4, 5]. The underlying mechanism might be the migration of SO droplets into the anterior chamber, which could directly obstruct the trabecular meshwork or cause inflammation in it [6]. In addition, long-term contact between the emulsified SO and the trabecular meshwork may result in sclerosis and collapse of the trabecular meshwork. Silicone-laden macrophages have been found within the trabecular meshwork of pathologic specimens, suggesting their role in the obstruction of the outflow tract [7]. Medical control of IOP is the first choice treatment. Budenz et al. [8] reported a success rate of 69% for medical IOP control at 6 months, which dropped to 48% at 24 months. If IOP cannot be satisfactorily controlled, silicone removal is recommended. Additional invasive procedures include trabeculectomy, cycloablation, and implantation of glaucoma drainage devices.

Considering that trabeculectomy has a poor prognosis due to conjunctival scarring from previous vitreoretinal surgery, glaucoma drainage devices could be an alternative treatment approach. Widely used glaucoma drainage devices include the EX-PRESS glaucoma filtration device (Alcon Laboratories, Inc., Nevellan, Israel) and the Ahmed glaucoma valve (AGV) (New World Medical, Inc., Rancho Cucamonga, CA, USA). Errico et al. [9] reported an overall success rate of 73% with the

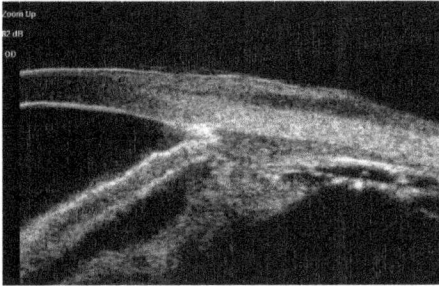

FIGURE 1: Image of UBM of a patient with glaucoma after PPV and SO injection showed an open chamber angle and several dotted high-echoes in the angle suggesting the SO emulsification.

EX-PRESS implanted in patients who were diagnosed with glaucoma with SO emulsification in a 24-month follow-up period. Reports of AGV use for glaucoma with SO emulsification are limited. Ishida et al. [10] reported successful control of IOP in 47% of patients with SO endotamponade over 4 years.

In the current study, we retrospectively reviewed a series of patients who were diagnosed with glaucoma secondary to SO emulsification and received EX-PRESS or AGV implants. We recorded their ocular data and evaluated the surgery results for OAG secondary to SO emulsification.

2. Methods

2.1. Participants. This was a retrospective case-control study. A total of 23 eyes from 23 patients who were diagnosed with OAG secondary to SO emulsification at the Department of Ophthalmology, Eye, Ear, Nose and Throat Hospital, affiliated with Shanghai Fudan University, from January 2012 to June 2015, were included in the study. Patients with high IOP before pars plana vitrectomy (PPV) or whose IOP elevation was thought to be caused by other factors, including synechial angle closure, rubeosis iridis, SO overfilling, pupillary block, inflammation, or steroid-induced glaucoma, were excluded from the study. Not only eyes with rhegmatogenous retinal detachment (RRD) but also cases with ocular trauma, foreign body, or endophthalmitis were included. The previous surgery was PPV and SO injection in all of the eyes. SO with a viscosity of 5,000 centistokes was used. The diagnosis of glaucoma secondary to SO emulsification was confirmed by the presence of SO emulsion droplets in the anterior chamber and high IOP. The appearance of SO microglobules in the chamber angle was determined via a gonioscope and an ultrasound biomicroscope (Figure 1). In all of the eyes, SO removal was performed and IOP-reducing medication (≥ 2 types) was administered but was ineffective. Data on the general characteristics of included patients were compared between the AGV and EX-PRESS groups. Detailed ophthalmological examinations were performed 1 day before antiglaucoma surgery, including best-corrected VA, Goldmann applanation tonometry, slit-lamp examination, and fundus examination. VA was measured via a decimal chart. Previous ocular history and the use of topical or general antiglaucoma medications were recorded. In our study, all of

the participants signed informed consent forms. The study was approved by the institutional review board of the Eye, Ear, Nose and Throat Hospital of Fudan University and was performed in accordance with the tenets of the Declaration of Helsinki.

2.2. Surgical Techniques and Measurements. Both the EX-PRESS P200 implant (Alcon Laboratories) and the AGV implant model FP7 (New World Medical, Inc.) were used in all 23 eyes. All surgeries were performed under peribulbar anesthesia by the same surgeon.

For EX-PRESS shunt implantation, a limbal-based conjunctival dissection was created after a sub-Tenon injection of 1% lidocaine. A 4.0 mm × 3.5 mm partial thickness trapezoidal scleral flap was created, and a sponge soaked with 0.4 mg/mL of MMC was applied under the conjunctival and scleral flaps for 3 min followed by rinsing with 20 mL of 0.9% sodium chloride. A 26-gauge needle was then used to make a microincision under the scleral flap in the center of the blue-gray transition zone, and the EX-PRESS drainage device was inserted into the anterior chamber. The scleral flap and the conjunctiva were then closed as in a trabeculectomy.

In the AGV group, a conjunctival incision was made at the limbus, and 0.4 mg/mL of MMC was applied under the conjunctival flap for 3 min and then washed out. The AGV was inserted through the conjunctiva and Tenon's capsule and sutured to the sclera approximately 8 mm behind the limbus. The tube was trimmed to an appropriate length and inserted into the anterior chamber with the bevel facing anteriorly through a scleral track 2 mm behind the limbus created using a 23-gauge needle. A rectangular donor scleral patch graft was created and then fixed over the exposed part of the tube using 10-0 nylon sutures. The conjunctiva and Tenon's capsule were repaired using absorbable sutures.

The postoperative follow-up visits were scheduled at 1 day, 1 month, 3 months, 6 months, and 12 months after surgery. Ocular parameters, including VA and IOP, and the number of medications used were recorded at each visit. Three outcomes were defined for this study: eyes with normal IOP (<21 mmHg) at the 12-month follow-up were considered successes, and among these, those controlled by glaucoma medications (≤ 3) or needle revision were considered qualified successes and those not requiring any medication or needle revision were regarded as complete successes. Eyes with high IOP that could not be controlled with medication and that underwent other surgical intervention, such as surgical scar removal and cyclocryotherapy, were considered failures and were removed from the follow-up sample. In eyes classified as failures, IOP, medication, and VA data were collected beyond the failure date until the last available follow-up. Data on the IOP and medications at each visit were compared between the AGV and EX-PRESS groups.

2.3. Statistical Analysis. The independent sample *t*-test and Mann–Whitney *U* test (SPSS, Inc., Chicago, IL, USA) were used for the comparison of data between the two groups depending on whether the data followed a normal distribution.

TABLE 1: Baseline characteristics of the study patients.

Characteristic	AGV Patients ($n = 14$)	EX-PRESS Patients ($n = 9$)	P value
Age (years), mean ± SD (range)	46.8 ± 13.5 (15–65)	44.3 ± 17.4 (14–75)	0.708
Gender, n (%)			
Male	11 (78.6)	7 (77.8)	
Female	3 (21.4)	2 (22.2)	
Indication for PPV, n (%)			
RRD	11 (78.6)	7 (77.8)	
Giant retinal hole or multiple retinal holes	4 (28.6)	3 (33.3)	
Macular hole caused by high myopia	2 (14.3)	2 (22.2)	
Associated with choroidal detachment	2 (14.3)	1 (11.1)	
PVR after failed PPV	2 (14.3)	2 (22.2)	
Ocular injury	3 (21.4)	2 (22.2)	
Penetrating injury	3 (17.4)	1 (11.1)	
With endophthalmitis	1 (8.7)	1 (11.1)	
With IOFB	2 (14.3)	0 (0)	
Rupture	0 (0)	1 (11.1)	
Tamponade duration (months), mean ± SD (range)	11.3 ± 8.2 (3–31)	10.0 ± 13.7 (3–46)	0.153
Duration between removal of silicone oil and antiglaucoma surgery (months), mean ± SD (range)	2.8 ± 1.6 (1–5)	3.6 ± 1.6 (1–6)	0.240
Axial length of the eye (mm), mean ± SD (range)	25.5 ± 2.4 (23.3–30.7)	26.9 ± 3.0 (24.2–31.1)	0.208
Anterior chamber depth (mm), mean ± SD (range)	3.1 ± 0.5 (2.3–3.8)	3.0 ± 0.5 (2.1–3.5)	0.801

AGV: Ahmed glaucoma valve; EX-PRESS: EX-PRESS glaucoma filtration device; SD: standard deviation; PPV: pars plana vitrectomy; RRD: rhegmatogenous retinal detachment; PVR: proliferative vitreoretinopathy; IOFB: intraocular foreign body.

The K–S test was used to determine the normality of data. Kaplan–Meier survival analysis was performed for the entire group and for each type of surgical procedure. Categorical variables were compared using the log-rank test, taking into account the time of failure and time of loss to follow-up for each subject. $P < 0.05$ was considered statistically significant.

3. Results

A total of 23 eyes from 23 patients (18 males and 5 females) with a mean age of 46.0 ± 14.8 years (range 14–75 years) were included in this study. The surgical indications of PPV were RRD in 18 eyes and ocular injury or consequent ocular infection in 5 eyes. Among the eyes with RRD, fundus manifestations were giant retinal hole, multiple retinal holes, high myopia with macular holes, choroidal detachment, and severe proliferative vitreoretinopathy (PVR) after PPV failure. Ocular injuries included intraocular foreign bodies caused by penetrating injuries and ocular rupture. Two eyes were diagnosed with traumatic endophthalmitis. The mean silicone tamponade duration was 10.8 ± 10.4 months (range 3–46 months). Ten eyes underwent extended tamponade due to a high risk of retinal redetachment. The other 13 eyes were lost to follow-up after PPV surgery until the patients felt eye pain and were diagnosed with high IOP. All of the eyes underwent surgery for SO removal with good retinal adhesion. The mean duration between SO removal and antiglaucoma surgery was 3.1 ± 1.6 months (range 1–6 months). There were no significant differences in the data between the AGV and EX-PRESS groups. The characteristics of the AGV and EX-PRESS groups are shown in Table 1. The mean preoperative IOP was 34.3 ± 7.6 mmHg (range 25–49 mmHg), and visual acuity (VA) ranged from "hand

motion" to 0.25. The mean number of topical antiglaucoma drops used before surgery was 3.4 ± 0.9.

Among the 23 eyes, 14 underwent AGV implantation and 9 underwent EX-PRESS shunt implantation. After a mean follow-up of 8.4 ± 4.8 months, IOP and the number of antiglaucoma medications decreased (Figure 2). In the AGV group, the mean IOP was 15.8 ± 9.2 mmHg the day after surgery and 17.7 ± 1.5 mmHg 12 months after surgery, and in the EX-PRESS group, the corresponding values were 10.0 ± 4.3 mmHg and 18.3 ± 0.6 mmHg, respectively. The mean numbers of glaucoma medications in use at the 12-month visit were 1.0 ± 1.2 in the AGV group and 1.0 ± 1.7 in the EX-PRESS group. There were no significant differences in IOP and the number of medications between the AGV and EX-PRESS groups at each visit except in the number of medications at the 3-month visit ($P = 0.033$). Table 2 shows a summary of IOPs and the numbers of glaucoma medications in the AGV and EX-PRESS groups before surgery and at each follow-up time-point thereafter and the statistical results. At 12 months, 14 of the 23 eyes (60.9%) were considered a success, of which 7 (30.4%) were a complete success and 7 (30.4%) were a qualified success. Nine eyes still exhibited high IOP after the administration of more than 3 antiglaucoma medications and were judged as failures. At 1, 3, 6, and 12 months after surgery, the respective cumulative success rates were 100%, 82.6%, 69.6%, and 60.9%. At the end of follow-up, the success rates were 78.6% in the AGV group and 33.3% in the EX-PRESS group, and this difference was statistically significant ($P = 0.022$). Figure 3 shows the Kaplan–Meier survival curves for all eyes based on surgical procedures. The main reason for surgical failure was thought to be scar formation. Two eyes in the AGV group were judged as failure after 3-month follow-up. In the EX-PRESS

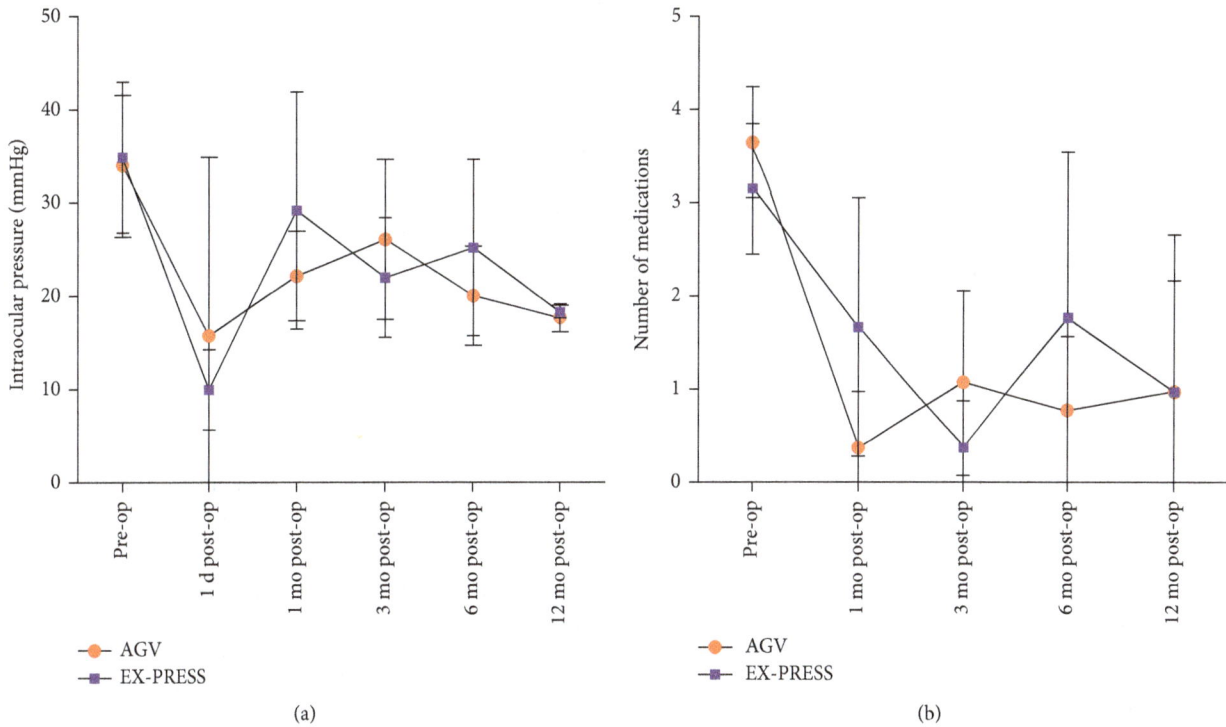

FIGURE 2: (a) The line graph of intraocular pressure before surgery and one day, one month, three months, six months, and twelve months after surgery. (b) The line graph of the number of medications used before surgery and one day, one month, three months, six months, and twelve months after surgery.

TABLE 2: Preoperative and follow-up outcomes.

		Preoperative	1 day	1 month	3 months	6 months	12 months	P1 value
AGV	Number of patients	14	14	14	14	11	11	—
	IOP	34.0 ± 7.6 (25–49)	15.8 ± 9.2 (7.9–42)	22.2 ± 4.8 (15–30)	26.1 ± 8.6 (16–42)	20.1 ± 5.3 (9.1–30)	17.7 ± 1.5 (15–20)	0.000 —
	Medications	3.7 ± 0.6 (3–5)	0	0.4 ± 0.6 (0–2)	1.1 ± 1.0 (0–3)	0.8 ± 0.0 (0–2)	1.0 ± 1.2 (0–3)	0.000 —
EX-PRESS	Number of patients	9	9	9	5	5	3	—
	IOP	34.9 ± 8.1 (27–49)	10.0 ± 4.3 (5.4–17)	29.2 ± 12.7 (8–41)	22.0 ± 6.4 (17–30)	25.2 ± 9.4 (17–39)	18.3 ± 0.6 (18–19)	0.000 —
	Medications	3.2 ± 0.7 (2–4)	0	1.7 ± 1.4 (0–3)	0.4 ± 0.5 (0–1)	1.8 ± 1.8 (0–4)	1.0 ± 1.7 (0–3)	0.000 —
P2 value	IOP	0.792	0.051	0.195	0.485	0.307	0.524	—
	Medications	0.100	—	0.033	0.138	0.314	0.801	—

AGV: Ahmed glaucoma valve; EX-PRESS: EX-PRESS glaucoma filtration device; IOP: intraocular pressure. The values shown are means ± standard deviation, with the range in brackets. P1 value: comparison between preoperative and 12 months. P2 value: comparison between AGV group and EX-PRESS group at each time-point.

group, four eyes and 2 eyes were judged as failure after 1-month and 6-month follow-up, respectively. The conjunctiva was reopened, and fibrous scarring around the filtering bleb or Tenon cyst encapsulating the valve body was removed in 8 patients. Another eye with uncontrollable high IOP had no light perception at the 6-month follow-up, and cyclocryotherapy treatment was administered to relieve the ocular pain. The distribution of all failure cases in the study is presented in Table 3.

After surgery, 11 eyes underwent needling revision with 5-fluorouracil within 1 to 3 months. Complications encountered in our study included AGV tube obstruction by

inflammatory exudation and consequent high IOP (up to 42 mmHg) in 1 eye, which was treated using a yttrium aluminum garnet laser and transient hypotony soon after surgery, which resolved spontaneously in 2 eyes in the EX-PRESS group. No corneal decompensation or endophthalmitis was encountered.

4. Discussion

SO is the favored material for tamponade in eyes with PVR or giant retinal tears [11]. Elevation of IOP is a common complication of PPV with SO injection. Emulsification of the

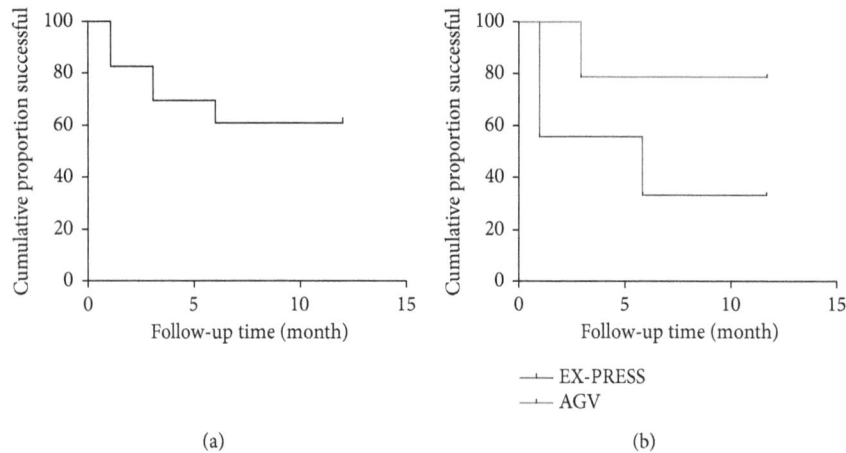

FIGURE 3: (a) The Kaplan–Meier survival curve for all of the eyes (all data referred to total success rate). (b) The Kaplan–Meier survival curve based on surgical procedures (Ahmed glaucoma valves or EX-PRESS) (all data referred to total success rate).

TABLE 3: Distribution of surgical failures in this study.

	EX-PRESS	AGV	Treatment
1 month postoperative	4	0	Surgical scar removal
3 months postoperative	0	3	Surgical scar removal
6 months postoperative	2	0	Surgical scar removal/cyclocryotherapy

AGV: Ahmed glaucoma valve; EX-PRESS: EX-PRESS glaucoma filtration device.

SO has been reported to be associated with a rise in IOP in the late period [12], the associated factors of which are mentioned in Introduction. In our study, two different glaucoma drainage implants, the EX-PRESS P200 and the AGV model FP7, were used as alternative surgery options to treat glaucoma secondary to SO emulsification. The success rate over a 12-month period in the AGV model FP7 group was 78.6%, and that in the EX-PRESS P200 group was 33.3%. The results were statistically significant (log-rank test, $P < 0.05$). The AGV model FP7 showed a likely better clinical outcome than the EX-PRESS P200.

SO emulsification is a multifactorial process in which the biochemical properties of SO, endotamponade duration and ocular inflammation all play roles. It has been reported that 1000 centistokes of oil is more likely to cause elevated IOP than 5000 centistokes of oil [13]. A previous study reported that SO emulsification is independent of the duration of SO endotamponade [14]. In our opinion, a long SO tamponade duration might lead to the elevation of IOP. In our study, the SO endotamponade ranged from 3 months to 46 months with a mean duration of 10.8 months, which was longer than a normal SO tamponade period of 3–6 months.

SO removal is performed to reduce IOP when there is a low risk of retinal redetachment. Budenz et al. [8] reported a success rate of 64% in patients who underwent SO removal alone in a study involving a 36-month follow-up period. At the stage when SO removal alone plays no role, trabeculectomy—a

conventional filtration surgery—can be used. However, this approach produces limited results in the management of glaucoma secondary to SO emulsification. Conjunctival scarring from previous PPV surgery always results in a poor prognosis [6]. Gedde et al. [15] reported a multicenter randomized clinical trial in which patients with previous ocular surgery underwent a tube shunt placement or a trabeculectomy, and in that trial, the tube shunt yielded a higher success rate than trabeculectomy with mitomycin C (MMC) over a 5-year follow-up period.

In our EX-PRESS group, the surgical success rate was 33.3%, which is much lower than the 80% success rate reported by Mendoza-Mendieta et al. [16] for eyes with primary OAG. In our opinion, this major difference could be due to the previous ocular surgery in the cases in our study. AGV is a widely used implant in refractory glaucoma. Ishida et al. [10] reported a success rate of 80% with AGV implants in eyes with SO endotamponade, which is similar to the rate of 78.6% observed in our study. In all cases included in our study, the anterior conjunctiva was opened in previous interventions, which rendered the formation of subconjunctival scarring inevitable. Given that the main reasons for the failure of implant surgery are reportedly bleb encapsulation and the proliferation of subconjunctival fibrous tissue [17], we considered the previous conjunctival scarring of each patient when choosing the type of implant. We preferred to use the AGV in patients with more serious anterior conjunctival scarring because EX-PRESS implants are placed just behind the corneal limbus, whereas AGV implants are placed 8–10 mm behind the limbus, where previous surgical disturbances were fewer. Although we considered these factors, we still observed a better result in the AGV group at the 12-month follow-up time-point, which strongly supports the use of AGV in eyes with a history of previous ocular surgery. Success rate Kaplan–Meier survival curves also indicated that there was minimal change in scar formation in the AGV group or the EX-PRESS group between 6 and 12 months.

We applied bleb needling with 5-fluorouracil in 11 eyes with IOP elevation during the follow-up period, and IOP was lowered effectively in 6 of these eyes. Needling seemed most likely to succeed in eyes with IOP lower than 30 mmHg, possibly because in these eyes, fibrosis formation was not particularly severe and needling together with antimetabolite treatment could therefore be effective. The relationship between patient age and the success rate of needling reported by Quaranta et al. [17] was not apparent in our study, possibly because the number of patients who received needling in our study was limited.

During the surgical process, we identified an additional advantage of AGV implantation compared to EX-PRESS implantation. In our study, all of the eyes had previously undergone PPV, and aqueous fluid had filled the vitreous cavity. The straightforward aqueous outflow procedure adopted in the EX-PRESS group caused large IOP fluctuations during surgery and hypotony soon after surgery. Conversely, the AGV is a restrictive valve device designed to prevent hypotony during and after surgery, which renders the surgical process safer [18].

In our study, although VA was recorded at each follow-up visit, these data were not used in the statistical analysis because all of the eyes had previous retinal disease and preoperative vision was poor in most of them (ranging from "hand motion" to "counting fingers"). We believe that the change in VA during the follow-up period might not be completely attributable to IOP fluctuation.

The limitations of this study include the small sample sizes of both groups, which may challenge the validity of the survival analysis in our study, and the retrospective nature of the study. Given that IOP can be reduced and stabilized to a large extent after the extraction of silicone oil in conjunction with the administration of one or two medicines, glaucoma surgery is only required in relatively few cases. In the past 4 years, as the largest eye institute in the east of China, we have encountered 23 cases based on strict exclusion criteria. More prospective studies with larger cohorts of subjects are needed to support the present findings.

5. Conclusions

In summary, in this retrospective study, glaucoma implants were effective in lowering IOP for eyes with glaucoma secondary to SO emulsification, and AGVs might produce better outcomes than EX-PRESS devices. These results might provide some insight for clinical practice.

Conflicts of Interest

The authors declare that there are no known conflicts of interest associated with this publication.

Authors' Contributions

Zhuyun Qian and Kai Xu contributed equally and should be considered as co-first authors.

Acknowledgments

The authors were supported by the Surface Project of National Natural Science Foundation of China (Grant no. 81770922, China), the Project of Shanghai Municipal Commission of Health and Family Planning (Grant no. 201740204, China), and the Clinical Science and Technology Innovation Project of Shanghai Shenkang Hospital Development Center (SHDC12017X18).

References

[1] K. H. Lucke, M. H. Foerster, and H. Laqua, "Long-term results of vitrectomy and silicone oil in 500 cases of complicated retinal detachments," *American Journal of Ophthalmology*, vol. 104, no. 6, pp. 624–633, 1987.

[2] L. L. Burk, M. B. Shields, A. D. Proia, and B. W. McCuen II, "Intraocular pressure following intravitreal silicone oil injection," *Ophthalmic Surgery*, vol. 19, no. 8, pp. 565–569, 1988.

[3] Q. H. Nguyen, M. A. Lloyd, D. K. Heuer et al., "Incidence and management of glaucoma after intravitreal silicone oil injection for complicated retinal detachments," *Ophthalmology*, vol. 99, no. 10, pp. 1520–1526, 1992.

[4] A. M. Al-Jazzaf, P. A. Netland, and S. Charles, "Incidence and management of elevated intraocular pressure after silicone oil injection," *Journal of Glaucoma*, vol. 14, no. 1, pp. 40–46, 2005.

[5] L. R. de Corral, S. B. Cohen, and G. A. Peyman, "Effect of intravitreal silicone oil on intraocular pressure," *Ophthalmic Surgery*, vol. 18, no. 6, pp. 446–449, 1987.

[6] J. B. Miller, T. D. Papakostas, and D. G. Vavvas, "Complications of emulsified silicone oil after retinal detachment repair," *Seminars in Ophthalmology*, vol. 29, no. 5-6, pp. 312–318, 2014.

[7] L. Wickham, R. H. Asaria, R. Alexander, P. Luthert, and D. G. Charteris, "Immunopathology of intraocular silicone oil: enucleated eyes," *British Journal of Ophthalmology*, vol. 91, no. 2, pp. 253–257, 2007.

[8] D. L. Budenz, K. E. Taba, W. J. Feuer et al., "Surgical management of secondary glaucoma after para plana vitrectomy and silicone oil injection for complex retinal detachment," *Ophthalmology*, vol. 108, no. 9, pp. 1628–1632, 2001.

[9] D. Errico, F. L. Scrimieri, R. Riccardi, and G. Iarossi, "Trabeculectomy versus Ex-Press glaucoma filtration device in silicomacrophagocytic open angle glaucoma secondary to silicone oil emulsification," *Middle East African Journal of Ophthalmology*, vol. 23, no. 2, pp. 177–182, 2016.

[10] K. Ishida, I. I. Ahmed, and P. A. Netland, "Ahmed glaucoma valve surgical outcomes in eyes with and without silicone oil endotamponade," *Journal of Glaucoma*, vol. 18, no. 4, pp. 325–330, 2009.

[11] C. C. Barr, M. Y. Lai, J. S. Lean et al., "Postoperative intraocular pressure abnormalities in the silicone study. Silicone study report 4," *Ophthalmology*, vol. 100, no. 11, pp. 1629–1635, 1993.

[12] P. Ichhpujani, A. Jindal, and L. Jay Katz, "Silicone oil induced glaucoma: a review," *Graefe's Archive for Clinical and Experimental Ophthalmology*, vol. 247, no. 12, pp. 1585–1593, 2009.

[13] J. Petersen and U. Ritzau-Tondrow, "Chronic glaucoma following silicone oil implantation: a comparison of two oils of differing viscosity," *Fortschritte der Ophthalmologie*, vol. 85, no. 6, pp. 632–634, 1988, in German.

[14] J. B. Jonas, H. L. Knorr, R. M. Rank, and W. M. Budde, "Intraocular pressure and silicone oil endotamponade," *Journal of Glaucoma*, vol. 10, no. 2, pp. 102–108, 2001.

[15] S. J. Gedde, J. C. Schiffman, W. J. Feuer, L. W. Herndon, J. D. Brandt, and D. L. Budenz, "Treatment outcomes in the Tube Versus Trabeculectomy (TVT) study after five years of follow-up," *American Journal of Ophthalmology*, vol. 153, pp. 789–803, 2012.

[16] M. E. Mendoza-Mendieta, A. P. López-Venegas, and G. Valdés-Casas, "Comparison between the EX-PRESS P-50 implant and trabeculectomy in patients with open-angle glaucoma," *Clinical Ophthalmology*, vol. 10, pp. 269–276, 2016.

[17] L. Quaranta, I. Floriani, L. Hollander, D. Poli, A. Katsanos, and A. G. P. Konstas, "Needle revision with 5-fluorouracil for the treatment of Ahmed glaucoma valve filtering blebs: 5-fluorouracil needling revision can be a useful and safe tool in the management of failing Ahmed glaucoma valve filtering blebs," *Journal of Glaucoma*, vol. 25, no. 4, pp. 367–371, 2016.

[18] K. Hille, B. Moustafa, A. Hille, and K. W. Ruprecht, "Drainage devices in glaucoma surgery," *Klinika Oczna*, vol. 106, no. 4-5, pp. 670–681, 2004.

21

The Effect of Corneal Refractive Surgery on Glaucoma

Vassilios Kozobolis, Aristeidis Konstantinidis, Haris Sideroudi, and G. Labiris

University Eye Clinic, University Hospital of Alexandroupolis, 68131 Alexandroupolis, Greece

Correspondence should be addressed to Vassilios Kozobolis; vkozompo@med.duth.gr

Academic Editor: Antonio M. Fea

Laser-assisted refractive procedures have become very popular in the last two decades. As a result, a "generation" of patients with altered corneal properties is emerging. These patients will require both cataract extraction and glaucoma follow-up in the future. Since the glaucoma examination largely depends on the corneal properties, the reshaped postrefractive surgery cornea poses a challenge in the diagnosis, follow-up, and management of the glaucomatous patient. In order to overcome this problem, every patient who is planned to undergo corneal refractive surgery must have a thorough glaucoma examination in order for the ophthalmologist to be able to monitor their patients for possible glaucoma development and/or progression. Some examinations such as tonometry are largely affected by the corneal properties, while others such as the evaluation of the structures of the posterior pole remain unaffected. However, the new imaging modalities of the anterior segment in combination with the most recent advances in tonometry can accurately assess the risk for glaucoma and the need for treatment.

1. Introduction

Laser-assisted refractive corrections constitute a large part of the ophthalmic surgeries that take place every year. It is estimated that about 4 million refractive procedures were performed in 2014 throughout the world. On the other hand, glaucoma is an optic neuropathy, the incidence of which is increasing steadily over time. In 2013, the number of glaucoma patients was estimated at about 64.3 million and is expected to reach 118.3 million by 2040 [1]. Given the frequency of refractive corrections and the incidence of glaucoma in the general population, it becomes necessary for the ophthalmologist to assess the risks of a laser-assisted refractive operation in a glaucoma patient or a patient at a high risk of developing glaucoma in the future.

2. Preoperative Assessment

Every patient who is planned to undergo laser-assisted refractive correction should be evaluated for the risk of developing glaucoma in the future. Among others, the following factors should be taken into consideration.

2.1. Family History of Glaucoma. Epidemiological studies have shown that people with familiar predisposition for glaucoma (especially with first-degree relative) have increased risk of developing ocular hypertension (OHT) and glaucoma. Moreover, these individuals tend to develop glaucoma/OHT at a younger age than the general population [2, 3]. The assessment of the presence of glaucoma in a patient's family is therefore of great importance in order to estimate the risk of developing glaucoma in the future.

2.2. Intraocular Pressure (IOP). Elevated IOP remains the most important, modifiable, risk factor for developing glaucoma [4, 5]. However, a single IOP measurement is not sufficient to assess the actual risk of glaucoma, especially when there are other coexisting risk factors. A better understanding of the characteristics of the IOP (average IOP, highest reading, and diurnal fluctuation) is achieved by taking more than one measurements of the IOP in a 24-hour period. Large diurnal fluctuations of the IOP and/or IOP asymmetry between the two eyes are an indication of increased likelihood of developing glaucoma [6, 7].

2.3. Myopia. Myopia is a risk factor of developing glaucoma, and most patients undergoing refractive surgery are potentially glaucoma patients. High myopes (>6.00 D) have a higher risk [8]. Furthermore, tilted discs and peripapillary atrophy are more often seen in high myopes and this can complicate the clinical assessment of the glaucomatous optic neuropathy and monitor changes of the disc structure and the retina over time. As the modern imaging tools do not include high myopes in their database (high myopes are rather excluded), the measurements that they provide are unreliable. In these cases, preoperative photography of the disc is of great value.

2.4. High Vertical Cup-to-Disc Ratio. Although the cup-to-disc ratio in the vertical axis shows great diversity, a high vertical C/D ratio is a risk factor of developing glaucoma [9]. The parameters of the optic disc and the thickness of peripapillary layer of nerve fibers play a pivotal role in the postoperative follow-up of patients who have undergone refractive surgery.

2.5. Central Corneal Thickness. It is well known that a thin cornea is not only a limiting factor for laser-assisted surface ablations but also an independent risk factor for developing glaucoma [9, 10].

2.6. Race. People of Afro-Caribbean origin develop open-angle glaucoma more often and at an earlier age than white people [11], although this may be partly due to the fact that black people have thinner corneas [12].

2.7. Other Ophthalmic Diseases. Pseudoexfoliation syndrome [13–15] and pigment dispersion syndrome [16] are known risk factors for secondary open-angle glaucoma. A study of 12 patients (22 eyes) with pigment dispersion syndrome showed that its presence does not affect the results of refractive surgery, but the authors indicate that the final refractive outcome in patients who receive topical antiglaucoma medication before surgery is less predictable and the healing process of the corneal wound can last longer [17].

2.8. Hypermetropia. Hypermetropes are more likely to have narrow anterior chamber angles and a case of acute angle closure after LASIK in a hypermetropic patient has been reported [18]. Preoperative gonioscopy will help the surgeon to recognize patients with narrow angles.

2.9. Previous Antiglaucoma Procedure. Photorefractive keratectomy (PRK) is the safest surgical option in patients with previous antiglaucoma filtering operation [19]. The creation of the corneal flap with the mechanical keratome or the femto-second laser (docking) during LASIK may damage the filtering bleb and compromise its function. The new refractive lenticule extraction surgery still requires docking of the femto-laser operating system on the eye and should be carefully used in eyes with thin blebs.

2.10. Visual Fields. Preoperative visual fields help the surgeon identify the following:

(i) The presence of established glaucomatous damage

(ii) The extent of glaucomatous damage

(iii) The risk of developing glaucoma. Patients with high PSD have a greater chance of developing glaucoma,

even in the absence of visual fields scotomas [20]. Consequently, the preoperative examination of the visual fields, especially in patients with predisposing factors for glaucoma, is a useful tool for the future monitoring of refractive patients.

2.11. Modern Imaging Modalities. Modern imaging methods (OCT, HRT, and GDx) provide quantitative analysis of the peripapillary optic nerve fibers at a particular distance from the center of the optic disc. They also provide information for several structural parameters of the optic nerve head. In order to differentiate between the disc cup and the nerve fiber rim, they use a reference plane. The structures above the reference plane are read as the rim of the nerve fibers, and the structures below it are recognized by the device as the disc cup. The advantages include objective and reproducible measurements that can be compared with future measurements. The disadvantage is that their databases (although constantly enriched) include limited number of people, while "unusual" discs (tilted, high ametropias) are excluded from the databases. Unfortunately, many candidates for refractive surgery have optic discs with "unusual" appearance that cannot be meaningfully compared with the "normal" optic discs of the databases. In these cases, the digital photographing of the optic disc and the comparison with future photos will give valuable information about the changes of both the optic nerve and retinal nerve fibers.

The red-free imaging of the optic disc is as valuable in differentiating between normal and glaucomatous patients as the OCT (optical coherence tomography), the SLP (scanning laser polarimetry), and the CSLO (confocal scanning laser ophthalmoscope) [21–24].

3. Intraoperative Risk Factors for Glaucoma Progression

During the corneal flap creation in LASIK, the intraocular pressure can go as high as 90 mmHg [25, 26]. The effect of high IOP on the vascular perfusion of the retina has been studied experimentally in pigs but not in glaucoma patients. Research has shown that increased IOP significantly lowers the blood flow through the vessels. The point at which the flow stops completely depends not only on the level of the IOP but also on the blood pressure as well [27]. LASIK surgery does not seem to affect the structure and function of the optic nerve (visual fields, color perception, contrast sensitivity, and pupillary reflex) despite the transient significant elevation of the IOP during surgery [28]. Additionally, it has not been shown that the LASIK affects the structure of the optic nerve or the thickness of the layer of nerve fibers [29–31]. Some studies have reported a reduction of the nerve fiber layer after LASIK [32] with the SLP technology used by the GDx machines, but these effects are probably due to the change of the corneal birefringence and are not real damage of the retinal nerve fibers [33–35]. The new GDx machines with enhanced corneal compensator (ECC) seem to overcome this issue [36].

However, cases of ischaemic optic neuropathy following LASIK and epi-LASIK that can cause permanent damage to the optic nerve have been reported [37–39].

The visual fields, as assessed by automated static perimetry, do not seem to be affected after refractive surgery in the glaucoma and normal population [40]. Nevertheless, there have been reports of visual field deterioration in people with and without glaucoma [41, 42]. It is possible that a small group of glaucoma patients are prone to develop optic nerve damage following an elevation of the IOP during LASIK, but the visual field defects are either very mild or masked by the learning effect of the visual field examination [40]. There have also been reports of loss of the contrast sensitivity and scotoma development from the transition zone [43, 44].

In summary, although the sudden increase of the IOP during LASIK surgery does not appear to affect significantly the structure and function of the optic nerve, it is recommended that the PRK is the preferred method of refractive surgery in the case of the glaucoma patient [19].

4. Postoperative Patient Assessment

4.1. The Effect of the Central Corneal Thickness on the Measurement of the IOP. Goldmann applanation tonometry is still the gold standard method of measuring the IOP. This tonometer was first described by Hans Goldmann and Theo Schmidt in 1957 [45], and it is based on the Imbert-Fick principle.

Both PRK [46–48] and LASIK [49–52] cause a reduction of the postoperative IOP. This reduction (and consequently the clinical underestimation of the actual postoperative IOP) depends on the depth of the ablation and the preoperative IOP. The deeper the ablation and the higher the preoperative IOP, the greater the postoperative reduction of the IOP will be. In addition, the myopic refractive surgery causes larger underestimation of IOP compared to the hypermetropic corrections which are thought to cause negligible IOP change. The postoperative reduction of the IOP is due to the thinning of the corneal stroma, the change in corneal curvature, the instability of the corneal flap (LASIK) [50, 51], and the removal of the Bowman's layer (PRK) [46]. In order to calculate the reduction of the postoperative IOP, Kohlhaas et al. [51] proposed an algorithm that computes the actual IOP after myopic LASIK [IOP (real) = IOP (measured) + $(540 - CCT)/71 + (43 - K - value)/1.7 + 0.75$ mmHg], where IOP (real) is the actual IOP; IOP (measured) is the measured IOP; CCT is the central corneal thickness postoperatively; and K is the average of keratometry readings postoperatively. However, there is not still a commonly accepted algorithm that can calculate with high accuracy the level of the actual postoperative IOP [52].

In order to overcome the problem of the postoperative IOP underestimation with the Goldmann tonometer, some authors suggest that the measurement (in myopic eyes) is done in the periphery of the cornea where less corneal tissue is removed.

The pneumatonometer applanates a smaller area of the corneal surface than the Goldmann tonometer does. It also records a lower IOP postoperatively [50, 53, 54], but some writers argue that the underestimation is lower than that of the Goldmann tonometer [48, 55].

Tonopen is a popular applanation tonometer based on the Mackay-Marg principle. Compared to the Goldmann tonometer, its measurements are less influenced by the thinning of the stroma and the reduction of the corneal curvature [56]. The advantage is that it can record IOP measurements from the periphery of the cornea where the measurement is considered more representative of the true intraocular pressure as the stromal thinning and the change of curvature are smaller there [57–59].

The Pascal Dynamic Contour Tonometer (DCT) is based on contour matching. Its advantage lies on the fact that the measurements are not influenced by the viscoelastic properties of the cornea. It is generally thought that the DCT understates to a lesser extent of the IOP compared to the Goldmann tonometer after both LASIK and PRK [60, 61]. It is also more accurate than the pneumatonometer [62, 63].

4.2. Effect on the Corneal Viscoelastic Properties. Several studies have shown that the viscoelastic properties of the cornea are reduced after LASIK και PRK [64–66] because of the corneal thinning and the creation of the corneal flap. IOPcc is affected to a lesser extent than the IOPg [65], while the IOPg and the IOP estimations with the Goldmann tonometer are reduced to the same extent [67].

The corneal viscoelastic properties have shown a reduction after LASIK [68], which can be attributed to the corneal thinning and the formation of the corneal flap. The IOP measurement with the Corvis ST seems to underestimate the IOP reduction less than the IOPg reading of the ORA and the IOP measurement with the Goldmann tonometer. The postoperative estimation of the IOP with the ORA's IOPcc reading and Corvis ST are the most accurate methods.

The biomechanical properties of the cornea can also be measured with the Corvis ST tonometer which applanates the cornea with a jet of air and the surface deformation is recorded by a high speed and high resolution Scheimpflug camera [69]. The deformation pattern as captured by the Scheimpflug also changes after corneal refractive surgery which is attributed to the corneal changes incurred by the stromal ablation and flap formation [70].

4.3. Interface Fluid Syndrome, IFS. This syndrome is due to fluid accumulation between the corneal flap and the underlying stroma after LASIK surgery. This fluid may act as a "cushion" resulting in a falsely low IOP reading as measured with the Goldmann tonometer, while the IOP with other tonometers may be measured correctly high [71–75]. If this condition remains undiagnosed and the IOP is not assessed correctly with a different type of tonometer (other than the Goldmann tonometer), visual capacity may be threatened due to a continuous deterioration of the glaucomatous damage. Pham et al. [76] report a case of this syndrome that appeared 6 years after LASIK following an eye injury with a substantial increase of the IOP. The patient showed signs of ischemic optic neuropathy as the rise of the IOP were not detected by the Goldmann tonometer. Rehany et al. describe a patient with high IOP after LASIK where the Tonopen and the Goldmann tonometers failed to unveil a high IOP which was measured correctly with the Schiøtz tonometer [77]. Najman-Vainer et al. [78] and Shaikh et al. [79] warn even for end-stage glaucoma risk if the IOP is not measured correctly and the ophthalmologist does not rely on functional tests (visual field). This syndrome should be distinguished from the diffuse lamellar keratitis (DLK) as it does not respond to topical steroids and requires treatment aqueous suppressants.

4.4. Steroid Responders. The international literature [80] has shown that the use of topical steroids postoperatively can lead to a significant rise of the IOP especially in patients with the following:

(i) Primary open-angle glaucoma (POAG)

(ii) Glaucoma suspects

(iii) People with first-degree relatives suffering from POAG

(iv) Diabetes mellitus type I

(v) High myopia

(vi) People with a previous episode of steroid responsiveness

(vii) Patients with rheumatic diseases (e.g., rheumatoid arthritis)

(viii) Advanced age.

Increased IOP leads to a spectrum of clinical manifestations in the cornea that ranges from a simple rise of the IOP to pressure induced stromal keratitis (PISK) and to IFS [81, 82]. In the early stages of the IOP rise, there is stromal swelling which causes corneal haze. The corneal swelling then leads to fluid accumulation between the corneal flap and the stroma [83, 84]. If there is fluid accumulation under the flap, the IOP should be measured with a tonometer other than the Goldmann tonometer so as not to miss the diagnosis of IFS. In this case, topical steroids must be stopped and treatment with topical aqueous suppressants must be initiated.

4.5. Corneal Permeability after Refractive Surgery. Studies in patients have shown that the corneal permeability increases after PRK and LASIK surgery. Specifically, the corneal permeability to fluorescein increased the first 2 months postoperatively and then decreased gradually from the second until the sixth month postoperatively when it returned to normal levels. Indeed, the deeper the ablation, the higher the corneal permeability [85]. Chung and Feder [86] also noted that three months after LASIK instillation of tropicamide drops caused greater pupil mydriasis 10, 15, and 20 minutes after instillation. Unlike the above reports, the experimental PRK and LASIK in hares caused nonsignificant increase of corneal permeability to timolol 1 month after surgery [87]. The concentration of timolol in the aqueous was measured by liquid chromatography.

4.6. Topical Antiglaucoma Medication after Refractive Surgery. Unfortunately, little evidence exists about the effectiveness of the topical antiglaucoma drops in refractive patients. The combination of timolol 0.5% twice a day and dorzolamide 3 times a day is more effective in lowering the IOP after PRK in ocular hypertensive patients compared to timolol twice daily alone or dorzolamide 3 times a day alone [88]. Latanoprost and timolol have the same hypotensive effect in ocular hypertension due to steroid responsiveness [89].

5. Conclusions

The preoperative assessment of glaucoma patients who are candidates for refractive surgery should be based on a set of tests which starts from the family history, IOP measuring (even performing a 24-hour IOP phasing in some cases), visual field test, and imaging of the optic nerve and the peripapillary nerve fiber layer. Because age is a strong risk factor [90], it is easily understood that all young refractive patients are potentially glaucoma patients over time. Therefore, the preoperative glaucoma risk assessment should be performed in every patient.

The preoperative imaging of the structures of the posterior pole can be done with digital photography or/and with one of the newer imaging methods (OCT, HRT, and GDx). Fundus photography does not give objective measurements of the structures but enables us to monitor the changes over time even in "unusual" discs (tilted and myopic discs). The other imaging modalities provide detailed measurements of various parameters of the structures of the posterior pole. They also compare the parameters of each individual patient to a database of normal individuals. However, these comparisons may not be entirely reliable in patients with "unusual" discs as occurs in many myopic patients who are excluded from the database of these machines.

The correct measurement of the postoperative IOP is an important challenge for the ophthalmologist. The changes in the corneal thickness, curvature, viscoelastic properties, and the creation of the corneal flap (in LASIK and epi-LASIK) make the assessment of IOP with the Goldmann tonometer unreliable. The clinician should not rely only on the IOP measurement for the diagnosis and monitoring of glaucoma suspects or true glaucoma patients. Visual field tests and imaging of the optic nerve are needed to monitor these patients. In order to accurately estimate the true IOP, the measurements should be done with the Tonopen (which has a smaller applanation surface than the Goldmann tonometer) from the periphery of the cornea or with the DCT whose measurements are not affected by the viscoelastic properties of the cornea. The ORA's IOPcc, which is less affected by the corneal changes, and the Corvis ST are thought to estimate more accurately the true level of the IOP following a refractive procedure.

The clinician should always bear in mind the possible diagnosis of PISK which has a similar clinical picture with DLK but does not respond to topical steroids and should be treated with aqueous suppressants. PISK can be complicated by fluid accumulation under the corneal flap, in which case, the Goldmann tonometer can significantly underestimate the true IOP. As a consequence, the IOP must be monitored with more than one tonometer.

In summary, every young glaucoma patient should be treated as a future glaucoma patient and baseline tests should be carried out preoperatively. In this way, the ophthalmologist will be able to recognize the development of glaucomatous optic neuropathy in the future.

Conflicts of Interest

The authors declare that there is no conflict of interest regarding the publication of this paper.

References

[1] Y. C. Tham, X. Li, T. Y. Wong, H. A. Quigley, T. Aung, and C. Y. Cheng, "Global prevalence of glaucoma and projections of glaucoma burden through 2040: a systematic review and meta-analysis," *Ophthalmology*, vol. 121, no. 11, pp. 2081–2090, 2014.

[2] M. C. Leske, B. Nemesure, Q. He, S. Y. Wu, J. Fielding Hejtmancik, and A. Hennis, "Patterns of open-angle glaucoma in the Barbados family study," *Ophthalmology*, vol. 108, no. 6, pp. 1015–1022, 2001.

[3] R. C. Wolfs, C. C. Klaver, R. S. Ramrattan, C. M. van Duijn, A. Hofman, and P. T. de Jong, "Genetic risk of primary open-angle glaucoma. Population-based familial aggregation study," *Archives of Ophthalmology*, vol. 116, no. 12, pp. 1640–1645, 1998.

[4] M. C. Leske, S. Y. Wu, A. Hennis, R. Honkanen, B. Nemesure, and BESs Study Group, "Risk factors for incident open-angle glaucoma: the Barbados eye studies," *Ophthalmology*, vol. 115, no. 1, pp. 85–93, 2008.

[5] M. O. Gordon, J. A. Beiser, J. D. Brandt et al., "The ocular hypertension treatment study: baseline factors that predict the onset of primary open-angle glaucoma," *Archives of Ophthalmology*, vol. 120, no. 6, pp. 714–712, 2002.

[6] S. Asrani, R. Zeimer, J. Wilensky, D. Gieser, S. Vitale, and K. Lindenmuth, "Large diurnal fluctuations in intraocular pressure are an independent risk factor in patients with glaucoma," *Journal of Glaucoma*, vol. 9, no. 2, pp. 134–142, 2000.

[7] A. L. Williams, S. Gatla, B. E. Leiby et al., "The value of intraocular pressure asymmetry in diagnosing glaucoma," *Journal of Glaucoma*, vol. 22, no. 3, pp. 215–218, 2013.

[8] L. Xu, Y. Wang, S. Wang, Y. Wang, and J. B. Jonas, "High myopia and glaucoma susceptibility the Beijing eye study," *Ophthalmology*, vol. 114, no. 2, pp. 216–220, 2007.

[9] B. L. Lee, "Wilson MR; ocular hypertension treatment study (OHTS). Ocular hypertension treatment study (OHTS) commentary," *Current Opinion in Ophthalmology*, vol. 14, no. 2, pp. 74–77, 2003.

[10] A. L. Coleman and S. Miglior, "Risk factors for glaucoma onset and progression," *Survey of Ophthalmology*, vol. 53, Supplement 1, pp. S3–10, 2008.

[11] J. M. Tielsch, A. Sommer, J. Katz, R. M. Royall, H. A. Quigley, and J. Javitt, "Racial variations in the prevalence of primary open-angle glaucoma. The Baltimore eye survey," *Jama.*, vol. 266, no. 3, pp. 369–374, 1991.

[12] E. Aghaian, J. E. Choe, S. Lin, and R. L. Stamper, "Central corneal thickness of Caucasians, Chinese, Hispanics, Filipinos, African Americans, and Japanese in a glaucoma clinic," *Ophthalmology*, vol. 111, no. 12, pp. 2211–2219, 2004.

[13] R. Ritch, "Exfoliation syndrome," *Current Opinion in Ophthalmology*, vol. 12, no. 2, pp. 124–130, 2001.

[14] V. P. Kozobolis, "Epidemiology of pseudoexfoliation in the island of Crete (Greece)," *Acta Ophthalmologica Scandinavica*, vol. 75, no. 6, pp. 726–729, 1997.

[15] A. G. Konstas, D. A. Mantziris, and W. C. Stewart, "Diurnal intraocular pressure in untreated exfoliation and primary open-angle glaucoma," *Archives of Ophthalmology*, vol. 115, no. 2, pp. 182–185, 1997.

[16] Y. Siddiqui, R. D. Ten Hulzen, J. D. Cameron, D. O. Hodge, and D. H. Johnson, "What is the risk of developing pigmentary glaucoma from pigment dispersion syndrome?" *American Journal of Ophthalmology*, vol. 135, no. 6, pp. 794–799, 2003.

[17] N. S. Jabbur, S. Tuli, I. S. Barequet, and T. P. O'Brien, "Outcomes of laser in situ keratomileusis in patients with pigment dispersion syndrome," *Journal of Cataract and Refractive Surgery*, vol. 30, no. 1, pp. 110–114, 2004.

[18] M. Paciuc, C. F. Velasco, and R. Naranjo, "Acute angle-closure glaucoma after hyperopic laser in situ keratomileusis," *Journal of Cataract and Refractive Surgery*, vol. 26, no. 4, pp. 620–623, 2000.

[19] K. P. Bashford, G. Shafranov, S. Tauber, and M. B. Shields, "Considerations of glaucoma in patients undergoing corneal refractive surgery," *Survey of Ophthalmology*, vol. 50, no. 3, pp. 245–251, 2005.

[20] European Glaucoma Prevention Study (EGPS) Group, S. Miglior, N. Pfeiffer et al., "Predictive factors for open-angle glaucoma among patients with ocular hypertension in the European glaucoma prevention study," *Ophthalmology*, vol. 114, no. 1, pp. 3–9, 2007

[21] F. Badalà, K. Nouri-Mahdavi, D. A. Raoof, N. Leeprechanon, S. K. Law, and J. Caprioli, "Optic disk and nerve fiber layer imaging to detect glaucoma," *American Journal of Ophthalmology*, vol. 144, no. 5, pp. 724–732, 2007.

[22] L. M. Zangwill, J. Williams, C. C. Berry, S. Knauer, and R. N. Weinreb, "A comparison of optical coherence tomography and retinal nerve fiber layer photography for detection of nerve fiber layer damage in glaucoma," *Ophthalmology*, vol. 107, no. 7, pp. 1309–1315, 2000.

[23] J. E. Deleón-Ortega, S. N. Arthur, G. McGwin Jr, A. Xie, B. E. Monheit, and C. A. Girkin, "Discrimination between glaucomatous and nonglaucomatous eyes using quantitative imaging devices and subjective optic nerve head assessment," *Investigative Ophthalmology & Visual Science*, vol. 47, no. 8, pp. 3374–3380, 2006.

[24] M. J. Greaney, D. C. Hoffman, D. F. Garway-Heath, M. Nakla, A. L. Coleman, and J. Caprioli, "Comparison of optic nerve imaging methods to distinguish normal eyes from those with glaucoma," *Investigative Ophthalmology & Visual Science*, vol. 43, no. 1, pp. 140–145, 2002.

[25] J. L. Hernández-Verdejo, L. de Benito-Llopis, and M. A. Teus, "Comparison of real-time intraocular pressure during laser in situ keratomileusis and epithelial laser in situ keratomileusis in porcine eyes," *Journal of Cataract and Refractive Surgery*, vol. 36, no. 3, pp. 477–482, 2010.

[26] N. Kasetsuwan, R. T. Pangilinan, L. L. Moreira et al., "Real time intraocular pressure and lamellar corneal flap thickness in keratomileusis," *Cornea*, vol. 20, no. 1, pp. 41–44, 2001.

[27] C. T. Dollery, P. Henkind, E. M. Kohner, and J. W. Paterson, "Effect of raised intraocular pressure on the retinal and choroidal circulation," *Investigative Ophthalmology*, vol. 7, no. 2, pp. 191–198, 1968.

[28] T. M. McCarty, D. R. Hardten, N. J. Anderson, K. Rosheim, and T. W. Samuelson, "Evaluation of neuroprotective qualities of brimonidine during LASIK," *Ophthalmology*, vol. 110, no. 8, pp. 1615–1625, 2003.

[29] M. Iester, P. Tizte, and A. Mermoud, "Retinal nerve fiber layer thickness changes after an acute increase in intraocular pressure," *Journal of Cataract and Refractive Surgery*, vol. 28, no. 12, pp. 2117–2122, 2002.

[30] J. Y. Nevyas, H. J. Nevyas, and A. Nevyas-Wallace, "Change in retinal nerve fiber layer thickness after laser in situ keratomileusis," *Journal of Cataract and Refractive Surgery*, vol. 28, no. 12, pp. 2123–2128, 2002.

[31] J. T. Whitson, J. P. McCulley, H. D. Cavanagh, J. Song, R. W. Bowman, and L. Hertzog, "Effect of laser in situ keratomileusis on optic nerve head topography and retinal nerve fiber layer thickness," *Journal of Cataract and Refractive Surgery*, vol. 29, no. 12, pp. 2302–2305, 2003.

[32] T. V. Roberts, M. A. Lawless, C. M. Rogers, G. L. Sutton, and Y. Domniz, "The effect of laser-assisted in situ keratomileusis on retinal nerve fiber layer measurements obtained with scanning laser polarimetry," *Journal of Glaucoma*, vol. 11, no. 3, pp. 173–176, 2002.

[33] P. Sony, R. Sihota, N. Sharma, A. Sharma, and R. B. Vajpayee, "Influence of LASIK on retinal nerve fiber layer thickness," *Journal of Refractive Surgery*, vol. 21, no. 3, pp. 303–305, 2005.

[34] R. Gürses-Ozden, M. E. Pons, C. Barbieri et al., "Scanning laser polarimetry measurements after laser-assisted in situ keratomileusis," *American Journal of Ophthalmology*, vol. 129, no. 4, pp. 461–464, 2000.

[35] A. P. Aristeidou, G. Labiris, E. I. Paschalis, N. C. Foudoulakis, S. C. Koukoula, and V. P. Kozobolis, "Evaluation of the retinal nerve fiber layer measurements after PRK and LASIK, using scanning laser polarimetry (GDX VCC). Effect of laser in situ keratomileusis on retinal nerve fiber layer thickness measurements by scanning laser polarimetry," *Graefe's Archive for Clinical and Experimental Ophthalmology*, vol. 248, no. 5, pp. 731–736, 2010.

[36] M. Tóth and G. Holló, "Evaluation of enhanced corneal compensation in scanning laser polarimetry: comparison with variable corneal compensation on human eyes undergoing LASIK," *Journal of Glaucoma*, vol. 15, no. 1, pp. 53–59, 2006.

[37] S. R. Montezuma, S. Lessell, and R. Pineda, "Optic neuropathy after epi-LASIK," *Journal of Refractive Surgery*, vol. 24, no. 2, pp. 204–208, 2008.

[38] A. G. Lee, T. Kohnen, R. Ebner et al., "Optic neuropathy associated with laser in situ keratomileusis," *Journal of Cataract and Refractive Surgery*, vol. 26, no. 11, pp. 1581–1584, 2000.

[39] B. D. Cameron, N. A. Saffra, and M. B. Strominger, "Laser in situ keratomileusis-induced optic neuropathy," *Ophthalmology*, vol. 108, no. 4, pp. 660–665, 2001.

[40] K. C. Chan, A. Poostchi, T. Wong, E. A. Insull, N. Sachdev, and A. P. Wells, "Visual field changes after transient elevation of intraocular pressure in eyes with and without glaucoma," *Ophthalmology*, vol. 115, no. 4, pp. 667–672, 2008.

[41] H. S. Weiss, R. S. Rubinfeld, and J. F. Anderschat, "Case reports and small case series: LASIK-associated visual field loss in a glaucoma suspect," *Archives of Ophthalmology*, vol. 119, no. 5, pp. 774–775, 2001.

[42] D. M. Bushley, V. C. Parmley, and P. Paglen, "Visual field defect associated with laser in situ keratomileusis," *American Journal of Ophthalmology*, vol. 129, no. 5, pp. 668–671, 2000.

[43] R. Montés-Micó and T. Ferrer-Blasco, "Contrast sensitivity loss in the peripheral visual field following laser in situ keratomileusis," *Journal of Cataract and Refractive Surgery*, vol. 33, no. 6, pp. 1120–1122, 2007.

[44] S. M. Brown and J. Morales, "Iatrogenic ring scotoma after laser in situ keratomileusis," *Journal of Cataract and Refractive Surgery*, vol. 28, no. 10, pp. 1860–1863, 2002.

[45] H. Goldmann, "Applanation tonometry," in *Glaucoma Transactions of the Second Conference*, F. Newell, Ed., pp. 167–220, Josiah Mercy Jr. Foundation, New York, 1957.

[46] M. J. Doughty and M. L. Zaman, "Human corneal thickness and its impact on intraocular pressure measures: a review and meta-analysis approach," *Survey of Ophthalmology*, vol. 44, no. 5, pp. 367–408, 2000.

[47] C. Tamburrelli, A. Giudiceandrea, A. S. Vaiano, C. G. Caputo, F. Gullà, and T. Salgarello, "Underestimate of tonometric readings after photorefractive keratectomy increases at higher intraocular pressure levels," *Investigative Ophthalmology & Visual Science*, vol. 46, no. 9, pp. 3208–3213, 2005.

[48] O. E. Abbasoglu, R. W. Bowman, H. D. Cavanagh, and J. P. McCulley, "Reliability of intraocular pressure measurements after myopic excimer photorefractive keratectomy," *Ophthalmology*, vol. 105, no. 12, pp. 2193–2196, 1998.

[49] D. H. Chang and R. D. Stulting, "Change in intraocular pressure measurements after LASIK the effect of the refractive correction and the lamellar flap," *Ophthalmology*, vol. 112, no. 6, pp. 1009–1016, 2005.

[50] J. M. Schallhorn, S. C. Schallhorn, and Y. Ou, "Factors that influence intraocular pressure changes after myopic and hyperopic LASIK and photorefractive keratectomy: a large population study," *Ophthalmology*, vol. 122, no. 3, pp. 471–479, 2015.

[51] M. Kohlhaas, E. Spoerl, A. G. Boehm, and K. Pollack, "A correction formula for the real intraocular pressure after LASIK for the correction of myopic astigmatism," *Journal of Refractive Surgery*, vol. 22, no. 3, pp. 263–267, 2006.

[52] E. Chihara, H. Takahashi, K. Okazaki, M. Park, and M. Tanito, "The preoperative intraocular pressure level predicts the amount of underestimated intraocular pressure after LASIK for myopia," *The British Journal of Ophthalmology*, vol. 89, no. 2, pp. 160–164, 2005.

[53] Q. Fan, J. Zhang, L. Zheng, H. Feng, and H. Wang, "Intraocular pressure change after myopic laser in situ keratomileusis as measured on the central and peripheral cornea," *Clinical & Experimental Optometry*, vol. 95, no. 4, pp. 421–426, 2012.

[54] M. A. El Danasoury, A. El Maghraby, and S. J. Coorpender, "Change in intraocular pressure in myopic eyes measured with contact and non-contact tonometers after laser in situ keratomileusis," *Journal of Refractive Surgery*, vol. 17, no. 2, pp. 97–104, 2001.

[55] D. Zadok, D. B. Tran, M. Twa, M. Carpenter, and D. J. Schanzlin, "Pneumotonometry versus Goldmann tonometry after laser in situ keratomileusis for myopia," *Journal of Cataract and Refractive Surgery*, vol. 25, no. 10, pp. 1344–1348, 1999.

[56] Y. Levy, D. Zadok, Y. Glovinsky, D. Krakowski, and P. Nemet, "Tono-Pen versus Goldmann tonometry after excimer laser photorefractive keratectomy," *Journal of Cataract and Refractive Surgery*, vol. 25, no. 4, pp. 486–491, 1999.

[57] I. Schipper, P. Senn, K. Oyo-Szerenyi, and R. Peter, "Central and peripheral pressure measurements with the Goldmann tonometer and Tono-Pen after photorefractive keratectomy for myopia," *Journal of Cataract and Refractive Surgery*, vol. 26, no. 6, pp. 929–933, 2000.

[58] H. J. Garzozi, H. S. Chung, Y. Lang, L. Kagemann, and A. Harris, "Intraocular pressure and photorefractive keratectomy: a comparison of three different tonometers," *Cornea*, vol. 20, no. 1, pp. 33–36, 2001.

[59] H. J. Park, K. B. Uhm, and C. Hong, "Reduction in intraocular pressure after laser in situ keratomileusis," *Journal of Cataract and Refractive Surgery*, vol. 27, no. 2, pp. 303–309, 2001.

[60] A. P. Aristeidou, G. Labiris, A. Katsanos, M. Fanariotis, N. C. Foudoulakis, and V. P. Kozobolis, "Comparison between Pascal dynamic contour tonometer and Goldmann applanation tonometer after different types of refractive surgery," *Graefe's Archive for Clinical and Experimental Ophthalmology*, vol. 249, no. 5, pp. 767–773, 2011.

[61] J. S. Pepose, S. K. Feigenbaum, M. A. Qazi, J. P. Sanderson, and C. J. Roberts, "Changes in corneal biomechanics and intraocular pressure following LASIK using static, dynamic, and non-contact tonometry," *American Journal of Ophthalmology*, vol. 143, no. 1, pp. 39–47, 2007.

[62] H. Burvenich, E. Burvenich, and C. Vincent, "Dynamic contour tonometry (DCT) versus non-contact tonometry (NCT): a comparison study," *Bulletin de la Société Belge d'Ophtalmologie*, vol. 298, pp. 63–69, 2005.

[63] D. S. Siganos, G. I. Papastergiou, and C. Moedas, "Assessment of the Pascal dynamic contour tonometer in monitoring intraocular pressure in unoperated eyes and eyes after LASIK," *Journal of Cataract and Refractive Surgery*, vol. 30, no. 4, pp. 746–751, 2004.

[64] W. Lau and D. Pye, "A clinical description of ocular response analyzer measurements," *Investigative Ophthalmology & Visual Science*, vol. 52, no. 6, pp. 2911–2916, 2011.

[65] S. Chen, D. Chen, J. Wang, F. Lu, Q. Wang, and J. Qu, "Changes in ocular response analyzer parameters after LASIK," *Journal of Refractive Surgery*, vol. 26, no. 4, pp. 279–288, 2010.

[66] J. Shin, T. W. Kim, S. J. Park, M. Yoon, and J. W. Lee, "Changes in biomechanical properties of the cornea and intraocular pressure after myopic laser in situ keratomileusis using a femtosecond laser for flap creation determined using ocular response analyzer and Goldmann applanation tonometry," *Journal of Glaucoma*, vol. 24, no. 3, pp. 195–201, 2015.

[67] C. Kirwan and M. O'Keefe, "Measurement of intraocular pressure in LASIK and LASEK patients using the Reichert ocular response analyzer and Goldmann applanation tonometry," *Journal of Refractive Surgery*, vol. 24, no. 4, pp. 366–370, 2008.

[68] A. Frings, S. J. Linke, E. L. Bauer, V. Druchkiv, T. Katz, and J. Steinberg, "Effects of laser in situ keratomileusis (LASIK) on corneal biomechanical measurements with the Corvis ST tonometer," *Clinical Ophthalmology*, vol. 9, pp. 305–311, 2015.

[69] J. Hong, J. Xu, A. Wei et al., "A new tonometer-the Corvis ST tonometer: clinical comparison with noncontact and Goldmann applanation tonometers," *Investigative Ophthalmology & Visual Science*, vol. 54, no. 1, pp. 659–665, 2013.

[70] H. Hashemi, S. Asgari, M. Mortazavi, and R. Ghaffari, "Evaluation of corneal biomechanics after excimer laser corneal refractive surgery in high myopic patients using dynamic Scheimpflug technology," *Eye & Contact Lens*, 2016.

[71] J. L. Ramos, S. Zhou, C. Yo, M. Tang, and D. Huang, "High-resolution imaging of complicated LASIK flap interface fluid syndrome," *Ophthalmic Surgery, Lasers & Imaging*, vol. 39, 4 Supplement, pp. S80–S82, 2008.

[72] S. Goto, S. Koh, R. Toda et al., "Interface fluid syndrome after laser in situ keratomileusis following herpetic keratouveitis," *Journal of Cataract and Refractive Surgery*, vol. 39, no. 8, pp. 1267–1270, 2013.

[73] W. A. Lyle, G. J. Jin, and Y. Jin, "Interface fluid after laser in situ keratomileusis," *Journal of Refractive Surgery*, vol. 19, no. 4, pp. 455–459, 2003.

[74] R. Fogla, S. K. Rao, and P. Padmanabhan, "Interface fluid after laser in situ keratomileusis," *Journal of Cataract and Refractive Surgery*, vol. 27, no. 9, pp. 1526–1528, 2001.

[75] S. Senthil, V. Rathi, and C. Garudadri, "Misleading Goldmann applanation tonometry in a post-LASIK eye with interface fluid syndrome," *Indian Journal of Ophthalmology*, vol. 58, no. 4, pp. 333–335, 2010.

[76] M. T. Pham, R. E. Peck, and K. R. Dobbins, "Nonarteritic ischemic optic neuropathy secondary to severe ocular hypertension masked by interface fluid in a post-LASIK eye," *Journal of Cataract and Refractive Surgery*, vol. 39, no. 6, pp. 955–957, 2013.

[77] U. Rehany, V. Bersudsky, and S. Rumelt, "Paradoxical hypotony after laser in situ keratomileusis," *Journal of Cataract and Refractive Surgery*, vol. 26, no. 12, pp. 1823–1826, 2000.

[78] J. Najman-Vainer, R. J. Smith, and R. K. Maloney, "Interface fluid after LASIK: misleading tonometry can lead to end-stage glaucoma," *Journal of Cataract and Refractive Surgery*, vol. 26, no. 4, pp. 471–472, 2000.

[79] N. M. Shaikh, S. Shaikh, K. Singh, and E. Manche, "Progression to end-stage glaucoma after laser in situ keratomileusis," *Journal of Cataract and Refractive Surgery*, vol. 28, no. 2, pp. 356–359, 2002.

[80] J. P. Kersey and D. C. Broadway, "Corticosteroid-induced glaucoma: a review of the literature," *Eye (London, England)*, vol. 20, no. 4, pp. 407–416, 2006.

[81] V. Galvis, A. Tello, M. L. Revelo, and P. Valarezo, "Post-LASIK edema-induced keratopathy (PLEK), a new name based on pathophysiology of the condition," *BMJ Case Reports*, vol. 2012, 2012.

[82] M. W. Belin, S. B. Hannush, C. W. Yau, and R. L. Schultze, "Elevated intraocular pressure-induced interlamellar stromal keratitis," *Ophthalmology*, vol. 109, no. 10, pp. 1929–1933, 2002.

[83] A. Galal, A. Artola, J. Belda et al., "Interface corneal edema secondary to steroid-induced elevation of intraocular pressure simulating diffuse lamellar keratitis," *Journal of Refractive Surgery*, vol. 22, no. 5, pp. 441–447, 2006.

[84] J. Frucht-Pery, D. Landau, F. Raiskup et al., "Early transient visual acuity loss after LASIK due to steroid-induced elevation of intraocular pressure," *Journal of Refractive Surgery*, vol. 23, no. 3, pp. 244–251, 2007.

[85] G. S. Polunin, V. V. Kourenkov, I. A. Makarov, and E. G. Polunina, "The corneal barrier function in myopic eyes after laser in situ keratomileusis and after photorefractive keratectomy in eyes with haze formation," *Journal of Refractive Surgery*, vol. 15, 2 Supplement, pp. S221–S224, 1999.

[86] H. S. Chung and R. S. Feder, "Pupil response to tropicamide following laser in situ keratomileusis," *Journal of Cataract and Refractive Surgery*, vol. 31, no. 3, pp. 553–556, 2005.

[87] N. Hamada, S. Amano, S. Yamagami et al., "Change in corneal permeability to timolol after laser in situ keratomileusis and photorefractive keratectomy in rabbit," *Japanese Journal of Ophthalmology*, vol. 49, no. 1, pp. 12–14, 2005.

[88] Z. Z. Nagy, A. Szabó, R. R. Krueger, and I. Süveges, "Treatment of intraocular pressure elevation after photorefractive keratectomy," *Journal of Cataract and Refractive Surgery*, vol. 27, no. 7, pp. 1018–1024, 2001.

[89] M. Vetrugno, A. Maino, G. M. Quaranta, and L. Cardia, "A randomized, comparative open-label study on the efficacy of latanoprost and timolol in steroid induced ocular hypertension after photorefractive keratectomy," *European Journal of Ophthalmology*, vol. 10, no. 3, pp. 205–211, 2000.

[90] B. Bengtsson and A. Heijl, "A long-term prospective study of risk factors for glaucomatous visual field loss in patients with ocular hypertension," *Journal of Glaucoma*, vol. 14, no. 2, pp. 135–138, 2005.

22

Capability of Ophthalmology Residents to Detect Glaucoma using High-Dynamic-Range Concept versus Color Optic Disc Photography

Mantapond Ittarat, Rath Itthipanichpong, Anita Manassakorn, Visanee Tantisevi, Sunee Chansangpetch, and Prin Rojanapongpun

Department of Ophthalmology, Chulalongkorn University and King Chulalongkorn Memorial Hospital,
1873 Rama IV Rd., Pathumwan, Bangkok 10330, Thailand

Correspondence should be addressed to Anita Manassakorn; animanassa@gmail.com

Academic Editor: Kazuyuki Hirooka

Background. Assessment of color disc photograph (C-DP) is affected by image quality, which decreases the ability to detect glaucoma. High-dynamic-range (HDR) imaging provides a greater range of luminosity. Therefore, the objective of this study was to evaluate the capability of ophthalmology residents to detect glaucoma using HDR-concept disc photography (HDR-DP) compared to C-DP. *Design.* Cross-sectional study. *Methods.* Twenty subjects were classified by 3 glaucoma specialists as either glaucoma, glaucoma suspect, or control. All C-DPs were converted to HDR-DPs and randomly presented and assessed by 10 first-year ophthalmology residents. Sensitivity and specificity of glaucoma detection were compared. *Results.* The mean ± SD of averaged retinal nerve fiber layer (RNFL) thickness was $74.0 \pm 6.1\,\mu m$, $100.2 \pm 9.6\,\mu m$, and $105.8 \pm 17.2\,\mu m$ for glaucoma, glaucoma suspect, and controls, respectively. The diagnostic sensitivity of HDR-DP was higher than that of C-DP (87% versus 68%, mean difference: 19.0, 95% CI: 4.91 to 33.1; $p = 0.014$). Regarding diagnostic specificity, HDR-DP and C-DP yielded 46% and 75% (mean difference: 29.0, 95% CI: 13.4 to 44.6; $p = 0.002$). *Conclusions.* HDR-DP statistically increased diagnostic sensitivity but not specificity. HDR-DP may be a screening tool for nonexpert ophthalmologists.

1. Introduction

Glaucoma is a chronic progressive optic neuropathy that is characterized by loss of retinal nerve tissue and field of vision. Due to the asymptomatic nature of the disease, most patients are not aware that they have glaucoma until the late stage of the disease. Currently, more than 8.4 million people worldwide are bilaterally blind from glaucoma [1]. It has been estimated that worldwide prevalence of glaucoma will rise to 111.8 million by 2040, with a high proportion in Asia and Africa [2, 3]. However, the actual prevalence of glaucoma may be higher than this estimation, because more than half of glaucoma patients are under diagnosed [4–6]. Early diagnosis and treatment is the key to preventing blindness from glaucoma. One of the highest sensitivity methods for

monitoring early glaucomatous change is detection of retinal nerve fiber layer (RNFL) defect [7–9]. Color optic disc photography (C-DP) is a standard tool for RNFL evaluation due to its convenient, low-cost, and noninvasive technique. However, the ability to detect glaucoma, especially by clinicians lacking expertise in glaucoma, has been hindered by the poor quality of C-DP images (e.g., light exposure, poor contrast, and color tone), which are frequently found in media opacity and tigroid fundus cases [10]. High-dynamic-range (HDR) imaging is a computerized technique that was developed to produce a greater dynamic range of luminosity, compensate for loss of detail by adapting different exposure levels, and integrate those exposure levels to reproduce a new image with broader tonal range [11, 12]. Accordingly, the aim of this study was to evaluate the capability of ophthalmology residents to detect glaucoma and peripapillary RNFL defect using HDR optic disc photography (HDR-DP), as compared to detection using C-DP.

2. Materials and Methods

This cross-sectional study was conducted at the Department of Ophthalmology, King Chulalongkorn Memorial Hospital (Bangkok, Thailand) and was approved by the Institutional Review Board of the Faculty of Medicine, Chulalongkorn University. This study was conducted in accordance with the Declaration of Helsinki and all of its subsequent amendments. There were 3 groups of participants in this study, including glaucoma patients, glaucoma suspect patients, and healthy volunteers. Color optic disc photographs were taken from the eyes of participants in all 3 subgroups. Evaluators consisted of 10 first-year ophthalmology residents. After receiving permission to access and retrieve images, color disc photographs of glaucoma and glaucoma suspect patients were recruited from our hospital's imaging database. Written informed consent was obtained from healthy volunteers prior to their participation in the study. All subjects were more than 18 years old and had a spherical refractive error between −6 diopters and +6 diopters and astigmatism of less than 3 diopters. Exclusion criteria were history of intraocular trauma, retinal disease, neurological disease, and uncooperative subject. All glaucoma and glaucoma suspect subjects had undergone C-DP (KOWA Company Ltd., Nagoya, Aichi, Japan), optical coherence tomography (OCT) (Cirrus-HD OCT; Carl Zeiss Meditec, Dublin, CA, USA), and standard automated perimetry (SAP) (Carl Zeiss Meditec, Dublin, CA, USA) within 6 months prior to the start of the study. All C-DPs from the glaucoma and glaucoma suspect groups were performed in dilated condition by a single experienced photographer at dimensions and settings of 1600×1216 pixels and RGB color space in JPEG format. Only qualified images were recruited. Glaucoma patient was defined as vertical cup-to-disc ratio greater than 97.5th percentile of normal population with presence of RNFL defect in OCT or disc photograph that correlated with visual field defect in SAP. Presence of vertical cup-to-disc ratio between 97.5th and 99.5th percentiles of normal population without RNFL defect or functional visual field loss and IOP of less than 21 mmHg were classified as glaucoma suspect subjects. Healthy volunteers who participated in this study had visual field tests and images taken following the same process by the same single photographer. Healthy participants had a vertical cup-to-disc ratio of less than 97.5th percentile with a normal reliable SAP result. Nonqualifying images, OCT, and visual fields included the following: (1) images with poor visualization of retinal blood vessels; (2) OCT scans with incorrect ONH detection, off-centered ONH, motion artifacts, wrong segmentation, or signal strength less than 6; and (3) unreliable SAP with fixation loss, false-positive or false-negative responses greater than 20%. Images from 10 glaucoma patients, 5 glaucoma suspect patients, and 5 healthy volunteers were taken, recorded, and included in the study. A total of 20 C-DPs from all subjects were recruited from April to October 2014. Three

glaucoma specialists (VT, AM, and SC) evaluated C-DP, OCT, and SAP to confirm the diagnosis and to identify the number and affected areas of peripapillary RNFL defect in six quadrants (nasal, superonasal, superotemporal, temporal, inferotemporal, and inferonasal) (Figure 1). The determinations reached by the 3 specialists were marked as references for further evaluation by the ophthalmology residents.

All recruited C-DPs were then processed into HDR photos by adjusting the light exposure as overexposed, normally exposed, or underexposed (Figure 2).

Image editing was performed using preview program for Mac OS X version 8.0. Three different exposure images were then combined using the following settings: strength −4.4, brightness 0.4, local contrast 8.4, white Clip 1.0, black Clip 0, midtone 0, and color saturation −1.5 (Figure 3).

After that, the ten first-year ophthalmology residents who volunteered to join the study provided written informed consent to participate as evaluators. All evaluators were trained in how to diagnose glaucoma and identify RNFL defect. Evaluators were blinded to patient clinical information and diagnosis. The ophthalmology resident evaluators independently assessed a set of 40 randomly sequenced disc photographs consisting of 20 C-DPs and 20 HDR-DPs. Images were projected onto a projector screen at a resolution of 1280×800 pixels with 32-bit color in a dark room, and all of the evaluators assessed the image within a period of 30 seconds. The residents were asked to answer 2 questions within 30 seconds, as follows: determine whether the presenting image is glaucoma or not and identify the number and location of RNFL defect.

3. Statistical Analysis

All statistical analyses were performed using SPSS version 17.0 (SPSS Inc., Chicago, IL, USA). Paired t-test was used to test statistical differences of sensitivity and specificity between C-DP and HDR-DP, as evaluated by the residents when using the glaucoma specialists' references. The primary outcomes were mean difference $\pm$ SD of sensitivity and specificity of the test. p values less than 0.05 were considered statistically significant.

4. Results

Demographic and clinical data of study subjects are shown in Table 1.

All subjects had best-corrected visual acuity better than 20/30. Distribution of sensitivity and specificity of glaucoma diagnosis using C-DP and HDR-DP by the 10 ophthalmology residents is shown in Figure 4. The scatter plot graph shows high level of distribution for sensitivity in HDR-DP, compared to medium level of distribution for specificity.

The average sensitivity of glaucoma detection in HDR-DP was better than that in C-DP (87% $\pm$ 13.4% and 68% $\pm$ 19.3%, resp.). The mean difference of sensitivity was 19.0 $\pm$ 19.7 (95% CI: 4.91 to 33.1). The average specificity of glaucoma detection in HDR-DP and C-DP was 46% $\pm$ 28.8% and 75% $\pm$ 17.2%, respectively. The mean difference in specificity was 29.0 $\pm$ 21.8 (95% CI: 13.4 to 44.6) (Table 2).

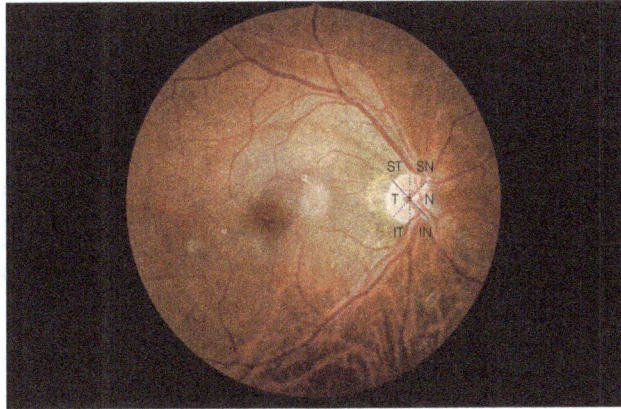

FIGURE 1: Locations of peripapillary retinal nerve fiber layer. N: nasal; SN: superonasal; ST: superotemporal; T: temporal; IT: inferotemporal; IN: inferonasal.

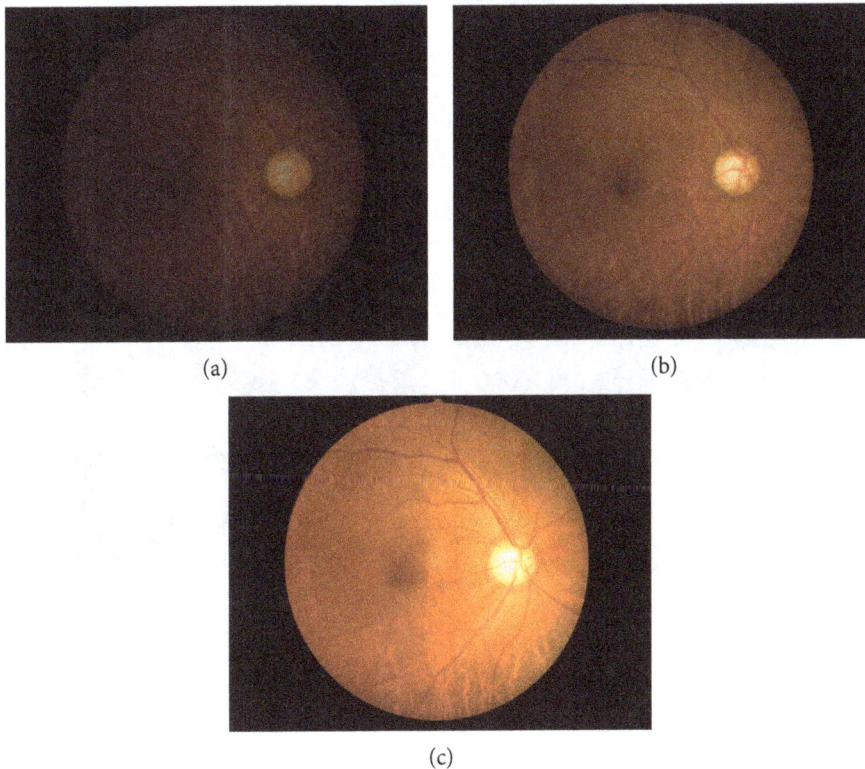

(a)

(b)

(c)

FIGURE 2: High-dynamic-range image processing of color disc photography with three different exposure levels. (a) Underexposed image; (b) normally exposed image; (c) overexposed image.

The average sensitivity of RNFL defect detection between C-DP and HDR-DP in each quadrant of the glaucoma group was analyzed, but no statistical significant difference was observed (Table 3). Interobserver agreement in our study was 0.33 (95% CI: 0.21 to 0.45) and 0.43 (95% CI: 0.31 to 0.56) for HDR-DP and C-DP, respectively.

5. Discussion

In this study, we applied the HDR technique and evaluated diagnostic accuracy compared with original C-DP in nonexperienced trainees. We found that HDR-DP had higher sensitivity for detecting glaucoma than C-DP, but specificity for detection of glaucoma using HDR-DP was lower than that using C-DP. RNFL defect detection was similar between the two techniques.

Color disc photograph is the backbone diagnostic method for glaucoma diagnosis and is widely used in clinical practice. To improve the visualization of optic disc characteristics, stereoscopic disc photograph for three-dimensional evaluation is normally recommended. Many studies have compared the diagnostic ability of using stereoscopic versus

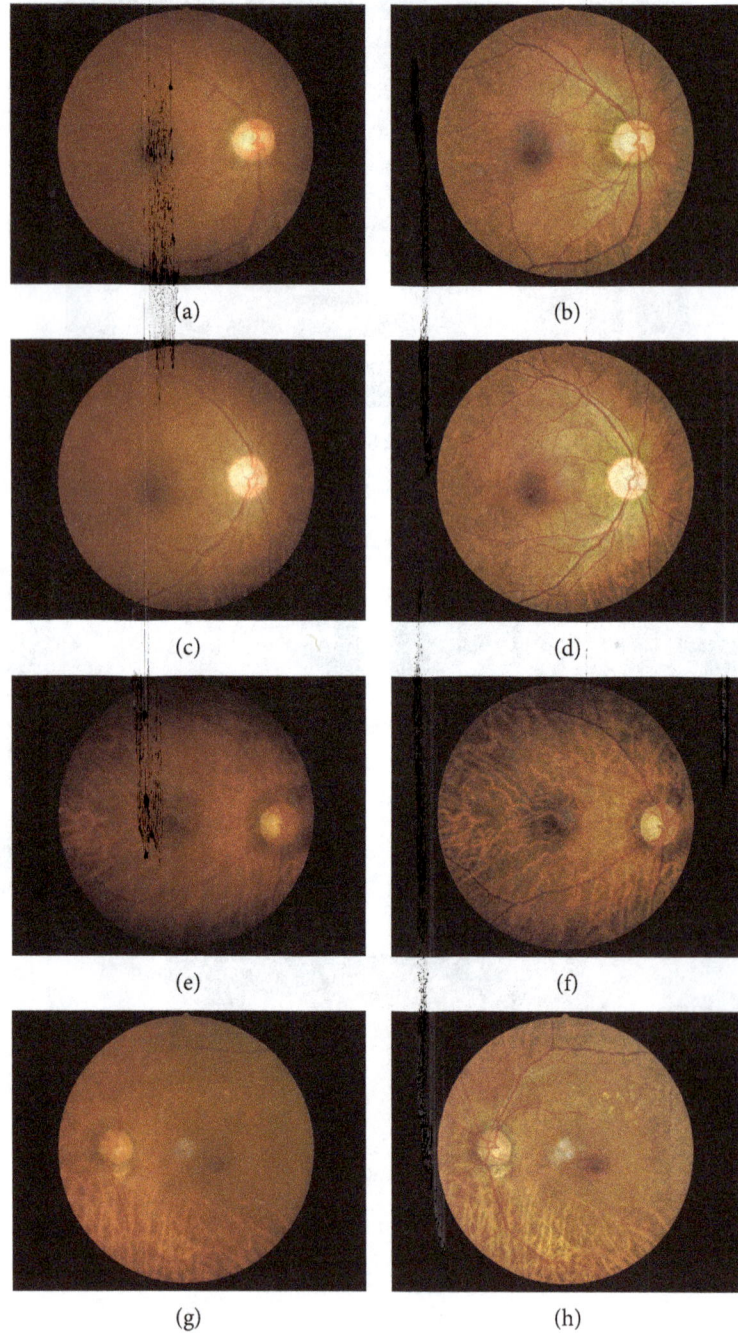

FIGURE 3: Examples of color and high-dynamic-range disc photographs of 2 normal controls (a, b and c, d) and 2 glaucoma patients (e, f and g, h). Left column (a, c, e, and g) color disc photograph and right column (b, d, f, and h) high-dynamic-range concept disc photograph.

monoscopic disc photographs to detect multiple optic disc characteristics, and they have reported varying and sometimes controversial results [13, 14]. A recent paper by the Glaucomatous Optic Neuropathy Evaluation (GONE) Project found that intraobserver and interobserver agreements for determining glaucoma, including vertical cup-to-disc ratio and RNFL defect detection, were similar between monoscopic and stereoscopic disc photographs in experienced observers [15, 16]. They then explored the factors associated with underdiagnosis of glaucoma in trainees using monoscopic disc photograph. The most common factor was

inability to identify RNFL defect, followed by unseen disc hemorrhage, neural rim loss, and vertical cup-to-disc ratio [17]. These results were more pronounced in ophthalmology trainees than in fully trained ophthalmologists. In our study, two-thirds of glaucoma patients were diagnosed using C-DP by trainees, with approximately 32% of the confirmed glaucoma being missed. This reflected the limitation of identifying RNFL defect and detecting glaucoma using only C-DP.

To highlight RNFL visualization, red-free disc photograph and blue reflectance RNFL with confocal scanning

TABLE 1: Demographic and clinical data of study subjects.

Demographic and clinical data	Glaucoma ($N = 10$)	Glaucoma suspect ($N = 5$)	Normal ($N = 5$)
Age (y), mean ± SD	61.0 ± 9.8	55.8 ± 12.1	47.6 ± 1.8
Female (eyes)	7	3	5
Laterality (right eye)	5	3	3
Lens status			
Clear	0	3	3
Nuclear sclerosis grade 1	7	2	2
Nuclear sclerosis grade 2	2	0	0
Pseudophakia	1	0	0
Cup-to-disc ratio, mean ± SD	0.7 ± 0.1	0.7 ± 0.1	0.3 ± 0.0
Spherical equivalent (D), mean ± SD	0.1 ± 0.1	2.2 ± 0.2	0.1 ± 0.7
Intraocular pressure (mmHg), mean ± SD	14.0 ± 3.2	12.2 ± 2.9	15.6 ± 3.7
Average RNFL thickness (μm), mean ± SD	74.0 ± 6.1	100.2 ± 9.6	105.8 ± 17.2
Mean deviation (dB), mean ± SD	−4.1 ± 2.9	−1.5 ± 1.9	−0.4 ± 0.7
Pattern standard deviation (dB), mean ± SD	4.1 ± 2.1	2.4 ± 0.9	1.5 ± 0.3

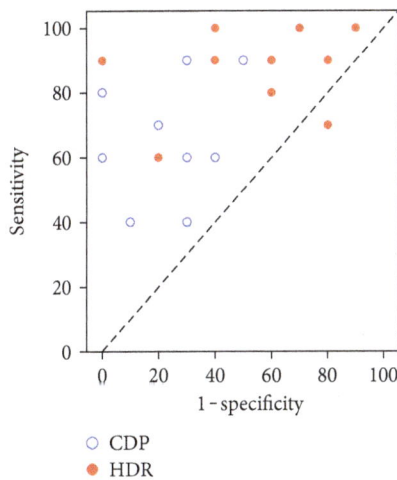

○ CDP
● HDR

FIGURE 4: Scatter plot of distribution of sensitivity and specificity in glaucoma diagnosis between C-DP and HDR-DP.

TABLE 2: Comparison of averaged sensitivity and specificity between C-DP and HDR-DP.

	Mean ± SD (95% CI)		Mean difference ± SD (95% CI)	p value*
	C-DP	HDR-DP		
Sensitivity (%)	68.0 ± 19.3 [54.2, 81.8]	87.0 ± 13.4 [77.4, 96.6]	19.0 ± 19.7 [4.91, 33.1]	0.014
Specificity (%)	75.0 ± 17.2 [62.7, 87.3]	46.0 ± 28.8 [25.4, 66.6]	−29.0 ± 21.8 [44.6, −13.4]	0.002
PPV (%)	75.0 ± 15.1 [64.2, 85.8]	64.4 ± 15.4 [53.3, 75.4]	−10.6 ± 16.2 [−22.2, 0.9]	0.068
NPV (%)	72.1 ± 12.3 [63.3, 81.0]	79.7 ± 19.7 [65.6, 93.7]	7.5 ± 23.3 [9.1, 24.2]	0.332

*p values less than 0.05 indicate statistical significance. SD: standard deviation; CI: confidence interval; C-DP: color optic disc photography; HDR-DP: high dynamic-range concept optic disc photography; PPV: positive predictive value; NPV: negative predictive value. Mean difference is the comparison of each item between HDR-DP and C-DP (HDR − C).

laser ophthalmoscopy were assessed and compared with C-DP [18]. They found that both red-free and blue reflectance images provided better sensitivity than C-DP; however, specificity was not statistically significantly different from C-DP. Marlow et al. applied an image-processing technique to analyze glaucoma progression [19]. Baseline and subsequent optic disc photographs were autoaligned and subtracted to show differences in optic disc characteristics. For glaucoma detection, the objective of our study, this technique could also be applied. However, this technique is unable to deliver prompt glaucoma diagnosis, since it requires at least 2 photographs to detect changes. In addition, this method requires good quality images and complicated manual processes. In this study, we applied HDR concept using a wide range of luminosities to create a final image with more visible details, especially to highlight the RNFL and the characteristics of the optic disc. There are several advantages of HDR concept over original disc photograph. First, HDR does not require a good

quality image, as HDR can enhance image quality by adjusting parameters. As a result, images with media opacity will benefit from this technique (Figures 3(c), 3(d), 3(g) and 3(h)). In addition, the background of fundus in high myopia and tigroid fundus usually interfere with the evaluation of RNFL. HDR can emphasize the visualization of RNFL in such cases (Figures 3(e) and 3(f)). Furthermore, HDR requires no special device other than software that is autoadjustable and normally available free of charge. Using the HDR application, the sensitivity of glaucoma detection was significantly higher than using C-DP. In this study, HDR-DP was created by adjusting the light exposure from 1 original C-DP image, because true HDR technology is difficult to obtain due to motion artifact. While not true for HDR technology, HDR-DP modification facilitates the creation of final images with broader dynamic ranges than those of C-DP images [11].

However, HDR-DP had lower specificity than C-DP, as well as average sensitivity for RNFL defect in each quadrant

TABLE 3: Comparison of averaged sensitivity of RNFL defect detection between C-DP and HDR-DP in each quadrant of the glaucoma group.

Area	Method	Mean ± SD	Mean difference* ± SD (95% CI)	p value of mean difference
Nasal	C-DP	72.0 ± 9.2	10.0 ± 16.3 (−1.7, 21.7)	0.085
	HDR-DP	62.0 ± 14.8		
Superonasal	C-DP	58.0 ± 7.9	3.0 ± 6.7 (−1.8, 7.8)	0.193
	HDR-DP	55.0 ± 9.7		
Superotemporal	C-DP	59.0 ± 17.9	7.0 ± 18.9 (−6.5, 20.5)	0.271
	HDR-DP	52.0 ± 11.4		
Temporal	C-DP	78.0 ± 4.2	6.0 ± 11.7 (−2.4, 14.4)	0.140
	HDR-DP	72.0 ± 10.3		
Inferotemporal	C-DP	41.0 ± 16.6	−6.0 ± 22.7 (−22.2, 10.2)	0.425
	HDR-DP	47.0 ± 17.0		
Inferonasal	C-DP	57.0 ± 15.7	1.0 ± 13.7 (−8.8, 10.8)	0.823
	HDR-DP	56.0 ± 15.1		

*Mean difference is the comparison of each item between HDR-DP and C-DP (HDR − C).

in the glaucoma group. This finding was possibly due to the higher false-positive rate among normal disc photographs and glaucoma suspect photographs. Both slit defect mimicking true wedge-shaped RNFL defect and unrecognized defect in diffuse RNFL loss images could be the explanation for high false-positive results. Differences between the HDR-DP and C-DP techniques for RNFL defect detection in each quadrant were not observed. This may be explained by the fact that HDR potentially improved visualization of not only the RNFL but also the disc characteristics, which may have led to the bias of RNFL defect at the corresponding disc area.

Interobserver agreement in our study was 0.33 (95% CI: 0.21 to 0.45) and 0.43 (95% CI: 0.31 to 0.56) for HDR-DP and C-DP, respectively. This was similar to Callewaert et al. that reported interobserver variability on fundus images of 0.29 for trainees and 0.37 for residents [20]. Even after training, nonexpert ophthalmologists demonstrated interobserver agreement of 0.27 [10]. Although definitions of nonexperienced clinicians/evaluators varied among studies, glaucoma experts always showed better interobserver agreement [21].

There were some limitations in our study. First, low specificity was found due to overestimation of RNFL defect in the HDR-DP group. The RNFL pattern in HDR-DP of normal and glaucoma suspect patients mimicked slit RNFL defect and may have induced false-positive results. Improvement in HDR program parameters may improve overall specificity and increase sensitivity of RNFL defect, when compared to C-DP. Secondly, we performed the study using first-year residents that had only 3 months of clinical ophthalmology training. Although we had briefly trained them on how to evaluate optic disc photograph in glaucoma, their lack of experience remained the predominant drawback. In addition, the residents may have had added difficulty with HDR interpretation, because this was the first time HDR concept was applied to disc photograph. These factors resulted in the high interobserver variations found in our study. Further study is needed using evaluators with different levels of experience. Moreover, we did not explore other specific

characteristics of the optic disc that affect or may affect glaucoma detection. These optic disc characteristics should also be further investigated.

In summary, HDR-DP provided better sensitivity for glaucoma detection than C-DP, but specificity was not improved. HDR-DP might be an effective alternative glaucoma screening tool for general practitioners, nonexpert ophthalmologists, and trainees.

Disclosure

This paper was delivered as a poster presentation at the 6th World Glaucoma Congress, 6–9 June, 2015, Hong Kong.

Conflicts of Interest

The authors declare that they have no conflicts of interest.

Acknowledgments

This study was supported by the Ratchadapisak Sompotch Fund, Faculty of Medicine, Chulalongkorn University.

References

[1] H. A. Quigley and A. T. Broman, "The number of people with glaucoma worldwide in 2010 and 2020," *The British Journal of Ophthalmology*, vol. 90, no. 3, pp. 262–267, 2006.

[2] Y. C. Tham, X. Li, T. Y. Wong, H. A. Quigley, T. Aung, and C. Y. Cheng, "Global prevalence of glaucoma and projections of glaucoma burden through 2040: a systematic review and meta-analysis," *Ophthalmology*, vol. 121, no. 11, pp. 2081–2090, 2014.

[3] J. W. Cheng, Y. Zong, Y. Y. Zeng, and R. L. Wei, "The prevalence of primary angle closure glaucoma in adult Asians: a systematic review and meta-analysis," *PloS One*, vol. 9, no. 7, article e103222, 2014.

[4] R. Robinson, J. Deutsch, H. S. Jones et al., "Unrecognised and unregistered visual impairment," *The British Journal of Ophthalmology*, vol. 78, no. 10, pp. 736–740, 1994.

[5] A. J. King, A. Reddy, J. R. Thompson, and A. R. Rosenthal, "The rates of blindness and of partial sight registration in glaucoma patients," *Eye (London, England)*, vol. 14, Part 4, pp. 613–619, 2000.

[6] Y. Shaikh, F. Yu, and A. L. Coleman, "Burden of undetected and untreated glaucoma in the United States," *American Journal of Ophthalmology*, vol. 158, no. 6, pp. 1121–1129, 2014, e1.

[7] A. Sommer, N. R. Miller, I. Pollack, A. E. Maumenee, and T. George, "The nerve fiber layer in the diagnosis of glaucoma," *Archives of Ophthalmology*, vol. 95, no. 12, pp. 2149–2156, 1977.

[8] H. A. Quigley, N. R. Miller, and T. George, "Clinical evaluation of nerve fiber layer atrophy as an indicator of glaucomatous optic nerve damage," *Archives of Ophthalmology*, vol. 98, no. 9, pp. 1564–1571, 1980.

[9] A. Sommer, J. Katz, H. A. Quigley et al., "Clinically detectable nerve fiber atrophy precedes the onset of glaucomatous field loss," *Archives of Ophthalmology*, vol. 109, no. 1, pp. 77–83, 1991.

[10] C. Breusegem, S. Fieuws, I. Stalmans, and T. Zeyen, "Agreement and accuracy of non-expert ophthalmologists in assessing glaucomatous changes in serial stereo optic disc photographs," *Ophthalmology*, vol. 118, no. 4, pp. 742–746, 2011.

[11] B. Přibyl, A. Chalmers, and P. Zemčík, "Feature point detection under extreme lighting conditions," in *Proceedings of the 28th Spring Conference on Computer Graphics ACM*, pp. 143–150, New York, USA, 2012.

[12] G. Kontogianni, A. Georgopoulos, and A. Doulamis, "HDR imaging for feature detection on detailed architectural scenes," *The International Archives of the Photogrammetry, Remote Sensing and Spatial Information Sciences Architectures Avila, Spain*, vol. 40, no. 5, pp. 325–330, 2015.

[13] B. Parkin, G. Shuttleworth, M. Costen, and C. Davison, "A comparison of stereoscopic and monoscopic evaluation of optic disc topography using a digital optic disc stereo camera," *The British Journal of Ophthalmology*, vol. 85, no. 11, pp. 1347–1351, 2001.

[14] E. L. Lamoureux, K. Lo, J. G. Ferraro et al., "The agreement between the Heidelberg Retina Tomograph and a digital non-mydriatic retinal camera in assessing area cup-to-disc ratio," *Investigative Ophthalmology & Visual Science*, vol. 47, no. 1, pp. 93–98, 2006.

[15] Y. X. Kong, M. A. Coote, E. C. O'Neill et al., "Glaucomatous optic neuropathy evaluation project: a standardized internet system for assessing skills in optic disc examination," *Clinical and Experimental Ophthalmology*, vol. 39, no. 4, pp. 308–317, 2011.

[16] H. H. Chan, D. N. Ong, Y. X. Kong et al., "Glaucomatous optic neuropathy evaluation (GONE) project: the effect of monoscopic versus stereoscopic viewing conditions on optic nerve evaluation," *American Journal of Ophthalmology*, vol. 157, no. 5, pp. 936–944, 2014.

[17] E. C. O'Neill, L. U. Gurria, S. S. Pandav et al., "Glaucomatous Optic Neuropathy Evaluation Project: factors associated with underestimation of glaucoma likelihood," *JAMA Ophthalmology*, vol. 132, no. 5, pp. 560–566, 2014.

[18] H. W. Bae, N. Lee, C. Y. Kim, M. Choi, S. Hong, and G. J. Seong, "Comparison of three types of images for the detection of retinal nerve fiber layer defects," *Optometry and Vision Science*, vol. 92, no. 4, pp. 500–505, 2015.

[19] E. D. Marlow, M. M. McGlynn, and N. M. Radcliffe, "A novel optic nerve photograph alignment and subtraction technique for the detection of structural progression in glaucoma," *Acta Ophthalmologica*, vol. 92, no. 4, pp. e267–e272, 2014.

[20] S. Callewaert, S. Fieuws, I. Stalmans, and T. Zeyen, "Appraisal of optic disc stereo photos pre- and post-training session," *Bulletin de la Societe Beige d'Ophthalmologie*, vol. 316, pp. 27–32, 2010.

[21] J. Scheetz, K. Koklanis, M. Long, K. Lawler, L. Karimi, and M. E. Morris, "Validity and reliability of eye healthcare professionals in the assessment of glaucoma - a systematic review," *International Journal of Clinical Practice*, vol. 69, no. 6, pp. 689–702, 2015.

23

Outcome of Primary Nonpenetrating Deep Sclerectomy in Patients with Steroid-Induced Glaucoma

Abdelhamid Elhofi⑩ and **Hany Ahmed Helaly**⑩

Ophthalmology Department, Faculty of Medicine, Alexandria University, Alexandria, Egypt

Correspondence should be addressed to Hany Ahmed Helaly; hany209209@yahoo.com

Academic Editor: Ciro Costagliola

Purpose. To evaluate the outcome of primary nonpenetrating deep sclerectomy (NPDS) in patients with steroid-induced glaucoma. *Methods.* This was a retrospective interventional clinical study that included 60 eyes of 60 steroid-induced glaucoma patients that had undergone NPDS. Patients were followed up for 4 years. Data from the records was retrieved as regards corrected distance visual acuity (CDVA), intraocular pressure (IOP), visual field mean defect (dB), and number of antiglaucoma medications needed if any. Complete success of the surgical outcome was considered an IOP ≤ 21 mmHg with no antiglaucoma medications. Qualified success was considered an IOP ≤ 21 mmHg using antiglaucoma medications. *Results.* The mean age was 21.2 ± 8.5 years (ranged from 12 to 35 years). At 48 months, mean IOP was 13.6 ± 2.8 mmHg (range 11–23 mmHg). This represented 60% reduction of mean IOP from preoperative levels. One case had YAG laser goniopuncture. Three cases required needling followed by ab interno revision. Using ANOVA test, there was a statistically significant difference between preoperative and postoperative mean IOP values ($P = 0.032$). Twelve, 16, and 20 patients required topical antiglaucoma medications at 24, 26, and 48 months postoperative, respectively. *Conclusion.* Primary nonpenetrating deep sclerectomy is a safe and an effective method of treating eyes with steroid-induced glaucoma. No major complications were encountered. After 4 years of follow-up, complete success rate was 56.7% and qualified success rate was 70%.

1. Introduction

Steroid-induced glaucoma (SIG) is considered as a secondary open-angle glaucoma. It can occur with topical, periocular, or systemic routes of administration of steroids [1, 2]. Like primary open-angle glaucoma, the main problem is pathology of the trabecular meshwork. The exact pathogenesis is not fully understood, but it is suggested that corticosteroids decrease the conventional trabecular outflow and thus increase the intraocular pressure (IOP). Corticosteroids cause accumulation of glycosaminoglycans in the trabecular meshwork, which leads to increasing outflow resistance [3–6].

The MYOC gene is equally expressed in the trabecular meshwork cells. Normal myocilin increases in response to trabecular meshwork stress, increased IOP, or dexamethasone, suggesting it has a protective role. Mutations in this gene cause the formation of an abnormal TIGR/MYOC protein that causes trabecular meshwork (TM) clogging and increases outflow resistance [6–8]. Also, the effect of steroids on inhibiting phagocytosis of TM endothelial cells and decreasing the expression of extracellular proteinases may play a role in the pathogenesis of SIG [9–11].

Nonpenetrating deep sclerectomy (NPDS) is a nonpenetrating glaucoma procedure that involves the removal of a deep scleral flap [12, 13]. This leads to the formation of a scleral space where the aqueous humor is collected and then drained either to the subconjunctival space or to the suprachoroidal space. It works by deroofing Schlemm's canal (SC) and the removal of juxtacanalicular trabecular meshwork as well as a part of the corneoscleral trabecular meshwork [14–17]. The main resistance to aqueous humor outflow lies in those membranes. Yet, NPDS maintains an intact part of the TM which allows gradual decrease in the IOP preventing the sudden hypotony that occurs with the penetrating glaucoma surgery. Space-maintaining devices, such as collagen and hydrophilic acrylic implants, are used with the NPDS to maintain the scleral space during the period of maximal healing. This augments the IOP lowering effect of the surgery [18, 19].

The aim of the current study was to evaluate the outcome of primary nonpenetrating deep sclerectomy in patients with steroid-induced glaucoma.

2. Subjects and Methods

This was a retrospective interventional clinical study that included 60 eyes of 60 steroid-induced glaucoma patients. Records of the patients were revised, and the patients were recalled for a final follow-up visit. The included patients were nonresponsive or had intolerance to maximal medical treatment and had undergone a primary nonpenetrating deep sclerectomy with a collagen implant. All cases were operated upon by the same surgeon (A.E.). Included patients had complete records covering a follow-up period of at least 4 years. Patients were excluded if they had other ocular pathology or comorbidity, for example, had complicated cataract, had congenital glaucoma, or had previous laser or surgical intervention before NPDS. Patients with incomplete data or follow-up period were also excluded.

The current study was approved by the local ethics committee of the Faculty of Medicine, Alexandria University, Egypt. Tenets of the Declaration of Helsinki were followed. All patients signed an informed consent at the final follow-up visits.

2.1. Surgical Technique. The cases were operated upon using general anesthesia. A fornix-based superior conjunctival flap was done. Dissection of a superficial scleral flap (one-third of the scleral depth) was continued until a clear cornea is reached anteriorly; the dimensions of the rectangular flap were 5×5 mm. This was followed by the application of 0.02% of mitomycin C for 2 minutes using soaked sponges under the scleral flap and the conjunctiva, then a thorough wash with a balanced salt solution. A 4×4 mm deeper scleral flap was dissected anteriorly to Schlemm's canal and continued further anterior in the cornea to create a trabeculo-Descemet's window. The deep scleral flap was excised. A collagen implant was used to maintain the space created and fixed with a single 10-0 suture. The superficial scleral flap was then sutured using 10-0 nylon sutures. The conjunctiva was sutured with 8-0 absorbable sutures. Postoperative topical antibiotic and steroid were prescribed 5 times daily for the first month, and then steroid eye drops were tapered slowly. Any complications were recorded. Also, any further intervention needed was recorded such as yttrium aluminum garnet (YAG) laser goniopuncture, needling, or ab interno revision plus subconjunctival 5-fluouracil injection.

Needling was performed under topical anesthesia using 27-gauge needle. The needle was used to dissect adhesion under the superficial scleral flap. At the end of the procedure, subconjunctival injection of 0.5 ml of 5-flourouracil was done. The technique of ab interno revision was as follows: In the operating room under topical anesthesia using methyl cellulose injection in the anterior chamber through a side port, a spatula was inserted either temporally or nasally until the tip of the spatula is seen under the conjunctiva doing

synechiolysis with a sweeping to and fro movement attacking the contralateral side of the scleral flap. This was followed by removing the methyl cellulose by washing the anterior chamber by balanced saline solution. This would form the bleb ensuring success of the procedure converting it into a penetrating trabeculectomy. Finally, subconjunctival injection of 0.5 ml of 5-flourouracil was done.

Patients were followed up for 4 years. Data from the records was retrieved as regards corrected distance visual acuity (CDVA), IOP, visual field mean defect (dB), and number of antiglaucoma medications needed if any.

Corrected distance visual acuity was measured and expressed in logMAR units for statistical analysis preoperative and up to 48 months following surgery. Rules mentioned by Holladay [20] for calculating average visual acuity were followed. Haag-Streit Goldmann applanation tonometer AT 900 (Haag-Streit, Berne, Switzerland) was used for IOP measurements. Intraocular pressure measurements were taken while the patient was seated at a slit lamp. All measurements were obtained during the daily office work hours by the same operator to minimize the variations. An average of 3 reliable measurements was recorded. Care was taken to avoid squeezing of the eyelids to avoid false rise in the IOP. Visual field testing was done using Humphrey field analyzer (Humphrey Instruments, San Leandro, Calif) automated perimetry. The 24-2 test was performed using white stimulus on white background. Patients were instructed before taking the visual field exam. The first visual field test result was discarded to avoid the learning curve effect. All visual field tests were done by the same operator. Also, an average visual field mean defect of 3 reliable tests was recorded. Unreliable visual field tests (e.g., presence of artifacts or sleepy patients) were excluded and repeated.

Complete success of the surgical outcome was considered an IOP ≤ 21 mmHg with no antiglaucoma medications. Qualified success was considered an IOP ≤ 21 mmHg using antiglaucoma medications. Failure was defined as an IOP > 21 mmHg despite the use of medications, an IOP < 4 mmHg (hypotony), or a need for another glaucoma intervention was present.

Data analysis was performed using the software SPSS for Windows version 20.0 (SPSS Inc., Chicago, USA). Quantitative data were described using range, mean, and standard deviation. Normality of data samples was evaluated using the Kolmogorov-Smirnov test. ANOVA test was used to compare between different means. Paired *t*-test was used for comparisons between means of the preoperative and postoperative data. Kaplan-Meier method was used for survival analysis to report complete success and qualified success percentages along time. Chi-square test was used to compare between different percentages. Differences were considered statistically significant when the associated P value was less than 0.05.

3. Results

The study included 60 eyes of 60 patients. Thirty-four patients (57%) were males and 36 patients (43%) were females. The mean age was 21.2 ± 8.5 years (ranged from 12 to 35 years). Most of the patients were exposed to steroids for a long duration of time (6 months or more). Prolonged use of topical steroids was the cause in 52 patients representing 87% of the cases while prolonged use of systemic steroids was the cause in 8 patients representing 13% of the cases.

The mean preoperative CDVA was 0.37 ± 0.13 logMAR (range 0.1–0.7 logMAR). The mean preoperative IOP was 34.22 ± 6.90 mmHg (range 27–45 mmHg). The mean deviation of preoperative visual field defect was -12.51 ± 7.33 dB (range −23.44 to −2.2 dB). The average number of preoperative anti glaucoma medications was 2.47 ± 0.51.

Mean postoperative IOP at 6 months was 12.3 ± 2.1 mmHg (range 8–15 mmHg). This represented 64% reduction of mean IOP from preoperative levels. No cases needed YAG laser goniopuncture or ab interno revision. Two cases had needling with subconjunctival injection of 5-fluorouracil. At 12 months, mean IOP was 12.3 ± 2.6 mmHg (range 8–17 mmHg). Two patients needed YAG laser goniopuncture. Three cases required needling and no cases needed ab interno revision. Mean postoperative IOP at 24 months was 12.8 ± 3.2 mmHg (range 9–18 mmHg). Another two patients needed YAG laser goniopuncture. Three cases required needling and one case needed ab interno revision. Mean postoperative IOP at 36 months was 13.3 ± 3.1 mmHg (range 10–23 mmHg). No other cases had YAG laser goniopuncture. Two cases required needling followed by ab interno revision. At 48 months, mean IOP was 13.6 ± 2.8 mmHg (range 11–23 mmHg). This represented 60% reduction of mean IOP from preoperative levels. One case had YAG laser goniopuncture. Three cases required needling followed by ab interno revision. Using ANOVA test, there was a statistically significant difference between preoperative and postoperative mean IOP values ($P = 0.032$). Using paired t-test to compare each postoperative mean IOP to the preoperative levels, the difference was statistically significant ($P < 0.001$) (Table 1). Using paired t-test to compare final 48 months mean IOP with previous means, it was significantly higher than that of 6 months, 12 months, and 24 months ($P < 0.05$) but was not statistically different from that of 36 months ($P = 0.621$).

Total number of cases that required YAG laser goniopuncture along the 48 months follow-up was 5 cases. As regards needling with subconjunctival injection of 5-fluorououracil, it was done in 13 cases. Ab interno revision was required in 6 cases. Figure 1 shows a survival analysis curve for YAG laser goniopuncture, needling, and ab interno revision. No major postoperative complications were detected. However, cheese wiring of the conjunctival sutures was detected in 8 cases.

Four patients required topical antiglaucoma medications by the end of the 6th month. By the end of the 1st year, eight patients in total required antiglaucoma medications. Twelve, 16, and 20 patients required topical antiglaucoma medications at 24, 26, and 48 months, respectively. Table 2 shows the mean values for topical antiglaucoma medications required at different time intervals. Using ANOVA test, there was a statistically significant difference between preoperative and postoperative mean number of topical medications required ($P = 0.021$). Using multiple paired t-tests, mean number of topical medications required was significantly higher than the mean number of medications required at 6 months, 12 months, 24 months, and 36 months.

TABLE 1: The mean preoperative and postoperative intraocular pressure values among the study group.

	Intraocular pressure (mmHg) (mean ± SD)	P value
Preoperative	34.2 ± 6.9	N/A
At 6 months	12.3 ± 2.1	0.001*
At 12 months	12.3 ± 2.6	0.001*
At 24 months	12.8 ± 3.2	0.001*
At 36 months	13.3 ± 3.1	0.001*
At 48 months	13.6 ± 2.8	0.001*

*Significant using paired t-test to compare with mean preoperative levels.

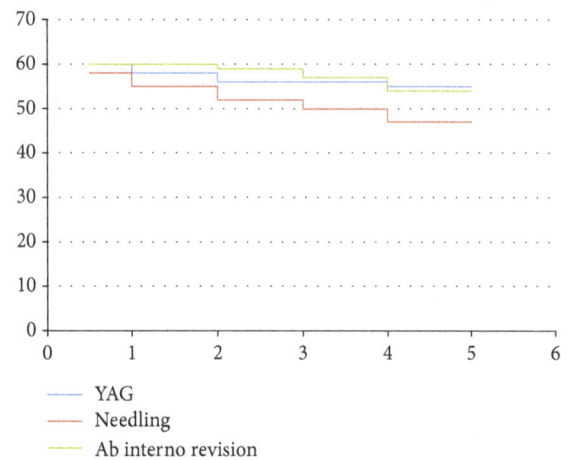

FIGURE 1: Survival analysis for YAG laser goniopuncture, needling, and ab interno revision. y-axis: number of patients; x-axis: time interval in years.

TABLE 2: The mean preoperative and postoperative values for topical antiglaucoma medications required among the study group.

	Medications required (mean ± SD)	P value
Preoperative	2.47 ± 0.51	N/A
At 6 months	0.07 ± 0.25	0.001*
At 12 months	0.13 ± 0.34	0.001*
At 24 months	0.20 ± 0.40	0.001*
At 36 months	0.27 ± 0.45	0.001*
At 48 months	0.33 ± 0.48	0.001*

*Significant using paired t-test to compare with mean preoperative levels.

Table 3 shows the mean preoperative and postoperative CDVA values. Using ANOVA test, there is no statistically significant difference between different means ($P = 0.105$). Using paired t-test, there is no statistically significant difference between preoperative mean CDVA and postoperative levels at 6 months, 12 months, 24 months, 36 months, and 48 months. Table 3 shows the mean preoperative and postoperative visual field defect mean deviation. There is a statistically significant difference between the different means using ANOVA test ($P = 0.021$). Visual field defect mean

TABLE 3: The mean best-corrected visual acuity and the visual field defect mean deviation among the study group.

	CDVA (mean ± SD)	P value	Visual field defect mean deviation (dB) (mean ± SD)	P value
Preoperative	0.37 ± 0.13	N/A	−12.51 ± 7.33	N/A
At 6 months	0.39 ± 0.11	0.112	−12.54 ± 7.12	0.210
At 12 months	0.35 ± 0.14	0.121	−12.65 ± 7.45	0.122
At 24 months	0.39 ± 0.12	0.111	−13.51 ± 8.76	0.038*
At 36 months	0.42 ± 0.12	0.089	−14.77 ± 7.13	0.001*
At 48 months	0.44 ± 0.15	0.067	−15.51 ± 6.83	0.001*

*Significant using paired t-test to compare with mean preoperative levels. CDVA: corrected distance visual acuity; dB: decibel.

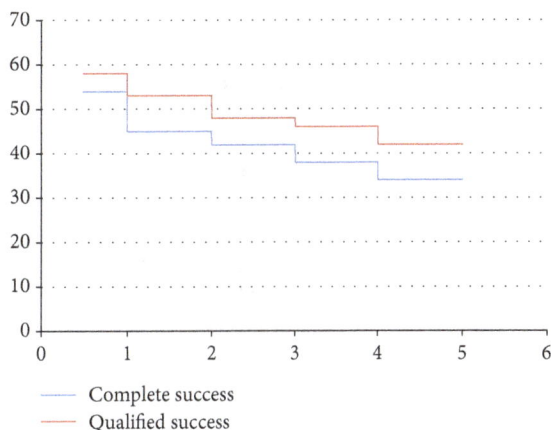

FIGURE 2: Survival analysis curve for complete and qualified success rates. y-axis: number of patients; x-axis: time interval in years.

deviation at 24 months, 36 months, and 48 months was statistically significantly higher than that of preoperative level.

Complete success rate at 6 months was 90% (54 eyes), and qualified success rate at 6 months was 96.7% (58 eyes). Complete success rate was 75% (45 eyes), 70% (40 eyes), and 63.3% (38 eyes) at 12 months, 24 months, and 36 months, respectively. Qualified success rate was 88.3% (53 eyes), 80% (48 eyes), and 76.7% (46 eyes) at 12 months, 24 months, and 36 months, respectively. At 48 months, complete success rate was 56.7% (34 eyes), and qualified success rate was 70% (42 eyes). Figure 2 shows survival curves for complete and qualified success rates at different time intervals.

4. Discussion

Steroid-induced glaucoma can theoretically occur after any route of administration of steroids. This can be troublesome in some cases when the discontinuation of steroid is harmful or when we cannot remove the already injected steroids, for example, in the case of intravitreal injection or the use of an intravitreal dexamethasone implant. The two main routes of administration in the current study were either topical route especially in cases of allergy and post laser vision correction surgery or systemic route in cases of immune disorders. None of the included cases had intravitreal dexamethasone implant. This yielded a relatively young age group in the current study. Males were slightly higher than females. Steroid-induced glaucoma has no gender or racial predilection [21]. The reported incidence of SIG may be underestimated because many cases went undiagnosed especially patients receiving systemic steroids. Most of these patients do not follow up their intraocular pressure. Also, frequent use of topical steroid eye drops without advice from the doctor to relieve chronic eye symptoms leads to increased incidence of SIG among our patients in Egypt. The reported incidence of marked increase of IOP after 4 to 6 weeks of using topical corticosteroids is 5–6% [22].

Nonpenetrating glaucoma surgery avoids the complications of trabeculectomy and yields comparable effect on lowering IOP especially if combined with other step, for example, use of mitomycin C, trabeculotomy, collagen implant, viscocanalostomy [23], or Ex-PRESS mini shunt

[24] (Alcon Inc., Fort Worth, TX). Trabeculectomy has many reported complications such as choroidal effusion, hypotony maculopathy, hyphema, blebitis, and bleb leakage. In 2016, a published study reported an incidence of 30% of hypotony in the follow-up period of trabeculectomy [25].

The current study focuses on reporting 4-year follow-up results of primary deep sclerectomy in SIG patients. The limitations of the study were the retrospective nature and lack of a control group. It had the advantages of long-term follow-up and focusing on steroid-induced glaucoma patients in a relatively young age group. All the NPDS surgeries were performed by the same surgeon with a reproducible technique to minimize variations among different patients. The depth of dissection and the anterior extension of dissection can vary the postoperative results.

In all included eyes, mitomycin C and a collagen implant were used during NPDS to enhance the IOP lowering effect and to prevent fibrosis that would obstruct the aqueous outflow. The relatively younger age population has higher healing capability with more tendencies to subconjunctival fibrosis and expected more difficult control of IOP without augmentation of the effect of NPDS. Also, the high preoperative mean IOP necessitated higher percentage of reduction to reach optimum target IOP levels. In the current study, we achieved 60–64% reduction from the high preoperative IOP levels that were maintained during the 4 years of follow-up periods. Some authors did not use mitomycin C with NPDS like Shaarawy et al. [26] while others (similar to the current study) used mitomycin C 0.2 mg/ml for two minutes [27].

As regards the safety of the procedure among the included patients, no major complications were detected and not a single case of hypotony. Shaarawy et al. [26] reported that no patient developed a shallow/flat anterior chamber, endophthalmitis, or surgery-induced cataract in a 5-year follow-up report of NPDS with collagen implant. During record scanning, 5 cases were transformed into full penetrating trabeculectomy due to accidental perforation during dissection and those cases were excluded from the study. During the follow-up period, the mean CDVA did not statistically differ from the preoperative levels despite a minor drop noticed at

3rd and 4th years. Five patients lost 1 line of CDVA, and none of the patients lost ≥2 lines. This may be attributed to the development of a complicated cataract due to steroids itself or progression of the glaucoma. However, visual acuity is not a good indicator for the success or the follow-up of a glaucoma surgery because there might be other confounding factors affecting the vision. Harju et al. [28] reported long-term results of NPDS with or without mitomycin C in normal tension glaucoma. They also did not report any major complications. They reported that 4 out of 37 eyes had lost 2 or more lines of CDVA, and they reported that those eyes had other pathologies that explained the drop in vision.

At the end of the follow-up period of 4 years, complete success rate was 56.7% (34 eyes). This represented eyes with IOP ≤ 21 mmHg with no additional medications or interventions. Qualified success rate was 70% (42 eyes). This represented eyes with IOP ≤ 21 mmHg with topical medications with no additional interventions. Unlike others [29–31], we considered further interventions such as needling a surgical failure and excluded those eyes from the complete success. They considered needling as an enhancement to reestablish a good filtration in a preexisting bleb. However, there are no standards for this subject as Heuer et al. [32] opposed this like our study. When the postoperative IOP level was unsatisfactory (either >21 mmHg or there was a progression in the mean deviation of the visual field defect), an intervention in the form of YAG laser goniopuncture, needling, or ab interno revision was resorted to. The authors preferred ab interno revision over needling because the latter is a blind procedure, whereas in ab interno revision, the surgeon can see what he/she is doing. When needling failed once, we resorted to ab interno revision. Koukkoulli et al. [33] reported 64% 1 year success after needling post NPDS and 40% 5-year success. The rate of YAG laser goniopuncture was minimal in the current study (5 eyes representing 8.3%) which was much lower than that reported in other studies [26]. Anand and Pilling [34] reported an annual rate of YAG laser goniopuncture around 20%. Topical medications were tried first to control IOP before the decision to intervene.

The authors preferred ab interno revision under vision and subconjunctival 5 fluorouracil injections over YAG laser goniopuncture because in many cases the trabeculo-Descemet's membrane could not be easily visualized besides the unfamiliarity of this technique to us. Also, YAG laser goniopuncture might lead to iris incarceration into the trabeculo-Descemet's membrane as a complication in up to 32% of the cases [28, 34].

Eksioglu et al. [35] evaluated the outcomes of Ahmed glaucoma valve (AGV) in the management of elevated IOP secondary to steroid use. They retrospectively evaluated 9 eyes of 5 patients. The mean age of their included patients was comparable to the current study (25.0 ± 8.3 years), and the mean follow-up period was 38.4 ± 13.2 months. The preoperative mean IOP level was 41.0 ± 8.3 mmHg and 12.8 ± 4.2 mmHg at 48th month. The degree of IOP reduction using AGV was comparable to our results using deep sclerectomy. They reported a decrease of mean topical antiglaucomatous medications used from 2.8 ± 0.4 preoperative to 0.4 ± 0.9 at 48 months postoperative, which was also comparable

to our results. Complete success rate was obtained in 7 (77%) eyes with no cases with failure. They reported 2 eyes with hypotony with choroidal detachment in one eye. Hyphema was reported in one eye. In our study, we had no case of hypotony despite the larger number of included patients in the current study. Ahmed glaucoma valve can provide comparable success as regards IOP management but somehow more liable to complication especially hypotony and the related complications like choroidal detachment. Nonpenetrating deep sclerectomy appears to be a more safe option with similar effect.

Trabeculectomy is considered the gold standard surgical procedure for most glaucoma cases. However, it is associated with a high incidence of early and late complications and surgical failure often observed over time [36]. Honjo et al. [37] investigated the effect of trabeculectomy on the eyes suffering from SIG. They retrospectively analyzed the results of 14 eyes of 7 patients with an average follow-up period of 60.6 ± 33.5 months. They concluded that intraocular pressure was well controlled ≤ to 21 mmHg at the final examinations. However, they reported the usual hypotony-related and bleb-related complications associated with trabeculectomy.

In conclusion, primary nonpenetrating deep sclerectomy is a safe and an effective method of treating eyes with steroid-induced glaucoma. No major complications were encountered. After 4 years of follow-up, complete success rate was 56.7%, and qualified success rate was 70%.

Abbreviations

SIG: Steroid-induced glaucoma
IOP: Intraocular pressure
TM: Trabecular meshwork
NPDS: Nonpenetrating deep sclerectomy
SC: Schlemm's canal
YAG: Yttrium aluminum garnet
CDVA: Corrected distance visual acuity
dB: Decibel
AGV: Ahmed glaucoma valve.

Conflicts of Interest

The authors declare that they have no conflicts of interest.

Authors' Contributions

Dr. Abdelhamid Elhofi contributed the following: the idea and concept of the study, shared in writing the manuscript, and collection of data. Dr. Hany Ahmed Helaly contributed the following: shared in the idea of the study, writing the manuscript, and analysis of the data. All authors contributed equally to the drafting, critical revision, and final approval of the manuscript.

References

[1] Y. Dang, K. Kaplowitz, H. A. Parikh et al., "Steroid-induced glaucoma treated with trabecular ablation in a matched comparison with primary open-angle glaucoma," *Clinical & Experimental Ophthalmology*, vol. 44, no. 9, pp. 783–788, 2016.

[2] B. M. Braunger, R. Fuchshofer, and E. R. Tamm, "The aqueous humor outflow pathways in glaucoma: a unifying concept of disease mechanisms and causative treatment," *European Journal of Pharmaceutics and Biopharmaceutics*, vol. 95, Part B, pp. 173–181, 2015.

[3] I. Rybkin, R. Gerometta, G. Fridman, O. Candia, and J. Danias, "Model systems for the study of steroid-induced IOP elevation," *Experimental Eye Research*, vol. 158, pp. 51–58, 2017.

[4] S. Phulke, S. Kaushik, S. Kaur, and S. S. Pandav, "Steroid-induced glaucoma: an avoidable irreversible blindness," *Journal of Current Glaucoma Practice with DVD*, vol. 11, no. 2, pp. 67–72, 2017.

[5] C. Kopczynski, F. Ahmed, D. Bharali, K. Torrejon, and C. W. Lin, "Anti-fibrotic effects of AR-13324 in a 3D bioengineered human trabecular meshwork model of steroid-induced glaucoma," *Investigative Ophthalmology & Visual Science*, vol. 57, no. 12, p. 5639, 2016.

[6] J. P. Kersey and D. C. Broadway, "Corticosteroid-induced glaucoma: a review of the literature," *Eye*, vol. 20, no. 4, pp. 407–416, 2006.

[7] J. H. Fingert, E. Heon, J. M. Liebmann et al., "Analysis of myocilin mutations in 1703 glaucoma patients from five different populations," *Human Molecular Genetics*, vol. 8, no. 5, pp. 899–905, 1999.

[8] J. H. Fingert, A. F. Clark, J. E. Craig et al., "Evaluation of the myocilin (*MYOC*) glaucoma gene in monkey and human steroid-induced ocular hypertension," *Investigative Ophthalmology & Visual Science*, vol. 42, no. 1, pp. 145–152, 2001.

[9] R. Jones III and D. J. Rhee, "Corticosteroid-induced ocular hypertension and glaucoma: a brief review and update of the literature," *Current Opinion in Ophthalmology*, vol. 17, no. 2, pp. 163–167, 2006.

[10] W. R. Lo, L. Leigh Rowlette, M. Caballero, P. Yang, M. R. Hernandez, and T. Borrás, "Tissue differential microarray analysis of dexamethasone induction reveals potential mechanisms of steroid glaucoma," *Investigative Ophthalmology & Visual Science*, vol. 44, no. 2, pp. 473–485, 2003.

[11] M. R. Razeghinejad and L. J. Katz, "Steroid-induced iatrogenic glaucoma," *Ophthalmic Research*, vol. 47, no. 2, pp. 66–80, 2012.

[12] G. Greifner, S. Roy, and A. Mermoud, "Results of CO2 laser-assisted deep sclerectomy as compared with conventional deep sclerectomy," *Journal of Glaucoma*, vol. 25, no. 7, pp. e630–e638, 2016.

[13] T. Takmaz, H. E. Akmeşe, and N. Onursever, "Comparison of combined phacoemulsification-non-penetrating deep sclerectomy and phacoemulsification-trabeculectomy," *Guoji Yanke Zazhi*, vol. 15, no. 11, pp. 1851–1856, 2015.

[14] A. S. G. Mousa, "Preliminary evaluation of nonpenetrating deep sclerectomy with autologous scleral implant in open-angle glaucoma," *Eye*, vol. 21, no. 9, pp. 1234–1238, 2007.

[15] S. A. Al Obeidan, "Nonpenetrating deep sclerectomy," *Expert Review of Ophthalmology*, vol. 4, no. 3, pp. 299–315, 2009.

[16] J. Cheng, K. Hu, and N. Anand, "Nonpenetrating glaucoma surgery (deep sclerectomy, viscocanaloplasty, and canaloplasty)," in *Managing Complications in Glaucoma Surgery*, pp. 51–72, Springer, Cham, 2017.

[17] S. A. Al-Obeidan, E. E.-D. A. Osman, A. S. Dewedar, P. Kestelyn, and A. Mousa, "Efficacy and safety of deep sclerectomy in childhood glaucoma in Saudi Arabia," *Acta Ophthalmologica*, vol. 92, no. 1, pp. 65–70, 2014.

[18] C. Dalmasso, J. A. Urcola, E. Vecino, J. Cabrerizo, and G. Saracibar, "Postoperative IOP is not related to intrascleral lake morphology after non penetrating deep sclerectomy without scleral implant," *Investigative Ophthalmology & Visual Science*, vol. 55, no. 13, p. 6131, 2014.

[19] S. Yazgan, H. Ates, S. Guven Yilmaz, and T. Celik, "Long-term results of up to 6 years of mitomycin-c augmented non-penetrating deep sclerectomy for pseudoexfoliation glaucoma," *Acta Ophthalmologica*, vol. 94, no. S256, 2016.

[20] J. T. Holladay, "Proper method for calculating average visual acuity," *Journal of Refractive Surgery*, vol. 13, no. 4, pp. 388–391, 1997.

[21] B. Z. Biedner, R. David, A. Grudsky, and U. Sachs, "Intraocular pressure response to corticosteroids in children," *British Journal of Ophthalmology*, vol. 64, no. 6, pp. 430–431, 1980.

[22] M. F. Armaly, "Statistical attributes of the steroid hypertensive response in the clinically normal eye I. The demonstration of three levels of response," *Investigative Ophthalmology & Visual Science*, vol. 4, pp. 187–197, 1965.

[23] S. Bylsma, "Nonpenetrating deep sclerectomy: collagen implant and viscocanalostomy procedures," *International Ophthalmology Clinics*, vol. 39, no. 3, pp. 103–119, 1999.

[24] K. Rao, I. Ahmed, D. A. Blake, and R. S. Ayyala, "New devices in glaucoma surgery," *Expert Review of Ophthalmology*, vol. 4, no. 5, pp. 491–504, 2009.

[25] S. K. Schultz, S. M. Iverson, W. Shi, and D. S. Greenfield, "Safety and efficacy of achieving single-digit intraocular pressure targets with filtration surgery in eyes with progressive normal-tension glaucoma," *Journal of Glaucoma*, vol. 25, no. 2, pp. 217–222, 2016.

[26] T. Shaarawy, M. Karlen, C. Schnyder, F. Achache, E. Sanchez, and A. Mermoud, "Five-year results of deep sclerectomy with collagen implant," *Journal of Cataract & Refractive Surgery*, vol. 27, no. 11, pp. 1770–1778, 2001.

[27] N. Anand, A. Kumar, and A. Gupta, "Primary phakic deep sclerectomy augmented with mitomycin C: long-term outcomes," *Journal of Glaucoma*, vol. 20, no. 1, pp. 21–27, 2011.

[28] M. Harju, S. Suominen, P. Allinen, and E. Vesti, "Long-term results of deep sclerectomy in normal-tension glaucoma," *Acta Ophthalmologica*, vol. 96, no. 2, pp. 154–160, 2018.

[29] B. Jongsareejit, A. Tomidokoro, T. Mimura, G. Tomita, S. Shirato, and M. Araie, "Efficacy and complications after trabeculectomy with mitomycin C in normal-tension glaucoma," *Japanese Journal of Ophthalmology*, vol. 49, no. 3, pp. 223–227, 2005.

[30] S. J. Gedde, J. C. Schiffman, W. J. Feuer et al., "Treatment outcomes in the tube versus trabeculectomy (TVT) study after five

years of follow-up," *American Journal of Ophthalmology*, vol. 153, no. 5, pp. 789–803.e2, 2012.

[31] H. Jayaram, N. G. Strouthidis, and D. S. Kamal, "Trabeculectomy for normal tension glaucoma: outcomes using the Moorfields Safer Surgery technique," *British Journal of Ophthalmology*, vol. 100, no. 3, pp. 332–338, 2015.

[32] D. K. Heuer, K. Barton, F. Grehn, T. Shaarawy, and M. Sherwood, "Consensus on definitions of success," in *World Glaucoma Association Guidelines on Design and Reporting of Glaucoma Surgical Trials*, T. Shaarawy, F. Grehn, and M. Sherwood, Eds., pp. 15–24, Kugler, The Hague, Amsterdam, Netherlands, 2009.

[33] A. Koukkoulli, F. Musa, and N. Anand, "Long-term outcomes of needle revision of failing deep sclerectomy blebs," *Graefe's Archive for Clinical and Experimental Ophthalmology*, vol. 253, no. 1, pp. 99–106, 2015.

[34] N. Anand and R. Pilling, "Nd:YAG laser goniopuncture after deep sclerectomy: outcomes," *Acta Ophthalmologica*, vol. 88, no. 1, pp. 110–115, 2010.

[35] U. Eksioglu, C. Oktem, G. Sungur, M. Yakin, G. Demirok, and F. Ornek, "Outcomes of Ahmed glaucoma valve implantation for steroid-induced elevated intraocular pressure in patients with retinitis pigmentosa," *International Ophthalmology*, pp. 1–6, 2017.

[36] T. HaiBo, K. Xin, L. ShiHeng, and L. Lin, "Comparison of Ahmed glaucoma valve implantation and trabeculectomy for glaucoma: a systematic review and meta-analysis," *PLoS One*, vol. 10, no. 2, article e0118142, 2015.

[37] M. Honjo, H. Tanihara, M. Inatani, and Y. Honda, "External trabeculotomy for the treatment of steroid-induced glaucoma," *Journal of Glaucoma*, vol. 9, no. 6, pp. 483–485, 2000.

24

Peripapillary Vessel Density Reversal after Trabeculectomy in Glaucoma

Jung Hee In ⓘD, So Yeon Lee ⓘD, Seok Ho Cho ⓘD, and Young Jae Hong ⓘD

Glaucoma Center, Nune Eye Hospital, Seoul, Republic of Korea

Correspondence should be addressed to Young Jae Hong; youngjhong@gmail.com

Academic Editor: Ciro Costagliola

Purpose. To evaluate the microvascular changes at the peripapillary area and optic disc in glaucomatous eyes after IOP lowering by trabeculectomy using OCT angiography. *Methods.* 25 patients with primary open-angle glaucoma (POAG) who underwent trabeculectomy by a single surgeon were evaluated. Using optical coherence tomography angiography, vessel density was evaluated within the whole image, peripapillary, nasal region, and temporal region. Peripapillary vessel density was measured preoperative, 1 week, 1 month, and 3 months postoperatively in POAG patients. Reversal of vessel density was calculated for all analyzed areas. *Results.* The intraocular pressure (IOP) decreased from 30.92 ± 6.32 mmHg (range, 18–44) to 12.64 ± 3.35 mmHg (range, 8–22) at 3-month postoperatively. Compared with the preoperative baseline value, whole vessel density, peripapillary vessel density (PvD), and PvD in nasal region and temporal region were significantly increased at 3-month postoperatively. The magnitude of the vessel density reversal was significantly associated with higher preoperative IOP and greater IOP reduction. *Conclusions.* A significant increase in the peripapillary vessel density was demonstrated after trabeculectomy using OCT angiography. The reversal of peripapillary vessel density was associated with higher preoperative IOP and greater IOP reduction. Our postoperative results suggest that the ocular perfusion impairment by high intraocular pressure can be improved by IOP reduction, and the reversal of microvasculature may contribute to the rate of glaucoma progression.

1. Introduction

Although intraocular pressure- (IOP-) related stress and strain play a central role in glaucoma [1, 2], the potential role of the ocular blood flow in the pathophysiology of glaucoma has been debated and extensively investigated [3, 4].

The association between ocular perfusion and glaucoma has been investigated using several imaging modalities such as fluorescein angiography (FA), Heidelberg retina flowmeter, color Doppler imaging, laser Doppler flowmetry (LDF), and laser speckle flowgraphy (LSFG).

FA has been extensively used to investigate vascular abnormalities in glaucoma, and previous studies reported absolute disc filling defects in glaucoma eyes [5–15].

Optical coherence tomography angiography (OCTA) is a new imaging technique that enables visualization of the retinal and choroidal microvasculatures. It enables visualization of retinal and choroidal blood flow that are not detectable with conventional angiography.

Recent studies using OCTA in which the majority of study population had primary open-angle glaucoma (POAG) demonstrated decreased optic disc and peripapillary perfusion in glaucoma eyes [14, 15]. Structural reversibility after glaucoma treatment is well documented. Reversible optic disc cupping following acute IOP lowering has been known to occur for decades [16–21]. Quigley [16] described an improvement of the optic disc cupping appearance in 40% of children with successful IOP lowering after trabeculectomy.

Also, lamina cribrosa depth can be reduced after surgical IOP lowering in patients with POAG, and the degree of that reduction was associated with the degree of IOP lowering achieved [22].

However, the reversal of the microvasculature in glaucoma has so far not been investigated using OCT angiography.

The present study evaluates the microvascular changes at the peripapillary area in glaucomatous eyes after IOP lowering by trabeculectomy using OCT angiography.

2. Methods

2.1. Subjects. This prospective study followed the principles of the Declaration of Helsinki and was approved by the Institutional Review Board of the Nune Eye Hospital.

Indications for trabeculectomy were IOP deemed to be associated with a high risk for progression or glaucomatous progression of the visual field or optic disc despite maximally tolerated medications.

Primary open-angle glaucoma (POAG) who were on maximum tolerable medical therapy showed progressive visual loss and judged by glaucoma specialist (YJH) in our center to require trabeculectomy were included.

All participants underwent comprehensive ophthalmic examinations that included best-corrected visual acuity (BCVA), slit-lamp biomicroscopy, gonioscopy, Goldmann applanation tonometry, and dilated stereoscopic examination of the optic disc. They also underwent central corneal thickness measurement using the Pentacam (OCULUS, Wetzlar, Germany), spectral-domain OCT (Cirrus HD-OCT; Carl Zeiss Meditec), standard automated perimetry (Humphrey Field Analyzer II 750; 30-2 Swedish interactive threshold algorithm; Carl-Zeiss Meditec, Dublin, CA), and OCT angiography using the RTVue-XR Avanti scanner (Optovue Inc., Fremont, CA, USA).

For inclusion, all the participants had to meet the following criteria at the initial assessment: best-corrected visual acuity of 20/40 or better, spherical refractive error between −6.0 and +3.0D, cylinder correction within +3D, and a normal anterior chamber and open-angle on slit-lamp and gonioscopic examination.

We defined POAG as the presence of glaucomatous optic nerve damage and associated visual field defects without ocular diseases or conditions that may elevate the IOP. A glaucomatous visual field change was defined as (1) outside normal limit on glaucoma Hemifield test or (2) 3 abnormal points with $P < 0.05$ probability of being normal and 1 point with a $P < 0.01$ by pattern deviation, or (3) pattern standard deviation of $P < 0.05$. A visual field measurement was considered as reliable when false-positive/negative results were <25% and fixation losses were <20%.

Eyes that had undergone previous intraocular surgery or coexisting retinal or neurologic diseases that could affect the visual field were excluded from this study.

All surgeries were performed under pin-point anesthesia. Limbus-based trabeculectomy involving the use of a 2×3 mm rectangular half-thickness scleral flap was performed by a single experienced surgeon (YJH) and the same method. All eyes received MMC application intraoperatively. A thin cellulose sponge (approximately 6×12 mm) soaked with MMC, concentration of 0.2 to 0.4 mg/cc, was placed over the intended site of the sclera flap for 1-2 min. The concentration and duration were based on the preoperative evaluation of each patient's risk factors for failure (conjunctival hyperaemia, inflammation, and scarring).

The postoperative regimen included topical gatifloxacin 4 times a day for 4 weeks and prednisolone every 2 hours in the first 1 week and then tapered over the next 4 weeks.

All the ocular hypotensive medications were continued up to the time of surgery. The preoperative IOP was defined as the average of 2 measurements within 2 weeks before trabeculectomy. We recorded IOP measurements by Goldmann applanation tonometry at each follow-up visit.

2.2. Optical Coherence Tomography Angiography. The OCTA imaging system provides a noninvasive method for visualizing the optic nerve head (ONH) and retinal vasculature. The image acquisition technique is optimized for the split-spectrum amplitude-decorrelation angiography (SSADA) algorithm described in detail by Jia et al. [23].

The system uses an SSADA method to distinguish the movement of red blood cells within the lumen of retinal and choroidal vessels and provide a high-resolution 3-dimensional visualization of retinal microvasculature.

The OCTA characterizes vascular information at each retinal layer as an en face angiogram, a vessel density map, and quantitatively as vessel density (percentage), calculated as the percentage area occupied by flowing blood vessels in the selected region.

The software automatically fits an ellipse to the optic disc margin and calculates the average vessel density within the ONH (referred to as the inside disc vessel density).

The peripapillary region was defined as a 0.75 mm-wide elliptical annulus extending from the optic disc boundary, using the intrinsic software provided by Optovue.

Whole en face image vessel density was measured in the entire 4.5×4.5 mm image, and peripapillary vessel density (PvD) was calculated in the region defined as a 0.75 mm-wide elliptical annulus extending from the optic disc boundary (Figure 1).

The peripapillary vessels were analyzed in superficial retinal layers from the radial peripapillary capillary (RPC) segment. The RPC segment extends from the internal limiting membrane to the nerve fiber layer. The peripapillary region was also divided into 6 sectors based on the Garway-Heath map [24] and vessel densities for the entire peripapillary area (average) and each sector were determined.

To compare the changes in the vessel density of the nasal and temporal areas, we defined the average of superotemporal, temporal, and inferotemporal sectors as the temporal region and the average of superonasal, nasal, and inferonasal sectors as the nasal region (Figure 1).

We reviewed scans, and those with poor image quality, as defined by the following criteria, were excluded: (1) a signal strength index <48 (1 = minimum, 100 = maximum), (2) poor clarity, (3) residual motion artifacts visible as an irregular vessel pattern or disc boundary on the en face angiogram, (4) a local weak signal, and (5) RNFL segmentation errors.

The delineation of the disc margin was reviewed for accuracy and adjusted manually, if required.

PvD was examined at 1 day before surgery and 1 week, 1 month, and 3 months postoperatively.

2.3. Statistical Analysis. Paired *t*-tests were used to compare preoperative and 3-month postoperative IOP and vessel density.

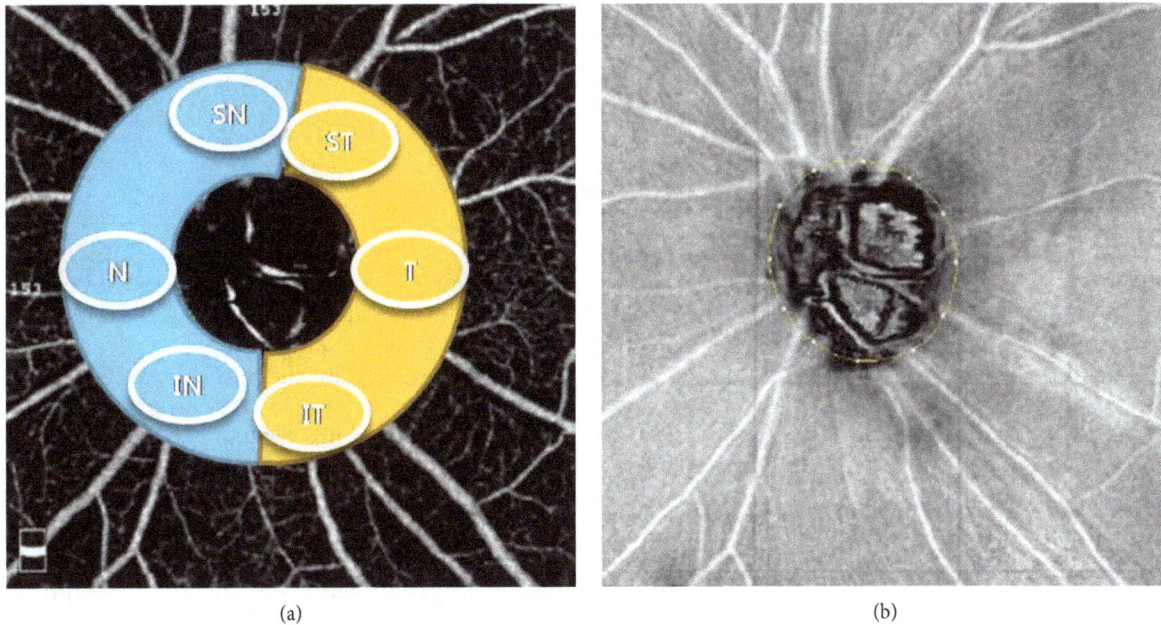

FIGURE 1: Peripapillary vessel density. Peripapillary vessel density was categorized into superonasal, nasal, inferonasal, superotemporal, temporal, and inferotemporal sectors. Peripapillary vessel density map measurement region defined.

Logistic regression analysis was used to determine the factors associated with the change of the PvD. Statistical analyses were performed using SPSS 22.0 software (SPSS Inc, Chicago, IL). $P < 0.05$ was considered significant.

3. Results

25 patients with POAG who underwent trabeculectomy were included.

The mean age was 61.12 ± 11.85 years (range, 37–82), and 10 subjects were women and 15 subjects were men. The mean refractive error (spherical equivalent) was -1.20 ± 1.70 diopters (range, -6.00 to $+1.50$), and the visual field mean deviation was -13.35 ± 6.23 dB (range, -20.82 to -2.28 dB) (Table 1).

The IOP decreased from 30.92 ± 6.32 mmHg (range, 18–44) to 12.64 ± 3.35 mmHg (range, 8–22) at 3-month postoperatively. Compared with the preoperative baseline value, whole vessel density, PvD, and PvD in nasal region and temporal region were significantly increased at 3-month postoperatively (whole image: 36.71 ± 5.81 preoperatively and 38.13 ± 6.21 at 3-month postoperatively ($P = 0.05$); PvD: 43.02 ± 6.83 preoperatively and 45.11 ± 6.89 at 3-month postoperatively ($P < 0.001$); PvD in nasal region: 41.59 ± 6.89 preoperatively and 43.43 ± 7.11 at 3-month postoperatively ($p < 0.008$); PvD in temporal region: 43.94 ± 8.13 preoperatively and 45.83 ± 7.60 at 3-month postoperatively ($P < 0.02$)) (Table 2).

The PvD decreased slightly at 1-week postoperatively, and thereafter, vessel density increased gradually after postoperative 1 week. At 3 months postoperatively, there was a significant increase compared to preoperative vessel density (Figure 2).

Linear regression showed significant influence of greater IOP reduction on the change of the whole and peripapillary

TABLE 1: Patients' clinical demographics ($N = 25$).

Variables	Mean ± standard deviation
Age (years)	61.12 ± 11.85
Gender (male/female)	15/10
Baseline IOP (mmHg)	30.92 ± 6.32
Spherical equivalent	-1.20 ± 1.70
Central corneal thickness (μm)	558.8 ± 47.23
Average RNFL thickness (μm)	65.4 ± 18.13
Visual field MD (dB)	-13.35 ± 6.23

Values are presented as mean + SD unless otherwise indicated. n = number of eyes; RNFL = retinal nerve fiber layer; IOP = intraocular pressure; MD = mean deviation.

vessel density. And, there were significant influences of higher preoperative IOP and greater IOP reduction on the change of the PvD of nasal and temporal region. In the multivariate analysis, none of the factors were associated with the reversal of PvD (Table 3).

3.1. Representative Case. Figure 3 shows 1 case that underwent trabeculectomy. Top row image indicated the preoperative PvD and bottom row image indicated the postoperative 3-month PvD. The IOP decreased from 32 to 15 mmHg. The IOP was controlled below 18 mmHg after the surgery. There was significant increase of whole and peripapillary vessel density. Note the reversal of the PvD on color-coded peripapillary vessel density map.

4. Discussion

This study investigated the reversal of the PvD after trabeculectomy in glaucomatous eyes.

TABLE 2: Pre- and postoperative (3-month) measurements of the IOP and peripapillary vessel density.

		Preoperative (mean ± SD)	Postoperative, 3 months (mean ± SD)	P value
	IOP (mmHg)	30.92 ± 6.32	12.64 ± 3.35	<0.001
Vessel density (%)	Whole image	36.71 ± 5.81	38.13 ± 6.21	0.05
	Peripapillary	43.02 ± 6.83	45.11 ± 6.89	<0.001
	Nasal sector	41.59 ± 6.89	43.43 ± 7.11	0.008
	Temporal sector	43.94 ± 8.13	45.83 ± 7.60	0.02

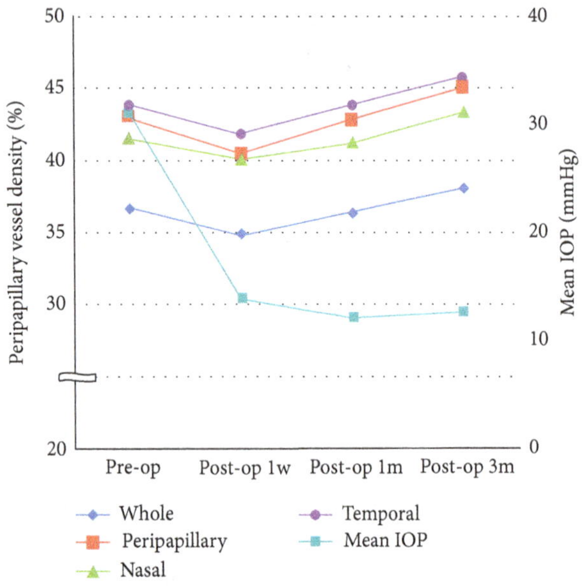

FIGURE 2: Change in peripapillary vessel density and mean IOP after trabeculectomy.

The results of this study demonstrated that the PvD decreased slightly at 1-week postoperatively and thereafter vessel density increased gradually after postoperative 1 week. At 3 months postoperatively, there was a significant increase compared to preoperative vessel density.

The vessel density reversal was expected in the nasal region where the RNFL defect was not mainly found, but vessel density reversal was similar in the nasal and temporal regions.

A significant reduction of the vessel density in sectors with RNFL defect has been reported [15, 25, 27], but reversal of vessel density has not been associated with RNFL defect location.

As mentioned earlier, the association between ocular perfusion and glaucoma has been investigated using several imaging modalities. Disc blood flow of glaucoma patients was previously investigated by fluorescein angiography, and fluorescein filling defects in the disc have been found in glaucoma patients [5–8].

In previous laser Doppler flowmetry (LDF) and laser speckle flowgraphy (LSFG) studies [9, 13, 26, 28] peripapillary and ONH blood flow decreased in patients with glaucoma compared with controls.

Also, Liu et al. [15] demonstrated higher repeatability and reproducibility of OCT angiography compared with other noninvasive techniques, such as LDF and LSFG. Several studies have suggested that vascular factors can play

a pathogenic role in glaucoma, and decreased peripapillary retinal vasculature identified by OCTA is clinically useful to observe the glaucoma progression.

In the present study, the preoperative IOP and the IOP reduction were related to the reversal of PvD postoperatively. This means that the higher preoperative IOP and the greater IOP reduction, the greater the PvD reversal.

Our postoperative results suggest that the ocular perfusion impairment by high intraocular pressure can be improved by IOP reduction and the reversal of microvasculature may contribute to the rate of glaucoma progression.

Recently, Zeboulon et al. [29] measured the influence of IOP lowering by filtering surgery on peripapillary and macular vessel density in glaucoma patients using OCT angiography. They demonstrated a very limited effect of surgically induced IOP reduction on peripapillary and macular vessel density. These results are contradictory to those of this study. The discrepancy between the 2 studies may be attributable to several factors. Firstly, in the study by Zeboulon et al. [29], patients were observed for only up to 1 month after trabeculectomy, so the degree of IOP reduction was maintained for a relatively short period. Secondly, the amount of IOP change differs between the studies. In the study by Zeboulon et al. [29], their patients had lower baseline IOP and lower IOP reduction (baseline IOP: 23.7 mmHg; mean IOP reduction: 11.5 mmHg). In contrast, the baseline IOP was 30.9 mmHg and the mean IOP reduction was 18.3 mmHg at 3 months postoperatively in our study.

And, Holló [30] showed that PvD increased in 6 patients after a medical reduction of IOP of at least 50% from baseline in patients with IOP higher than 35 mmHg.

Furthermore, Alnawaiseh et al. [31] demonstrated the improvement of the flow density of the macular and ONH after cataract surgery with iStent. In the iStent group, the mean IOP was 18.2 ± 3.3 mmHg prior to surgery and 13.2 ± 2.3 at follow-up. Despite the small amount of IOP change, the flow density of the macular and ONH improved after surgery.

Also, Shin et al. [32] evaluated the microvascular improvement after trabeculectomy. In the study, microvascular improvement in OCT angiography was arbitrarily defined as a reduction >30% of the area of vascular dropout on the color-coded vessel density map.

In this study, we evaluated the vessel density reversal on the peripapillary vessel density map.

At 1-week postoperatively, vessel density decreased rather than preoperative vessel density. We speculated that extremely low postoperative IOP after trabeculectomy often cause axial length reduction and change in corneal curvature

TABLE 3: Factors associated with change of peripapillary vessel density.

	Angio vessel density (P value)							
	Whole		Peripapillary		Nasal region		Temporal region	
	Univariate	Multivariate	Univariate	Multivariate	Univariate	Multivariate	Univariate	Multivariate
Age (years)	0.187		0.082		0.239		0.124	
Preoperative IOP (mmHg)	0.367		0.197		0.023	0.097	0.036	0.06
IOP reduction	0.028	0.084	0.05	0.178	0.024	0.09	0.05	0.073
Spherical equivalent	0.06		0.069		0.07		0.121	
Central corneal thickness (μm)	0.436		0.236		0.057		0.372	
Average RNFL thickness (μm)	0.227		0.476		0.109		0.162	
Visual field MD (dB)	0.267		0.288		0.284		0.168	

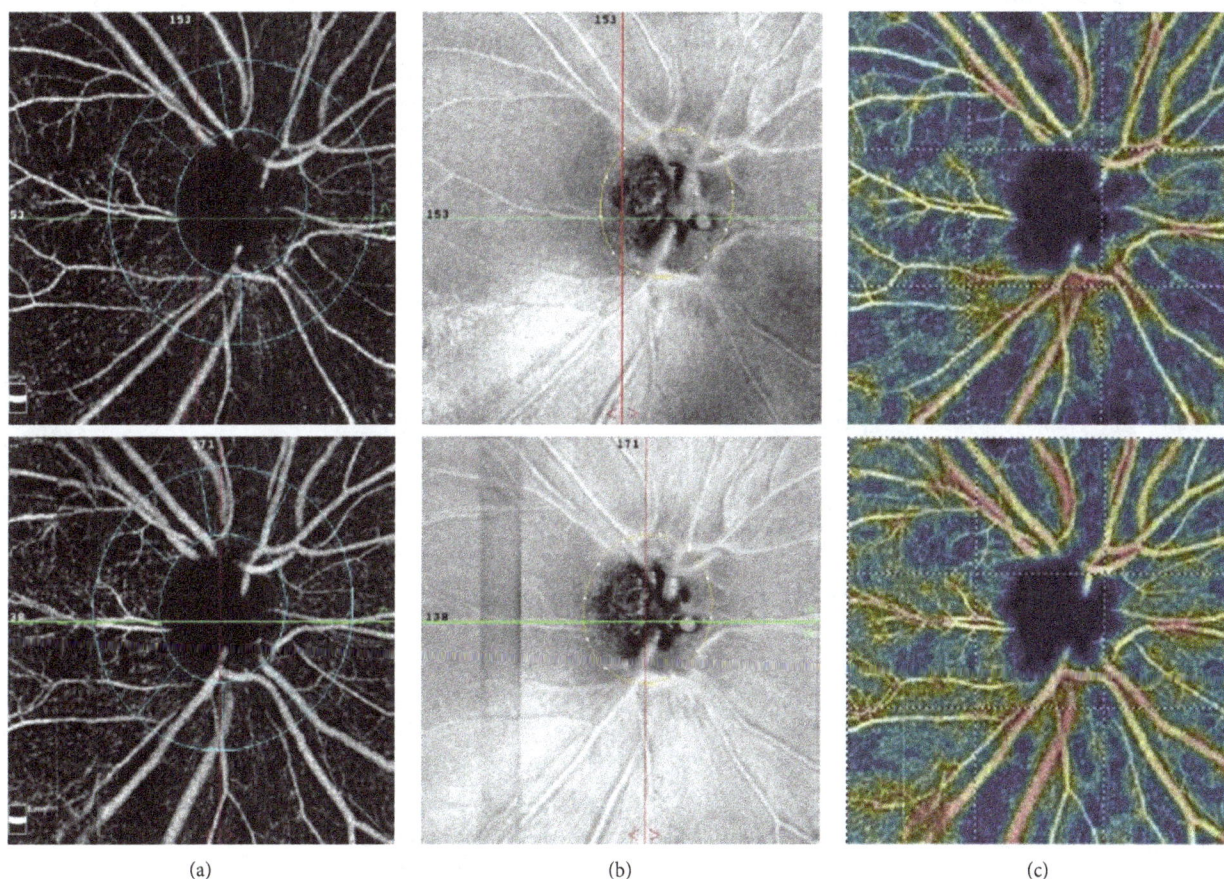

(a)	(b)	(c)

FIGURE 3: Change in peripapillary vessel density and mean IOP after trabeculectomy. Right eye of a 48-year-old female patient. Top row: preoperative peripapillary vessel density; bottom row: postoperative 3-month peripapillary vessel density. Peripapillary vessel density map of the radial peripapillary capillary layers with the measuring ellipse (a), en face retinal nerve fiber layer image (b), and color-coded peripapillary vessel density map (c). Note the change of the peripapillary vessel density.

[33, 34], and this may affect the signal strength of vessel density image in the early postoperative period. Also, postoperative inflammation, postoperative corneal edema, anterior chamber reaction, and hyphema may be variables.

4.1. Study Limitation. Our study has several limitations. Firstly, patients were observed for only up to 3 months after trabeculectomy. This was mainly because the IOP commonly re-elevates after this period. It is possible that reversal of the PvD may persist after this period if IOP remained well controlled.

Second, the small number of patients included is explained by the relative difficulty of performing an OCTA scan on the peripapillary area in glaucoma patients.

Third, the limitation inherent to the OCTA technique is that vessel density cannot differentiate large vessels from small capillaries. Thus, if a change in density is observed, it is unclear as to which vascular network is concerned. By observing the color-coded peripapillary vessel density map, nonetheless, we can hypothesize that capillaries are responsible for the vessel density reversal rather than arterioles and venules.

5. Conclusion

In conclusion, we demonstrated the reversal of PvD after trabeculectomy in patients with glaucoma.

It seems that reduced ocular perfusion induced by high IOP can be improved by IOP reduction, and the vessel density reversal may contribute to glaucoma progression.

The PvD reversal was affected by preoperative IOP and magnitude of IOP lowering. Further study is required to confirm the influence of the vessel density reversal after IOP reduction on glaucoma prognosis.

Conflicts of Interest

The authors do not have any proprietary interests or conflicts of interest.

References

[1] R. N. Weinreb, T. Aung, and F. A. Medeiros, "The pathophysiology and treatment of glaucoma: a review," *JAMA*, vol. 311, no. 18, pp. 1901–1911, 2014.

[2] H. A. Quigley, "Glaucoma," *The Lancet*, vol. 377, no. 9774, pp. 1367–1377, 2011.

[3] J. Flammer, "The vascular concept of glaucoma," *Survey of Ophthalmology*, vol. 38, pp. S3–S6, 1994.

[4] L. Bonomi, G. Marchini, M. Marraffa et al., "Vascular risk factors for primary open angle glaucoma: The Egna-Neumarkt Study," *Ophthalmology*, vol. 107, no. 7, pp. 1287–1293, 2000.

[5] B. Schwartz, J. C. Rieser, and S. L. Fishbein, "Fluorescein angiographic defects of the optic disc in glaucoma," *Archives of Ophthalmology*, vol. 95, no. 11, pp. 1961–1974, 1977.

[6] R. A. Hitchings and G. L. Spaeth, "Fluorescein angiography in chronic simple and low-tension glaucoma," *British Journal of Ophthalmology*, vol. 61, no. 2, pp. 126–132, 1977.

[7] G. Adam and B. Schwartz, "Increased fluorescein filling defects in the wall of the optic disc cup in glaucoma," *Archives of Ophthalmology*, vol. 98, no. 9, pp. 1590–1592, 1980.

[8] N. Plange, M. Kaup, A. Weber et al., "Fluorescein filling defects and quantitative morphologic analysis of the optic nerve head in glaucoma," *Archives of Ophthalmology*, vol. 122, no. 2, pp. 195–201, 2004.

[9] P. Hamard, H. Hamard, J. Dufaux et al., "Optic nerve head blood flow using a laser Doppler velocimeter and haemorheology in primary open angle glaucoma and normal pressure glaucoma," *British Journal of Ophthalmology*, vol. 78, pp. 449–453, 1994.

[10] A. Martinez and M. Sanchez, "Predictive value of color Doppler imaging in a prospective study of visual field progression in primary open-angle glaucoma," *Acta Ophthalmologica Scandinavica*, vol. 83, no. 6, pp. 716–723, 2005.

[11] F. Galassi, A. Sodi, F. Ucci et al., "Ocular hemodynamics and glaucoma prognosis: a color Doppler imaging study," *Archives of Ophthalmology*, vol. 121, no. 12, pp. 1711–1715, 2003.

[12] M. Satilmis, S. Orgul, B. Doubler et al., "Rate of progression of glaucoma correlates with retrobulbar circulation and intraocular pressure," *American Journal of Ophthalmology*, vol. 135, no. 5, pp. 664–669, 2003.

[13] K. Yaoeda, M. Shirakashi, S. Funaki et al., "Measurement of microcirculation in the optic nerve head by laser speckle flowgraphy and scanning laser Doppler flowmetry," *American Journal of Ophthalmology*, vol. 129, no. 6, pp. 734–739, 2000.

[14] Y. Jia, E. Wei, X. Wang et al., "Optical coherence tomography angiography of optic disc perfusion in glaucoma," *Ophthalmology*, vol. 121, no. 7, pp. 1322–1332, 2014.

[15] L. Liu, Y. Jia, H. L. Takusagawa et al., "Optical coherence tomography angiography of the peripapillary retina in glaucoma," *JAMA Ophthalmology*, vol. 133, no. 9, pp. 1045–1052, 2015.

[16] H. A. Quigley, "Childhood glaucoma: results with trabeculotomy and study of reversible cupping," *Ophthalmology*, vol. 89, no. 3, pp. 219–226, 1982.

[17] A. Aydin, G. Wollstein, L. L. Price, J. G. Fujimoto, and J. S. Schuman, "Optical coherence tomography assessment of retinal nerve fiber layer thickness changes after glaucoma surgery," *Ophthalmology*, vol. 110, no. 8, pp. 1506–1511, 2003.

[18] J. Funk, "Increase of neuroretinal rim area after surgical intraocular pressure reduction," *Ophthalmic Surgery*, vol. 21, no. 8, pp. 585–588, 1990.

[19] L. J. Katz, G. L. Spaeth, L. B. Cantor, E. M. Poryzees, and W. C. Steinmann, "Reversible optic disk cupping and visual field improvement in adults with glaucoma," *American Journal of Ophthalmology*, vol. 107, no. 5, pp. 485–492, 1989.

[20] M. R. Lesk, G. L. Spaeth, A. Azuara-Blanco et al., "Reversal of optic disc cupping after glaucoma surgery analyzed with a scanning laser tomography," *Ophthalmology*, vol. 106, no. 5, pp. 1013–1018, 1999.

[21] D. H. Shin, M. Bielik, Y. J. Hong et al., "Reversal of glaucomatous optic disc cupping in adult patients," *Archives of Ophthalmology*, vol. 107, no. 11, pp. 1599–1603, 1989.

[22] E. J. Lee, T. W. Kim, and R. N. Weinreb, "Reversal of lamina cribrosa displacement and thickness after trabeculectomy in glaucoma," *Ophthalmology*, vol. 119, no. 7, pp. 1359–1366, 2012.

[23] Y. Jia, O. Tan, J. Tokayer et al., "Split-spectrum amplitude decorrelation angiography with optical coherence tomography," *Optics Express*, vol. 20, no. 4, pp. 4710–4725, 2012.

[24] D. F. Garway-Heath, D. Poinoosawmy, F. W. Fitzke, and R. A. Hitchings, "Mapping the visual field to the optic disc in normal tension glaucoma eyes," *Ophthalmology*, vol. 107, no. 10, pp. 1809–1815, 2000.

[25] E. J. Lee, K. M. Lee, S. H. Lee, and T. W. Kim, "OCT angiography of the peripapillary retina in primary open-angle glaucoma," *Investigative Opthalmology & Visual Science*, vol. 57, no. 14, pp. 6265–6270, 2016.

[26] J. R. Piltz-Seymour, J. E. Grunwald, S. M. Hariprasad, and J. Dupont, "Optic nerve blood flow is diminished in eyes of primary open angle glaucoma suspects," *American Journal of Ophthalmology*, vol. 132, no. 1, pp. 63–69, 2001.

[27] M. H. Suh, L. M. Zangwill, P. I. C. Manalastas et al., "Optical coherence tomography angiography vessel density in glaucomatous eyes with focal lamina cribrosa defects," *Ophthalmology*, vol. 123, no. 11, pp. 2309–2317, 2016.

[28] A. S. Hafez, R. L. Bizzarro, and M. R. Lesk, "Evaluation of optic nerve head and peripapillary retinal blood flow in glaucoma patients, ocular hypertensives, and normal subjects," *American Journal of Ophthalmology*, vol. 136, no. 6, pp. 1022–1031, 2003.

[29] P. Zeboulon, P.-M. Levéque, E. Brasnu et al., "Effect of surgical intraocular pressure lowering on peripapillary and macular vessel density in glaucoma patients: an optical coherence tomography angiography study," *Journal of Glaucoma*, vol. 26, no. 5, pp. 466–472, 2017.

[30] G. Holló, "Influence of large intraocular pressure reduction on peripapillary OCT vessel density in ocular hypertensive and glaucoma eyes," *Journal of Glaucoma*, vol. 26, no. 1, pp. e7–e10, 2016.

[31] M. Alnawaiseh, V. Müller, L. Lahme et al., "Changes in flow density measured using optical coherence tomography angiography after istent insertion in combination with phacoemulsification in patients with open-angle," *Journal of Ophthalmology*, vol. 2018, Article ID 2890357, 5 pages, 2018.

[32] J. W. Shin, K. R. Sung, K. B. Uhm et al., "Peripapillary microvascular improvement and lamina cribrosa depth reduction after trabeculectomy in primary open-angle glaucoma," *Investigative Opthalmology & Visual Science*, vol. 58, no. 13, p. 5993, 2017.

[33] B A Francis, M Wang, H Lei et al., "Changes in axial length following trabeculectomy and glaucoma drainage device surgery," *British Journal of Ophthalmology*, vol. 89, no. 1, pp. 17–20, 2005.

[34] M. S. Kook, H. B. Kim, and S. U. Lee, "Short-term effect of mitomycin-C augmented trabeculectomy on axial length and corneal astigmatism," *Journal of Cataract & Refractive Surgery*, vol. 27, no. 4, pp. 518–523, 2001.

25

Ahmed Glaucoma Valve Implantation in Vitrectomized Eyes

Nimet Yeşim Erçalık ⓘ **and Serhat İmamoğlu**

Haydarpaşa Numune Research and Training Hospital, Istanbul, Turkey

Correspondence should be addressed to Nimet Yeşim Erçalık; dryercalik@gmail.com

Academic Editor: Paolo Fogagnolo

Purpose. To evaluate the outcomes of Ahmed glaucoma valve (AGV) implantation in vitrectomized eyes. *Materials and Methods.* The medical records of 13 eyes that developed glaucoma due to emulsified silicon oil or neovascularization following pars plana vitrectomy and underwent AGV implantation were retrospectively reviewed. The main outcome measures were intraocular pressure (IOP), best-corrected visual acuity (BCVA), number of antiglaucoma medications, and postoperative complications. Surgical success was defined as last IOP ≤21 mmHg or ≥6 mmHg and without loss of light perception. *Results.* The mean follow-up duration was 11.7 ± 5.5 (range, 6–23) months. The mean IOP before the AGV implantation was 37.9 ± 6.7 mmHg with an average of 3.5 ± 1.2 drugs. At the final visit, the mean IOP was 15.9 ± 4.6 mmHg ($p = 0.001$) and the mean number of glaucoma medications decreased to 2.3 ± 1.3 ($p = 0.021$). At the last visit, 11 eyes (84.4%) had stable or improved VA and one eye (7.7%) had a final VA of no light perception. Surgical success was achieved in 11 of the 13 eyes (84.4%). Postoperative complications were bleb encapsulation (69.2%), early hypotony (38.5%), hyphema (23.1%), decompression retinopathy (23.1%), choroidal detachment (15.4%), intraocular hemorrhage (7.7%), and late endophthalmitis (7.7%). One eye (7.7%) was enucleated because of late endophthalmitis. *Conclusions.* Despite complications necessitating medical and surgical interventions, vitrectomized eyes were effectively managed with AGV implantation.

1. Introduction

Secondary glaucoma is not a rare complication following vitreoretinal surgery. It develops due to surgery and tamponading agents, is usually transient, and is generally managed with antiglaucoma therapy [1, 2]. Refractory glaucoma indicates surgical treatment, such as silicone oil (SO) removal, anterior chamber washout of emulsified SO, trabeculectomy, and valve implants [3, 4].

Vitreoretinal procedures can cause scarring and alteration of the wound healing of the conjunctiva, which can make any glaucoma surgery challenging. Furthermore, an ischemic intraocular environment due to retinal disease may deteriorate the surgical outcomes. Therefore, conventional filtering surgery in such cases has a poor prognosis. Glaucoma drainage devices (GDD) provide advantages when there is a high risk of failure with standard filtering surgery [5]. Among them, the Ahmed glaucoma valve (AGV) is easy to insert, has a wide filtration area, and prevents low IOP by functioning only when the IOP is over 8 mmHg [6, 7].

Previous studies have reported that AGV implantation has a high success rate in IOP control and a low complication rate [8, 9]. However, there are only a few studies reporting these results in the eyes that underwent vitreoretinal surgery. This study aims at evaluating the results and complications of AGV implantation in the vitrectomized eyes.

2. Materials and Methods

The medical records of 13 patients with a history of pars plana vitrectomy (PPV) who underwent AGV implantation between 2014 and 2016 were retrospectively reviewed. Written informed consent was obtained from each patient. The study followed the tenets of the Declaration of Helsinki.

Patients with a postoperative follow-up less than 6 months after AGV implantation, patients with a pre-AGV implantation vision of no light perception, eyes filled with SO, and eyes with a history of primary open angle glaucoma (OAG) before PPV were excluded from the study. Surgical success was defined as last IOP ≤21 mmHg or ≥6 mmHg and without loss of light perception. Failure caused by hypotony was defined as IOP of ≤5 mmHg.

Before the surgical procedure, all patients underwent an ophthalmologic examination including measurement of best-corrected visual acuity (BCVA) with the Snellen chart, biomicroscopy, gonioscopy, fundus examination, and Goldmann applanation tonometry (Haag-Streit, Köniz, Switzerland). All examinations and surgical procedures were performed by a single glaucoma specialist (SI). Demographic information, BCVA, IOP, number of glaucoma medications, history of prior vitreoretinal surgery, and postoperative complications were recorded. Postoperative visits were performed at 1 day, 1 week, 1 month, and 3 months later, and every 3 months thereafter. More frequent examinations were done when clinically necessary. After Ahmed glaucoma valve implantation, elevation of IOP was treated either medically or surgically when necessary.

2.1. Surgical Procedure. The AGV-FP7 model (New World Medical, Rancho Cucamonga, CA, USA) was used in all eyes. Under local or general anesthesia, the plate was implanted at the superior temporal or superior nasal quadrant by the long scleral tunnel technique. A fornix-based conjunctival flap was created at 90–120 degrees. With care to the rectus muscles, a posterior dissection was performed and the sclera was exposed for the implantation of the plate. Three scleral incisions, 10–12 mm, 6–8 mm, and 1.5–2 mm away from the limbus, respectively, were performed. The incisions, which were 2.5 mm in length and one-half to two-thirds the thickness of the sclera in depth, were made parallel to the limbus. The incisions were bonded using a 60-degree bevel-up 2.0 mm crescent knife. By bonding these three incisions, a scleral tunnel was created. An episcleral plate was inserted behind the rectus muscles and behind the equator. The plate was secured to the sclera with two absorbable 6/0 vicryl sutures. Then, the silicone tube of the device was placed in the scleral tunnel. Using the third scleral incision, parallel to the iris, a partial paracentesis was made with a 23-gauge microvitreoretinal knife. The tube was inserted 1–2 mm into the anterior chamber in 9 eyes and the ciliary sulcus in 4 eyes. The tube was shortened to prevent crystalline lens touch when necessary. The scleral incision close to the limbus was closed with an 8/0 vicryl suture to avoid leakage. The conjunctiva was sutured with 8/0 vicryl. After AGV implantation, all patients received a standard topical therapy including moxifloxacin and prednisolone for 6–8 weeks.

3. Statistical Analysis

Statistical analyses were performed using the IBM SPSS Statistics software (SPSS, Chicago, IL). The variables were investigated using visual (histograms, probability plots) and analytical methods (Kolmogorov–Smirnov/Shapiro–Wilk test) to determine whether or not they were normally distributed. Descriptive analyses were presented using medians and interquartile range (IQR) for the nonnormally distributed and ordinal variables. The Wilcoxon test was performed to test the significance of pairwise differences. A

TABLE 1: Characteristics of the study patients.

Age (years)	53.93 ± 16 (23–78)
Gender (female/male), number (%)	3 (23.1), 10 (76.9)
Preoperative BCVA (LogMAR)	1.58 ± 0.91
Preoperative IOP (mmHg)	37.9 ± 6.7
Preoperative number of glaucoma medications	3.5 ± 1.2
Lens status (eyes/%)	
Phakia	2 (15.4)
Pseudophakia	9 (69.2)
Aphakia	2 (15.4)

Intraocular pressure (IOP); best-corrected visual acuity (BCVA).

p value of less than 0.05 was considered to show a statistically significant result.

4. Results

Thirteen eyes of 13 patients with medically uncontrolled glaucoma after 23-gauge PPV were included in the study. The characteristics of the patients are summarized in Table 1. The mean follow-up duration was 11.7 ± 5.5 (range, 6–23) months. The mean interval between the PPV and AGV implantation was 24.1 ± 17.3 months. Indications for performing 23-gauge PPV included retinal detachment (61.5%) and neovascular glaucoma (NVG) (38.5%).

Four eyes (30.8%) had undergone glaucoma surgeries (trabeculectomy in 1 eye and cyclophotocoagulation in 3 eyes) before AGV implantation. We injected intracameral antivascular endothelial growth factor (anti-VEGF) agent, 3 days–1 week prior to the AGV implantation into 3 eyes with stage 3 of NVG (marked by secondary angle closure glaucoma) of the 5 NVG cases. One eye (7.7%) underwent combined phacoemulsification and AGV implantation.

The mean IOP before the AGV implantation was 37.9 ± 6.7 mmHg with an average of 3.5 ± 1.2 drugs. At the final visit, the mean IOP was 15.9 ± 4.6 mmHg ($p = 0.001$) and the mean number of glaucoma medications had decreased to 2.3 ± 1.3 ($p = 0.021$). Preoperative BCVA increased from 1.58 ± 0.91 LogMAR to 1.46 ± 1.06 LogMAR at the last visit ($p = 0.7$). At the final follow-up, 11 eyes (84.4%) had stable or improved VA and one eye (7.7%) had a final VA of no light perception. Figure 1 shows the visual gain/loss of the study patients postoperatively.

We also evaluated the results separately in NVG and non-NVG cases. In the NVG group, the mean IOP before the AGV implantation was 38.4 ± 2.6 mmHg with an average of 3.8 ± 0.8 drugs. At the final visit (mean follow-up time = 11.7 months), the mean IOP was 18 ± 6.8 mmHg ($p = 0.042$). We achieved the IOP control in all except one of our NVG patients following AGV implantation. We had not used anti-VEGF in that patient with uncontrolled IOP elevation. In the non-NVG group, preoperative IOP was 37.6 ± 8.6 mmHg. At the final visit (mean follow-up time = 11.7 months), the mean IOP decreased to 14.6 ± 2.2 mmHg ($p = 0.012$).

Postoperative complications were bleb encapsulation (69.2%), early hypotony (38.5%), hyphema (23.1%), decompression retinopathy (23.1%), choroidal detachment

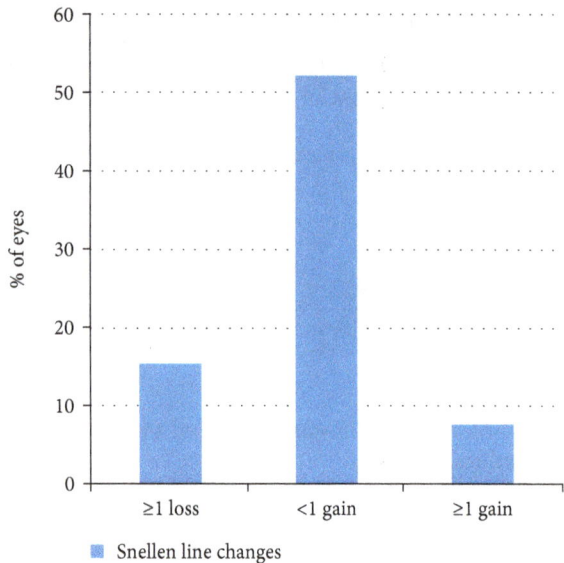

FIGURE 1: Visual gain/loss of the study patients postoperatively.

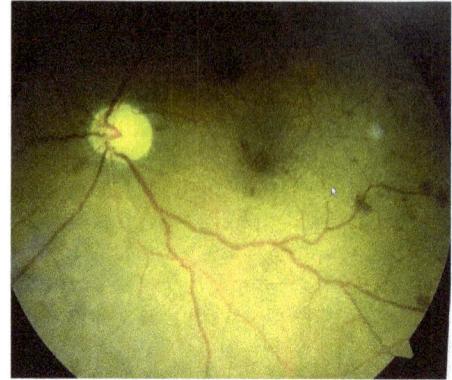

FIGURE 2: Fundus examination showing scattered retinal hemorrhages in the periphery and posterior pole typical for decompression retinopathy.

(15.4%), intraocular hemorrhage (7.7%), and late endophthalmitis (7.7%). Figure 2 shows the fundus photo of one case with decompression retinopathy. The most commonly encountered problem was a hypertensive phase due to bleb encapsulation over the plate. Six of the 9 eyes with a hypertensive phase due to bleb encapsulation necessitated needling with 0.1 cc 5-fluorouracil (5-FU) (50 mg/ml). The mean intervention time for needling was 70.8 ± 20.2 days. One eye (7.7%) was enucleated because of late endophthalmitis. One eye (7.7%) resulted in vision with no light perception postoperatively. Except for these 2 cases, surgical success was achieved in 11 of the 13 eyes (84.6%).

5. Discussion

Despite several studies reporting the early transient increase in IOP after vitrectomy, limited information is available in the literature on late glaucoma after vitreoretinal surgery. Late IOP elevation after PPV was reported as 26–41% in the previous studies [10, 11].

It has been reported that PPV causes an increase in oxygen levels in the vitreous chamber that remain elevated for at least 10 months [12]. Increased oxidative damage to the trabecular meshwork [13] and small lesions created during vitrectomy leading to secondary scarring to the trabecular meshwork [14] were the two hypothesized mechanisms associated with the risk of glaucoma after PPV. In addition to these two theories, other mechanisms responsible for the IOP elevation after PPV include intraocular gas expansion, inflammation, hemorrhagic complications, silicone oil complications, pupillary block, response to steroids, and progression of the neovascularization and ciliary body edema [11, 15].

Ischemic retinal environment, conjunctival scarring, increased inflow of vasoformative factors from the vitreous cavity into the anterior chamber, and inflammation after vitreoretinal surgery were thought to result in a worse prognosis after trabeculectomy in the eyes with NVG [16, 17]. Therefore, the GDD may be preferred as the primary choice for refractory glaucoma in the eyes with previous vitreoretinal surgery. Successful long-term results were reported after AGV implantation in the eyes with NVG [18].

Inoue et al. [19] assumed that NVG may be a more significant risk factor in the vitrectomized eyes than in the nonvitrectomized eyes because vasoformative factors in the vitreous cavity could easily diffuse into the anterior chamber in the vitrectomized eyes, leading to a more severe neovascularization and inflammation. Intravitreal and intracameral bevacizumab injection have been reported to be a safe and effective adjuvant for GDD in NVG [20, 21]. In three eyes of the five cases, we used an intracameral anti-VEGF agent. We encountered hyphema in three eyes and intraocular hemorrhage in one eye, but these hemorrhages were slight and disappeared without therapy. The use of anti-VEGF agent may have prevented severe hemorrhages in our study.

It has been reported that 7.1–10% of patients who underwent PPV and SO injection developed uncontrolled glaucoma despite medical therapy and removal of SO [22]. Gupta et al. [23] reported that long-term success of AGV implantation after PPV with SO injection and subsequent removal was better than that reported for trabeculectomy. They observed 62% success at 12 months after implantation of AGV in these eyes [23]. In our series, we excluded eyes that were filled with SO and included only cases with droplets of emulsified SO. Surgical success was achieved in all of these eyes with emulsified SO, except in one eye, which was enucleated because of endophthalmitis.

The Ahmed glaucoma valve has a built-in valve mechanism which allows immediate postoperative flow and prevents hypotony but may require more glaucoma medications in the long term. We preferred to implant the AGV FP7 model in our vitrectomized eyes. A study reported that eyes with the Baerveldt tube implantation had a higher risk of refractory hypotony when compared to the eyes with AGV implantation [24]. Therefore, the AGV may be preferred for the eyes that are at risk of hypotony such as the vitrectomized eyes. However, the rate of bleb encapsulation was found to be higher in AGV compared to the Baerveldt tube in the previous studies. The use of a valve within the tube as well as the early conjunctival exposure to the proinflammatory mediators from the aqueous or the uneven surface texture of the Ahmed base plate and the small base plate area of the Ahmed valve design may be the reasons for this high encapsulation rate [25–27].

Bleb encapsulation is one of the main reasons for glaucoma valve failure [28]. Souza et al. [29] reported that previous conjunctival surgery changed the conjunctival surface, and the subsequent operation can induce a proliferation of fibrous cells leading to bleb encapsulation. It has also been reported that SO migration can occur through the tube into the subconjunctival space, causing an inflammatory reaction [30, 31]. If bleb encapsulation is encountered, needling of the bleb may help, with the aim of outflow resistance [32]. Six of the nine eyes in our study group with bleb encapsulation necessitated needling with 5-FU. In these eyes, the control of IOP was achieved in the early period following needling.

Exposure of the implant's tube with conjunctival erosion has been suggested as the main risk factor for endophthalmitis after GDD implantation [33, 34]. Also, in our case with late endophthalmitis, the conjunctival erosion was the reason for infection. We used the long scleral tunnel technique in all of the eyes in our study group. Kugu et al. [35] reported that AGV implantation performed with the long scleral tunnel technique is more effective in preventing tube exposure. They detected tube exposure in 2.5% of their patients after a mean follow-up period of 46 months.

Hypotony, hyphema, decompression retinopathy, and choroidal detachment in our patients were successfully treated with medical therapy. Intraocular hemorrhage was resolved in the early postoperative period without therapy.

Decompression retinopathy can occur after laser or medical therapy for acute glaucoma [36–38], trabeculectomy [39], and valve implantation [40, 41]. To the best of our knowledge, no study reported decompression retinopathy after AGV implantation in the vitrectomized eyes. We found the rate of decompression retinopathy as 23.1% in our series; this may be due to initial high IOP in these eyes. Operating surgeons should be aware of this complication and avoid sudden drop of IOP. Previous vitreoretinal surgery was not reported among the predisposing factors for decompression retinopathy after AGV implantation in the literature. We suspect that previous PPV may have increased the rate for decompression retinopathy in our series.

The reduction in IOP and the number of medications used postoperatively were both statistically and clinically significant in our patients. These results are consistent with previous studies evaluating AGV implantation in the vitrectomized eyes. Hong and Choi [42] found the success rate after the AGV implantation in the vitrectomized eyes as 83.4% at 6 months and 76.4% at the final visit. Preoperative IOP decreased from 47.5 mmHg with 1.76 drugs to 13.8 mmHg with 0.35 drug at 6 months. Park et al. [43] reported the success rate of AGV implantation as 83.8% at 1 year in their vitrectomized patients. Final visual acuity improved or stabilized in 78.6% of their cases, which is consistent with our results. Cheng et al. [44] evaluated the effect of AGV implantation in diabetic vitrectomized eyes. Postoperatively, IOP

decreased from 49.4 mmHg to 17.5 mmHg. Sixty-six point seven percent of the eyes still needed average 0.8 drug.

Limitations of this study are retrospective design, small sample size, short follow-up time, variation of the etiologic factors for PPV, and the lack of a control group. Despite complications necessitating medical and surgical interventions, vitrectomized eyes were effectively managed with AGV implantation. A larger series with a longer follow-up is required.

Conflicts of Interest

The authors declare that they have no conflicts of interest.

References

[1] Q. H. Nguyen, M. A. Lloyd, D. K. Heuer, G. Baerveldt, J. S. Lean, and P. E. Liggett, "Incidence and management of glaucoma after intravitreal silicone oil injection for complicated retinal detachments," *Ophthalmology*, vol. 99, no. 10, pp. 1520–1526, 1992.

[2] C. Nowack, K. Lucke, and H. Laqua, "Removal of silicone oil in treatment of so-called emulsification glaucoma," *Der Ophthalmologe*, vol. 89, no. 6, pp. 462–464, 1992.

[3] S. J. Gedde, "Management of glaucoma after retinal detachment surgery," *Current Opinion in Ophthalmology*, vol. 13, no. 2, pp. 103–109, 2002.

[4] D. V. Vasconcelos-Santos, P. G. Nehemy, A. P. Schachat, and M. B. Nehemy, "Secondary ocular hypertension after intravitreal injection of 4 mg of triamcinolone acetonide incidence and risk factors," *Retina*, vol. 28, no. 4, pp. 573–580, 2008.

[5] I. U. Scott, S. J. Gedde, D. L. Budenz et al., "Baerveldt drainage implants in eyes with a pre-existing buckle," *Archives of Ophthalmology*, vol. 118, no. 11, pp. 1509–1513, 2000.

[6] A. L. Coleman, R. Hill, M. R. Wilson et al., "Initial clinical experience with the Ahmed glaucoma valve implant," *American Journal of Ophthalmology*, vol. 120, no. 1, pp. 23–31, 1995.

[7] K. C. Huh and C. W. Kee, "A clinical analysis of the Ahmed glaucoma valve implant with or without partial ligation of silicone tube," *Journal of the Korean Ophthalmological Society*, vol. 41, pp. 2611–2617, 2000.

[8] N. H. Joseph, M. B. Sherwood, G. Trantas, R. A. Hitchings, and L. A. Lattimer, "A one-piece drainage system for glaucoma surgery," *Transactions of the Ophthalmological Societies of the United Kingdom*, vol. 105, pp. 657–664, 1986.

[9] J. H. Lee, S. S. Kim, and Y. J. Hong, "A clinical study of the Ahmed valve implant in refractory glaucoma," *Journal of the Korean Ophthalmological Society*, vol. 42, pp. 1003–1010, 2001.

[10] J. J. Hwang, Y. Y. Kim, and K. Huk, "Risk factors of intraocular pressure elevation after pars plana vitrectomy," *Journal of the Korean Ophthalmological Society*, vol. 41, pp. 945–950, 2000.

[11] D. P. Han, H. Lewis, F. H. Lambrou Jr., W. F. Mieler, and A. Hartz, "Mechanisms of intraocular pressure elevation after pars plana vitrectomy," *Ophthalmology*, vol. 96, no. 9, pp. 1357–1362, 1989.

[12] N. M. Holekamp, Y. B. Shui, and D. Beebe, "Vitrectomy surgery increases oxygen exposure to the lens: a possible mechanism for nuclear cataract formation," *American Journal of Ophthalmology*, vol. 139, no. 2, pp. 302–310, 2005.

[13] S. Chang, "LXII Edward Jackson lecture: open angle glaucoma after vitrectomy," *American Journal of Ophthalmology*, vol. 141, no. 6, pp. 1033–1043, 2006.

[14] E. Van Aken, H. Lemij, Y. Vander Haeghen, and P. de Waard, "Baerveldt glaucoma implants in the management of refractory glaucoma after vitreous surgery," *Acta Ophthalmologica*, vol. 88, no. 1, pp. 75–79, 2010.

[15] A. Goto, M. Inatani, T. Inoue et al., "Frequency and risk factors for neovascular glaucoma after vitrectomy in eyes with proliferative diabetic retinopathy," *Journal of Glaucoma*, vol. 22, no. 7, pp. 572–576, 2013.

[16] Y. Kiuchi, R. Sugimoto, K. Nakae, Y. Saito, and S. Ito, "Trabeculectomy with mitomycin C for treatment of neovascular glaucoma in diabetic patients," *Ophthalmologica*, vol. 220, pp. 383–388, 2006.

[17] Y. Takihara, M. Inatani, M. Fukushima, K. Iwao, M. Iwao, and H. Tanihara, "Trabeculectomy with mitomycin C for neovascular glaucoma: prognostic factors for surgical failure," *American Journal of Ophthalmology*, vol. 147, no. 5, pp. 912.e1–918.e1, 2009.

[18] I. S. Yalvac, U. Eksioglu, B. Satana, and S. Duman, "Long-term results of Ahmed valve and Molteno implant in neovascular glaucoma," *Eye*, vol. 21, no. 1, pp. 65–70, 2007.

[19] T. Inoue, M. Inatani, Y. Takihara, N. Awai-Kasaoka, M. Ogata-Iwao, and H. Tanihara, "Prognostic risk factors for failure of trabeculectomy with mitomycin C after vitrectomy," *Japanese Journal of Ophthalmology*, vol. 56, no. 5, pp. 464–469, 2012.

[20] J. P. Shin, J. W. Lee, B. J. Sohn, H. K. Kim, and S. Y. Kim, "In vivo corneal endothelial safety of intracameral bevacizumab and effect in neovascular glaucoma combined with Ahmed valve implantation," *Journal of Glaucoma*, vol. 18, no. 8, pp. 589–594, 2009.

[21] T. M. Eid, A. Radwan, W. el-Manawy, and I. el-Hawary, "Intravitreal bevacizumab and aqueous shunting surgery for neovascular glaucoma: safety and efficacy," *Canadian Journal of Ophthalmology*, vol. 44, no. 4, pp. 451–456, 2009.

[22] D. L. Budenz, K. E. Taba, W. J. Feuer et al., "Surgical management of secondary glaucoma after pars plana vitrectomy and silicone oil injection for complex retinal detachment," *Ophthalmology*, vol. 108, no. 9, pp. 1628–1632, 2001.

[23] S. Gupta, A. K. Chaurasia, R. Chawla et al., "Long-term outcomes of glaucoma drainage devices for glaucoma post-vitreoretinal surgery with silicone oil insertion: a prospective evaluation," *Graefe's Archive for Clinical and Experimental Ophthalmology*, vol. 254, no. 12, pp. 2449–2454, 2016.

[24] D. L. Budenz, K. Barton, S. J. Gedde et al., "Five-year treatment outcomes in the Ahmed Baerveldt comparison study," *Ophthalmology*, vol. 122, no. 2, pp. 308–316, 2015.

[25] A. C. Molteno, M. Fucik, A. G. Dempster, and T. H. Bevin, "Otago Glaucoma Surgery Outcome Study: factors controlling capsule fibrosis around Molteno implants with histopathological correlation," *Ophthalmology*, vol. 110, no. 11, pp. 2198–2206, 2003.

[26] L. Choritz, K. Koynov, G. Renieri, K. Barton, N. Pfeiffer, and H. Thieme, "Surface topographies of glaucoma drainage devices and their influence on human tenon fibroblast adhesion," *Investigative Opthalmology and Visual Science*, vol. 51, no. 8, pp. 4047–4053, 2010.

[27] M. A. Lloyd, G. Baerveldt, P. S. Fellenbaum, P. A. Sidoti, D. S. Minckler, and J. F. Martone, "Intermediate-term results of a randomized clinical trial of the 350 versus the 500 mm² Baerveldt implant," *Ophthalmology*, vol. 101, no. 8, pp. 1456–1464, 1994.

[28] M. Eibschitz-Tsimhoni, R. M. Schertzer, D. C. Musch, and S. E. Moroi, "Incidence and management of encapsulated cysts following Ahmed glaucoma valve insertion," *Journal of Glaucoma*, vol. 14, no. 4, pp. 276–279, 2005.

[29] C. Souza, D. H. Tran, J. Loman, S. K. Law, A. L. Coleman, and J. Caprioli, "Long-term outcomes of Ahmed glaucoma valve implantation in refractory glaucomas," *American Journal of Ophthalmology*, vol. 144, no. 6, pp. 893–900, 2007.

[30] S. M. Hyung and J. P. Min, "Subconjunctival silicone oil drainage through the Molteno implant," *Korean Journal of Ophthalmology*, vol. 12, no. 1, pp. 73–75, 1998.

[31] C. K. Chan, D. G. Tarasewicz, and S. G. Lin, "Subconjunctival migration of silicone oil through a Baerveldt pars plana glaucoma implant," *British Journal of Ophthalmology*, vol. 89, no. 2, pp. 240-241, 2005.

[32] I. Riva, G. Roberti, F. Oddone, A. G. Konstas, and L. Quaranta, "Ahmed glaucoma valve implant: surgical technique and complications," *Clinical Ophthalmology*, vol. 11, pp. 357–367, 2017.

[33] S. J. Gedde, I. U. Scott, H. Tabandeh et al., "Late endophthalmitis associated with glaucoma drainage implants," *Ophthalmology*, vol. 108, no. 7, pp. 1323–1327, 2001.

[34] A. A. Al-Torbak, S. Al-Shahwan, I. Al-Jadaan, A. Al-Hommadi, and D. P. Edward, "Endophthalmitis associated with the Ahmed glaucoma valve implant," *British Journal of Ophthalmology*, vol. 89, no. 4, pp. 454–458, 2005.

[35] S. Kugu, G. Erdogan, M. S. Sevim, and Y. Ozerturk, "Efficacy of long scleral tunnel technique in preventing Ahmed glaucoma valve tube exposure through conjunctiva," *Seminars in Ophthalmology*, vol. 30, no. 1, pp. 1–5, 2015.

[36] G. Nah, T. Aung, and C. C. Yip, "Ocular decompression retinopathy after resolution of acute primary angle closure glaucoma," *Clinical and Experimental Ophthalmology*, vol. 28, no. 4, pp. 319-320, 2000.

[37] J. S. Lai, V. Y. Lee, D. Y. Leung, and T. C. Chung, "Decompression retinopathy following laser peripheral iridoplasty for acute primary angle-closure," *Eye*, vol. 19, no. 12, pp. 1345–1347, 2005.

[38] J. Landers and J. Craig, "Decompression retinopathy and corneal oedema following Nd:YAG laser peripheral iridotomy," *Clinical and Experimental Ophthalmology*, vol. 34, no. 2, pp. 182–184, 2006.

[39] A. Bansal and U. Ramanathan, "Ocular decompression retinopathy after trabeculectomy with mitomycin-C for angle recession glaucoma," *Indian Journal of Ophthalmology*, vol. 57, no. 2, pp. 153-154, 2009.

[40] D. F. Dudley, M. M. Leen, J. L. Kinyoun, and R. P. Mills, "Retinal hemorrhages associated with ocular decompression after glaucoma surgery," *Ophthalmic Surgery and Lasers*, vol. 27, no. 2, pp. 147–150, 1996.

[41] I. S. Yalvac, H. Kocaoglan, U. Eksioglu, N. Demir, and S. Duman, "Decompression retinopathy after Ahmed glaucoma valve implantation in a patient with congenital aniridia and pseudophakia," *Journal of Cataract and Refractive Surgery*, vol. 30, no. 7, pp. 1582–1585, 2004.

[42] J. W. Hong and G. J. Choi, "Ahmed valve implantation for refractory glaucoma following pars plana vitrectomy," *Korean Journal of Ophthalmology*, vol. 19, no. 4, pp. 293–296, 2005.

[43] U. C. Park, K. H. Park, D. M. Kim, and H. G. Yu, "Ahmed glaucoma valve implantation for neovascular glaucoma after vitrectomy for proliferative diabetic retinopathy," *Journal of Glaucoma*, vol. 20, no. 7, pp. 433–438, 2011.

[44] Y. Cheng, X. H. Liu, X. Shen, and Y. S. Zhong, "Ahmed valve implantation for neovascular glaucoma after 23-gauge vitrectomy in eyes with proliferative diabetic retinopathy," *International Journal of Ophthalmology*, vol. 6, no. 3, pp. 316–320, 2013.

26

Effects of Oral Supplementation with Docosahexaenoic Acid (DHA) plus Antioxidants in Pseudoexfoliative Glaucoma: A 6-Month Open-Label Randomized Trial

Stéphanie Romeo Villadóniga ⓘ,[1] Elena Rodríguez García,[1] Olatz Sagastagoia Epelde,[2] M. Dolores Álvarez Díaz,[1] and Joan Carles Domingo Pedrol[3]

[1]

Service of Ophthalmology, Complejo Hospitalario Universitario de Ferrol, Ferrol, A Coruña, Spain
[2]*Clinical Analysis Laboratory, Complejo Hospitalario Universitario de Ferrol, Ferrol, A Coruña, Spain*
[3]*Department of Biochemistry and Molecular Biomedicine, Faculty of Biology, University of Barcelona, Barcelona, Spain*

Correspondence should be addressed to Stéphanie Romeo Villadóniga; stephimed@hotmail.com

Academic Editor: Tomasz Zarnowski

Purpose. To assess the effects of antioxidant oral supplementation based on docosahexaenoic acid (DHA) in pseudoexfoliative (PEX) glaucoma. *Patients and Methods.* A prospective 6-month open-label randomized controlled trial was conducted in patients with PEX glaucoma and adequate intraocular pressure (IOP) control. Patients in the DHA group received a high-rich DHA (1 g) nutraceutical formulation. Ophthalmological examination, DHA erythrocyte membrane content (% total fatty acids), plasma total antioxidant capacity (TAC), plasma malondialdehyde (MDA), and plasma IL-6 levels were assessed. *Results.* Forty-seven patients (DHA group 23, controls 24; mean age 70.3 years) were included. In the DHA group, the mean IOP in the right eye decreased from 14.7 [3.3] mmHg at baseline to 12.1 [1.5] mmHg at 6 months ($P = 0.01$). In the left eye, IOP decreased from 15.1 [3.3] mmHg at baseline to 12.2 [2.4] mmHg at 6 months ($P = 0.007$). DHA erythrocyte content increased in the DHA group, with significant differences versus controls at 3 months and 6 months (8.1% [0.9] vs. 4.4% [0.7]; $P < 0.0001$). At 6 months and in the DHA group only, TAC levels as compared with baseline increased significantly (919.7 [117.9] vs. 856.9 [180.3] μM copper-reducing equivalents; $P = 0.01$), and both MDA (4.4 [0.8] vs. 5.2 [1.1] nmol/mL; $P = 0.02$) and IL-6 (2.8 [1.3] vs. 4.7 [2.3] pg/mL; $P = 0.006$) levels were lower than in controls. *Conclusions.* Targeting pathophysiology mechanisms of PEX glaucoma by reducing oxidative stress and inflammation with a high-rich DHA supplement might be an attractive therapeutic approach. Despite the short duration of treatment, decrease in IOP supports the clinical significance of DHA supplementation.

1. Introduction

Pseudoexfoliative (PEX) glaucoma has been widely described as the result of the accumulation of pseudoexfoliative material, which obstructs the trabecular meshwork (TM) leading to an increase in intraocular pressure (IOP) levels. PEX glaucoma is the most common identifiable secondary form of open-angle glaucoma, accounting for up to 25% of glaucoma cases in the world [1, 2]. Compared with primary open-angle glaucoma, PEX glaucoma is associated with greater mean IOP, more advanced visual field loss at diagnosis, and poorer treatment response [3].

The etiopathogenetic mechanisms of pseudoexfoliation syndrome/PEX glaucoma are still not well understood. Decreased levels of antioxidant capacity might be involved in glaucomatous TM and neuronal damage as a result of local inadequate defense against oxidative stress [4, 5]. In the presence of reactive oxygen species (ROS), nitric oxide produces toxic metabolites (peroxynitrites) and the associated oxidative-nitrative stress induces sustained inflammation, cell proliferation, and/or neurotoxicity [5]. Oxidative DNA damage is significantly increased in the ocular epithelium regulating aqueous humor outflow in the TM. Oxidative damage constitutes an important pathogenetic step–triggering

TM degeneration, which results in intraocular hypertension [6]. Also, the transcriptional factor NF-kappaB (NF-kB) can be activated by increased IOP, increased age, vascular disease, and oxidative stress [7, 8]. Overstimulation of NF-kB is also involved in the amplification of the inflammatory cascade [8]. Other studies have shown that interleukin-6 (IL-6) is linked to the pathogenesis of glaucoma [9]. Dysregulation of proinflammatory cytokines seems to be implicated in pseudoexfoliation syndrome, with high production of IL-6 at early stages of the disease inducing production of TGF-β_1 and fibrotic proteins [10]. Moreover, the IL-6 family and their signal transducer glycoprotein (gp130) have been shown to be involved in inflammation and cell survival in glaucoma [11], as well as to play a specific role in the progression of retinal ganglion cell axonopathy from functional deficits to structural degeneration [12].

In recent years, there has been growing interest of the health benefits of omega-3 long-chain polyunsaturated fatty acids (ω-3 PUFAs), particularly docosahexaenoic acid (DHA), the pleiotropic actions of which may affect molecular pathways involved in the pathogenesis of ocular diseases, such as age-related macular edema [13], diabetic retinopathy and diabetic macular edema [14, 15], and dry eye syndrome in glaucoma patients [16]. The rationale of the use of DHA for improving retinal function is based on the inhibitory effect of DHA on the activation NF-κB and synthesis of inflammatory cytokines [17, 18], generation of eicosanoids and stimulation of inflammation resolving docosanoids (resolvins and protectins) [19], antiangiogenic effects of ω-3 PUFAs in human endothelial cells, and antioxidant protective effects on retinal pigment epithelium and photoreceptors [20, 21]. Recently, dietary consumption of PUFAs in glaucoma has been proposed as a modifiable factor for IOP regulation through docosanoids-driven increase of aqueous outflow [22], reversal of ω-3 and ω-6 imbalance in red blood cell membranes [23, 24], and improvement of glaucomatous optic neuropathy [25]. However, the clinical experience with dietary intake of ω-3 PUFAs in glaucoma is very limited [26, 27].

Therefore, a midterm prospective open-label randomized controlled trial was conducted to assess the effects of oral supplementation with a nutraceutical formulation based on high-rich DHA plus vitamins and minerals in patients with PEX glaucoma. It was hypothesized that DHA supplementation improves antioxidant protection and ameliorates subclinical inflammation in PEX glaucoma.

2. Methods

2.1. Study Design. A prospective, randomized, open-label controlled study was conducted at the Service of Ophthalmology of an acute-care hospital in Ferrol, A Coruña, Spain. The duration of the study was 6 months. The objective of the study was to determine the effects of daily supplementation with a nutraceutical formulation rich in DHA plus vitamins and minerals on clinical and biochemical parameters in patients with PEX glaucoma. Ethical approval for this study was provided by the Clinical Research Ethics Committee of the autonomous community of Galicia, Spain. All participants

provided written informed consent before enrollment. The study was conducted in accordance with principles of the Declaration of Helsinki and guidelines for Good Clinical Practice. The study was registered in the European Clinical Trials Database (EudraCT) (EudraCT trial number 2014-001104-21 for the Sponsor's protocol code number: GLAUPIO).

2.2. Participants. Between July 2016 and February 2017, all consecutive patients of both sexes aged between 18 and 70 years diagnosed with initial or moderate PEX glaucoma (stages 1 and 2 of the Hodapp-Parrish-Anderson classification) [28] were invited to participate in the study during an ophthalmologic appointment at the study center. Good control of IOP with IOP-lowering medications was an inclusion criterion. Patients unable to participate in the study according to the criteria of the ophthalmologist, pregnant women, and those who refused to sign the written consent were excluded. Patients using nutritional supplement including vitamins, minerals, fatty acids, and trace elements and those with hypersensitivity to these compounds were also excluded. Patients were specifically asked if they were already supplementing their diet with DHA (i.e., fish or flax seed oil).

2.3. Study Intervention. Each participant contributed 2 study eyes to the protocol. Study patients were consecutively assigned with a 1:1 sequential allocation to the DHA supplementation (experimental) group or to the control group using www.random.org (Randomness and Integrity Services Ltd., Dublin, Ireland). Patients assigned to the control group met all eligibility conditions, so that the selection criteria (inclusion and exclusion) were identical for all study patients. Subjects in the control group were masked regarding the existence of the experimental group. Patients in the DHA group received a high-rich DHA (1,050 mg/day) nutraceutical formulation (BrudyPio 1.5 g; Brudy Lab, S.L., Barcelona, Spain). This is a concentrated DHA triglyceride having a high antioxidant activity patented to prevent cellular oxidative damage [29, 30]. Table 1 shows the composition of the nutraceutical formulation, which includes a high dose of DHA (1 g), eicosapentaenoic acid (EPA), and a mixture of B vitamins, vitamins C, E, lutein, zeaxanthin, and minerals. All fatty acids were present in the form of triglycerides (>95%) or ethyl esters (<5%). Patients were instructed to take 3 capsules of BrudyPio 1.5 g once daily. Also, patients were told not to change glaucoma medications during the study.

2.4. Study Procedures. The duration of the study was 6 months. All patients were evaluated at baseline and at 3 and 6 months thereafter. At each visit, patients underwent a complete ophthalmologic examination, including slit-lamp examination, best corrected visual acuity (BCVA) (in decimals), IOP, corneal pachymetry, and retinal nerve fiber layer thickness (RNFLT) using by spectral-domain optical coherence tomography (SD-OCT) (Topcon 3D OCT-1000,

TABLE 1: Composition of BrudyPio 1.5 g (Brudy Lab S.L., Barcelona, Spain) per capsule.

Composition	Per capsule	% recommended daily amount in one capsule	Per three capsules	% recommended daily amount in three capsules
Concentrated oil in ω-3 fatty acids (mg)	500		1,500	
TG-DHA 70%	350	—	1,050	—
EPA 8.5%	42.5	—	127.5	—
DPA 6%	30	—	90	—
Vitamins				
Vitamin A (retinol, μg)	133.3	17	400	50
Vitamin C (ascorbic acid, mg)	26.7	33	80	100
Vitamin E (d-α-tocopherol, mg)	4	33	12	100
Vitamin B1 (thiamine, mg)	0.36	33	1.1	100
Vitamin B2 (riboflavin, mg)	0.46	33	1.4	100
Vitamin B3 (niacin equivalent, mg)	5.33	33	16	100
Vitamin B6 (pyridoxine, mg)	0.46	33	1.4	100
Vitamin B9 (folic acid, μg)	66.7	33	200	100
Vitamin B12 (cobalamin, μg)	0.83	33	2.5	100
Essential trace elements				
Zinc, mg	3.33	33	10	100
Copper, mg	0.33	33	1	100
Selenium, μg	18.3	33	55	100
Manganese, mg	0.66	33	2	100
Other components				
Lutein, mg	3.33	—	10	—
Zeaxanthin, mg	0.33	—	1	—
Glutathione, mg	2	—	6	—
Lycopene, mg	2	—	6	—
Coenzyme Q10, mg	2	—	6	—
Anthocyanins, mg	5	—	15	—
Oleuropein, μg	67	—	200	—

TG-DHA: triglyceride-bound DHA; EPA: eicosapentaenoic acid; DPA: docosapentaenoic acid. Note: The dosage is tested is three capsules per day, which corresponds to 100% of the recommended daily amounts of the included vitamins and minerals.

de Topcon Cooperation, Tokyo, Japan). In all participants, IOP was measured by the same investigator (SRV) using a Perkins handheld applanation tonometer and during morning hours between 9:00 and 12:00 AM. Biochemical analyses included DHA erythrocyte membrane content, plasma total antioxidant capacity (TAC), plasma malondialdehyde (MDA), and plasma IL-6 levels.

At the baseline visit, eligibility criteria were checked and patients were fully informed of the purpose of the study and were requested to sign the informed consent. At the baseline visit, the nutraceutical formulation was delivered to the patient for 30-day treatment. The same assessments as in the baseline visit were performed at 1, 3, and 6 months (final visit), except for TAC, MDA, and IL-6 levels which were measured at baseline and at 6 months. At the 1-month and 3-month visits, the nutraceutical formulation was provided for the following 60 and 90 days, respectively. Compliance with DHA supplementation was assessed at the study visits by return of supplementation tablet counts and analytical data especially erythrocyte membrane DHA content. Ophthalmologists paid special care to insist on the importance of compliance with the dietary supplement and the benefit that the patient may receive from the supplement. At study visits, adverse events were recorded by questioning the patient. Patients could withdraw from the study of their own free will or be removed according to the ophthalmologist's criteria due to adverse events, concomitant diseases, or any other medical reasons.

2.5. Biochemical Analyses. Biochemical measurements included the composition of fatty acids on the erythrocyte membrane (ω 3 DHA) and levels of TAC, MDA, and IL-6 I plasma samples. The methods used for assessment of ω-3 DHA in the erythrocyte membrane and plasma TAC and IL-6 levels have been previously described in detail [31]. The content of ω-3 DHA of the erythrocyte membrane was expressed in percentages as relative amounts of total fatty acids (FA), plasma TAC as μM copper-reducing equivalent values, and plasma IL-6 as pg/mL. The level of MDA was measured colorimetrically in a Synergy™ H1M, Hybrid Multi-Mode Microplate Reader (BioTek Instruments, Inc., Winooski, VT, USA). The absorbance was detected at 532 nm. MDA quantitation results are expressed as μmol/L (μM) concentration using the MDA standard curve obtained during processing the plasma samples.

2.6. Statistical Analysis. The sample size of 27 patients per group (total 54) was calculated based on a variance of 0.048 of TAC plasma levels in PEX glaucoma, with a difference of 0.15, a power of 80%, and a type I error of 0.05. The sample size was increased to 30 patients per arm (total 30 patients) to account for a 10% loss. Categorical variables are expressed as frequencies and percentages, and continuous variables as mean and standard deviation (SD). The chi-squared (χ^2) test or the Fisher's exact test was used for the analysis of categorical variables and the Student's t-test or the Wilcoxon signed-rank test or the Friedman test for the comparison of quantitative variables according to the conditions of application. The analysis of variance (ANOVA) for repeated measures (within subject factor: baseline, 3 and 6 months; between subject factor: experimental or control), with Bonferroni's correction was used for the comparison of study variables collected from the participants throughout the study. Changes of IOP were analyzed for the right and left eyes separately, and also as one group (both eyes together). Statistical significance was set at $P < 0.05$. Statistical analyses were performed using the Statistical Package for the Social Sciences (SPSS®) program (IBM, Armonk, New York, USA) version 21.0.

3. Results

During the study period, a total of 47 patients met the inclusion criteria and were included in the study, 23 of which were randomized to the experimental group and 24 to the control group. There were 25 men and 22 women, with a mean (SD) of 70.3 (5.0) years. Statistically significant differences between patients in the study groups regarding baseline characteristics were not found (Table 2). The distribution of comorbid diseases was also similar in the two study groups.

Patients in the experimental group showed decreases of IOP from 14.7 (3.3) mmHg at baseline to 13.0 (2.7) mmHg at 3 months ($P = 0.072$) and 12.1 (1.5) mmHg at 6 months ($P = 0.01$) in the right eye. In the left eye, the mean IOP decreased from 15.1 (3.3) mmHg at baseline to 12.8 (2.6) mmHg at 3 months ($P = 0.042$) and 12.2 (2.4) mmHg at 6 months ($P = 0.007$). In controls, decreased IOP at 6 months as compared with baseline was not statistically significant neither in the right or left eyes. Between group differences for changes of IOP throughout the study were statistically significant ($P = 0.033$) for the left eye only (Figures 1 and 2). The analysis of both eyes together showed statistically significant differences of mean IOP values between 3 and 6 months versus baseline in the experimental group, whereas in controls decreases of IOP were only significant at 3 months (Table 3). Changes in BCVA and RNFLT during the study period were not observed in any of the study groups.

The content of DHA in the erythrocyte membrane (% total fatty acids) increased in the experimental group only, with significant differences as compared with controls at 3 (7.7 [1.4] vs. 4.4 [0.7] and 6 months (8.1 [0.9] vs. 4.4 [0.7] (between group differences $P < 0.0001$). At 6 months and in the experimental group only, TAC levels as compared with baseline increased significantly (919.7 [117.9] vs. 856.9 [180.3] μM copper-reducing equivalents; $P = 0.01$) (between group differences $P = 0.02$) (Figure 3).

Also, as shown in Figures 4 and 5, both MDA and IL-6 levels decreased significantly at 6 months versus baseline in the experimental group only (MDA 4.4 [0.8] vs. 5.0 (0.9) μm, $P = 0.001$; and IL-6 2.8 [1.3] versus 4.7 [2.3] pg/mL, $P = 0.006$). Between group differences were significant for both MDA ($P = 0.0002$) and IL-6 ($P = 0.02$).

The nutraceutical formulation was well tolerated, and no adverse events were registered. In relation to compliance

with the nutraceutical supplement, all patients in the DHA supplementation group reported having taken the three capsules each day of the study. Also, none of the patients had their medications changed during the study.

4. Discussion

In the present series of patients with early or moderate PEX glaucoma, daily ingestion of a nutraceutical supplement based on high-rich DHA triglyceride plus vitamins and minerals for 6 months was associated with a trend of amelioration of IOP and clear improvement of biochemical parameters related to oxidative stress, lipid peroxidation, and inflammation. These midterm results are encouraging since a simple dietary intervention may provide an adjunct therapeutic option for patients with PEX glaucoma.

The benefits derived from omega-3 supplementation in patients with glaucoma highlight the potential targets underlying the action of DHA in response to the pathophysiological mechanisms of oxidative stress and inflammation present in open-angle glaucoma. Patients with open-angle glaucoma exhibit low levels of circulating glutathione, suggesting a general compromise of the antioxidative defense [32]. Glutathione plays a critical role in many biological processes in mammalian cells, providing a defense system for the protection of cells against reactive oxygen species. During aging, glutathione levels decline, thereby putting cells at increased risk of succumbing to oxidative stress [33]. Furthermore, glaucoma patients also show significant serum and aqueous humor increase in lipid peroxidation levels [34, 35]. Thus, oxidative stress may play a significant role during glaucoma course, initially damaging the trabecular meshwork, and then contributing to the alteration of the homeostasis in ganglionary cells, facilitating their death [36]. A significant correlation has been shown among human trabecular meshwork DNA oxidative damage, visual field damage, and IOP [37]. It has also been proved that the specific activity of superoxide dismutase demonstrates an age-dependent decline [38]. Moreover, apoptosis in glaucoma is triggered by endothelial dysregulation and dysfunction, hypoxia, and subclinical inflammation. All these conditions might contribute to accelerate the trabecular meshwork sclerosis favoring IOP increase and the apoptosis of retinal ganglion cells. Accordingly, an intervention affecting these mechanisms especially by decreasing oxidative stress and inflammation supports the rationale for the study.

However, little is known about the effect of antioxidant intake and prevention or amelioration of IOP in glaucoma. In an experimental study carried out in rats, an association between dietary omega-3 fatty acid intake and decrease in IOP caused by altered aqueous outflow was found [22]. The authors of this study suggested that dietary manipulation may provide a modifiable factor for IOP regulation. Data of clinical studies, however, are sparse. Kant et al. [39] used a food frequency questionnaire to assess the relation between the intake of a variety of antioxidants derived from food and dietary supplements in 474 glaucoma patients

TABLE 2: Baseline characteristics of the study patients.

Variables	Total patients (n = 47)	Study group Experimental (n = 23)	Control (n = 24)	P value
Men/women	25/22	11/12	14/10	0.470
Age, years, mean (SD)	70.3 (5.0)	70.7 (4.5)	69.9 (5.6)	0.563
Comorbid diseases	—	—	—	—
Hypertension	19	10	9	—
Dyslipidemia	21	10	11	—
Diabetes mellitus	4	2	2	—
Chronic obstructive pulmonary disease	6	2	4	—
Osteoporosis	5	2	3	—
Ischemic heart disease	2	2	—	—
Depression	2	—	2	—
Arthrosis	2	1	1	—
PEX glaucoma	—	—	—	0.765
Right eye	14 (29.8)	7 (30.4)	7 (29.2)	—
Left eye	13 (27.6)	5 (21.7)	7 (29.2)	—
Both eyes	21 (44.7)	11 (47.8)	10 (41.7)	—
BCVA, decimals, mean (SD)	—	—	—	—
Right eye	0.90 (0.19)	0.91 (0.22)	0.89 (0.16)	0.735
Left eye	0.86 (0.21)	0.87 (0.19)	0.85 (0.22)	0.776
IOP, mmHg, mean (SD)	—	—	—	—
Right eye	14.8 (3.5)	14.7 (3.3)	15.0 (3.7)	0.769
Left eye	14.9 (4.2)	15.1 (3.3)	14.7 (4.9)	0.732
Central corneal thickness, μm, mean (SD)	—	—	—	—
Right eye	535.9 (38.6)	543.2 (36.6)	529.0 (40.0)	0.214
Left eye	535.5 (37.5)	540.1 (36.0)	531.1 (39.0)	0.416
RNFLT, μm, mean (SD)	—	—	—	—
Right eye	67.8 (22.1)	67.2 (20.5)	68.3 (23.8)	0.880
Left eye	74.5 (19.2)	71.7 (16.4)	76.7 (21.2)	0.416

PEX: pseudoexfoliative; BCVA: best corrected visual acuity; IOP: intraocular pressure; RNFLT: retinal nerve fiber layer thickness.

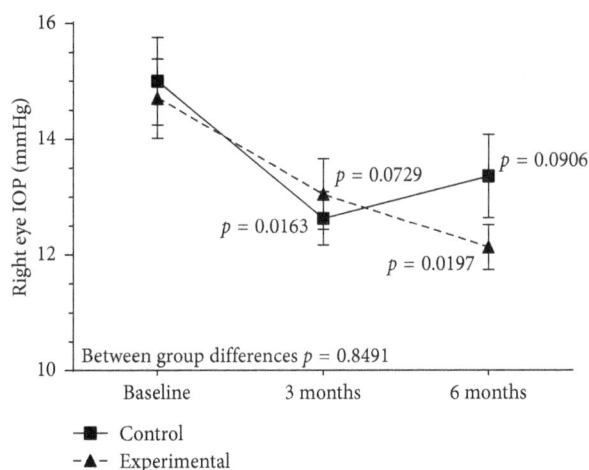

FIGURE 1: Changes of IOP values in the right eye in the experimental and control groups throughout the study.

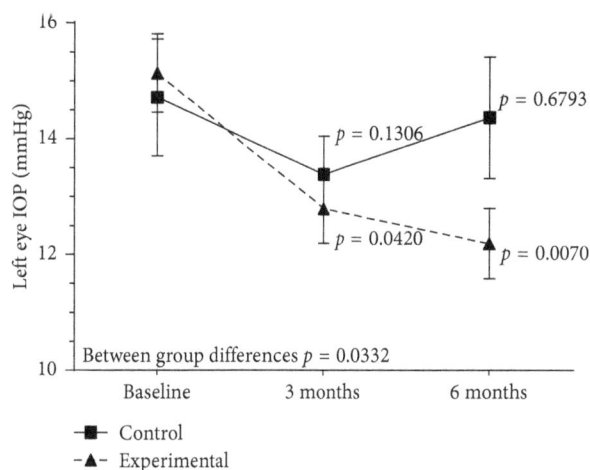

FIGURE 2: Changes in IOP values in the left eye in the experimental and control groups throughout the study.

selected from the Nurses' Health Study and the Health Professionals Follow-up Study and followed for more than 10 years and did not observe any strong associations between antioxidant consumption and the risk of primary open-angle glaucoma. In a systematic review of 46 articles in which the effect of nutrients on open-angle glaucoma was studied,

nitric oxide present in dark green leafy vegetables seemed to have a beneficial effect [27]. Interestingly, Wang et al. [26] analyzed the association between glaucoma and daily intake of PUFAs, including ω-3 fatty acids, in 3865 participants in the National Health and Nutrition Examination Survey 2005–2008 database who were 40 years or older and has

TABLE 3: Changes of intraocular pressure (IOP) during the study.

Study group	IOP, mmHg, mean (SD)					
	Right eye	P value*	Left eye	P value*	Both eyes	P value*
Experimental						
Baseline	14.7 (3.3)	—	15.1 (3.3)		14.9 (3.3)	—
3 months	13.0 (2.7)	0.072	12.8 (2.6)	0.04	12.9 (2.6)	0.006
6 months	12.1 (1.5)	0.01	12.2 (2.4)	0.007	12.2 (2.0)	0.0003
Control						
Baseline	15.0 (3.7)	—	14.7 (4.9)	—	14.8 (4.3)	—
3 months	12.6 (2.2)	0.016	13.4 (3.2)	0.130	13.0 (2.8)	0.004
6 months	13.4 (3.4)	0.090	14.4 (4.9)	0.679	13.9 (4.2)	0.110

*P values versus baseline for all comparisons.

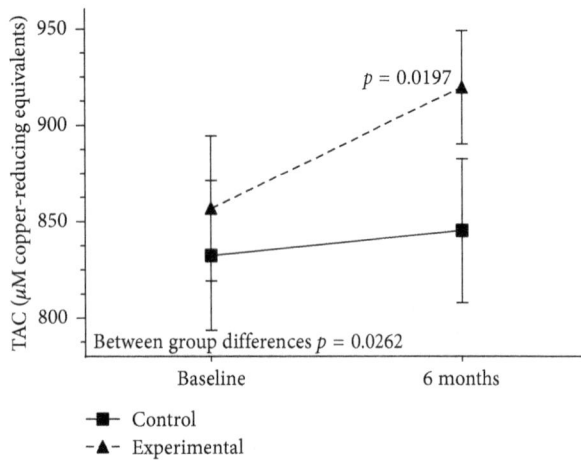

FIGURE 3: Changes of plasma total antioxidant capacity (TAC) levels in the experimental and control groups throughout the study.

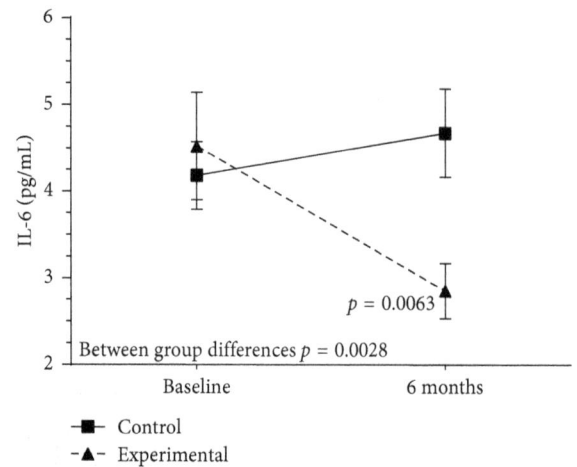

FIGURE 5: Changes of plasma interleukin- (IL-) 6 values in the experimental and control groups throughout the study.

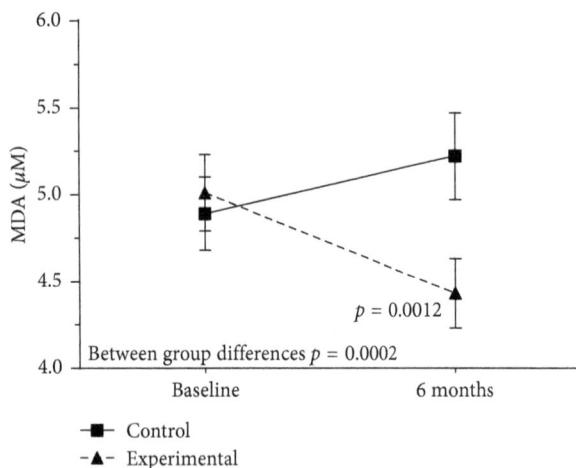

FIGURE 4: Serum malondialdehyde (MDA) values decreased significantly in the experimental group throughout the study.

available results of eye examinations. Increased levels of daily dietary intake of EPA (odds ratio [OR] 0.06, 95% CI 0.00–0.73) and DHA (OR 0.06, 95% CI 0.01–0.87) were associated with significantly lower odds of having glaucoma. In a previous open study of 1255 patients with glaucoma and dry eye syndrome treated for 12 weeks with the same nutritional supplement, a significant decrease in IOP values in

both eyes as compared with baseline was observed [16]. These findings are consistent with a potential beneficial role of DHA supplementation in glaucoma patients. The nutraceutical product also includes minerals, vitamins, and other compounds, but the high DHA content is a remarkable characteristic of the supplement.

Finally, recent studies provided evidence of the association between systemic redox status and visual field damage in glaucoma patients, suggesting that lower systemic antioxidant capacity is associated with more severe visual field damage in glaucoma disease. Tanito et al. [40] assessed the correlation between the visual field sensitivity value and systemic levels of pro-oxidants and antioxidants by analyzing the blood biochemistry in 202 patients with open-angle glaucoma (OAG). Univariate and multivariate analyses suggested a positive correlation between mean value of visual field sensitivity and systemic levels of antioxidants, which may indicate that lower systemic antioxidant capacity is associated with more severe visual field damage in OAG. In another study, Asano et al. [41] examined the association between biological antioxidant potential (BAP), a biomarker of systemic antioxidative capacity, and glaucoma severity in 247 patients (480 eyes) with OAG and 66 healthy controls. Mixed-effect regression analysis showed that BAP was an independent contributing factor to glaucomatous damage, particularly in young males, suggesting that antioxidant therapy might be more effective in these patients. Biomarkers of systemic oxidative stress should therefore be regarded as valuable complementary information sources in glaucoma care.

Although our findings should be interpreted according to the small sample size and the limited duration of the study, further statistically significant reduction of IOP in patients assigned to the experimental group, who had otherwise good control of IOP at entry, supports the potential clinical usefulness of DHA supplementation in daily practice. More studies (longitudinal and randomized clinical trials) are needed to make the present results clinically applicable, but they may help ophthalmologists to suggest their patients an advice on high dietary intake of omega-3 fatty acids.

Disclosure

This study was presented as a poster at the 13th EGS Congress, Florence, Italy, May 19–22, 2018.

Conflicts of Interest

The authors declare that they have no conflicts of interest.

Acknowledgments

The authors thank Jaume Borrás, MD, for his coordination and monitoring of the study and to Marta Pulido, MD, PhD, for editing the manuscript and for her editorial assistance.

References

[1] R. Ritch and U. Schlötzer-Schrehardt, "Exfoliation syndrome," *Survey of Ophthalmology*, vol. 45, no. 4, pp. 265–315, 2001.

[2] P. Plateroti, A. M. Plateroti, S. Abdolrahimzadeh, and G. Scuderi, "Pseudoexfoliation syndrome and pseudoexfoliation glaucoma: a review of the literature with updates on surgical management," *Journal of Ophthalmology*, vol. 2015. Article ID 370371, pp. 1–9, 2015.

[3] R. Ritch, "The management of exfoliative glaucoma," *Progress in Brain Research*, vol. 173, pp. 211–224, 2008.

[4] M. Tanito, S. Kaidzu, Y. Takai, and A. Ohira, "Status of systemic oxidative stress in patients with primary open-angle glaucoma and pseudoexfoliation syndrome," *PLoS One*, vol. 7, no. 11, Article ID e49680, 2012.

[5] M. D. Pinazo-Durán, V. Zanón-Moreno, J. J. vGarcía-Medina, and R. Gallego-Pinazo, "Evaluation of presumptive biomarkers of oxidative stress, immune response and apoptosis in primary open-angle glaucoma," *Current Opinion in Pharmacology*, vol. 13, no. 1, pp. 98–107, 2013.

[6] A. Izzotti, A. Bagnis, and S. C. Saccà, "The role of oxidative stress in glaucoma," *Mutation Research/Reviews in Mutation Research*, vol. 612, no. 2, pp. 105–114, 2006.

[7] S. K. Srivastava and K. V. Ramana, "Focus on molecules: nuclear factor-kappaB," *Experimental Eye Research*, vol. 88, no. 1, pp. 2-3, 2009.

[8] C. Erb, "Importance of the nuclear factor kappaB for the primary-open angle glaucoma—a hypothesis," *Klinische Monatsblätter für Augenheilkunde*, vol. 227, no. 2, pp. 120–127, 2010.

[9] C. Y. Wang, C. Y. Liang, S. C. Feng et al., "Analysis of the interleukin-6 (-174) locus polymorphism and serum IL-6 levels with the severity of normal tension glaucoma," *Ophthalmic Research*, vol. 57, no. 4, pp. 224–229, 2017.

[10] F. Zahir-Jouzdani, F. Atyabi, and N. Mojtabavi, "Interleukin-6 participation in pathology of ocular diseases," *Pathophysiology*, vol. 24, no. 3, pp. 123–131, 2017.

[11] F. D. Echevarria, A. E. Rickman, and R. M. Sappington, "Interleukin-6: a constitutive modulator of glycoprotein 130, neuroinflammatory and cell survival signaling in retina," *Journal of Clinical & Cellular Immunology*, vol. 7, no. 4, p. 439, 2016.

[12] F. D. Echevarria, C. R. Formichella, and R. M. Sappington, "Interleukin-6 deficiency attenuates retinal ganglion cell axonopathy and glaucoma-related vision loss," *Frontiers in Neuroscience*, vol. 11, p. 318, 2017.

[13] H. Wang and B. P. Daggy, "The role of fish oil in inflammatory eye diseases," *Biomedicine Hub*, vol. 2, no. 1, Article ID 455818, 6 pages, 2017.

[14] M. Sasaki, R. Kawasaki, S. Rogers et al., "The associations of dietary intake of polyunsaturated fatty acids with diabetic retinopathy in well-controlled diabetes," *Investigative Ophthalmology & Visual Science*, vol. 56, no. 12, pp. 7473–7479, 2015.

[15] M. Lafuente, L. Ortín, M. Argente et al., "Three-year outcomes in a randomized single-blind controlled trial of intravitreal ranibizumab and oral supplementation with docosahexaenoic acid and antioxidants for diabetic macular edema," *Retina*, p. 1, 2018, In press.

[16] J. Tellez-Vazquez, "Omega-3 fatty acid supplementation improves dry eye symptoms in patients with glaucoma: results of a prospective multicenter study," *Clinical Ophthalmology*, vol. 10, pp. 617–626, 2016.

[17] J. Dawczynski, S. Jentsch, D. Schweitzer, M. Hammer, G. E. Lang, and J. Strobel, "Long term effects of lutein, zeaxanthin and omega-3-LCPUFAs supplementation on optical density of macular pigment in AMD patients: the LUTEGA study," *Graefe's Archive for Clinical and Experimental Ophthalmology*, vol. 251, pp. 2711–2723, 2013.

[18] W. Chen, W. J. Esselman, D. B. Jump et al., "Anti-inflammatory effect of docosahexaenoic acid on cytokine-induced adhesion molecule expression in human retinal vascular endothelial cells," *Investigative Opthalmology & Visual Science*, vol. 46, no. 11, pp. 4342–4347, 2005.

[19] P. C. Calder, "Omega-3 fatty acids and inflammatory processes," *Nutrients*, vol. 2, no. 3, pp. 355–374, 2010.

[20] M. V. Simón, D. L. Agnolazza, O. L. German et al., "Synthesis of docosahexaenoic acid from eicosapentaenoic acid in retina neurons protects photoreceptors from oxidative stress," *Journal of Neurochemistry*, vol. 136, no. 5, pp. 931–946, 2016.

[21] N. P. Rotstein, L. E. Politi, O. L. German, and R. Girotti, "Protective effect of docosahexaenoic acid on oxidative stress-induced apoptosis of retina photoreceptors," *Investigative Opthalmology & Visual Science*, vol. 44, no. 5, pp. 2252–2259, 2003.

[22] C. T. Nguyen, B. V. Bui, A. J. Sinclair, and A. J. Vingrys, "Dietary omega 3 fatty acids decrease intraocular pressure with age by increasing aqueous outflow," *Investigative Opthalmology & Visual Science*, vol. 48, no. 2, pp. 756–762, 2007.

[23] H. Ren, N. Magulike, K. Ghebremeskel, and M. Crawford, "Primary open-angle glaucoma patients have reduced levels of blood docosahexaenoic and eicosapentaenoic acids," *Prostaglandins, Leukotrienes and Essential Fatty Acids*, vol. 74, no. 3, pp. 157–163, 2006.

[24] N. Acar, O. Berdeaux, P. Juaneda et al., "Red blood cell plasmalogens and docosahexaenoic acid are independently reduced in primary open-angle glaucoma," *Experimental Eye Research*, vol. 89, no. 6, pp. 840–853, 2009.

[25] C. T. Nguyen, A. J. Vingrys, and B. V. Bui, "Dietary ω-3 deficiency and IOP insult are additive risk factors for ganglion cell dysfunction," *Journal of Glaucoma*, vol. 22, no. 4, pp. 269–277, 2013.

[26] Y. E. Wang, V. L. Tseng, J. Caprioli, and A. L. Coleman, "Association of dietary fatty acid intake with glaucoma in the United States," *JAMA Ophthalmology*, vol. 136, no. 2, pp. 141–147, 2018.

[27] W. D. Ramdas, "The relation between dietary intake and glaucoma: a systematic review," *Acta Ophthalmologica*, 2018, In press.

[28] E. Hodapp, R. K. Parrish, and D. R. Anderson, *Clinical Decisions in Glaucoma*, C. V. Mosby, St. Louis, MO, USA, 1993.

[29] Brudy Technology, "Results shown in the (held by) related to the use of DHA for treating a pathology associated with cellular oxidative damage," European Patent EP 1 962 825 B1, 2014.

[30] P. Bogdanov and J. C. Domingo, "Docosahexaenoic acid improves endogenous antioxidant defense in ARPE-19 cells," in *Proceedings of Association for Research in Vision and Ophthalmology*, Fort Lauderdale, FL, USA, May, 2008, poster 5932/A306.

[31] M. E. Rodríguez González-Herrero, M. Ruiz, F. J. López Román, J. M. Marín Sánchez, and J. C. Domingo, "Supplementation with a highly concentrated docosahexaenoic acid plus xanthophyll carotenoid multivitamin in nonproliferative diabetic retinopathy: prospective controlled study of macular function by fundus microperimetry," *Clinical Ophthalmology*, vol. 12, pp. 1011–1020, 2018.

[32] D. Gherghel, H. R. Griffiths, E. J. Hilton, I. A. Cunliffe, and S. L. Hosking, "Systemic reduction in glutathione levels occurs in patients with primary open-angle glaucoma," *Investigative Opthalmology & Visual Science*, vol. 46, no. 3, pp. 877–883, 2005.

[33] P. Maher, "The effects of stress and aging on glutathione metabolism," *Ageing Research Reviews*, vol. 4, no. 2, pp. 288–314, 2005.

[34] O. Yildirim, N. A. Ateş, B. Ercan et al., "Role of oxidative stress enzymes in open-angle glaucoma," *Eye*, vol. 19, no. 5, pp. 580–583, 2005.

[35] V. Zanon-Moreno, P. Marco-Ventura, A. Lleo-Perez et al., "Oxidative stress in primary open-angle glaucoma," *Journal of Glaucoma*, vol. 17, no. 4, pp. 263–268, 2008.

[36] S. C. Saccà, A. Izzotti, P. Rossi, and C. Traverso, "Glaucomatous outflow pathway and oxidative stress," *Experimental Eye Research*, vol. 84, no. 3, pp. 389–399, 2007.

[37] S. C. Saccà, A. Pascotto, P. Camicione, P. Capris, and A. Izzotti, "Oxidative DNA damage in the human trabecular meshwork: clinical correlation in patients with primary open-angle glaucoma," *Archives of Ophthalmology*, vol. 123, no. 4, pp. 458–463, 2005.

[38] S. C. Saccà, S. Gandolfi, A. Bagnis et al., "From DNA damage to functional changes of the trabecular meshwork in aging and glaucoma," *Ageing Research Reviews*, vol. 29, pp. 26–41, 2016.

[39] J. H. Kang, L. R. Pasquale, W. Willett et al., "Antioxidant intake and primary open-angle glaucoma: a prospective study," *American Journal of Epidemiology*, vol. 158, no. 4, pp. 337–346, 2003.

[40] M. Tanito, S. Kaidzu, Y. Takai, and A. Ohira, "Association between systemic oxidative stress and visual field damage in open-angle glaucoma," *Scientific Reports*, vol. 6, no. 1, p. 25792, 2016.

[41] Y. Asano, N. Himori, H. Kunikata et al., "Age- and sex-dependency of the association between systemic antioxidant potential and glaucomatous damage," *Scientific Reports*, vol. 7, no. 1, p. 8032, 2017.

27

Is the Retinal Vasculature Related to β-Peripapillary Atrophy in Nonpathological High Myopia? An Optical Coherence Tomography Angiography Study in Chinese Adults

Jiao Sun📷, Jialin Wang📷, Ran You, and Yanling Wang📷

Department of Ophthalmology, Beijing Friendship Hospital Affiliated to Capital Medical University, Beijing, China

Correspondence should be addressed to Yanling Wang; wangyanl@ccmu.edu.cn

Academic Editor: Lawrence S. Morse

Purpose. The association between β-peripapillary atrophy and the retinal vasculature in nonpathological high myopia is unclear. The aim of this study is to investigate whether β-peripapillary atrophy contribute to the changes of the retinal vasculature using optical coherence tomography angiography. *Methods.* In a cross-sectional study, one hundred and thirty eyes with nonpathological high myopia were included. β-peripapillary atrophy was analysed using Image J software based on fundus photographs. A $3.0 \times 3.0 \, mm^2$ grid and a $4.5 \times 4.5 \, mm^2$ grid were used to scan parafoveal and peripapillary regions using optical coherence tomography angiography, respectively. Vessel density and fractal dimensions of the retina and foveal avascular zone were analysed and quantified using en face projection images. Correlations between the vascular density, foveal avascular zone, and β-peripapillary atrophy were determined. *Results.* Using multivariate analysis, β peripapillary atrophy was negatively correlated with the vessel density in radial peripapillary capillaries ($p = 0.002$) even after adjusting for other variables. This relationship was also confirmed in the macula (superficial retinal plexus: $p < 0.05$; deep retinal plexus: $p < 0.05$). The vessel densities in the nasal and inferior sectors were more strongly correlated with β-peripapillary atrophy. *Conclusions.* There was a negative correlation between β-peripapillary atrophy and the retinal vasculature in highly myopic eyes, especially in radial peripapillary capillaries and deep retinal plexus. β-peripapillary atrophy can be visualized and is a convenient structural feature that can benefit the early diagnosis and detection of chorioretinal atrophy in high myopia.

1. Introduction

The prevalence of myopia has markedly increased over the past three decades, especially in China [1]. In myopic eyes, there are morphological changes in the optic disc, such as β-peripapillary atrophy (β-PPA), tilt, and rotation [2]. The myopic β-PPA, also known as the optic disc crescent, is a white area with a well-defined boundary and visible sclera due to uncovering of the retinal pigment epithelium (RPE), a common structure in myopic eyes [3]. One study demonstrated that myopic β-PPA eyes showed a thinner ganglion cell-inner plexiform layer and macular thickness than myopic eyes without β-PPA [4]. Another study found that the quadrantal alterations in myopic eyes were uneven, with the greatest changes noted in the inferior nasal sector [5]. Moreover, Wang and associates [6] found a decrease in peripapillary perfusion in highly myopic eyes and inferred that β-PPA may play a role in the decreased peripapillary blood flow in myopic eyes. Therefore, we hypothesized that β-PPA might be associated with macular and peripapillary perfusion. Additionally, as β-PPA is a common finding in normal-tension glaucoma (NTG) and the pathogenesis between myopia and NTG remains unclear, focusing on a potential shared pathway between the retinal vasculature and NTG could improve our understanding of the pathophysiology and expand therapies for each condition.

Optical coherence tomography angiography (OCTA) is a novel quantitative method used to analyse the retinal microvasculature. Previous studies using different imaging modalities have demonstrated a reduction in retinal and choroidal perfusion in high myopia. In addition, a growing body of evidence suggests that vascular dysfunction is a complication of myopia [3, 7, 8]. Thus, it is important to study retinal perfusion in myopic eyes because this information is helpful for the early diagnosis and monitoring of chorioretinal atrophy in eyes with high myopia [9].

The aims of the present study were to quantify vasculature parameters using OCTA to determine whether retinal vasculature is associated with β-PPA and to characterize differences in β-PPA with macular perfusion in each sector in highly myopic eyes.

2. Methods and Materials

2.1. Participants. Patients from the Beijing Friendship Hospital (Beijing, China) were recruited. This cross-sectional study was approved by the Ethics Committee of the Beijing Friendship Hospital (Beijing, China) and was conducted in accordance with the ethical standards stated in the Declaration of Helsinki. Written informed consent was obtained from all examined patients and volunteer participants prior to OCTA imaging. Each subject underwent a complete ocular examination, including best-corrected visual acuity (BCVA), intraocular pressure (IOP) by automatic tonometer, slit-lamp examination, fundus colour photography, and axial length (AL) measurement by optical biometry (IOL Master; Carl Zeiss Meditec, Jena, Germany). Subjects with a refraction of greater than 6 diopters (D) or ALs longer than 26.5 mm were included in this study. The exclusion criteria were myopic maculopathy, any prior history or clinical evidence of vitreoretinal conditions or surgery, IOP > 21 mmHg, visual field defects, and systemic diseases potentially affecting the eyes (Figure 1).

2.2. Image Acquisition and Analysis. The OCTA instrument, RTVue XR Avanti with AngioVue (Optovue Inc., Fremont, California, USA), was used at a scanning speed of 70,000 A-scans per second by a single operator (JS). The scan protocol examined a $3.0 \times 3.0\,mm^2$ area focused on the macula and a $4.5 \times 4.5\,mm^2$ area focused on the optic disc and obtained a horizontal priority (X-scan) and a vertical priority (Y-scan) in approximately 2.9 s for each of the two raster scans. The RTVue instrument was used to segment superficial and deep inner retinal vascular plexuses (Figure 2). The superficial retinal plexus (SRP) was segmented from the outer boundary of the inner limiting membrane (ILM) to the outer boundary of the inner plexiform layer (IPL), which extends from 3 μm below the ILM to 15 μm below the IPL. The deep retinal plexus (DRP) was segmented from the outer boundary of the IPL to the outer boundary of the outer plexiform layer (OPL), which extends from 15 to 70 μm below the IPL. The split-spectrum amplitude decorrelation angiography (SSADA) algorithm was used to segment the vessels. The superficial retinal layer comprises ganglion cell and inner plexiform layers, whereas the deep

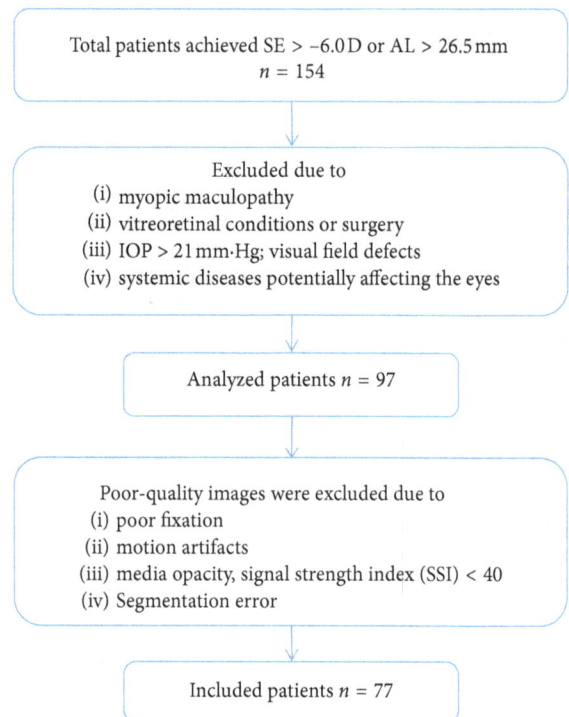

FIGURE 1: Study population. SE = spherical equivalent; AL = axial length.

retinal layer comprises inner nuclear and outer plexiform layers. These layers encompass the entire retinal vascular network. Furthermore, OCTA images of the superficial and deep retinal layers were divided into 5 parts: fovea, nasal, temporal, inferior, and superior sectors. The resolution of the exported OCTA images was 304×304 pixels. The motion correction technology (MCT) function was used to correct the horizontal and vertical scans. Because the magnification is different in myopic eyes, the imaging sampling density used in myopic eyes must be lower than that used in normal eyes [10]. Therefore, images obtained from highly myopic eyes were corrected for magnification using Bennett's formula. The RTVue instrument was also used to measure the retinal nerve fiber layer (RNFL) thickness and cup-to-disc ratio (CDR) from the OCT B-scans. Two independent examiners (XMM, FZ) reviewed the images. Poor-quality images were excluded based on the following criteria: (1) evidence of poor fixation, including a double vessel pattern and motion artefacts; (2) the presence of motion artefacts that could not be corrected by MCT; (3) media opacity, as marked by shadowing or obscuration of the vessel signal in the field of view or a signal strength index (SSI) of less than 40; and (4) a segmentation error in defining vascular layers (Figure 1).

High-resolution digital colour fundus photographs were taken using a digital retina camera (Kowa Nonmyd WX; Kowa Company Ltd., Japan). β-PPA is defined as the area in a fundus colour photograph characterized by a marked atrophy of retinal photoreceptors, RPE, and the choriocapillaris, along with the distinct visibility of large choroidal vessels and the sclera (Figure 3). When there was disagreement between the graders, we outlined the area with the help of OCT.

(a)

(b)

(c)

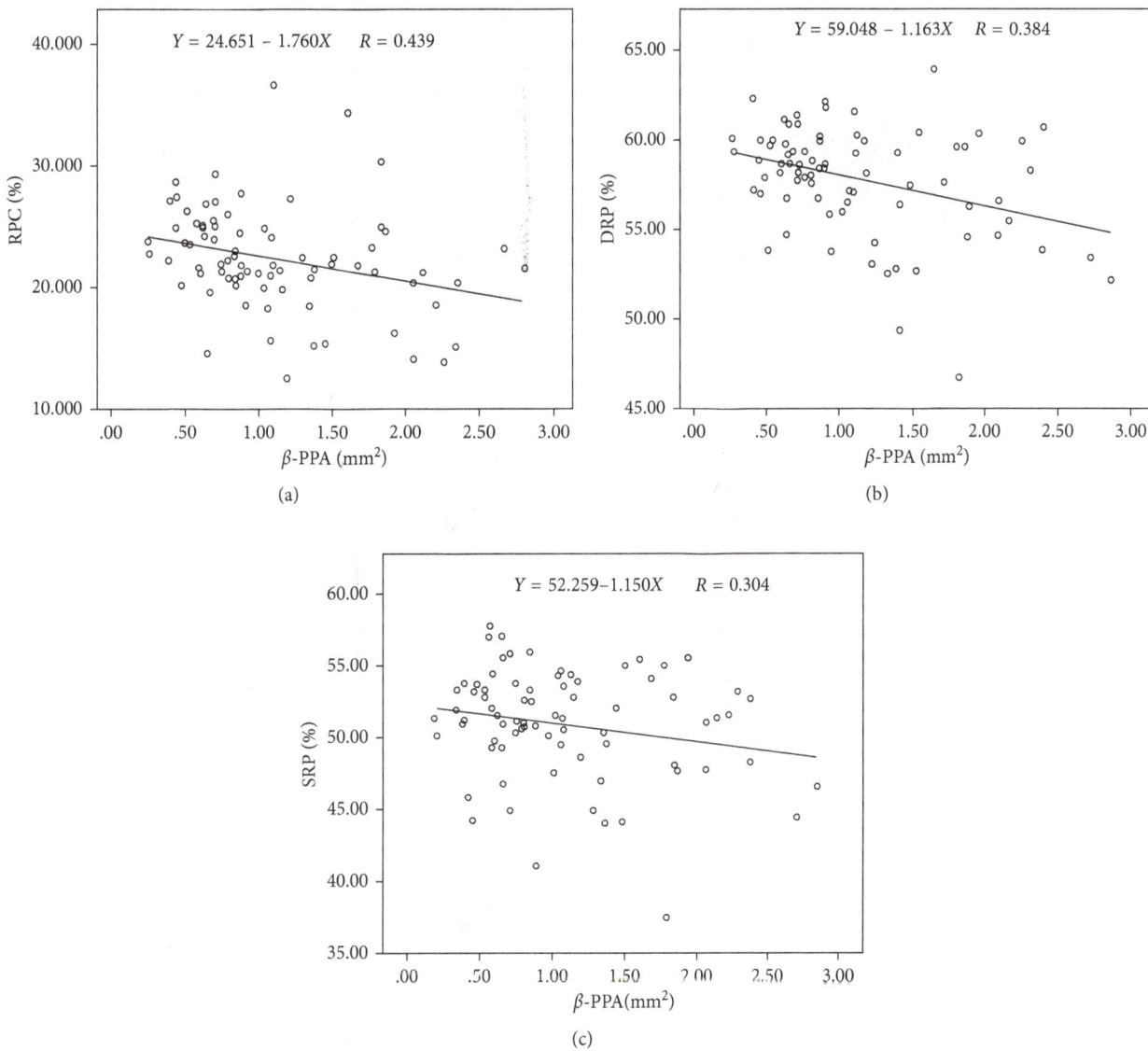

Figure 2: Correlation analyses between vessel density and β-peripapillary atrophy in the retina. (a) Radial peripapillary capillaries. (b) Deep retinal plexus. (c) Superficial retinal plexus.

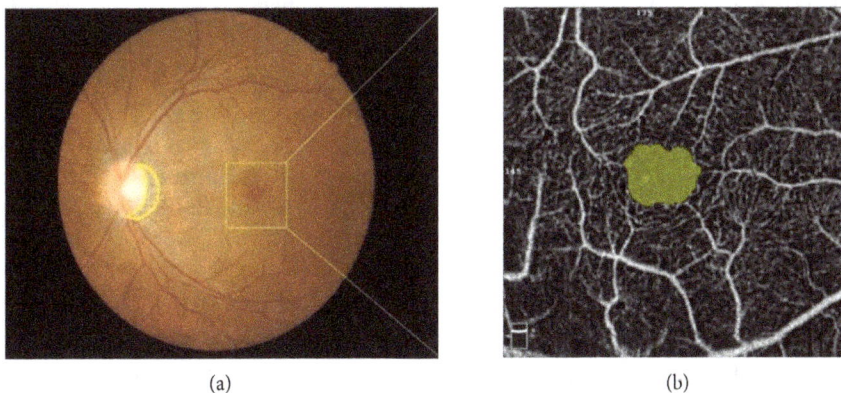

(a)

(b)

Figure 3: Continued.

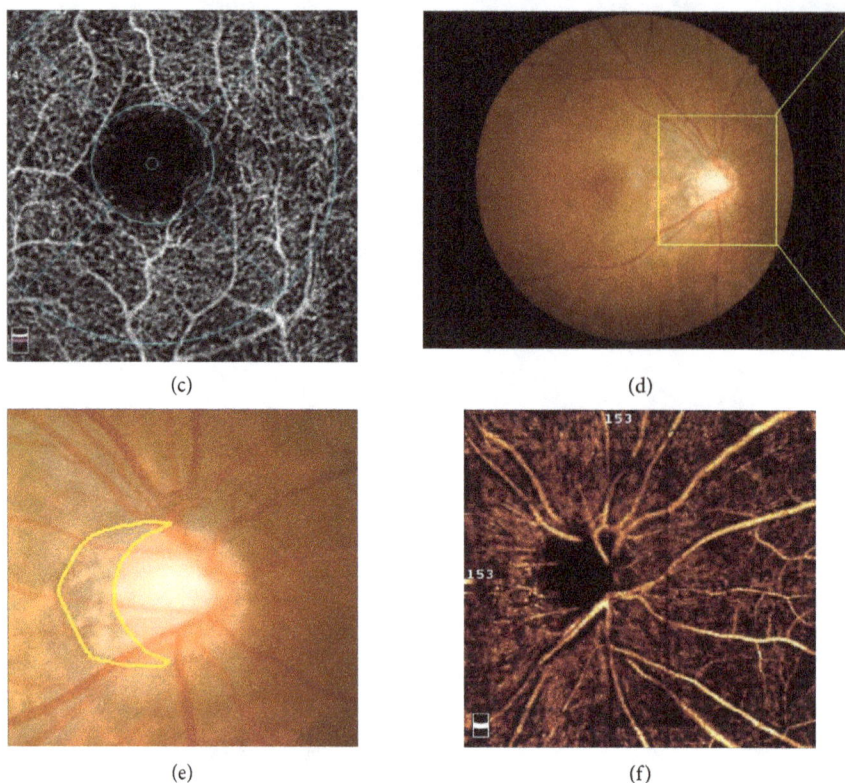

FIGURE 3: Images of β-peripapillary atrophy in a fundus colour paragraph (a, d, e), foveal avascular zone and vessel images of the superficial retinal plexus (b), deep retinal plexus (c), and radial peripapillary capillaries (f) using optical coherence tomography angiography in areas of $3.0 \times 3.0 \, \text{mm}^2$ and $4.5 \times 4.5 \, \text{mm}^2$.

OCTA data were analysed using Optovue software (RTVue XR version 2016.2.0.35). The foveal avascular zone (FAZ) area for each superficial plexus image was found and measured using the built-in nonflow automatic measurement tool of the AngioVue review software. Image processing of the radial peripapillary capillary (RPC) vascular density and β-PPA area measurements were performed using the public domain software Image J, version 1.50i (National Institutes of Health, Bethesda, Maryland, USA) (Figure 3). Binary images of the vascular networks were created using an automated thresholding algorithm. Vessel density was defined as the percentage area occupied by blood vessels, with the blood vessels being defined as pixels having values above the threshold level [11]. To assess the reproducibility of the technique, two examiners (XMM, FZ) measured each image 3 times.

2.3. Statistical Analysis.

Statistical analysis was performed using a commercially available statistics software programme (SPSS for Microsoft, version 24.0; IBM/SPSS, Chicago, Illinois, USA). First, we calculated the means and standard deviations of the main outcome parameters. Second, we carried out multivariate regression models, modelling the vasculature parameters as the dependent variable, and all parameters that were associated with the vasculature parameters as independent variables, taking a p value < 0.05 as the cutoff value. Third, we performed a linear regression of potential associations between β-PPA and macular vessel density in each sector.

Finally, we calculated the standardized regression coefficient beta and the nonstandardized regression coefficient B together with its 95% confidence interval (CI).

3. Results

3.1. Demographics. Among the 97 participants recruited, 20 were excluded from the analysis because of poor signal quality (SSI < 45) or blink artefacts. A total of 130 eyes from 77 participants with nonpathological high myopia were analysed in this study. The mean age at the initial visit was 35.24 ± 8.45 years, and the mean spherical equivalent (SE) refractive error was -10.03 ± 3.57 D. The demographics of these participants are shown in Table 1.

3.2. Association between β-PPA and RPC Parameters. Using linear regression analysis, β-PPA was shown to be negatively associated with the RPC (Figure 2(a), Table 2, $p < 0.001$). After adjusting for the compounding factors of age, IOP, CDR, and RNFL thickness, the parameter AL was still significantly negatively correlated with RPC ($\beta = -1.472$, $p = 0.002$) (Table 2). Specifically, a $1.0 \, \text{mm}^2$ increase in β-PPA was associated with 1.472% lower in RPC density.

3.3. Association between β-PPA and Macular Perfusion Parameters. Using linear regression analysis, β-PPA was shown to be negatively associated with SRP and DRP (Figures 2(b) and 2(c), Table 3, $p < 0.001$ and $p = 0.005$,

TABLE 1: Demographic and ocular characteristics of the participants.

	Mean ± SD ($n = 77$)	Male ($n = 37$)	Female ($n = 40$)	p value
Age (y)	35.24 ± 8.45	36.29 ± 9.54	34.47 ± 7.55	0.339
SE (D)	10.03 ± 3.57	0.97 ± 0.13	0.98 ± 0.15	0.493
IOP (mmHg)	15.62 ± 3.25	16.60 ± 3.32	14.89 ± 3.03	0.017
β-PPA (mm²)	1.09 ± 0.62	1.06 ± 0.62	1.10 ± 0.63	0.760
AL (mm)	27.43 ± 1.68	27.67 ± 1.54	27.25 ± 1.77	0.259
SP (mmHg)	119.95 ± 11.90	125.34 ± 12.32	115.94 ± 8.91	<0.001
DP (mmHg)	74.67 ± 8.75	79.43 ± 7.86	71.13 ± 7.70	<0.001
HR	76.11 ± 8.33	74.00 ± 7.23	77.68 ± 8.82	0.047
RNFL (μm)	95.69 ± 0.49	94.58 ± 8.56	96.47 ± 10.11	0.383

SE, spherical equivalent; D, diopters; IOP, intraocular pressure; β-PPA, β-peripapillary atrophy; AL, axial length; SP, systolic pressure; DP, diastolic pressure; HR, heart rate; RNFL, retinal nerve fiber layer.

TABLE 2: Multivariate regression analysis: association between β-PPA and retinal peripapillary capillary (RPC) plexus.

Variable	Model[a]	Unstandardized coefficients B	Std. Error	Standardized coefficients Beta	t	p	Adjusted R^2	95.0% CI for B Lower bound	Upper bound
β-PPA	1	−1.760	0.455	−0.397	−3.871	<0.001	0.147	−2.665	−0.855
β-PPA	2	−1.469	0.475	−0.332	−3.094	0.003	0.172	−2.414	−0.524
β-PPA	3	−1.277	0.438	−0.293	−2.913	0.005	0.305	−2.150	−0.404
β-PPA	4	−1.472	0.459	−0.337	−3.207	0.002	0.313	−2.386	−0.557

[a]Model 1, crude; model 2, adjustment for age and gender; model 3, further adjustment for intraocular pressure, cup-to-disc ratio, and retinal nerve fiber layer thickness; model 4, further adjustment for axial length.

TABLE 3: Multivariate regression analysis: association between β-PPA and deep/superficial retinal plexus.

Variable	Model[a]	Unstandardized coefficients B	Std. Error	Standardized coefficients Beta	T	p	Adjusted R^2	95.0% CI for B Lower bound	Upper bound
DRP									
β-PPA	1	−1.163	0.312	0.384	−3.722	<0.001	0.137	−1.784	−0.541
β-PPA	2	−0.874	0.318	−0.289	−2.744	0.008	0.202	−1.507	−0.240
β-PPA	3	−0.836	0.310	−0.290	−2.697	0.009	0.209	−1.454	−0.218
β-PPA	4	−0.609	0.318	−0.211	−1.918	0.059	0.251	−1.242	0.024
SRP									
β-PPA	1	−1.150	0.403	−0.304	−2.854	0.005	0.081	−1.952	−0.348
β-PPA	2	−0.924	0.423	−0.244	−2.184	0.032	0.099	−1.765	−0.082
β-PPA	3	−0.855	0.421	−0.231	−2.029	0.046	0.101	−1.694	−0.015
β-PPA	4	−0.501	0.427	−0.135	−1.174	0.244	0.181	−1.351	0.350

β-PPA, β-peripapillary atrophy; DRP, deep retinal plexus; SRP, superficial retinal plexus. [a]Model 1, crude; model 2, adjustment for age and gender; model 3, further adjustment for intraocular pressure, cup-to-disc ratio, and retinal nerve fiber layer thickness; model 4, further adjustment for axial length.

respectively, for DRP and SRP). An increase in β-PPA by 1 mm² was associated with a decrease in the vessel density of DRP by 1.163%, whereas the SRP lessened by 1.150%. Using multiple linear regression analysis, β-PPA was shown to be negatively associated with DRP in model 2 when we adjusted age and gender (Table 3, $\beta = -0.874$, $p < 0.05$); when we added the factors of IOP, CDR, and RNFL thickness, β-PPA is still significantly correlated with SRP (Table 3, model 3: $\beta = -0.836$, $p < 0.05$). After adjusting AL in model 4, we found that the p value was very closely approaching the conventional significance level ($p = 0.059$, when we take a p value < 0.05 as the cutoff value).

3.4. Association between β-PPA and Macular Perfusion Parameters in Each Sector. Furthermore, we concluded the results of the regression analysis associating β-PPA with macular perfusion parameters in different sectors. As shown in Table 4, after we had adjusted the factors of age, gender, IOP, CDR, RNFL thickness, and AL, β-PPA is still significant negatively correlated with DRP in the nasal sector ($\beta = -1.029$, $p < 0.05$). Moreover, the p value of the DRP inferior sector is approaching the conventional significance level, although not reaching significance ($p = 0.083$). In SRP, the p value in the nasal sector nearly reached a significance level ($p = 0.090$). The nonsignificant results (with p values

TABLE 4: Multivariate regression analysis: association between β-PPA and macular perfusion parameters in each sector.

Dependent	Model 1 Coefficient (95% CI)	Model 2 Coefficient (95% CI)	Model 3 Coefficient (95% CI)	Model 4 Coefficient (95% CI)
SRP				
Nasal	**−1.786 (−2.097, −0.600)**	**−1.285 (−2.266, −0.303)**	**−1.274 (−2.270, −0.279)**	−0.868 (−1.877, 0.140)
Temporal	−1.018 (−1.871, −0.166)	−0.725 (−1.622, 0.171)	−0.667 (−1.573, 0.240)	−0.277 (−1.191, 0.637)
Superior	−1.023 (−1.952, 0.093)	−0.777 (−1.766, 0.213)	−0.788 (−1.802, 0.226)	−0.305 (−1.315, 0.705)
Inferior	**−1.669 (−2.799, −0.559)**	**−1.226 (−2.397, −0.058)**	**−1.198 (−2.387, 0.010)**	−0.754 (−1.967, 0.459)
Fovea	−0.019 (−1.150, 1.188)	−0.004 (−1.172, 1.162)	0.216 (−1.120, 1.293)	0.285 (−1.531, 0.962)
FAZ	−0.011 (−0.042, 0.020)	−0.006 (−0.029, 0.018)	−0.078 (−0.031, 0.015)	0.285 (−0.018, 0.028)
DRP				
Nasal	**−1.348 (−2.097, 0.600)**	**−1.043 (−1.817, −0.269)**	**−1.024 (−1.797, 0.252)**	**−1.029 (−1.847, −0.211)**
Temporal	−0.958 (−1.871, −0.166)	**−0.716 (−1.448, 0.015)**	**−0.640 (−1.352, 0.071)**	−0.474 (−1.217, 0.269)
Superior	−0.726 (−1.859, −1.750)	−0.624 (−2.309, 1.061)	−0.598 (−2.330, 1.134)	−0.377 (−2.204, 1.450)
Inferior	**−1.556 (−2.372, 0.741)**	**−1.161 (−1.989, −0.333)**	**−1.125 (−1.969, 0.281)**	−0.746 (−1.592, 0.101)
Fovea	0.281 (−1.12, 1.682)	0.323 (−1.190, 1.836)	0.005 (−1.331, 1.763)	−0.434 (−1.997, 1.130)

Model 1, crude; model 2, adjustment for age and gender; model 3, further adjustment for intraocular pressure, cup-to-disc ratio, and retinal nerve fiber layer thickness; model 4, further adjustment for axial length. β-PPA, β-peripapillary atrophy; DRP, deep retinal plexus; SRP, superficial retinal plexus.

larger than 0.05) in Table 4 may be explained by a single research center in this study. Further studies in multiple clinical research centers are needed to clarify the associations between β-PPA and retinal perfusion.

4. Discussion

The present study revealed a negative correlation between β-PPA and retinal vascular densities in the macula and RPC (Figure 2), although there was no correlation between β-PPA and foveal vascular density and FAZ. In the fractal analysis, this correlation was more significant in the nasal and inferior regions. Earlier work demonstrated that vessel density was reduced in high myopia compared with that in healthy subjects [12]. However, these studies did not consider β-PPA. To our knowledge, our analysis is the first to study the associations of β-PPA with the retinal vasculature and to characterize differences in β-PPA with macular fractal perfusion in highly myopic eyes.

The retina has three levels of blood supply (plexuses): the RPC plexus, superficial plexuses, and deep plexuses [13]. Half of the inner retina receives blood supply from three of these vascular plexuses, whereas choriocapillaries provide blood supply to the outer half of the retina and macula, and these are derived from the posterior ciliary artery (PCA) [14]. Histological findings have shown that photoreceptors, RPE, and choroid fall short and suffer even partial or complete loss at the temporal atrophic area of the crescent in myopia. Due to stretching forces and retinal degeneration, the vessels in β-PPA become straighter and thinner [15]; this may damage the endothelial cells and thus reduce the concentration of vascular endothelial growth factor (VEGF). The reduction in VEGF may also contribute to the possible loss of capillary networks [16, 17]. The chloride channels in RPE can regulate the choroid vasculature [18, 19]. Aakriti Garg and associates [20] showed that choroidal thinning is associated with β-PPA. Peripapillary intrachoroidal cavitation (PICC) often appears in myopic eyes with β-PPA, and patients with PICC have larger β-PPA than those without

PICC [21]. Furthermore, β-PPA in children is associated with extreme peripapillary thinning [22]. Chui and associates [23] reported that retinal stretching may not mirror scleral growth, and their results suggest that there could be slippage within the retina during eye growth. This may be the reason for retinoschisis and thus for the reduction in macular perfusion. Because of the separation tendency with the choroid, the retina cannot obtain enough nutrition. Moreover, thinning of the parafovea and macular ganglion cell-inner plexiform layer occurs in myopic eyes with β-PPA [4]. The thinning of the tissue may cause reduced oxygen demand, and as a result, blood circulation may decrease. Previous studies have demonstrated a reduction in the SCP and DCP of the macula in highly myopic eyes, and our results show that the vessel density parameters in both layers were correlated to β-PPA. Thus, it can be assumed that the macula is involved in the pathological process at the onset of disease due to the correlation with β-PPA.

AL appears to be significantly associated with both β-PPA [23] and decreased macular vasculature [24], and the latter two variables are affected by multiple factors. However, myopic disc changes are not always accompanied by axial elongation, which varies among individuals [25], suggesting that β-PPA also plays an important role in vasculature changes. In our study, the retinal vasculature parameters were all associated with AL and β-PPA. The AL was a confounder in the relationship with β-PPA and macular vasculature, while β-PPA was independently correlated with the RPC vessel density. Due to the direction of the traction force as AL is elongated, the macula is more strongly affected by AL than the optic disc.

Additionally, previous studies have reported an association between glaucoma and myopia; the mechanism by which myopia increases the risk of glaucoma remains unclear, and an understanding of myopia's role in glaucoma is important. β-PPA is a very common and characteristic structure in high myopia and glaucoma. Macular vessel density is decreased in glaucoma and high myopia and is correlated with the extent of disease. A previous study demonstrated that OCTA has the diagnostic value for determining macular vascular density for the early detection of glaucoma [14]. In patients with NTG, eyes with β-PPA demonstrated a significantly greater prevalence of retina pseudodrusen (RPD) than eyes without β-PPA [20]. A number of studies have reported an association between ocular circulation disorders and myopic morphological change. In the macular area, the GCC is thinner in high myopia, and this can be attributed to the vascular decline. In the peripapillary area, the reduced peripapillary perfusion can lead to the atrophy or lesion of the optic nerve head, RNFL thinning, and visual field defects. Together, these factors can increase the risk of NTG in high myopia. However, whether the reduced vascular perfusion in high myopia is a cause or result of NTG is not clear. Elucidating the effect of myopia on ocular circulation can lead to improved knowledge of the pathogenesis of myopia. However, these correlations require further study.

We observed that the fractal dimension representing vascular density in the whole retina was slightly higher than that in each of the individual layers. Moreover, the strength of the correlation was different in the fractal dimension. Our study further showed that the nasal and inferior sectors were more strongly related than other sectors in the SCP and DCP. This relationship could contribute to the direction of β-PPA and the structures related to it. β-PPA normally presents temporally or inferotemporally to the disc and must be differentiated from the congenital tilted disc, which normally occurs inferiorly [26]. The PICC is more easily found in the temporal and inferior sectors [21], and the RNFL is thinner in the temporal sector of the optic disc. Inferior subfoveal scleral thickness was lower than that for other regions around the posterior pole. However, further investigation is needed to reveal the pathogenesis underlying the relationship identified in this study. Furthermore, the vessel density in the nasal and inferior sectors may serve as a sensitive indicator of myopic retinopathy, thus explaining the mechanism of the myopia process.

Our study demonstrated that the FAZ of the fovea was not correlated with β-PPA. This might occur because most of the oxygen supplied to the retina from the FAZ is derived from the choroidal vessel rather than the retinal circulation, and changes in the FAZ may not be evident in the early stages of high myopia. Hence, we did not observe a correlation between the FAZ and β-PPA. Wang et al. [27] found that the FAZ was not significantly associated with the vessel densities of the retina and choroid in normal subjects. The FAZ has been reported to be enlarged in patients with diabetic retinopathy [28] and retinal vein occlusion [29]. However, the FAZ area did not significantly differ between highly myopic eyes and control group eyes [5] and did not change significantly in response to hyperoxia [30]. This result might also indicate that the regulatory response of the vasculature to hyperoxia differs between the retinal and choroidal circulations, suggesting that the FAZ may not be an ideal location for studying changes in microvessel network density in myopic eyes. Similarly, our study found that the fovea was not correlated with β-PPA. This result may be attributable to the thickness of the fovea because the average macular thickness of the foveal and parafoveal regions of myopic patients did not change with the degree of myopia, although the parafovea was thinner and the fovea was thicker due to traction by the vitreous [31]. In addition, measurement of the fovea in OCTA might also have been affected by the FAZ.

There is some strength in this study. First, previous studies demonstrated that vessel density was reduced in high myopia compared with that in healthy subjects. However, these studies did not consider β-PPA. To our knowledge, our analysis is the first to study the associations of β-PPA with the retinal vasculature in highly myopic eyes. Second, we specially involved young participants with no pathologically myopic change in our study. Third, it is an originally statistical analysis to study the association between β-PPA and vessel density in high myopia using a novel quantitative method OCTA. Our findings can increase the clinical significance of β-PPA and benefit the early diagnosis and detection of chorioretinal atrophy in high myopia.

There are several potential limitations to the current study. First, this study was limited by its cross-sectional design; in that, the number of participants was not very large. Additional studies with close follow-up of these patients are therefore warranted. Second, to better characterize the relationship between myopia and β-PPA, future studies should assess different directional PPA, diffuse PPA, and other types of PPA, such as alpha, gamma, and delta zone and optic disc torsion. Third, we assume that all the eyes are independent from each other in our study; however, there is limitation that some eyes are from same patient. Thus, our findings must be confirmed by further research.

In summary, this study demonstrated a correlation between β-PPA and the retinal vasculature in highly myopic eyes using OCTA, thereby presenting a possible reason for the reduced retinal vessel density. However, attention should be given to the AL because when we adjusted for this in the model, the relationship in the macula was not significant. Considering this relationship, retinal fundus photography may be an economic and convenient method for evaluating vessel density in clinical practice, especially for the nasal and inferior sectors. This information is helpful for understanding the pathogenic relationship between myopia and NTG and for the early diagnosis of chorioretinal atrophy in eyes with high myopia. Additionally, β-PPA should be adjusted while analysing retinal perfusion using OCTA in future studies.

Conflicts of Interest

The authors declare that there are no conflicts of interest regarding the publication of this paper.

Authors' Contributions

JS and J-LW contributed equally to this work.

References

[1] J. B. Jonas, L. Xu, W. B. Wei et al., "Myopia in China: a population-based cross-sectional, histological, and experimental study," *The Lancet*, vol. 388, p. S20, 2016.

[2] M. S. Sung, H. Heo, Y. S. Ji, and S. W. Park, "Predicting the risk of parafoveal scotoma in myopic normal tension glaucoma: role of optic disc tilt and rotation," *Eye*, vol. 31, no. 7, pp. 1051–1059, 2017.

[3] F. E. Fantes and D. R. Anderson, "Clinical histologic correlation of human peripapillary anatomy," *Ophthalmology*, vol. 96, no. 1, pp. 20–25, 1989.

[4] S. Seo, C. E. Lee, J. H. Jeong, K. H. Park, D. M. Kim, and J. W. Jeoung, "Ganglion cell-inner plexiform layer and retinal nerve fiber layer thickness according to myopia and optic disc area: a quantitative and three-dimensional analysis," *BMC Ophthalmology*, vol. 17, no. 1, p. 22, 2017.

[5] M. Li, Y. Yang, H. Jiang et al., "Retinal microvascular network and microcirculation assessments in high myopia," *American Journal of Ophthalmology*, vol. 174, pp. 56–67, 2017.

[6] X. Wang, X. Kong, C. Jiang, M. Li, J. Yu, and X. Sun, "Is the peripapillary retinal perfusion related to myopia in healthy eyes? A prospective comparative study," *BMJ Open*, vol. 6, no. 3, article e010791, 2016.

[7] A. Benavente-Perez, S. L. Hosking, N. S. Logan, and D. C. Broadway, "Ocular blood flow measurements in healthy human myopic eyes," *Graefe's Archive for Clinical and Experimental Ophthalmology*, vol. 248, no. 11, pp. 1587–1594, 2010.

[8] N. Shimada, K. Ohno-Matsui, S. Harino et al., "Reduction of retinal blood flow in high myopia," *Graefe's Archive for Clinical and Experimental Ophthalmology*, vol. 242, no. 4, pp. 284–288, 2004.

[9] K. Ohno-Matsui, T. Y. Lai, C. C. Lai, and C. M. Cheung, "Updates of pathologic myopia," *Progress in Retinal and Eye Research*, vol. 52, pp. 156–187, 2016.

[10] D. M. Sampson, P. Gong, D. An et al., "Axial length variation impacts on superficial retinal vessel density and foveal avascular zone area measurements using optical coherence tomography angiography," *Investigative Opthalmology & Visual Science*, vol. 58, no. 7, pp. 3065–3072, 2017.

[11] A. Shahlaee, W. A. Samara, J. Hsu et al., "In vivo assessment of macular vascular density in healthy human eyes using optical coherence tomography angiography," *American Journal of Ophthalmology*, vol. 165, pp. 39–46, 2016.

[12] Y. Yang, J. Wang, H. Jiang et al., "Retinal microvasculature alteration in high myopia," *Investigative Opthalmology & Visual Science*, vol. 57, no. 14, pp. 6020–6030, 2016.

[13] D. M. Snodderly, R. S. Weinhaus, and J. C. Choi, "Neural-vascular relationships in central retina of macaque monkeys (Macaca fascicularis)," *Journal of Neuroscience*, vol. 12, no. 4, pp. 1169–1193, 1992.

[14] N. I. Kurysheva, "Does OCT angiography of macula play a role in glaucoma diagnostics?," *Ophthalmology Open Journal*, vol. 2, no. 1, pp. 1–11, 2017.

[15] K. Sugiyama, *Myopia and Glaucoma*, Springer Japan KK, Tokyo, Japan, 2015.

[16] M. Zhang, T. S. Hwang, J. P. Campbell et al., "Projection-resolved optical coherence tomographic angiography," *Biomedical Optics Express*, vol. 7, no. 3, p. 816, 2016.

[17] G. Landa and R. B. Rosen, "New patterns of retinal collateral circulation are exposed by a retinal functional imager (RFI)," *British Journal of Ophthalmology*, vol. 94, no. 1, pp. 54–58, 2010.

[18] Y. Zhang and C. F. Wildsoet, "RPE and choroid mechanisms underlying ocular growth and myopia," *Progress in Molecular Biology and Translational Science*, vol. 134, pp. 221–240, 2015.

[19] H. Zhang, C. L. Wong, S. W. Shan et al., "Characterisation of Cl(-) transporter and channels in experimentally induced myopic chick eyes," *Clinical and Experimental Optometry*, vol. 94, no. 6, pp. 528–535, 2011.

[20] A. Garg, D. M. Blumberg, L. A. Al-Aswad et al., "Associations between beta-peripapillary atrophy and reticular pseudodrusen in early age-related macular degeneration," *Investigative Opthalmology & Visual Science*, vol. 58, no. 5, pp. 2810–2815, 2017.

[21] C. Qiuying, H. Jiangnan, H. Yihong, and F. Ying, "Exploration of peripapillary vessel density in highly myopic eyes with peripapillary intrachoroidal cavitation and its relationship with ocular parameters using optical coherence tomography angiography," *Clinical Experimental Ophthalmology*, vol. 45, no. 9, pp. 884–893, 2017.

[22] T. Yokoi, D. Zhu, H. S. Bi et al., "Parapapillary diffuse choroidal atrophy in children is associated with extreme thinning of parapapillary choroid," *Investigative Opthalmology & Visual Science*, vol. 58, no. 2, pp. 901–906, 2017.

[23] T. Y. Chui, Z. Zhong, and S. A. Burns, "The relationship between peripapillary crescent and axial length: implications for differential eye growth," *Vision Research*, vol. 51, no. 19, pp. 2132–2138, 2011.

[24] H. Fan, H. Y. Chen, H. J. Ma et al., "Reduced macular vascular density in myopic eyes," *Chinese Medical Journal*, vol. 130, no. 4, pp. 445–451, 2017.

[25] J. W. Kwon, J. A. Choi, J. S. Kim, and T. Y. La, "Ganglion cell-inner plexiform layer, peripapillary retinal nerve fiber layer, and macular thickness in eyes with myopic beta-zone parapapillary atrophy," *Journal of Ophthalmology*, vol. 2016, Article ID 3746791, 8 pages, 2017.

[26] J. Vongphanit, P. Mitchell, and J. J. Wang, "Population prevalence of tilted optic disks and the relationship of this sign to refractive error," *American Journal of Ophthalmology*, vol. 133, no. 5, pp. 679–685, 2002.

[27] Q. Wang, S. Chan, J. Y. Yang et al., "Vascular density in retina and choriocapillaris as measured by optical coherence tomography angiography," *American Journal of Ophthalmology*, vol. 168, pp. 95–109, 2016.

[28] J. Conrath, R. Giorgi, D. Raccah, and B. Ridings, "Foveal avascular zone in diabetic retinopathy: quantitative vs qualitative assessment," *Eye*, vol. 19, no. 3, pp. 322–326, 2005.

[29] M. B. Parodi, F. Visintin, R. P. Della, and G. Ravalico, "Foveal avascular zone in macular branch retinal vein occlusion," *International Ophthalmology*, vol. 19, no. 1, pp. 25–28, 1995.

[30] H. Xu, G. Deng, C. Jiang et al., "Microcirculatory responses to hyperoxia in macular and peripapillary regions," *Investigative Opthalmology & Visual Science*, vol. 57, no. 10, pp. 4464–4468, 2016.

[31] M. C. Lim, S. T. Hoh, P. J. Foster et al., "Use of optical coherence tomography to assess variations in macular retinal thickness in myopia," *Investigative Opthalmology & Visual Science*, vol. 46, no. 3, p. 974, 2005.

28

Risk Factors of Malignant Glaucoma Occurrence after Glaucoma Surgery

Karolina Krix-Jachym,[1] Tomasz Żarnowski,[2] and Marek Rękas[1]

[1]Department of Ophthalmology, Military Institute of Medicine, Szaserów Street 128, 04-141 Warsaw, Poland
[2]Department of Diagnostics and Microsurgery of Glaucoma, Medical University of Lublin, Chmielna Street 1, 20-079 Lublin, Poland

Correspondence should be addressed to Karolina Krix-Jachym; krixkarolina@gmail.com

Academic Editor: Ozlem G. Koz

Purpose. The aim of this study was twofold: first, to evaluate the predisposing factors for occurrence of malignant glaucoma and second, to compare frequency of malignant glaucoma depending on the type of primary glaucoma surgery. *Methods*. Retrospective analysis was performed in 1689 consecutive patients who underwent glaucoma surgery alone or combined with phacoemulsification. Data collected included the type of surgery, width of the filtration angle, presence or absence of malignant glaucoma in the postoperative period, and time from the primary surgery to malignant glaucoma occurrence. *Results*. Malignant glaucoma occurred in 22 eyes that amounted to 1.3% of cases among all surgery performed. Mean time from glaucoma surgery to malignant glaucoma occurrence was 61.4 ± 190.5 days. Among patients with penetrating surgery, malignant glaucoma occurred in 2.3% of patients, whereas after nonpenetrating operations, such complication was not found ($p = 0.00004$). Malignant glaucoma occurred more often in patients with shallow iridocorneal angle ($p = 0.0013$). *Conclusions*. The risk of malignant glaucoma development is associated with penetrating characteristic of glaucoma surgery, after which this complication appears and its occurrence is higher in eyes with shallow iridocorneal angle. The risk of malignant glaucoma after trabeculectomy compared to iridencleisis as well as after phacotrabeculectomy compared to phacoiridencleisis is equivalent.

1. Introduction

The problem of malignant glaucoma as a complication of glaucoma surgery appears to be rare enough that large randomized trials have not been conducted yet in order to determine the relationship between its occurrence and various types of treatments or to determine treatment strategy giving the best results in large populations of patients. At the same time, it is one of the most serious complications of intraocular surgery, which in the natural course results in, often irreversible, loss of vision in a short period of time.

So far, predisposition for malignant glaucoma was found in eyes with chronic angle closure glaucoma; nevertheless, cases in which open angle glaucoma was diagnosed prior to the surgery have also been reported [1, 2]. Malignant glaucoma is more frequent in small eyes, and anatomical abnormalities in the anterior chamber are also predisposing

[2, 3]. Its relationship to conditions such as hyperopia and microphthalmos (*nanophthalmos*) has been described [4–6]. It has also been determined that higher incidence of malignant glaucoma among women occurs presumably due to smaller dimensions of the anterior segment of the eye [3].

Symptoms of inflammation in the anterior segment of the eye and previous surgical procedures were also mentioned as predisposing to malignant glaucoma [1]. The high intraocular pressure prior to the surgery was suggested as a predisposing factor, but further observations have not confirmed it [7].

The aim of this study was to identify preoperative risk factors for malignant glaucoma and to assess its occurrence depending on the type and nature of the primarily conducted glaucoma surgery. Defining factors predisposing to malignant glaucoma is important due to the possibility of early diagnosis in the endangered eyes, which ultimately determines the final effect of the treatment. This is particularly important because persistent symptoms of malignant glaucoma lead to corneal oedema and its decompensation, severe anterior adhesions, cataract formation in phakic eyes, and structural and functional damage of the optic nerve associated with glaucomatous process. Unfortunately, there are no reliable methods to prevent complications such as malignant glaucoma in the predisposed eyes so far. As long as the causative factors and the aetiology of the process are not well understood, the treatment is an even greater problem.

2. Methods

This was a single-centre, retrospective study of glaucoma patients, and the study protocol was approved by the Institutional Review Board. Retrospective analysis was performed in 1689 consecutive patients (1061 women and 628 men) who underwent glaucoma surgery or combined cataract and glaucoma surgical treatment.

Among the procedures performed in the study group, there were methods of surgery: trabeculectomy, nonpenetrating deep sclerectomy, iridencleisis, Ahmed valve implantation, Gold Micro Shunt (GMS) implantation, Ex-Press implantation, and a group of "other" treatments that have been performed rarely and therefore analysed jointly: implantation of i-Stent, viscocanalostomy, CyPass implantation, and canaloplasty.

Iridencleisis is a quite old and rarely performed free-filtering procedure that creates a full-thickness fistula between the anterior chamber and the subconjunctival space through an anterior sclerostomy. The procedure involves entrapping a pillar of iris tissue into the sclerostomy to act as a wick to hold the sclerostomy open. From own experience, it is an efficacious surgical approach in patients with shallow iridocorneal angle when it comes to intraocular pressure (IOP) reduction. According to our observation, this type of surgery has favorable safety profile than trabeculectomy especially in eyes which are surgically challenging, in nanophthalmos and in eyes with crowded structures in the anterior chamber.

The decision to perform a combined procedure depended on vision loss connected with cataract development, the number of antiglaucoma medications used, and the stage of glaucoma. Subtype of glaucoma surgery was chosen individually for each patient.

Glaucoma surgery was classified as follows:

(i) Depending on the combination of glaucoma procedure with phacoemulsification:

(a) Glaucoma surgery without phacoemulsification

(b) Glaucoma surgery combined with phacoemulsification

(ii) Depending on the type of the aqueous humour main drainage pathway:

(a) Penetrating surgery (trabeculectomy, iridencleisis, seton implantation, surgery with implantation

of Ex-Press, and treatments mentioned above combined with phacoemulsification)

(b) Nonpenetrating surgery (nonpenetrating deep sclerectomy, i-Stent, CyPass and GMS implantation, viscocanalostomy, and canaloplasty both as a sole surgery and combined with phacoemulsification).

Collected data include the date and type of surgery, age and sex of the patient, operated eye, width of the chamber angle, the power of the implanted IOL for procedures combined with cataract surgery, and presence or absence of malignant glaucoma in the postoperative period. Consecutive patients who, after the primary surgery, experienced symptoms of malignant glaucoma, defined as a progressive increase in IOP associated with the axial shallowing of the anterior chamber in the presence of a patent iridotomy, were included into the analysed group. Medical history was collected regarding previous surgical and laser procedures; additional examinations included IOP, BCVA, anterior segment with anterior chamber depth assessment, ocular fundus with the evaluation of c/d, the measurements of CCT and AXL, ultrasound B-scan, and OCT examination of the anterior segment of the eye, if necessary. Iridocorneal angle was classified as shallow if it measures 0–20° (grade 0–2 according to Shaffer-Etienne Classification System) and wide if it measures 20–45° (grade 3-4 according to Shaffer-Etienne Classification System).

2.1. Statistical Analysis. Statistical analysis of the investigated variables was performed with the Shapiro-Wilk and paired Wilcoxon tests. Friedman ANOVA for matched groups and rank means and rank sums were also used for post hoc comparison. The Kaplan-Meier method was used to determine survival curves, and differences between them were tested by the log-rank test. A p value of 0.05 or less was considered significant. The calculations were performed with Statistica 10.0 PL.

3. Results

3.1. Demographic Data. The studied material included 1689 eyes treated with glaucoma surgery in a single clinic (Military Institute of Medicine in Warsaw), where 1061 accounted for women's eyes (62.8%) and 628 for men's eyes (37.2%). In the study group, 811 of the eyes were right, which accounted for 48.0% of the material, and the left eyes counted 878, which accounted for 52.0%. The number of 960 (56.8%) penetrating operations and 729 (43.2%) nonpenetrating operations have been conducted. The number of 1417 (83.9%) operations were combined with phacoemulsification, while glaucoma surgery without cataract surgery amounted to 272 cases (16.1%).

The filtration angle was wide opened in 1210 cases (71.6%), while it was shallow in 479 eyes (28.4%). Mean patients' age was 72.9 ± 10.6 years (Me 75) within the range of 16 to 95 years. Women's mean age was 73.2 ± 10.2 years (Me 75) within the range of 20 to 93 years. Men's mean age

Table 1: Patient's demographic data.

Demographic data	Mean ± SD (Me)
Sex n (%)	
Women	1061 (62.8%)
Men	628 (37.2%)
Together	1689 (100.0%)
Eye n (%)	
Right	811 (48.0%)
Left	878 (52.0%)
Surgery n (%)	
Penetrating	960 (56.8%)
Nonpenetrating	729 (43.2%)
Surgery n (%)	
Combined with phacoemulsification	1417 (83.9%)
Glaucoma surgery without phaco	272 (16.1%)
Iridocorneal angle n (%)	
Wide	1210 (71.6%)
Shallow	479 (28.4%)
Malignant glaucoma occurrence n (%)	
Malignant glaucoma	22 (1.3%)
Without malignant glaucoma	1667 (98.7%)
Age (years)	72.9 ± 10.6 Me 75 (69.80)
Range	16.0–95.0

Table 2: Percentage distribution of surgical methods in analysed material.

	Surgery	Number of surgeries (*n*)	%
1	Phacosclerectomy	545	32.3
2	Phacoiridencleisis	435	25.8
3	Phacotrabeculectomy	276	16.3
4	Deep sclerectomy	110	6.5
5	Phaco-ExPress	105	6.2
6	Trabeculectomy	61	3.6
7	Iridencleisis	45	2.7
8	Phaco-GMS	43	2.5
9	Seton valve implantation	21	1.2
10	Other	17	1.0
11	GMS	14	0.8
12	ExPress	14	0.8
13	Phaco-seton valve implantation	3	0.2
Together		1689	100.0

was 72.4 ± 11.3 years (Me 75) within the range of 16 to 95 years. The mean time elapsed from primary glaucoma surgery was 61.4 ± 190.5 days (Me 2.5; from 1 to 840 days). In the analysed material, malignant glaucoma occurred in 22 eyes, which accounted for 1.3% of the whole group (Table 1).

Analysis of the types of glaucoma surgery in whole group of patients is presented in Table 2.

In the group of patients with malignant glaucoma, 40.9% of eyes underwent surgical treatment with the method of phacoiridencleisis, 22.7% phacotrabeculectomy, 18.2% iridencleisis, 13.6% trabeculectomy, and 4.5% seton valve implantation before this complication occurred.

3.2. Analysis of the Types of Glaucoma Surgery

3.2.1. Analysis of Malignant Glaucoma Occurrence Depending on the Type of Glaucoma Surgery. Among patients with penetrating surgery, malignant glaucoma occurred in 2.3% of patients, whereas after nonpenetrating surgery, this complication was not found ($p = 0.00004$) (Table 3). The conclusion is that penetrating surgery is the risk factor of malignant glaucoma occurrence.

3.2.2. Analysis of Malignant Glaucoma Occurrence Depending on the Subtype of Glaucoma Surgery. The risk of malignant glaucoma after phacotrabeculectomy and phacoiridenclei-sis was equivalent ($p = 0.810$). When frequency of malig-nant glaucoma after trabeculectomy and iridencleisis was

compared, the difference was not statistically significant ($p = 0.416$) (Table 3).

3.2.3. Analysis of Malignant Glaucoma Occurrence Depending on Sex of the Patients. Malignant glaucoma was more frequent in women, but the difference was not statisti-cally significant ($p = 0.064$) (Table 3).

3.2.4. Analysis of Malignant Glaucoma Occurrence Depending on Iridocorneal Angle Width. This complication occurred more often in patients with shallow iridocorneal angle ($p = 0.001$). The risk of malignant glaucoma is 3 times higher in eyes with shallow filtration angle (Table 3).

4. Discussion

Understanding of malignant glaucoma since it was first reported in 1869 has extended, but still many questions remain unanswered.

The diagnostics of malignant glaucoma mechanisms enables using of specific treatment aimed at pathophysiolog-ical process being the underlying cause, but in fact different mechanisms may coexist, consequently complicating the diagnosis [8]. The theory of malignant glaucoma pathogen-esis involves reversed outflow of fluid towards or beyond the vitreous body, with subsequent increase in volume of the vitreous and shallowing of the posterior and anterior chamber [9].

In the initiation of this complication, both high lens: eye index (lens typically has a normal or increased thickness) [5] and abnormal histological structure of the sclera may play a role. A disproportionately large lens in relation to the ante-rior segment of the eye may indicate higher risk of malignant glaucoma incidence [10]; the relation between the size of the lens and the scleral ring or the top of the ciliary body is critical [1]. Disrupted structure of collagen fibres of the

TABLE 3: Analysis of malignant glaucoma occurrence depending on different factors.

Analysed data		Malignant glaucoma			p (Chi^2)
		Yes	No	Together	
Glaucoma surgery	Penetrating	22	938	960	0.00004
	Nonpenetrating	—	729	729	
	Together	22	1667	1689	
Subtype of glaucoma surgery	Phacotrabeculectomy	5	271	276	0.810
	Phacoiridencleisis	9	426	435	
	Together	14	697	711	
	Iridencleisis	4	41	45	0.416
	Trabeculectomy	3	58	61	
	Together	7	99	106	
Sex	Women	18	1041	1059	0.063
	Men	4	622	626	
	Together	22	1663	1685	
Iridocorneal angle	Wide	9	1201	1210	0.001
	Shallow	13	466	479	
	Together	22	1667	1689	

intercellular substance of the sclera's connective tissue [11] and increased levels of fibronectin have been found, as well as changes in the metabolism of glycosaminoglycans, which can cause compression of the collagen fibres and lead to thickening of the sclera. Thickening of the sclera may, on the other hand, cause partial narrowing of the vortex veins, impairing normal venous drainage [5], while its smaller surface decreases the transscleral protein transport. As a consequence of these predisposing factors, the choroidal bed becomes overflown (CE—*choroidal effusion*) [5, 12]. All of these features and increased oncotic pressure of the vitreous body may be associated with a higher risk of developing malignant glaucoma [5, 12]. It is important to recognize anatomical predisposing factors and pathophysiological changes leading to this process as a mechanism for introducing full-blown malignant glaucoma because the treatment of this complication is challenging.

In this group of patients when conservative management (mannitol intravenously, acetazolamide p.o., and locally: 1% atropine, 1% tropicamide, dorzolamide hydrochloride-timolol maleate ophthalmic solution, and 0.1% dexamethasone phosphate) was insufficient, laser treatment was recommended. Capsulotomy was performed using an energy of 1 to 4 mJ per pulse. The energy and pulses were modified according to the thickness of the capsule until an opening was achieved. 5–15 bursts with an energy of 1–3 mJ through iridotomy or iridectomy were usually effective in achieving communication, although some cases were refractory and symptoms of malignant glaucoma reappeared. The indication for surgical intervention was a lack of effectiveness of conservative and laser treatment. Partial PPV with peripheral lens capsule excision communicating anterior chamber and vitreous cavity was performed with satisfying results [13].

The occurrence of malignant glaucoma is most often a consequence of glaucoma surgery, although it was also reported in patients after laser and other ophthalmic procedures, even in the surgically nontreated eyes. In the analysed material encompassing eyes after glaucoma surgery, malignant glaucoma occurred in 22 eyes, which accounted for 1.3% of the whole group. Among the penetrating operations, prevalence of this complication was 2.3% in operated eyes, which is comparable with the observations other authors have made [7, 14]. In the analysed material, malignant glaucoma was not observed after nonpenetrating surgery.

Possibly, leaving TDM (trabeculo-Descemet's membrane) intact avoids sudden decompression associated with the opening of the anterior chamber, which causes its flattening and anterior displacement of the iridolenticular diaphragm. Such mechanism is regarded by some authors as the main intraoperative cause initiating malignant glaucoma development [15–17]. The movement of the diaphragm may occur as a result of leakage of filtering bleb, which initiates a vicious cycle mechanism leading ultimately to the development of malignant glaucoma [18]. Filtering bleb leakage may be associated with excessive filtration [19]. The problem that often occurs after full-thickness surgery and, in addition, the widespread use of antimetabolites significantly increases the incidence of this complication [20]. It is believed that the aqueous humour has lytic properties and inhibits the subconjunctival fibroblasts [21, 22], leading to persistent leakage of the filtering bleb [20]. In the controlled filtration surgery, an incomplete-thickness scleral flap may also become thin over time due to the lytic properties of aqueous humour and resemble effects of full-thickness filtration surgery, promoting the development of late bleb leakage. This process is enhanced by adjuvant antimetabolite therapy [20]. However, after nonpenetrating surgery, hypotension typically occurs without changing the anatomical relations, which may limit the incidence of malignant glaucoma. Karlen et al. described a case of malignant glaucoma occurring after NPDS (*nonpenetrating deep sclerectomy*) [23]. Thus, it is difficult to completely exclude the possibility of malignant glaucoma development after NPDS, especially since in many cases the microdamages of TDM happen, which facilitates aqueous humour outflow and causes it to perform similarly as in the classic penetrating surgery [24].

The study illustrates the incidence of malignant glaucoma in particular types of surgery. Among the procedures, where malignant glaucoma occurred as a complication, were trabeculectomy, iridencleisis, seton valve implantation, and surgery combined with phacoemulsification: phacoiridencleisis and phacotrabeculectomy. Penetrating nature of the operations allows us to formulate a general trend for the occurrence of this type of complication in this particular group of surgery. After iridencleisis, malignant glaucoma occurred in 8.9% of patients, which is highly interesting, as well as the fact that after trabeculectomy, this complication was observed in 4.9% of patients. The probable cause of this result was the fact that iridencleisis was performed in cases of narrow iridocorneal angle glaucoma as the operation of choice and predilection for malignant glaucoma are associated with this configuration [25].

When glaucoma coexisted with cataract, glaucoma operations were carried out combined with phacoemulsification. Phacotrabeculectomy was performed mainly in eyes with open iridocorneal angle glaucoma, while in the hyperopic eyes, microphthalmos, or relative anterior microphthalmos, the preferred surgical technique was iridencleisis combined with cataract surgery because of lower tendency of postoperative shallowing of the anterior chamber after mentioned procedure. In the analysed material, malignant glaucoma occurred in 1.81% of patients after phacotrabeculectomy, while after phacoiridencleisis, this complication was observed in 2.07% of patients. No differences were found in the incidence of malignant glaucoma, but it should be noted that the phacoemulsification with iridencleisis in the predisposed eyes could stabilize the anatomical relationships in the anterior segment of the eye.

The time of onset of malignant glaucoma symptoms from the primary glaucoma surgery differed significantly in the study group. Malignant glaucoma may have different dynamics of clinical manifestation immediately after surgery, when the causative factors cannot be compensated in a closed system of the eyeball. On the other hand, symptoms may be delayed if a relative balance between the volume of produced fluids and the drainage from the eyeball is established.

It appears that disturbed anatomical relations between the anterior and posterior segment of the eyeball underlie the pathogenesis of malignant glaucoma. According to some authors, eyes with malignant glaucoma tend to coexist with hyperopia with AXL < 22 mm [4]. Average AXL in patients with malignant glaucoma in our study was 21.79 ± 0.83. In the papers by Byrnes et al. (21 eyes) and Żarnowski et al. (10 eyes), the average AXL in malignant glaucoma patients was 21.15 mm and 21.30 mm, respectively [26, 27]. Among the examined patients, average anterior chamber depth was 2.0 ± 0.8 mm preoperatively, while in the normal adult population, the average chamber depth is 3.15 mm [28].

Taken together, assessment of factors that predispose to malignant glaucoma and knowledge of its occurrence depending on the type and nature of the primarily conducted glaucoma surgery might draw attention to the eyes at risk of developing this complication.

Filtration surgery in the predisposed eyes can be modified to reduce the incidence of this complication, where the aim is to keep the iridolenticular diaphragm in the anatomically correct position, which seems more probable when nonpenetrating procedures are used, although they are not always possible due to the anatomical relation occurring prior to the surgery. However, excessive filtration should be avoided as it may cause anterior chamber flattening and initiate the malignant process. Any inflammatory processes and a history of repeated surgical interventions in the eye prepared for the procedure should be taken into careful consideration, as well as a history of malignant glaucoma in the fellow eye.

Additional Points

Limitations of the Study. There are some limitations of the current study. First, retrospective data commonly has more sources of error due to confounding and bias. Second, the sample size was too small to detect slight differences between groups. It is difficult to collect a large number of cases since malignant glaucoma is a very rare disease. Prospective trials with greater statistical power will be needed to detect more detailed predisposing factors for malignant glaucoma. *Summary.* The risk of malignant glaucoma development is associated with eye anatomical relations and is particularly high in the eyes with shallow iridocorneal angle. Nonetheless, the complication does not occur in all cases of the eyes with anatomical predispositions. The cause may lie in the histological structure and existing biochemical features, which are not yet discovered. Malignant glaucoma occurrence is also linked to penetrating characteristic of glaucoma surgery, after which this complication appears. The risk of malignant glaucoma after trabeculectomy compared to iridencleisis as well as after phacotrabeculectomy compared to phacoiridencleisis is equivalent.

Disclosure

The authors have no proprietary interest in any of the materials, products, or methods mentioned in this article. The study sponsor had no involvement in the design and conduct of the study; collection, management, analysis, and interpretation of the data; and preparation, review, or approval of the manuscript.

Conflicts of Interest

The authors declare that there is no conflict of interests regarding the publication of this paper.

Acknowledgments

The study was supported with grant obtained from the Military Institute of Medicine (Grant no. 207).

References

[1] J. Lippas, "Mechanics and treatment of malignant glaucoma and the problem of a flat anterior chamber," *American Journal of Ophthalmology*, vol. 57, pp. 620–627, 1964.

[2] H. L. Birge, "Malignant glaucoma," *Transactions of the American Ophthalmological Society*, vol. 54, pp. 311–336, 1956.

[3] M. R. Razeghinejad, H. Amini, and H. Esfandiari, "Lesser anterior chamber dimensions in women may be a predisposing factor for malignant glaucoma," *Medical Hypotheses*, vol. 64, pp. 572–574, 2005.

[4] A. Sharma, F. Sii, P. Shah, and G. R. Kirkby, "Vitrectomy-phacoemulsification-vitrectomy for the management of aqueous misdirection syndromes in phakic eyes," *Ophthalmology*, vol. 113, pp. 1968–1973, 2006.

[5] A. Faucher, K. Hasanee, and D. S. Rootman, "Phacoemulsification and intraocular lens implantation in nanophthalmic eyes. Report of a medium-size series," *Journal of Cataract and Refractive Surgery*, vol. 28, pp. 837–842, 2002.

[6] R. Preetha, P. Goel, N. Patel et al., "Clear lens extraction with intraocular lens implantation for hyperopia," *Journal of Cataract and Refractive Surgery*, vol. 29, pp. 895–899, 2003.

[7] R. J. Simmons, "Malignant glaucoma," *The British Journal of Ophthalmology*, vol. 56, pp. 263–272, 1972.

[8] J. Tombran-Tink, C. J. Barnstable, and M. B. Shields, *Mechanisms of the Glaucomas*, Humana Press, New York, NY, USA, 2008.

[9] J. W. Harbour, P. E. Rubsamen, and P. Palmberg, "Pars plana vitrectomy in the management of phakic and pseudophakic malignant glaucoma," *Archives of Ophthalmology*, vol. 114, pp. 1073–1078, 1996.

[10] P. A. Chandler, "Malignant Glaucoma," *Transactions of the American Ophthalmological Society*, vol. 48, pp. 128–143, 1950.

[11] R. L. Trelstad, N. N. Silbermann, and R. J. Brockhurst, "Nanophthalmic sclera. Ultrastructural, histochemical, and biochemical observations," *Archives of Ophthalmology*, vol. 100, pp. 1935–1938, 1982.

[12] H. A. Quigley, D. S. Friedman, and N. G. Congdon, "Possible mechanisms of primary angle-closure and malignant glaucoma," *Journal of Glaucoma*, vol. 12, no. 2, pp. 167–180, 2003.

[13] M. Rękas, K. Krix-Jachym, and T. Żarnowski, "Evaluation of the effectiveness of surgical treatment of malignant glaucoma in pseudophakic eyes through partial PPV with establishment of communication between the anterior chamber and the vitreous cavity," *Journal of Ophthalmology*, vol. 2015, Article ID 873124, 6 pages, 2015.

[14] S. Ruben, J. Tsai, and R. Hitchings, "Malignant glaucoma and its management," *The British Journal of Ophthalmology*, vol. 81, pp. 163–167, 1997.

[15] G. E. Trope, C. J. Pavlin, A. Bau, C. R. Baumal, and F. S. Foster, "Malignant glaucoma. Clinical and ultrasound biomicroscopic features," *Ophthalmology*, vol. 101, no. 6, pp. 1030–1035, 1994.

[16] B. Francis, R. Wong, and D. S. Mincler, "Slit-lamp needle revision for aqueous misdirection after trabeculectomy," *Journal of Glaucoma*, vol. 11, no. 3, pp. 183–188, 2002.

[17] E. A. Ryan, J. Zwaan, and L. T. Chylack, "Nanophthalmos with uveal effusion. Clinical and embryologic considerations," *Ophthalmology*, vol. 89, pp. 1013–1017, 1982.

[18] K. F. Tomey, S. H. Senft, S. R. Antonios, I. V. Shammas, Z. M. Shihab, and C. E. Traverso, "Aqueous misdirection and flat chamber after posterior chamber implants with and without trabeculectomy," *Archives of Ophthalmology*, vol. 105, no. 6, pp. 770–773, 1987.

[19] G. L. Spaeth, *Chirurgia okulistyczna. Pooperacyjne spłycanie komory przedniej*, Urban & Partner, Wrocław, 2006.

[20] A. K. Mandal, "Management of the late leaking filtration blebs. A report of seven cases and a selective review of the literature," *Indian Journal of Ophthalmology*, vol. 49, p. 247, 2001.

[21] J. Herschler, A. J. Claflin, and G. Fiorentino, "The effects of aqueous humor on the growth of subconjunctival fibroblasts in tissue cultures and its implications for glaucoma surgery," *American Journal of Ophthalmology*, vol. 89, pp. 245–249, 1980.

[22] R. L. Radius, J. Herschler, A. Claflin, and G. Fiorentino, "Aqueous humor changes after experimental filtering surgery," *American Journal of Ophthalmology*, vol. 89, pp. 250–254, 1980.

[23] M. E. Karlen, E. Sanchez, C. C. Schnyder, M. Sickenberg, and A. Mermoud, "Deep sclerectomy with collagen implant: medium term results," *The British Journal of Ophthalmology*, vol. 83, no. 1, pp. 6–11, 1999.

[24] E. Sanchez, C. C. Schnyder, and M. Mermoud, "Résultats comparatives de la sclérectomie profonde transformée en trabéculectomie et de la trabéculectomie classique," *Klinische Monatsblätter für Augenheilkunde*, vol. 210, pp. 261–264, 1997.

[25] P. P. Ellis, "Malignant glaucoma occurring 16 years after successful filtering surgery," *Annals of Ophthalmology*, vol. 16, no. 2, pp. 177–179, 1984.

[26] G. A. Byrnes, M. M. Leen, T. P. Wong, and W. E. Benson, "Vitrectomy for ciliary block (malignant) glaucoma," *Ophthalmology*, vol. 102, pp. 1308–1311, 1995.

[27] T. Żarnowski, A. Wilkos-Kuc, M. Tulidowicz-Bielak et al., "Efficacy and safety of a new surgical method to treat malignant glaucoma in pseudophakia," *Eye (London, England)*, vol. 28, no. 6, pp. 761–764, 2014.

[28] P. J. Foster, D. C. Broadway, S. Hayat et al., "Refractive error, axial length and anterior chamber depth of the eye in British adults: the EPIC-Norfolk Eye Study," *The British Journal of Ophthalmology*, vol. 94, pp. 827–830, 2010.

29

Glaucomatous Optic Nerve Changes and Thyroid Dysfunction in an Urban South Korean Population

Yu Sam Won,[1] Da Yeong Kim,[2] and Joon Mo Kim[2]

[1]*Department of Neurosurgery, Kangbuk Samsung Hospital, Sungkyunkwan University School of Medicine, Seoul, Republic of Korea*
[2]*Department of Ophthalmology, Kangbuk Samsung Hospital, Sungkyunkwan University School of Medicine, Seoul, Republic of Korea*

Correspondence should be addressed to Joon Mo Kim; kjoonmo1@gmail.com

Academic Editor: Terri L. Young

Purpose. This study was performed to evaluate the relationship between intraocular pressure (IOP) and glaucomatous optic nerve change and thyroid factors in Korean population. *Materials and Methods.* The study included subjects who underwent health screening in Kangbuk Samsung Hospital. Detailed history taking and systemic and ocular examination including fundus photography were performed for all participants. All fundus photographs were divided into two groups based on disc and RNFL appearance: nonglaucoma and glaucoma group. Subjects were also divided into quartiles of each thyroid function parameter, and the relationship with IOP and glaucoma were analysed. *Results.* In univariate analysis, free T4, T3, and TSH in normal subjects and T3 in thyroid disease group were associated with the IOP. After adjusting for age and sex, the IOP tended to slightly decrease according to the level of the quartile of free T4 and T3 in normal subjects. In terms of glaucoma, on multivariate analysis, it did not show a significant correlation with any thyroid function tests. *Conclusions.* In normal subjects, the IOP tended to be decreased according to the level of free T4 and T3 but the amounts were clinically insignificant. Thyroid factors are not an independent risk factor for the development of glaucoma.

1. Introduction

Glaucoma is a chronic optic neuropathy caused by a variety of risk factors and characterized by the progressive loss of retinal ganglion cells (RGC). Intraocular pressure (IOP) is the most important risk factor; however, glaucoma can occur in a low IOP state, and glaucomatous progression can occur during IOP-lowering therapy [1–4]. Therefore, many studies have been conducted to investigate risk factors including IOP and other risk factors [5–7].

Hormones might affect the development of glaucoma and IOP through various mechanisms, and some studies have reported that thyroid hormone affects IOP. Thyroid hormones play a key role in metabolism and homeostasis [8]. Thyroid-associated ophthalmopathy has been described clinically; however, the relationship between thyroid function and glaucoma has remained controversial [9]. Some studies have reported a significant relationship, while others have not. Forte et al. [10] suggested that ocular hypertension

(OHT) patients with Graves' orbitopathy showed diffuse abnormalities of the VF and RNFL thinning.

Few studies have been conducted to reveal the relationship between thyroid dysfunction and glaucoma based on the large number of participants. The relationship between thyroid dysfunction and glaucoma is still under debate. In this study, we evaluated the association between IOP, glaucomatous optic nerve change, and thyroid dysfunction.

2. Materials and Methods

This study was conducted in two Kangbuk Samsung Hospital Screening Centers in Seoul and Suwon, South Korea, and followed a retrospective, cross-sectional design. This study followed the tenets of the Declaration of Helsinki and was approved by the institutional review board/ethics committee of Kangbuk Samsung Hospital. The study population consisted of individuals who participated in a comprehensive health screening programme at Kangbuk Samsung Hospital,

Seoul, Korea. The purpose of this screening programme was to promote health through early detection of chronic diseases and their risk factors. In addition, the Korean Industrial Safety and Health Law requires working individuals to participate in an annual or a biennial health examination. About 60% of the participants were employees of companies or local governmental organizations and their spouses. The remaining participants registered individually for the programme [11]. Subjects who underwent health screening from August 2012 to July 2013 and who were 20 years or older were enrolled in this study. Systemic examinations, including laboratory tests and sociodemographic and behavioural questionnaires, were administered to all subjects, and their medical histories were reviewed to determine the presence of associated systemic disease. Digital fundus images were collected with a digital fundus camera (CR6–45NM; Canon Inc., Tokyo, Japan). IOP was measured twice in each subject using a noncontact tonometer (TX–F; Canon Inc., Tokyo, Japan), and the mean value of two IOP readings was recorded. In cases of both eyes eligible, the right eye from each subject was considered in statistical analysis. Normal subjects were defined as the persons who did not show any glaucoma/glaucoma suspect findings in the fundus and did not have any medical or surgical history to effect on IOP including thyroid orbitopathy. Diabetes is diagnosed as previous diagnosis or treatment history and fasting plasma glucose level ≥ 7.0 mmol/L (126 mg/dL). Hypertension is diagnosed as a systolic blood pressure ≥ 140 mmHg, a diastolic blood pressure ≥ 90 mmHg, or current use of antihypertensive drugs. Hyperlipidaemia is diagnosed as abnormally elevated serum level of any or all lipids and/or lipoproteins. We all excluded glaucoma/glaucoma suspect patients and subjects who underwent glaucoma surgery or laser treatment from normal subjects. In glaucoma participants, data from the eyes with glaucoma were used. All fundus photographs were reviewed by two ophthalmologists, two glaucoma specialists, and one retina specialist who were all blinded to demographic features and laboratory findings. The grading was performed independently by ophthalmologists. Any discrepancies among the observers were resolved by consensus between two glaucoma specialists. First, each fundus photograph was classified into one of the two categories based on disc and RNFL appearance: nonglaucomatous or glaucomatous. A glaucomatous RNFL defect was defined as a localized wedge-shaped RNFL defect within 60 degrees running toward or touching the optic disc border. Nonglaucomatous RNFL defects included superior segmental optic hypoplasia and slit defect. A patient was defined as having a glaucomatous optic neuropathy if the vertical cup-disc ratio (VCDR) was ≥ 0.7 or if the VCDR asymmetry between the right and left eyes was ≥ 0.2. In cases with newly detected glaucomatous features, glaucoma evaluations were recommended and some of them were determined to have glaucoma or not after undergoing glaucoma evaluation at the hospital. Finally, subjects who had not been previously diagnosed with glaucoma or had not visited a hospital for glaucoma evaluation were placed into either category 2 or 3, according to the criteria set forth by the International Society of Geographical and Epidemiological

Ophthalmology (ISGEO) [12]. Category 1 requires a VF defect consistent with glaucoma and either a vertical cup-disc ratio (VCDR) ≥ 0.7 (97.5th percentile) or ≥ 0.2 VCDR asymmetry between the right and left eyes (97.5th percentile). Category 2 indicates that the VF results are not definitive, requiring a VCDR ≥ 0.9 (99.5th percentile) or VCDR asymmetry ≥ 0.3 (99.5th percentile). Category 3 indicates that there are no data available regarding VF testing or optic disc examination; therefore, visual acuity < 3/60 and an IOP greater than the 99.5th percentile for this population (IOP = 21 mmHg) are required.

Optic disc haemorrhage was defined as an isolated haemorrhage on or around the optic disc or in the peripapillary retina within 1-disc diameter. Subjects with alternative causes of retinal haemorrhage, such as ischemic optic neuropathy, papillitis, retinal vein occlusion, diabetic retinopathy, or posterior vitreous detachment, were excluded. We also excluded participants with low-quality fundus photographs due to media opacity or a small pupil in order to discriminate glaucoma patients, as well as patients who underwent glaucoma surgery and laser treatment and who were on systemic medications that could affect IOP, such as a β-blocker.

Subjects were divided equally into four groups (quartiles) based on thyroid laboratory testing as follows: thyroid-stimulating hormone (TSH, μIU/mL) quartiles, Q1 (TSH < 1.30), Q2 (1.30 $\leq$ TSH < 1.90), Q3 (1.90 $\leq$ TSH < 2.75), and Q4 (TSH $\geq$ 2.75); free thyroxine (free T4, ng/dL) quartiles, Q1 (free T4 < 1.15), Q2 (1.15 $\leq$ free T4 < 1.26), Q3 (1.26 $\leq$ free T4 < 1.38), and Q4 (free T4 $\geq$ 1.38); and tri-iodothyronine (T3, pg/mL) quartiles, Q1 (T3 < 2.87), Q2 (2.87 $\leq$ T3 < 3.12), Q3 (3.12 $\leq$ T3 < 3.40), and Q4 (T3 $\geq$ 3.40). This dividing analysis method was used to it at previous study with blood chemistry data [13]. History of thyroid abnormalities and newly diagnosed subjects were classified into hypothyroidism, hyperthyroidism, thyroid nodular cyst, and thyroid hormone treatment.

All statistical analyses were performed with PASW Statistics 18.0 (IBM, Armonk, New York, USA). Each variable was initially evaluated using the chi-square test, and significant variables ($p < 0.1$) were included in multivariate logistic regression. Multivariate logistic regression with stepwise selection while controlling for all confounding variables ($p < 0.1$) was used to evaluate the independent risk factors associated with glaucoma. Odds ratios (OR) with 95% confidence intervals (CI) were estimated using logistic regression models. In all cases, a $p < 0.05$ was considered statistically significant.

3. Results

Of 168,044 patients treated at the two screening centers, 164,029 (97.61%) were enrolled in this study. The remaining 4015 subjects were excluded because fundus photographs could not be obtained or because low-quality photographs could not be reliably evaluated due to media opacity or small pupil. Of the 164,029 participants, 93,559 (57.0%) were male and 70,470 (43.0%) were female. The mean age was 40.56 ± 8.51 years. Optic disc haemorrhage was noted

TABLE 1: Demographic and general health characteristics.

Characteristics	Glaucoma (+) ($n = 2431$)	Glaucoma (−) ($n = 161,598$)	p value
Age, years (mean ± SD)	44.10 ± 9.17	40.50 ± 8.50	<0.001*
Male (%)	1736 (71.4%)	91,823 (56.8%)	<0.001**
IOP (mmHg)	15.8 ± 3.1	15.0 ± 3.0	<0.001*
Diabetes (%)	157 (6.5)	4732 (2.9)	<0.001**
Hypertension (%)	497 (20.4)	13,998 (8.7)	<0.001**
Hyperlipidaemia (%)	473 (19.5)	22,332 (13.8)	<0.001**
Current smoker (%)	547 (22.5)	33,158 (20.5)	0.033**
TSH (μIU/mL)	2.39 ± 3.64	2.26 ± 2.67	0.089*
Free T4 (ng/dL)	1.27 ± 0.25	1.26 ± 0.23	0.080*
T3 (pg/mL)	3.21 ± 0.84	3.162 ± 0.65	<0.001*
Hyperthyroidism (%)	37 (1.5%)	2752 (1.7%)	<0.001**
Hypothyroidism (%)	36 (1.5%)	3086 (1.9%)	<0.001**
Nodular cyst (%)	138 (5.6%)	11,239 (6.7%)	<0.001**
Hormone treatment (%)	48 (2.0%)	3081 (1.8%)	<0.001**
Characteristic	Disc haemorrhage (+) ($n = 226$)	Disc haemorrhage (−) ($n = 163,803$)	p value
Age, years (mean ± SD)	44.68 ± 8.97	40.55 ± 8.51	<0.001*
Male (%)	151 (66.81%)	93,408 (57.02%)	0.003**

Continuous values are presented as mean ± standard deviation (SD).
Categorical values are presented as percentage (%).
*Student's t-test, **Chi-square test.

in 226 (0.14%) subjects. Of the total 164,029 participants, glaucomatous fundus photographs were obtained in 2454 (1.50%) subjects (apart from the ISGEO criteria, according to the results of optic disc and RNFL appearance in fundus photographs). 1477 subjects (60.2%) of 2454 had been previously diagnosed with glaucoma. Of the remaining 977 subjects, 313 subjects underwent glaucoma evaluations including red-free fundus photography, optical coherence tomography, and visual field testing in our glaucoma clinic. Among these 313 subjects, 162 and 128 were diagnosed as having definite and suspected glaucoma (early glaucoma with RNFL defect), respectively, whereas the remaining 23 did not have glaucoma. The remaining 664 subjects were considered to have glaucoma according to the ISGEO criteria and/or presence of RNFL defect. Glaucoma evaluation including visual field test was not available in 664 subjects; therefore, subjects were diagnosed as ISGEO category 3 (visual acuity < 3/60 and an IOP greater than the 99.5th percentile for this population are required). All eligible cases for glaucoma group showed RNFL defect. The demographic data are shown in Table 1.

On univariate analysis, there was a significant difference in T3 level ($p < 0.001$, chi-square test) between patients with and without glaucomatous optic neuropathy (Table 2). There was no relationship between disc haemorrhage and thyroid function on univariate analysis. The relationship between thyroid function and IOP was shown in Tables 3 and 4. On univariate analysis of normal population, as the quartile of free T4 and T3 increased, the IOP tended to increase slightly. On multivariate analysis adjusted for age, sex, and comorbidities (diabetes, hypertension, hyperlipidaemia, and current smoker), however, the IOP in the first quartile of free

T4 and T3 were higher than the second or other quartiles significantly (Table 5). In analysis of the odds ratio between thyroid dysfunction and glaucoma, thyroid function was not associated with glaucoma (Tables 6 and 7).

4. Discussion

Thyroid hormone affects the maintenance of homeostasis in the body and regulates the basal body metabolism [8]. Many studies have tried to determine the association between hypothyroidism and glaucoma. In our study, we did not find that thyroid dysfunction was an independent risk factor of glaucoma development. On univariate analysis, the presence of glaucomatous optic neuropathy was significantly influenced by the level of T3, but the association did not remain statistically significant on multivariate regression. Disc haemorrhage was not associated with thyroid dysfunction as well.

Considering previous reports about an association between IOP and thyroid function, there was a possible theoretical relationship between thyroid function and glaucoma. Hyperthyroidism might induce IOP increase through increased intraorbital pressure or contraction of enlarged extraocular muscles [14, 15]. The main mechanism could be elevation of episcleral venous pressure secondary to increasing of intraorbital content and pressure. The increased IOP in hypothyroidism could be due to the excessive accumulation of mucopolysaccharides in the trabecular meshwork [16, 17]. Smith et al. [16] reported that the prevalence of hypothyroidism in the primary open-angle glaucoma group was higher than those in the control subjects in their case-control study. They proposed that, in the untreated hypothyroid state, hyaluronic acid accumulates excessively in the

TABLE 2: Univariate analysis of glaucoma and thyroid function.

	Quartiles of thyroid hormone				p value
	1st quartile	2nd quartile	3rd quartile	4th quartile	
Glaucoma (+) (n = 2431)					
TSH (μIU/mL) (n = 2449) (0.01 ∼ 100)	635 (25.93%)	612 (24.99%)	604 (24.66%)	598 (24.42%)	0.943*
Free T4 (ng/dL) (n = 2442) (0.06 ∼ 7.70)	583 (23.87%)	638 (26.13%)	625 (25.59%)	596 (24.41%)	0.090*
T3 (pg/mL) (n = 2077) (0.34 ∼ 32.60)	438 (21.09%)	461 (22.20%)	612 (29.47%)	566 (27.25%)	<0.001*

*Chi-square test
TSH: 1st quartile < 1.30, 1.30 ≤ 2nd quartile < 1.90, 1.90 ≤ 3rd quartile < 2.75, 4th quartile ≥ 2.75; free T4: 1st quartile < 1.15, 1.15 ≤ 2nd quartile < 1.26, 1.26 ≤ 3rd quartile < 1.38, 4th quartile ≥ 1.38; T3: 1st quartile < 2.87, 2.87 ≤ 2nd quartile < 3.12, 3.12 ≤ 3rd quartile < 3.40, 4th quartile ≥ 3.40.

TABLE 3: Univariate analysis of thyroid function and IOP in a normal population without glaucoma.

Variables	IOP (mmHg)	p value
TSH (μIU/mL)		<0.001*
1st quartile (<1.30) (n = 39,894) (25.91%)	14.94 ± 2.96	
2nd quartile (1.30–1.90) (n = 39,402) (25.58%)	15.02 ± 2.96	
3rd quartile (1.90–2.75) (n = 38,013) (24.68%)	15.04 ± 2.94	
4th quartile (≥2.75) (n = 36,681) (23.83%)	15.02 ± 2.92	
Free T4 (ng/dL)		<0.001*
1st quartile (<1.15) (n = 39,071) (25.43%)	14.92 ± 2.94	
2nd quartile (1.15–1.26) (n = 39,972) (26.01%)	15.01 ± 2.95	
3rd quartile (1.26–1.38) (n = 39,268) (25.55%)	15.05 ± 2.95	
4th quartile (≥1.38) (n = 35,350) (23.01%)	15.05 ± 2.95	
T3 (pg/mL)		<0.001*
1st quartile (<2.87) (n = 33,064) (24.36%)	14.64 ± 2.95	
2nd quartile (2.87–3.12) (n = 31,796) (23.44%)	14.88 ± 2.95	
3rd quartile (3.12–3.40) (n = 35,356) (26.06%)	15.10 ± 2.96	
4th quartile (≥3.40) (n = 35,466) (26.14%)	15.19 ± 2.96	
Characteristics of disease	(+)	(−)	p value
Hypothyroidism	14.65 ± 2.93	15.01 ± 2.95	<0.001**
Hyperthyroidism	14.87 ± 2.92	15.01 ± 2.95	0.017**
Nodular cyst	14.92 ± 2.90	15.01 ± 2.95	0.003**
Hormone treatment	14.82 ± 2.93	15.01 ± 2.95	0.001**

Continuous values are presented as mean ± standard deviation (SD).
*One-way ANOVA, **Student's t-test.

TABLE 4: Univariate analysis of thyroid function and IOP in thyroid disease patients without glaucoma.

Variables	IOP (mmHg)	p value
TSH (μIU/mL)		0.128*
1st quartile (<1.30) (n = 3677) (32.32%)	14.79 ± 2.92	
2nd quartile (1.30–1.90) (n = 1788) (15.72%)	14.80 ± 2.80	
3rd quartile (1.90–2.75) (n = 2020) (17.75%)	14.68 ± 2.85	
4th quartile (≥2.75) (n = 3891) (34.21%)	14.87 ± 2.91	
Free T4 (ng/dL)		0.762*
1st quartile (<1.15) (n = 3755) (33.12%)	14.76 ± 2.89	
2nd quartile (1.15–1.26) (n = 2581) (22.76%)	14.81 ± 2.85	
3rd quartile (1.26–1.38) (n = 2101) (18.53%)	14.81 ± 2.88	
4th quartile (≥1.38) (n = 2901) (25.59%)	14.84 ± 2.92	
T3 (pg/mL)		<0.001*
1st quartile (<2.87) (n = 4171) (41.69%)	14.60 ± 2.92	
2nd quartile (2.87–3.12) (n = 2292) (22.91%)	14.77 ± 2.86	
3rd quartile (3.12–3.40) (n = 1818) (18.17%)	14.95 ± 2.88	
4th quartile (≥3.40) (n = 1724) (17.23%)	14.90 ± 2.91	
Characteristics of disease	(+)	(−)	p value
Hypothyroidism	14.65 ± 2.90	14.85 ± 2.88	0.001**
Hyperthyroidism	14.87 ± 2.94	14.78 ± 2.87	0.161**
Nodular cyst	14.88 ± 2.86	14.74 ± 2.91	0.016**
Hormone treatment	14.86 ± 2.95	14.78 ± 2.87	0.191**

Continuous values are presented as mean ± standard deviation (SD).
*One-way ANOVA, **Student's t-test.

TABLE 5: Adjusted coefficients and 95% confidence intervals of IOP stratified by each thyroid function parameter in a normal population without glaucoma.

Variables	Coefficients	95% confidence interval	p value*
Age	0.025	(0.024–0.027)	<0.001
Sex (male)	0.726	(0.693–0.759)	<0.001
Diabetes	0.697	(0.609–0.784)	<0.001
Hypertension	0.381	(0.326–0.436)	<0.001
Hyperlipidaemia	0.150	(0.106–0.194)	<0.001
Current smoker	0.234	(0.194–0.275)	<0.001
TSH (μIU/mL)			
1st quartile (<1.30)	0 (reference)		
2nd quartile (1.30–1.90)	0.074	(0.033–0.115)	<0.001
3rd quartile (1.90–2.75)	0.135	(0.094–0.177)	<0.001
4th quartile (≥2.75)	0.159	(0.117–0.200)	<0.001
Age	0.025	(0.023–0.026)	<0.001
Sex (male)	0.766	(0.732–0.801)	<0.001
Diabetes	0.702	(0.614–0.789)	<0.001
Hypertension	0.384	(0.329–0.439)	<0.001
Hyperlipidaemia	0.146	(0.102–0.190)	<0.001
Current smoker	0.220	(0.180–0.259)	<0.001
Free T4 (ng/dL)			
1st quartile (<1.15)	0 (reference)		
2nd quartile (1.15–1.26)	−0.025	(−0.066–0.016)	0.239
3rd quartile (1.26–1.38)	−0.087	(−0.129 to −0.044)	<0.001
4th quartile (≥1.38)	−0.176	(−0.221 to −0.131)	<0.001
Age	0.025	(0.023–0.027)	<0.001
Sex (male)	0.737	(0.702–0.773)	<0.001
Diabetes	0.693	(0.606–0.781)	<0.001
Hypertension	0.381	(0.326–0.436)	<0.001
Hyperlipidaemia	0.152	(0.108–0.196)	<0.001
Current smoker	0.216	(0.176 0.256)	<0.001
T3 (pg/mL)			
1st quartile (<2.87)	0 (reference)		
2nd quartile (2.87–3.12)	−0.102	(−0.143 to −0.060)	<0.001
3rd quartile (3.12–3.40)	−0.043	(−0.085 to −0.001)	0.045
4th quartile (≥1.38)	−0.050	(−0.094 to −0.006)	0.027
Hypothyroidism	−0.091	(−0.200–0.017)	0.099
Hyperthyroidism	0.042	(−0.071–0.156)	0.465
Nodular cyst	0.071	(0.011–0.130)	0.019
Hormone treatment	−0.004	(−0.113–0.104)	0.938

Adjusted for age, sex, diabetes, hypertension, hyperlipidaemia, and current smoker.
Diabetes is diagnosed as previous diagnosis or treatment history of diabetes or fasting plasma glucose level ≥ 7.0 mmol/L (126 mg/dL).
Hypertension is diagnosed as a systolic blood pressure ≥ 140 mmHg, a diastolic blood pressure ≥ 90 mmHg, or current use of antihypertensive drugs.
Hyperlipidaemia is diagnosed as abnormally elevated serum level of any or all lipids and/or lipoproteins.
*Multivariate linear regression analysis.

trabecular meshwork and/or aqueous, causing an obstruction to facility of outflow. This phenomenon was thought to be due to decreased enzyme activity in the hypothyroid state and decreased degradation of hyaluronic acid. After treatment of hypothyroidism, the outflow of aqueous humor was recovered. Some studies have reported that treating hypothyroidism decreases IOP through increasing aqueous

outflow. Centanni et al. [17] reported that the IOP of subjects who showed a significantly higher IOP than the control group of subclinical hypothyroidism were decreased approximately by 3 mmHg after treatment of hypothyroidism. Bahceci et al. [18] reported that hypothyroidism reversibly induced increasing IOP. On the other hand, Cheng and Perkins [19] did not find a statistically significant difference

TABLE 6: Adjusted odds ratio and 95% confidence intervals of glaucoma stratified by thyroid function.

Variables	Odds ratio	95% confidence interval	p value*
Age	1.029	(1.024–1.035)	<0.001
Sex (male)	1.783	(1.583–2.007)	<0.001
Diabetes	1.087	(0.878–1.345)	0.445
Hypertension	1.860	(1.632–21,192)	<0.001
Hyperlipidaemia	0.963	(0.850–1.090)	0.547
Current smoker	0.878	(0.781–0.988)	0.031
T3 (pg/mL)		(All subjects)	
1st quartile (<2.87)	1 (reference)		
2nd quartile (2.87–3.12)	1.008	(0.873–1.164)	0.915
3rd quartile (3.12–3.40)	1.134	(0.984–1.306)	0.082
4th quartile (≥3.40)	1.036	(0.892–1.203)	0.646
T3 (pg/mL)		(20 ~ 39 age subjects)	
1st quartile (<2.87)	1 (reference)		
2nd quartile (2.87–3.12)	0.912	(0.697–1.193)	0.500
3rd quartile (3.12–3.40)	1.065	(0.822–1.380)	0.634
4th quartile (≥3.40)	0.966	(0.740–1.260)	0.797
T3 (pg/mL)		(40 ~ 59 age subjects)	
1st quartile (<2.87)	1 (reference)		
2nd quartile (2.87–3.12)	1.071	(0.895–1.282)	0.452
3rd quartile (3.12–3.40)	1.153	(0.962–1.381)	0.123
4th quartile (≥3.40)	1.056	(0.871–1.280)	0.581
T3 (pg/mL)		(60 or older age subjects)	
1st quartile (<2.87)	1 (reference)		
2nd quartile (2.87–3.12)	0.823	(0.467–1.450)	0.500
3rd quartile (3.12–3.40)	1.200	(0.695–2.070)	0.514
4th quartile (≥3.40)	1.086	(0.565–2.087)	0.804

Adjusted for age, sex, diabetes, hypertension, hyperlipidaemia, and current smoker.
Characteristics of disease (hypothyroidism, hyperthyroidism, nodular cyst, hormone treatment) include both medical history review and currently diagnosed disease.
Diabetes is diagnosed as fasting plasma glucose level ≥ 7.0 mmol/L (126 mg/dL).
Hypertension is diagnosed as a systolic blood pressure ≥ 140 mmHg, a diastolic blood pressure ≥ 90 mmHg, or current use of antihypertensive drugs.
Hyperlipidaemia is diagnosed as abnormally elevated serum level of any or all lipids and/or lipoproteins.
*Multivariate logistic regression analysis.

TABLE 7: The odds ratio between thyroid factors and glaucoma.

Variables	Glaucoma (+)	(−)	Odds ratio	95% CI	p*
Hyperthyroidism			0.905	(0.653–1.255)	0.550
(+) (n = 2789)	37	2752			
(−) (n = 163,361)	2391	160,970			
Hypothyroidism			0.783	(0.563–1.091)	0.147
(+) (n = 3122)	36	3086			
(−) (n = 163,023)	2392	160,631			
Nodular cyst			0.817	(0.688–0.972)	0.022
(+) (n = 11,377)	138	11,239			
(+) (n = 154,949)	2293	152,656			
Hormone treatment			1.052	(0.789–1.403)	0.730
(+) (n = 3129)	48	3081			
(+) (n = 163,079)	2380	160,699			

*Chi-square test.

in the distribution of IOP between hypothyroidism and normal control groups. However, their study included thyroid hormone-treated patients, which could have affected the results due to the reversible effects of the treatment. McLenachan and Davies [20] reported that high IOP was associated with hypothyroidism due to changes in the quantity and quality of mucopolysaccharides in the trabecular meshwork.

Physiologically, TSH level and T3 and T4 levels are adjusted in relation to each other [8]. In the hyperthyroid state, blood tests typically show low thyroid-stimulating hormone (TSH) and elevated triiodothyronine (T3) and thyroxine (T4) levels. Otherwise, an elevated TSH indicates that the thyroid gland is not producing enough thyroid hormone (hypothyroid state). In our study, the IOP in the first quartile of free T4 and T3 were higher than those in the second or other quartiles. These results were statistically significant, but the changes were clinically insignificant. These results can be considered the several reasons that might appear. First, this study included a very large number of subjects and the results for each group might be distributed evenly. Due to very large number of the enrolled subjects in the study, statistically significant result was showed. However, the difference was very small and might not be noticeable. Second, in normal population, the structural abnormalities of the extraocular muscles or intraorbital tissues that could affect the IOP were less likely to appear. Therefore, the difference of IOP between groups was less likely to emerge.

Many studies have investigated the association between glaucoma and thyroid dysfunction. In the study of Smith et al. [16], 64 subjects with POAG and 64 controls were evaluated for hypothyroidism. About 23.4% of patients with POAG and 4.7% of controls had hypothyroidism, and the difference was statistically significant. Additionally, in POAG patients, 10.9% showed newly diagnosed hypothyroidism. Munoz-Negrete et al. [21] investigated the prevalence of hypothyroidism in 75 OAG patients and 75 controls. Although applying similar diagnostic criteria as Smith et al. [16], they did not find a statistically significant difference. Gillow et al. [22] investigated this relationship with 100 glaucoma patients using TSH level. Clinical hypothyroidism was present in 4% of participants, and subclinical hypothyroidism was present in 3% of participants. In this study, POAG patients did not show an association with hypothyroidism. Some previous studies about the association between glaucoma and thyroid function were based on their glaucoma diagnosis mainly on IOP, not optic disc evaluation [19, 20, 23, 24].

In the Namil study of Korean subjects, patients with a history of thyroid disease had a 7.4-fold higher risk of open-angle glaucoma than the control group [25]. In the Blue Mountain Eye Study, the incidence of glaucoma was 2.1-fold higher in the thyroxine treatment group than in the control group [26]. Cross et al. [27] reported that the incidence of glaucoma in the thyroid disease group was 1.4-fold higher than in the control group. Lin et al. [28] reported that the hypothyroidism group had a 1.9-fold higher incidence of glaucoma than the control group. Girkin et al. [29] showed significantly higher relative risk of glaucoma in the hypothyroidism group of male subjects that the average age of participants was 69 years.

On the other hand, Karadimas et al. reported a different result. In 100 patients of newly diagnosed hypothyroidism patients, there were no participants with glaucomatous optic nerve damage [30]. Motsko and Jones [31] investigated the risk of OAG with newly diagnosed OAG patients without hypothyroidism. Adjusted for other risk factors, they reported that OAG did not show significant association with hypothyroidism. Haefliger et al. [32] said that glaucoma prevalence does not seem to be significantly increased in thyroid eye disease. Kakigi et al. [33] reported a similar result with us. In this study, participants of National Health Interview Survey were relatively young age (no hypothyroidism; 57.0 ± 12.5, hypothyroidism; 61.5 ± 13.3). The unadjusted analysis showed a significant association between self-reported glaucoma and self-reported hypothyroidism. However, multivariate logistic regression analysis adjusted for age, gender, race, comorbidities, and health-related behavior showed no association between self-reported glaucoma and hypothyroidism or thyroid disease. This study was based on two US nationwide surveys and failed to confirm previously reported associations between hypothyroidism and glaucoma.

In some studies for racial characteristics of thyroid eye disease, the effects of thyroid factor on the eyes were different between races [34, 35]. In the study of the effect of smoking, the results showed tendency of higher prevalence of current smokers in subjects with larger orbital muscle volume in normal population [36]. Thyroid hormone might also have an effect on the extraocular muscles [14, 15]. The prevalence of thyroid eye disease between European and Asian populations and the overall risk for Europeans for developing thyroid eye disease were 6.4 times higher than for Asians [34]. The prevalence was 42% in Europeans compared to 7.7% in Asians [34]. Bednarczuk et al. [35] reported that smoking was a risk factor for thyroid eye disease in Polish people but not in Japanese people. There are reports as described above for the extraocular muscles; however, further studies are necessary to support our results. In our study, the percentage of current smoker did not show a significant difference between glaucoma and normal group.

In this study, glaucomatous optic neuropathy did not show a significant correlation with any thyroid factors. The age may be one of the causes of such results. In our study, the mean age of participants was 40.56 years. Other studies that reported the significant associations between glaucoma and thyroid factors had relatively older participants than in our study; the average age of participants was about 63 to 70 years for each study. The old age may have longer duration of thyroid disease than the young age, and thyroid factor may affect to the eye for a longer period of time in the old age. In addition to this, the number of enrolled subjects (164,029) in this study is a very huge data compared to other studies which have been conducted so far. This factor is thought to be able to level the results of statistics between the groups.

There are some limitations in the present study. The number 2431 that finally included in the glaucoma group is the remainder of 2454 which excluded the 23 subjects of non-glaucoma, finally confirmed. Therefore, glaucoma suspect might be included in the glaucoma group. The difference in prevalence of current smokers might influence the results. This study is not a population-based study. Also, patient selection based on participation in serial health screening might be biased toward higher economic and educational levels. Patients who worry about their health undergo medical examinations more frequently and, therefore, tend to be healthier than those who do not undergo frequent examinations. Our study was a cross-sectional study; however, considering the fact that glaucoma is a progressive disease, a longitudinal approach would also provide a valuable data. In addition, we did not perform glaucoma evaluation on all subjects, so it is difficult to fully evaluate the relationships between ophthalmic factors and other general factors. The use of non-contact tonometry rather than applanation tonometry may also be another limitation. Despite these limitations, this study was performed with a large number of participants and targeted a single race. Our data may be helpful to understand the pathophysiology of glaucoma.

In conclusion, our results showed that the IOP tend to be decreased slightly as the quartile of free T4 and T3 increased. However, the clinical significance may be limited. Our study also suggested that thyroid dysfunction was not an independent risk factor of glaucomatous optic neuropathy. These results may increase the understanding of risk factors of glaucoma. Further prospective study is needed to validate the results.

Conflicts of Interest

No conflicting relationships exist for any author.

References

[1] M. J. Kim, M. J. Kim, H. S. Kim, J. W. Jeoung, and K. H. Park, "Risk factors for open-angle glaucoma with normal baseline intraocular pressure in a young population: the Korea National Health and Nutrition Examination Survey," *Clinical & Experimental Ophthalmology*, vol. 42, no. 9, pp. 825–832, 2014.

[2] M. Kim, D. M. Kim, K. H. Park, T. W. Kim, J. W. Jeoung, and S. H. Kim, "Intraocular pressure reduction with topical medications and progression of normal-tension glaucoma: a 12-year mean follow-up study," *Acta Ophthalmologica*, vol. 91, no. 4, pp. e270–e275, 2013.

[3] M. C. Leske, A. Heijl, M. Hussein et al., "Factors for glaucoma progression and the effect of treatment: the early manifest glaucoma trial," *Archives of Ophthalmology*, vol. 121, no. 1, pp. 48–56, 2003.

[4] K. Nouri-Mahdavi, D. Hoffman, A. L. Coleman et al., "Predictive factors for glaucomatous visual field progression in the Advanced Glaucoma Intervention Study," *Ophthalmology*, vol. 111, no. 9, pp. 1627–1635, 2004.

[5] B. Chon, M. Qiu, and S. C. Lin, "Myopia and glaucoma in the South Korean population," *Investigative Ophthalmology & Visual Science*, vol. 54, no. 10, pp. 6570–6577, 2013.

[6] J. M. Kim, S. H. Kim, K. H. Park, S. Y. Han, and H. S. Shim, "Investigation of the association between Helicobacter pylori infection and normal tension glaucoma," *Investigative Ophthalmology & Visual Science*, vol. 52, no. 2, pp. 665–668, 2011.

[7] H. S. Kim, K. H. Park, J. W. Jeoung, and J. Park, "Comparison of myopic and nonmyopic disc hemorrhage in primary open-angle glaucoma," *Japanese Journal of Ophthalmology*, vol. 57, no. 2, pp. 166–171, 2013.

[8] E. A. McAninch and A. C. Bianco, "Thyroid hormone signaling in energy homeostasis and energy metabolism," *Annals of the New York Academy of Sciences*, vol. 1311, no. 1, pp. 77–87, 2014.

[9] K. I. Woo, Y. D. Kim, and S. Y. Lee, "Prevalence and risk factors for thyroid eye disease among Korean dysthyroid patients," *Korean Journal of Ophthalmology*, vol. 27, no. 6, pp. 397–404, 2013.

[10] R. Forte, P. Bonavolonta, and P. Vassallo, "Evaluation of retinal nerve fiber layer with optic nerve tracking optical coherence tomography in thyroid-associated orbitopathy," *Ophthalmologica*, vol. 224, no. 2, pp. 116–121, 2010.

[11] K. C. Sung, S. Ryu, Y. Chang, C. D. Byrne, and S. H. Kim, "C-reactive protein and risk of cardiovascular and all-cause mortality in 268 803 East Asians," *European Heart Journal*, vol. 35, no. 27, pp. 1809–1816, 2014.

[12] P. J. Foster, R. Buhrmann, H. A. Quigley, and G. J. Johnson, "The definition and classification of glaucoma in prevalence surveys," *The British Journal of Ophthalmology*, vol. 86, no. 2, pp. 238–242, 2002.

[13] H. T. Kim, J. M. Kim, J. H. Kim et al., "The relationship between vitamin D and glaucoma: a Kangbuk Samsung Health Study," *Korean Journal of Ophthalmology*, vol. 30, no. 6, pp. 426–433, 2016.

[14] K. Ohtsuka and Y. Nakamura, "Open-angle glaucoma associated with Graves disease," *American Journal of Ophthalmology*, vol. 129, no. 5, pp. 613–617, 2000.

[15] H. B. Lee, I. R. Rodgers, and J. J. Woog, "Evaluation and management of Graves' orbitopathy," *Otolaryngologic Clinics of North America*, vol. 39, no. 5, pp. 923–942, 2006, vi.

[16] K. D. Smith, B. P. Arthurs, and N. Saheb, "An association between hypothyroidism and primary open-angle glaucoma," *Ophthalmology*, vol. 100, no. 10, pp. 1580–1584, 1993.

[17] M. Centanni, R. Cesareo, O. Verallo et al., "Reversible increase of intraocular pressure in subclinical hypothyroid patients," *European Journal of Endocrinology*, vol. 136, no. 6, pp. 595–598, 1997.

[18] U. A. Bahceci, S. Ozdek, Z. Pehlivanli, I. Yetkin, and M. Onol, "Changes in intraocular pressure and corneal and retinal nerve fiber layer thicknesses in hypothyroidism," *European Journal of Ophthalmology*, vol. 15, no. 5, pp. 556–561, 2005.

[19] H. Cheng and E. S. Perkins, "Thyroid disease and glaucoma," *The British Journal of Ophthalmology*, vol. 51, no. 8, pp. 547–553, 1967.

[20] J. McLenachan and D. M. Davies, "Glaucoma and the thyroid," *The British Journal of Ophthalmology*, vol. 49, no. 8, pp. 441–444, 1965.

[21] F. J. Munoz-Negrete, G. Rebolleda, F. Almodovar, B. Diaz, and C. Varela, "Hypothyroidism and primary open-angle glaucoma," *Ophthalmologica*, vol. 214, no. 5, pp. 347–349, 2000.

[22] J. T. Gillow, P. Shah, and E. C. O'Neill, "Primary open angle glaucoma and hypothyroidism: chance or true association?" *Eye (London, England)*, vol. 11, no. Pt 1, pp. 113–114, 1997.

[23] K. D. Smith, G. J. Tevaarwerk, and L. H. Allen, "An ocular dynamic study supporting the hypothesis that hypothyroidism is a treatable cause of secondary open-angle glaucoma,"

Canadian Journal of Ophthalmology, vol. 27, no. 7, pp. 341–344, 1992.

[24] T. Krupin, L. S. Jacobs, S. M. Podos, and B. Becker, "Thyroid function and the intraocular pressure response to topical corticosteroids," *American Journal of Ophthalmology*, vol. 83, no. 5, pp. 643–646, 1977.

[25] M. Kim, T. W. Kim, K. H. Park, and J. M. Kim, "Risk factors for primary open-angle glaucoma in South Korea: the Namil study," *Japanese Journal of Ophthalmology*, vol. 56, no. 4, pp. 324–329, 2012.

[26] A. J. Lee, E. Rochtchina, J. J. Wang, P. R. Healey, and P. Mitchell, "Open-angle glaucoma and systemic thyroid disease in an older population: The Blue Mountains Eye Study," *Eye (London, England)*, vol. 18, no. 6, pp. 600–608, 2004.

[27] J. M. Cross, C. A. Girkin, C. Owsley, and G. McGwin Jr., "The association between thyroid problems and glaucoma," *The British Journal of Ophthalmology*, vol. 92, no. 11, pp. 1503–1505, 2008.

[28] H. C. Lin, J. H. Kang, Y. D. Jiang, and J. D. Ho, "Hypothyroidism and the risk of developing open-angle glaucoma: a five-year population-based follow-up study," *Ophthalmology*, vol. 117, no. 10, pp. 1960–1966, 2010.

[29] C. A. Girkin, G. McGwin Jr., S. F. McNeal, P. P. Lee, and C. Owsley, "Hypothyroidism and the development of open-angle glaucoma in a male population," *Ophthalmology*, vol. 111, no. 9, pp. 1649–1652, 2004.

[30] P. Karadimas, E. A. Bouzas, F. Topouzis, D. A. Koutras, and G. Mastorakos, "Hypothyroidism and glaucoma. A study of 100 hypothyroid patients," *American Journal of Ophthalmology*, vol. 131, no. 1, pp. 126–128, 2001.

[31] S. P. Motsko and J. K. Jones, "Is there an association between hypothyroidism and open-angle glaucoma in an elderly population? An epidemiologic study," *Ophthalmology*, vol. 115, no. 9, pp. 1581–1584, 2008.

[32] I. O. Haefliger, G. von Arx, and A. R. Pimentel, "Pathophysiology of intraocular pressure increase and glaucoma prevalence in thyroid eye disease: a mini-review," *Klinische Monatsblätter für Augenheilkunde*, vol. 227, no. 4, pp. 292–293, 2010.

[33] C. Kakigi, T. Kasuga, S. Y. Wang et al., "Hypothyroidism and glaucoma in the United States," *PloS One*, vol. 10, no. 7, e0133688 pages, 2015.

[34] M. Tellez, J. Cooper, and C. Edmonds, "Graves' ophthalmopathy in relation to cigarette smoking and ethnic origin," *Clinical Endocrinology*, vol. 36, no. 3, pp. 291–294, 1992.

[35] T. Bednarczuk, Y. Hiromatsu, T. Fukutani et al., "Association of cytotoxic T-lymphocyte-associated antigen-4 (CTLA-4) gene polymorphism and non-genetic factors with Graves' ophthalmopathy in European and Japanese populations," *European Journal of Endocrinology*, vol. 148, no. 1, pp. 13–18, 2003.

[36] N. I. Regensburg, W. M. Wiersinga, T. T. Berendschot, P. Saeed, and M. P. Mourits, "Effect of smoking on orbital fat and muscle volume in Graves' orbitopathy," *Thyroid*, vol. 21, no. 2, pp. 177–181, 2011.

Permissions

All chapters in this book were first published in JO, by Hindawi Publishing Corporation; hereby published with permission under the Creative Commons Attribution License or equivalent. Every chapter published in this book has been scrutinized by our experts. Their significance has been extensively debated. The topics covered herein carry significant findings which will fuel the growth of the discipline. They may even be implemented as practical applications or may be referred to as a beginning point for another development.

The contributors of this book come from diverse backgrounds, making this book a truly international effort. This book will bring forth new frontiers with its revolutionizing research information and detailed analysis of the nascent developments around the world.

We would like to thank all the contributing authors for lending their expertise to make the book truly unique. They have played a crucial role in the development of this book. Without their invaluable contributions this book wouldn't have been possible. They have made vital efforts to compile up to date information on the varied aspects of this subject to make this book a valuable addition to the collection of many professionals and students.

This book was conceptualized with the vision of imparting up-to-date information and advanced data in this field. To ensure the same, a matchless editorial board was set up. Every individual on the board went through rigorous rounds of assessment to prove their worth. After which they invested a large part of their time researching and compiling the most relevant data for our readers.

The editorial board has been involved in producing this book since its inception. They have spent rigorous hours researching and exploring the diverse topics which have resulted in the successful publishing of this book. They have passed on their knowledge of decades through this book. To expedite this challenging task, the publisher supported the team at every step. A small team of assistant editors was also appointed to further simplify the editing procedure and attain best results for the readers.

Apart from the editorial board, the designing team has also invested a significant amount of their time in understanding the subject and creating the most relevant covers. They scrutinized every image to scout for the most suitable representation of the subject and create an appropriate cover for the book.

The publishing team has been an ardent support to the editorial, designing and production team. Their endless efforts to recruit the best for this project, has resulted in the accomplishment of this book. They are a veteran in the field of academics and their pool of knowledge is as vast as their experience in printing. Their expertise and guidance has proved useful at every step. Their uncompromising quality standards have made this book an exceptional effort. Their encouragement from time to time has been an inspiration for everyone.

The publisher and the editorial board hope that this book will prove to be a valuable piece of knowledge for researchers, students, practitioners and scholars across the globe.

List of Contributors

Laia Jaumandreu, Francisco J. Muñoz–Negrete and Gema Rebolleda
Ophthalmology Service, University Hospital Ramón y Cajal, School of Medicine and Health Science, University of Alcalá, IRYCIS, Hospital Ramón y Cajal, Ctra. Colmenar Viejo km. 9100, 28034 Madrid, Spain

Noelia Oblanca
Ophthalmology Service, University Hospital Ramón y Cajal, IRYCIS, Hospital Ramón y Cajal, Ctra. Colmenar Viejo km. 9100, 28034 Madrid, Spain

Xiaomin Chen, Yue Wang, Fangfang Han and Min Ke
Department of Ophthalmology, Zhongnan Hospital, Wuhan University, Wuhan, China

Yong Un Shin, Eun HeeHong, Min Ho Kang, Heeyoon Cho and Mincheol Seong
Department of Ophthalmology, Hanyang University College of Medicine, Seoul, Republic of Korea

Vlad Diaconita and Cindy Hutnik
Ivey Eye Institute, London, ON, Canada
Schulich School of Medicine and Dentistry, Western University, London, ON, Canada

Monali S. Malvankar-Mehta
Ivey Eye Institute, London, ON, Canada
Department of Epidemiology and Biostatistics, Schulich School of Medicine and Dentistry, Western University, London, ON, Canada

Matthew Quinn
Schulich School of Medicine and Dentistry, Western University, London, ON, Canada
Queen's University, Ophthalmology Department, Kingston, ON, Canada

Dania Jamal
King Abdulaziz University, Saudi Arabia

Brad Dishan
St. Joseph's Health Care, London, ON, Canada

Wei-ran Niu, Chun-qiong Dong, Xi Zhang, Yi-fan Feng and Fei Yuan
Department of Ophthalmology, Zhongshan Hospital of Fudan University, Shanghai 200032, China

Tesfay Mehari Atey and Solomon Weldegebreal Asgedom
Clinical Pharmacy Unit, School of Pharmacy, College of Health Sciences, Mekelle University, Mekelle, Tigray, Ethiopia

Workineh Shibeshi
Department of Pharmacology and Clinical Pharmacy, School of Pharmacy, College of Health Sciences, Addis Ababa University, Addis Ababa, Ethiopia

Abeba T. Giorgis
Department of Ophthalmology, School of Medicine, College of Health Sciences, Addis Ababa University, Addis Ababa, Ethiopia

Enkelejda Kasneci
Department of Computer Science, University of Tübingen, Sand 14, 72076 Tübingen, Germany

Alex A. Black and Joanne M. Wood
School of Optometry and Vision Science, Institute of Health and Biomedical Innovation, Queensland University of Technology, Brisbane, QLD, Australia

Dongpeng Hu, Shu Tu, Chengguo Zuo and Jian Ge
State Key Laboratory of Ophthalmology, Zhongshan Ophthalmic Center, Sun Yat-sen University, 54 Xianlie Road, Guangzhou 510060, China

Alessio Martucci, Massimo Cesareo, Clarissa Giannini, Giulio Pocobelli, Raffaele Mancino and Carlo Nucci
Ophthalmology Unit, Department of Experimental Medicine, University of Rome Tor Vergata, Rome, Italy

Francesco Garaci
Department of Biomedicine and Prevention, University of Rome Tor Vergata, Rome, Italy

Nicola Toschi
Department of Biomedicine and Prevention, University of Rome Tor Vergata, Rome, Italy
Department of Radiology, Athinoula A. Martinos Center for Biomedical Imaging, Boston, MA, USA
Harvard Medical School, Boston, MA, USA

Félix Gil-Carrasco, Daniel Ochoa-Contreras and Marco A. Torres
Glaucoma Department, Hospital Luis Sánchez Bulnes, Asociaci'on para Evitar la Ceguera en México I.A.P, Mexico City, Mexico

Jorge Santiago-Amaya, Fidel W. Pérez-Tovar and Luis Nino-de-Rivera
Artificial Vision Laboratory, Instituto Politécnico Nacional, Mexico City, Mexico

Roberto Gonzalez-Salinas
Research Department, Asociación para Evitar la Ceguera en M'exico I.A.P, Mexico City, Mexico

Xinbo Gao, Qiongman Yang, Wenmin Huang, Tingting Chen, Chengguo Zuo, Xinyan Li, Wuyou Gao and Huiming Xiao
State Key Laboratory of Ophthalmology, Zhongshan Ophthalmic Center, Sun Yat-sen University, Guangzhou 510060, China

Mouna M. Al-Sa'ad
Department of Special Surgery, School of Medicine, e University of Jordan, Queen Rania Al-Abdullah Street, Amman 11942, Jordan

Amjad T. Shatarat and Darwish H. Badran
Department of Anatomy and Histology, School of Medicine, e University of Jordan, Queen Rania Al-Abdullah Street, Amman 11942, Jordan

Justin Z. Amarin
School of Medicine, e University of Jordan, Queen Rania Al-Abdullah Street, Amman 11942, Jordan

Jeffrey T. Y. Chow and Karla Solo
Department of Epidemiology and Biostatistics, Schulich School of Medicine and Dentistry, Western University, London, ON, Canada

Monali S. Malvankar-Mehta
Department of Epidemiology and Biostatistics, Schulich School of Medicine and Dentistry, Western University, London, ON, Canada
Department of Ophthalmology, Schulich School of Medicine and Dentistry, Western University, London, ON, Canada

Cindy M. L. Hutnik
Department of Ophthalmology, Schulich School of Medicine and Dentistry, Western University, London, ON, Canada

Elena Milla
Unidad de Glaucoma, Institut Clínic d'Oftalmologia (ICOF), Hospital Clínic, Barcelona, Spain
Unidad de Glaucoma y Genética, Institut Comtal d'Oftalmologia, Barcelona, Spain

Susana Duch
Unidad de Glaucoma y Genética, Institut Comtal d'Oftalmologia, Barcelona, Spain

Maria José Gamundi and Miguel Carballo
Servicio de Laboratorio, Hospital de Terrassa, Barcelona, Spain

Jose Rios
Servicio de Estadística, Hospital Clinic, Barcelona, Spain

Jin A Choi
Department of Ophthalmology, College of Medicine, St. Vincent's Hospital, Catholic University of Korea, Suwon, Republic of Korea

Hye-Young Shin
Department of Ophthalmology, College of Medicine, Uijeongbu St. Mary's Hospital, Catholic University of Korea, Uijeongbu, Republic of Korea

Hae-Young Lopilly Park and Chan Kee Park
Department of Ophthalmology, College of Medicine, Seoul St. Mary's Hospital, Catholic University of Korea, Seoul, Republic of Korea

Pedro C. Carricondo and Thais Andrade
Department of Ophthalmology, Hospital das Clínicas HCFMUSP, Faculdade de Medicina, Universidade de São Paulo, São Paulo, SP, Brazil

Lev Prasov, Bernadete M. Ayres and Sayoko E. Moroi
Department of Ophthalmology and Visual Sciences, Kellogg Eye Center, University of Michigan, 1000 Wall St., Ann Arbor, MI 48105, USA

Masako Sakamoto, Kazuyoshi Kitamura and Kenji Kashiwagi
Department of Ophthalmology, University of Yamanashi Faculty of Medicine, Chuo, Yamanashi, Japan

Lei Zuo and Jianhong Zhang
Department of Ophthalmology, Shanghai Fourth People's Hospital, Shanghai 200081, China

Xun Xu
Department of Ophthalmology, Shanghai General Hospital, Shanghai Jiao Tong University School of Medicine, Shanghai 200080, China

Handan Akil, Vikas Chopra, Alex S. Huang, Ramya Swamy and Brian A. Francis
Doheny Image Reading Center, Doheny Eye Institute, Los Angeles, CA, USA
Department of Ophthalmology, David Geffen School of Medicine, Los Angeles, CA, USA

Zhuyun Qian, Kai Xu and Huan Xu
Department of Ophthalmology and Visual Science, Eye, Ear, Nose, and roat Hospital, Shanghai Medical College, Fudan University, Shanghai, China

Xiangmei Kong
Department of Ophthalmology and Visual Science, Eye, Ear, Nose, and roat Hospital, Shanghai Medical College, Fudan University, Shanghai, China
Key Laboratory of Myopia, Ministry of Health, Fudan University, Shanghai, China
Shanghai Key Laboratory of Visual Impairment and Restoration, Fudan University, Shanghai, China

Vassilios Kozobolis, Aristeidis Konstantinidis, Haris Sideroudi and G. Labiris
University Eye Clinic, University Hospital of Alexandroupolis, 68131 Alexandroupolis, Greece

Mantapond Ittarat, Rath Itthipanichpong, Anita Manassakorn, Visanee Tantisevi, Sunee Chansangpetch and Prin Rojanapongpun
Department of Ophthalmology, Chulalongkorn University and King Chulalongkorn Memorial Hospital, 1873 Rama IV Rd., Pathumwan, Bangkok 10330, Thailand

Abdelhamid Elhofi and Hany Ahmed Helaly
Ophthalmology Department, Faculty of Medicine, Alexandria University, Alexandria, Egypt

Jung Hee In, So Yeon Lee, Seok Ho Cho and Young Jae Hong
Glaucoma Center, Nune Eye Hospital, Seoul, Republic of Korea

Nimet Yeşim Erçalık and Serhat İmamoğlu
Haydarpaşa Numune Research and Training Hospital, Istanbul, Turkey

Stéphanie Romeo Villadóniga, Elena Rodríguez García and M. Dolores Álvarez Díaz
Service of Ophthalmology, Complejo Hospitalario Universitario de Ferrol, Ferrol, A Coruña, Spain

Olatz Sagastagoia Epelde
Clinical Analysis Laboratory, Complejo Hospitalario Universitario de Ferrol, Ferrol, A Coruña, Spain

Joan Carles Domingo Pedrol
Department of Biochemistry and Molecular Biomedicine, Faculty of Biology, University of Barcelona, Barcelona, Spain

Jiao Sun, Jialin Wang, Ran You and Yanling Wang
Department of Ophthalmology, Beijing Friendship Hospital Affiliated to Capital Medical University, Beijing, China

Karolina Krix-Jachym and Marek Rękas
Department of Ophthalmology, Military Institute of Medicine, Szaserów Street 128, 04-141 Warsaw, Poland

Tomasz Żarnowski
Department of Diagnostics and Microsurgery of Glaucoma, Medical University of Lublin, Chmielna Street 1, 20-079 Lublin, Poland

Yu Sam Won
Department of Neurosurgery, Kangbuk Samsung Hospital, Sungkyunkwan University School of Medicine, Seoul, Republic of Korea

Da Yeong Kim and Joon Mo Kim
Department of Ophthalmology, Kangbuk Samsung Hospital, Sungkyunkwan University School of Medicine, Seoul, Republic of Korea

Index

www.ingramcontent.com/pod-product-compliance
Lightning Source LLC
Chambersburg PA
CBHW080526200326
41458CB00012B/4349